ANTIBODY Fc: LINKING ADAPTIVE AND INNATE IMMUNITY

ANTIBODY Fc: LINKING ADAPTIVE AND INNATE IMMUNITY

Margaret E. Ackerman
Thayer School of Engineering, Dartmouth College, NH, USA

Falk Nimmerjahn
Institute of Genetics, University of Erlangen-Nurnberg, Erlangen, Germany

ELSEVIER

AMSTERDAM • BOSTON • HEIDELBERG • LONDON
NEW YORK • OXFORD • PARIS • SAN DIEGO
SAN FRANCISCO • SINGAPORE • SYDNEY • TOKYO
Academic Press is an imprint of Elsevier

Academic Press is an imprint of Elsevier
32 Jamestown Road, London NW1 7BY, UK
225 Wyman Street, Waltham, MA 02451, USA
525 B Street, Suite 1800, San Diego, CA 92101-4495, USA

First edition 2014

British Library Cataloguing-in-Publication Data
A catalogue record for this book is available from the British Library

Library of Congress Cataloging-in-Publication Data
A catalog record for this book is available from the Library of Congress

ISBN: 978-0-12-394802-1

For information on all Academic Press publications
visit our website at elsevierdirect.com

Typeset by MPS Limited, Chennai, India
www.adi-mps.com

Short Contents

1

EFFECTOR MECHANISMS

2

EFFECTOR CELLS

3

FcR

4

VARIABILITY OF THE Fc DOMAIN

5

GENETIC ASSOCIATIONS

6

EVOLVING AREAS

Contents

5 Phagocytes and Immunoglobulins

LUISA MARTINEZ-POMARES

6 B Cells

ELIZABETH R. WALSH AND SILVIA BOLLAND

3

FcR

7 Structural Recognition of Immunoglobulins by Fcγ Receptors

PETER SUN

8 FcγRs Across Species

BRIAN MOLDT AND ANN J. HESSELL

4

VARIABILITY OF THE Fc DOMAIN

9 Human IgG Subclasses

THEO RISPENS AND GESTUR VIDARSSON

10 Antibody Glycosylation

XIAOJIE YU, KAVITHA BARUAH, CHRISTOPHER N. SCANLAN, AND MAX CRISPIN

List of Contributors

Shannon A. Allen Northwestern University Feinberg School of Medicine, Chicago, IL, USA

Robert M. Anthony Massachusetts General Hospital, Harvard Medical School, Boston, MA, USA

Kavitha Baruah University of Oxford, Oxford, United Kingdom

Carolyn M. Black National Center for Emerging and Zoonotic Infectious Diseases, Centers for Disease Control and Prevention, Atlanta, GA, USA

Wim K. Bleeker Genmab, Utrecht, The Netherlands

Silvia Bolland National Institute of Allergy and Infectious Diseases, National Institutes of Health, Rockville, MD, USA

Menna R. Clatworthy University of Cambridge School of Clinical Medicine, Cambridge, UK; National Institute of Allergy and Infectious Diseases, National Institutes of Health, Bethesda, MD, USA

Mattias Collin Lund University, Lund, Sweden

Max Crispin University of Oxford, Oxford, United Kingdom

Andreas Diefenbach Department of Medical Microbiology and Hygiene (IMMH), University of Freiburg, Freiburg, Germany

Victor Raúl Gómez Román International Vaccine Institute, Seoul, Korea

Scott B. Halstead Dengue Vaccine Initiative, International Vaccine Institute, Seoul, Korea

Ann J. Hessell Oregon Health & Science University, Beaverton, OR, USA

Thomas J. Hope Northwestern University Feinberg School of Medicine, Chicago, IL, USA

Joseph U. Igietseme National Center for Emerging and Zoonotic Infectious Diseases, Atlanta, GA, USA; Morehouse School of Medicine, Atlanta, GA, USA

Roy Jefferis University of Birmingham, Birmingham, United Kingdom

Jörg Köhla University of Lübeck, Lübeck, Germany; Cincinnati Children's Hospital and University, Cincinnati, OH, USA

Mogens Kilian Aarhus University, Aarhus, Denmark

Margaret A. Lindorfer University of Virginia Charlottesville, VA, USA

Luisa Martinez-Pomares Faculty of Medicine and Health Sciences, University of Nottingham, Nottingham, United Kingdom

Brian Moldt The Scripps Research Institute, La Jolla, CA, USA

Joseph C. Murray Georgetown University Medical Center, Washington, DC, USA

Falk Nimmerjahn University of Erlangen-Nürnberg, Erlangen, Germany

Marije B. Overdijk Genmab, Utrecht, The Netherlands

Annette Oxenius Institute of Microbiology, ETH Zürich, Zürich, Switzerland

Paul W.H.I. Parren Genmab, Utrecht, The Netherlands

Theo Rispens University of Amsterdam, The Netherlands

Christopher N. Scanlan University of Oxford, Oxford, United Kingdom

Peter Sun National Institutes of Health, Rockville, MD, USA

Ronald P. Taylor University of Virginia School of Medicine, Charlottesville, VA, USA

Sandra Verploegen Genmab, Utrecht, The Netherlands

Gestur Vidarsson University of Amsterdam, The Netherlands

Elizabeth R. Walsh National Institutes of Health, Rockville, MD, USA

Stefan S. Weber Institute of Microbiology, ETH Zürich, Zürich, Switzerland

George J. Weiner University of Iowa, Iowa City, IA, USA

Louis M. Weiner Georgetown University Medical Center, Washington, DC, USA

Xiaojie Yu University of Oxford, Oxford, United Kingdom

Xiaoping Zhu University of Maryland, College Park, MD, USA

CHAPTER

1

Antibody-Dependent Cellular Cytotoxicity (ADCC)

Victor Raúl Gómez Román[a,*], *Joseph C. Murray*[b,*] *and Louis M. Weiner*[b]

[a]International Vaccine Institute, Seoul, Korea, [b]Department of Oncology, Georgetown Lombardi Comprehensive Cancer Center, Georgetown Medical Center, Washington, DC, USA

BRIEF HISTORY OF ADCC

In the 1960s, several independent laboratory observations indicated that cells could be killed by other cells, yet the mechanisms of killing were unknown. Several hypotheses were formulated and experiments were conducted paving the way for the discovery and characterization of what we now know as cytotoxic T lymphocytes (CTLs) and natural killer (NK) cells. However, early experiments pointed to the hypothesis that immune serum was in some cases necessary for some types of effector cells to mediate killing of target cells. In 1965, Erna Möeller, a researcher working at the Karolinska Institute, showed that incubation of mouse tumor target cells with heat-inactivated anti-serum from rabbits immunized with these tumor cells, followed by incubation with lymphoid cells from unimmunized mice, resulted in cytotoxicity.[1] Such cytotoxicity required contact or "serum-induced aggregation" between the tumor targets and the lymphoid effectors. Experiments were subsequently performed to identify the aggregating and cytotoxicity-inducing factor contained in serum. In 1970, MacLennan, Loewi, and Harding, researchers working at the Canadian Red Cross Memorial Hospital, reported that the serum factor required for this type of cell-mediated cytotoxicity was an immunoglobulin with the "chemical properties of IgG."[2] Subsequent experiments confirmed this finding by showing that the antibody required belonged to the IgG class and that the mechanism of antibody-dependent killing of target cells by serum factors did not require the heat-labile components of complement, as heat inactivation of serum maintained the killing effect.[2] The phenomenon acquired the name of "antibody-dependent lymphocyte-mediated cytotoxicity"[3] and gradually became known as "antibody-dependent cell-mediated cytotoxicity," or ADCC. The three basic components of ADCC were recognized as being effector cells, antibodies, and target cells coated with antigen. "Targets" could refer to

* Corresponding Author

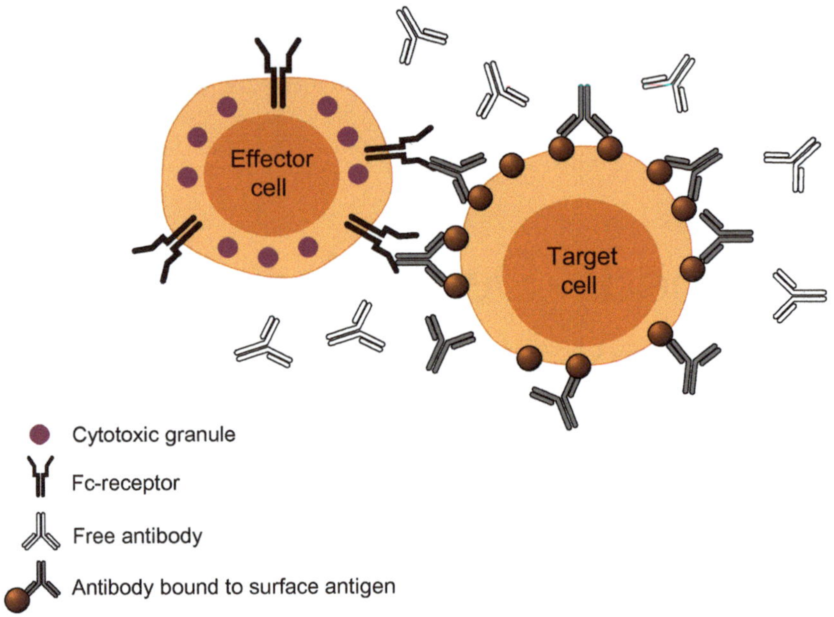

FIGURE 1.1 **Effector cells and targets.** ADCC involves the interplay between a granular effector cell and a target cell expressing antigens on its surface. The granular effector cell must express Fc receptors on its surface for ADCC to occur.

cells expressing tumor, viral, or bacterial antigens; therefore, ADCC became known as an immune mechanism that could be potentially protective against certain types of cancers as well as infectious diseases. Considerable progress has been made in characterizing the effector cells and the receptors involved in this phenomenon, and ADCC can now be defined as the immune mechanism through which Fc-receptor-bearing effector cells can kill target cells that have surface antigens complexed with antibody (Figure 1.1).

EFFECTOR CELLS

Although initial experiments focused on large granular lymphocytes as the main effector cells mediating ADCC, several groups have now characterized the types of cells that can mediate ADCC effector function. Table 1.1 describes the various types of effector cells that have been shown to mediate ADCC. Three common characteristics of these cells are that they are all leukocytes, they contain granules, and they express Fc receptors. Mononuclear leukocytes (NK cells, macrophages, γδ T cells) and polymorphonuclear leukocytes (neutrophils, basophils, eosinophils) can both mediate ADCC.[4] This diversity of effectors is worth emphasizing, as a significant proportion of ADCC experiments reported in the scientific literature are either "NK-centric" or focused on the use of the peripheral blood mononuclear cell (PBMC) fraction to obtain effector cells. This unintentional experimental bias tends to overlook the role of neutrophils and other polymorphonuclear leukocytes (PMNs or PMLs); it is probably a consequence of both the relative ease of working with peripheral NK cells and the practical difficulties associated with working with PMNs, which are rather short lived

TABLE 1.1 Peripheral Blood Effector Cells and Fc Receptors Involved in ADCC

Leukocyte Fraction	Effectors	Predominant Fc Receptors	Refs.
PBMC	NK cells	FcγRIIIA/CD16	Wallace et al.[4]
	Monocytes/macrophages	FcγRI/CD64 FcγRII/CD32	Wallace et al.,[4] Tudor and Bomsel[5]
	γδ T cells (subset)	FcγRIIIA/CD16	Chen and Freedman[120]
PMN	Granulocytes (neutrophils, basophils, eosinophils)	FcγRII/CD32 FcγRIIIb/CD16b FcαRI/CD89	Wallace et al.,[4] Horner et al.[6]

and may require isolation through cumbersome Percoll-gradient procedures or hypotonic lysis steps. While the effector cell phenotype of NK cells, phagocytes, and B are discussed in detail elsewhere in this book, cells contained in the PMN fraction may be equally important effectors involved in Fc-mediated functions, including ADCC.

RECEPTORS INVOLVED

Three types of Fc receptors are involved in mediating IgG-dependent ADCC: FcγRI (CD64), FCγRII (CD32), and FcγRIIIA (CD16). Of these, FcγRIIIA (CD16) is often invoked as the main receptor involved, as it is expressed predominantly by NK cells (Table 1.1); however, *in vitro* evidence indicates that monocytes and granulocytes can mediate equally potent ADCC via other Fc receptors.[4–6] In cancer and infectious disease research, all three FcγRs have been shown to mediate ADCC. Natural polymorphisms in the Fc receptors have been shown to have a clear impact on ADCC *in vitro* and an effect on ADCC-dependent cancer immunotherapy. Additionally, IgA-dependent ADCC has also been described in some models and is dependent on the Fc alpha receptor (FcαR, CD89), which is expressed primarily on PMN and monocytes (Table 1.1).

Our knowledge of Fc-receptor expression and ADCC function to date has been limited to the study of either immortalized effector cell lines or fresh effector cells circulating in peripheral blood. Less is known about Fc-receptor expression in cells residing in mucosal tissues, which represent the first line of defense against invading pathogens. For example, a recent study examining Fc-receptor expression in a limited number of patients (n=5) showed that CD16, CD32, and CD64 expression was virtually nonexistent on rectal macrophages compared to the levels of expression observed on peripheral blood monocytes.[7] Vaginal macrophages from the same patients, however, expressed very high levels of CD16. This may have important implications for ADCC, as it could suggest that ADCC (and other Fc-receptor-dependent mechanisms of immunity) may be relevant as a first line of mucosal defense in some compartments but not in others. In this regard, several studies have examined the role of mucosal antibody in mediating ADCC *in vitro* using effector cell lines or fresh effector cells derived from peripheral blood. In contrast, less is known about the ADCC function of effector cells recovered from mucosal tissues, and defining the expression of Fc receptors across mucosal tissues and assessing their *ex vivo* ADCC function might yield insights into the spatial and temporal role of ADCC in infection and immunity.

MECHANISMS OF ADCC

Recognition of the Target Cell and Cross-Linking of the Fc Receptor on the Effector Cell

An obvious prerequisite for ADCC to occur is the interaction of antibody bound to the target cell with Fc receptors on the effector cell. This interaction is both regulated and facilitated by conformational changes that occur in the antibody molecule only after it has bound to its cognate antigen (Figure 1.1). After binding to surface antigens on the target cell, conformational changes occur in the Fc region of the antibody, which result in its increased affinity for a single Fc receptor on the effector cell.[8] Glycosylation of the Fc region also plays an important role in modulating the affinity of antibody for Fc receptors; in particular, antibodies that are heavily fucosylated (during posttranslational modifications within the B cell) have decreased affinity for FcγRIIIA (CD16), whereas removal of fucose enhances their affinity for FcγRIIIA and their ability to mediate ADCC.[9] Recent evidence indicates that binding between IgG and FcγRIIIA involves tight carbohydrate–carbohydrate interactions that are weakened or obliterated when IgG is fucosylated.[10]

Compared to small, soluble antigens, the relatively larger size of tumors or virally infected cells coated with several antibody molecules on their surface can facilitate physical rearrangements and interactions between Fc receptors present on effector cells (Figure 1.2A). These interactions are often referred to as Fc-receptor ligation, agglutination, aggregation, or cross-linking. The main model to study "ADCC-like" signal transduction pathways relies on the assumption that the first step in generating an ADCC response is the ligation or cross-linking of Fc receptors on the surface of the effector cell as facilitated by a large, "particulate" antigen such as a viral-infected cell coated with surface antigen-specific antibody (Figure 1.2A). Experimentally, to simulate particulate antigen-induced Fc-receptor cross-linking, many researchers incubate NK cells with FcγRIIIA-specific antibodies, followed by incubation with a secondary antibody (Figure 1.2B).[11] Another method of simulating antigen-induced Fc-receptor cross-linking is by "reverse ADCC," an experimental setup in which the polarity of the bridging antibody is reversed (Figure 1.2C).[12] Using these two CD16-cross-linking simulation strategies, ADCC-like signal transduction pathways have been dissected in both human and murine NK cells.

Downstream Signals in the Effector Cell

For ADCC to occur, molecular signals must also be transduced when an FcγR-bearing effector cell recognizes an antibody-coated target cell.[13–15] Much of what we know about ADCC signal transduction is based on experiments using FcγRIIIA-bearing NK cells as effector cells. Less is known about signaling in other effector cells expressing other FcγRs.

In the current signaling model, the gamma (γ) subunit associated with the FcγRIIIA receptor plays a crucial role in signaling (Figure 1.3). It contains immunoreceptor tyrosine-based activation motifs (ITAMs), which are consensus sequences containing tyrosine residues that can be phosphorylated. ITAMs do not have intrinsic tyrosine kinase activity; instead, they become phosphorylated by cellular src kinases upon FcγRIIIA cross-linking. Phosphorylated ITAMs recruit the spleen tyrosine kinase (Syk) protein, which binds to the ITAMs via its SH2 domains and becomes activated (Figure 1.3). Recruitment and activation of Syk triggers three main pathways involved in ADCC: phospholipase C-gamma pathway (PLC-γ), phosphatidylinositol 3-kinase (PI-3K) pathway, and Vav/Rho-family G-proteins pathway.

The PLC-γ pathway involves the Syk-dependent phosphorylation of the PLC-γ isozymes. Activated PLC-γ cleaves membrane

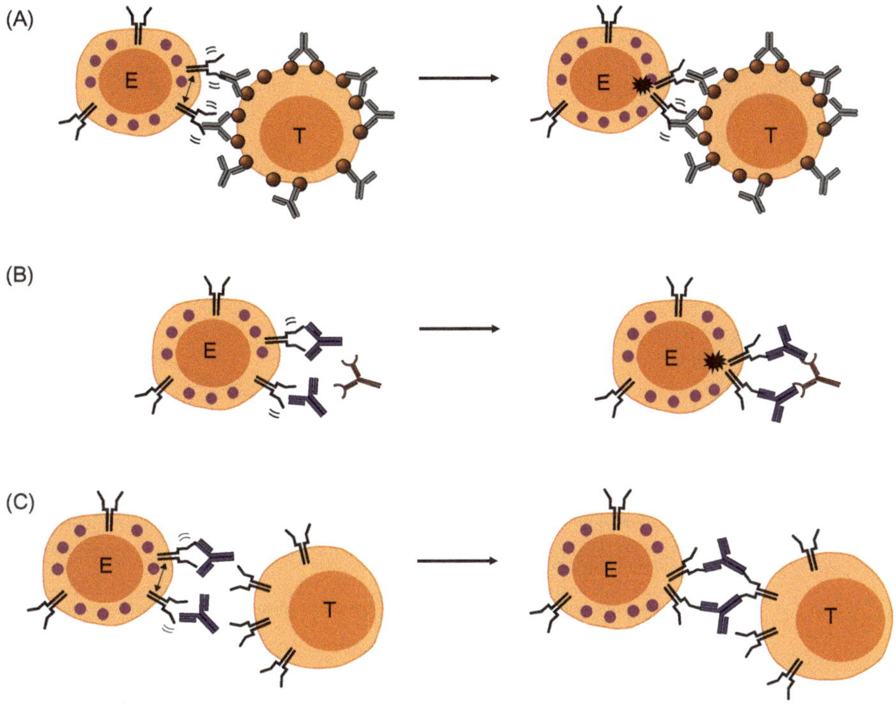

FIGURE 1.2 **Antibody and FcgR ligation.** ADCC involves cross-linking Fc receptors on the surface of effector cells. (A) The particulate nature of antibody complexed to antigens expressed on the surface of a target cell facilitates the physical rearrangement of Fc receptors, bringing them closer to each other and inducing their cross-linking (represented here by a black burst symbol). (B) ADCC in human NK cells can be simulated *in vitro* by incubating human NK effector cells with a mouse anti-human FcγRIIIA (mouse anti-human CD16) antibody (blue), followed by incubation with a secondary antibody (red), such as goat anti-mouse IgG. Addition of the secondary antibody will facilitate physical interactions between CD16 molecules, leading to their cross-linking. (C) ADCC in human NK cells can also be simulated *in vitro* via "reverse ADCC"—that is, by first incubating human NK effector cells with a mouse anti-human FcγRIIIA (mouse anti-human CD16) antibody (blue), followed by incubation with a mouse target cell expressing FcγRI receptors (gray). The particulate nature of the target cell will also facilitate physical interactions between CD16 molecules, leading to their cross-linking. Note the reversal in antibody polarity between (A) and (C). *E*, effector cell. *T*, target cell.

phosphatidylinositol 4,5-bisphosphate (PIP_2) to generate inositol-1,4,5-trisphosphate (IP_3) and diacylglycerol (DAG). IP_3 triggers an increase in intracellular free calcium, which is required for cytotoxic granule mobilization and exocytosis. DAG activates protein kinase C (PKC), which is necessary for other NK cell functions not directly related to ADCC. The PLC-γ pathway is required for ADCC function and can be blocked by herbimycin A, an antibiotic that inhibits tyrosine kinase activity and ADCC.

The PI-3K pathway involves the Syk-dependent activation of PI-3K. PI-3K is a heterodimer composed of an 85-kDa adaptor protein (facilitates interactions with other tyrosine kinases) and a 110-kDa catalytic subunit. PI-3K phosphorylates membrane PIP_2 into membrane phosphatidylinositol 3,4,5-triphosphate (PIP_3). PIP_3 mediates recruitment of pleckstrin homology (PH) domain-containing signaling proteins—that is, proteins (such as PLC-γ) that can be recruited to the membrane through binding

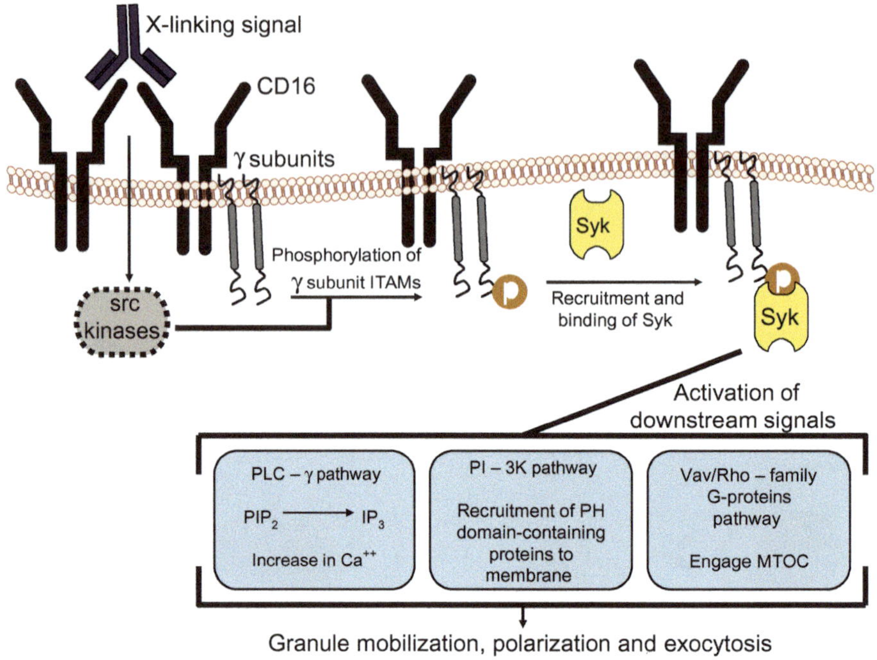

FIGURE 1.3 **ADCC signaling pathways.** ADCC mediated by NK cells involves three main signaling pathways. Following CD16 cross-linking, src kinases are activated and phosphorylate the ITAMs on the γ subunits associated with CD16. This is followed by recruitment of Syk and subsequent activation of the PLC-γ pathway, the PI-3K pathway and the Vav/Rho-family G-proteins pathway. The concerted action of these pathways leads to granule mobilization and exocytosis toward the target cell.

to membrane-bound PIP_3. Recruitment of PH domain-containing proteins to the membrane facilitates their interactions, thereby physically enhancing signal transduction pathways. The PI-3K pathway is also required for ADCC function and can be blocked by wortmannin, a fungal metabolite that inhibits ADCC and binds covalently to the p110 subunit of PI-3K.

The PH domain-containing Vav protein and the Rho family guanine nucleotide-binding proteins (G proteins) are also involved in NK cell granule polarization required for ADCC function. Syk is involved in the phosphorylation of Vav, although the precise mechanism remains unclear.[13,15] The cholera toxin A subunit (Ctx-A), a known inhibitor of G proteins, can inhibit ADCC activity; however, it is unclear where exactly this inhibition occurs, as Ctx-A may also have pleiotropic effects on IP_3 and GTP-binding proteins.[16]

For the sake of simplicity, it is tempting to limit the description of ADCC signaling mechanisms to the three Syk-related pathways outlined in Figure 1.3; however, we must bear in mind four important concepts to avoid oversimplifications or dogmatic views of the downstream signals involved in ADCC:

1. Signaling cascades do not work in isolation, and there is a considerable degree of cross-talk between Fc receptors and integrins,[17] surface receptors, and other intracellular proteins whose functions are still under investigation.[18]
2. There is a considerable degree of redundancy involving certain steps along these three pathways.
3. ADCC signaling mechanisms involving FcγRI, FcγRII, and FcγRIIIb have yet to be

characterized to the same extent as ADCC signaling involving FcγRIIIA.

4. Negative signals regulating each of the above-mentioned pathways exist.

With regard to the last point, we may cite the example of SH2-containing inositol phosphatase-1 (SHIP-1), a protein that modulates CD16-mediated ADCC in human NK cells. Whereas the three main ADCC signaling pathways described previously involve the phosphorylation of ITAMs present in the γ-subunit associated with FcγRIIIA, the SHIP-1 regulatory pathway engages the zeta (ζ) subunit associated with FcγRIIIA.[19]

Evidence supporting the role of these pathways in ADCC can be found in human immunodeficiency virus (HIV) infection and certain congenital abnormalities; for example, following CD16 cross-linking, NK cells from HIV-infected donors have significantly reduced levels of phosphorylated Syk in the cytoplasm compared to healthy controls.[20] This reduction correlates with a reduced ability of NK cells to degranulate and a reduced level in the number of CD16 molecules expressed per NK cell among HIV-infected donors. Similarly, NK cells from patients with congenital hemophagocytic syndromes have been shown to be impaired in their ability to degranulate due to loss-of-function mutations in genes whose corresponding proteins are involved in vesicle trafficking and/or cytotoxic granule formation and release.[21]

Mechanisms of Killing

CTLs and NK cells are able to kill target cells through three main pathways: the perforin/granzyme cell death pathway, the FAS-ligand (FAS-L) pathway, and the reactive oxygen intermediates/reactive oxygen species (ROI/ROS) or oxidative burst pathway. Of these three pathways, the perforin/granzyme cell death pathway, also known as the granule-exoctyosis pathway, has been the most widely investigated in the context of ADCC involving NK cells.

The Perforin/Granzyme Cell Death Pathway

Upon FcγRIIIA receptor cross-linking, the signaling pathways described earlier trigger the increase of intracellular calcium, the engagement of the microtubule-organizing center (MTOC) within the effector cell, and the polarization and release of cytotoxic granules containing perforin and granzyme.[13,15,22,23] These granules are highly organized dual-function organelles containing mainly perforin, granzyme, and granulysin within a dense core surrounded by a prelysosomal compartment of acidic pH containing lysosomal hydrolases. The content of cytotoxic granules in NK cells has been reviewed elsewhere.[23]

Killing of target cells via the perforin/granzyme cell death pathway essentially occurs in sequential stages involving the concerted action of perforin and granzyme. The most recent model for this pathway argues for the existence of a macromolecular complex containing perforin, granzyme, and other molecules being released by the effector cell. Granzyme B in this macromolecular complex interacts with the mannose 6-phosphate receptor (MPR) expressed on the surface of target cells, leading to MPR-mediated endocytosis of the macromolecular complex. Endosomes containing granzyme and perforin are formed within the target cell; endosome membrane disruption is achieved by perforin resulting in granzyme being released into the cytosol. Perforin by itself can mediate cell lysis and death but not apoptosis. For apoptosis to occur, granzyme B must either directly activate caspases that induce DNA fragmentation in the nucleus or cleave the Bid molecule, which, when truncated, can insert itself into mitochondria and release mitochondrial constituents that can in turn either potentiate caspase activation and nuclear DNA degradation or induce caspase-independent apoptosis.[22]

Experiments using human NK cells impaired in their ability to degranulate provide evidence that the perforin/granzyme cell death pathway is involved in ADCC. Such "degranuation-impaired" NK cells are obtained from patients with congenital immune disorders known as hemophagocytic syndromes. For example, Griscelli syndrome type 2 (GS2) and familial hemophagocytic lymphohistiocytosis type 3 (FHL3) are two congenital conditions associated with loss of function of the genes encoding the Rab27a and Munc13-4 proteins. While Rab27a is a member of the Rab GTPase family of proteins that regulate vesicle trafficking, Munc13-4 is a member of a family of proteins that regulate membrane fusion, including the fusion of perforin-containing granules with the plasma membrane. Cells derived from patients with these hemophagocytic syndromes express normal levels of Fc receptors; however, upon FcgRIIIA cross-linking, cells from GS2 and FHL3 patients cannot degranulate.[21]

In addition to these naturally occurring mutations affecting degranulation and ADCC, evidence for the involvement of the granule-exocytosis pathway in ADCC also stems from experiments in which perforin/granzyme granule polarization and release are blocked chemically. This can be achieved by the addition of calcium ion inhibitors interfering with microtubule rearrangement and granule polarization or, as briefly mentioned earlier, by the addition of herbimycin A, wortmannin, or cholera toxin A subunit—compounds that affect the three main signaling pathways leading to calcium increase and granule polarization and release.

Unlike previous models arguing for passive diffusion of cytotoxic granules into the target cell, the most recent model of the perforin/granzyme cell death pathway invokes a key role of novel receptors on the target cell that presumably mediate the uptake of the macromolecular complex containing perforin and granzyme. As mentioned above, the mannose 6-phosphate receptor (MPR) interacts with granzyme B and engages receptor-mediated endocytosis of the macromolecular complex.[22] There is also evidence that platelet-activating factor (PAF), a lysolipid that promotes platelet aggregation, is co-released with perforin when NK cells degranulate.[24] It has been postulated that this may potentiate lysis by allowing PAF released from the effector cell to form a molecular bridge with PAF receptors (PAF-Rs) present on target cells. Although the roles of MPR and PAF-R remain to be fully elucidated in the context of ADCC, it is conceivable that differences in MPR and PAF-R expression by target cells may translate into differences in target cell susceptibility to killing via ADCC and its associated perforin/granzyme pathway.

The FAS-L Pathway

Compared to the myriad of reports examining the role of the perforin/granzyme cell death pathway in ADCC, there is less but still substantial evidence to indicate that granule-independent mechanisms may also be involved in the killing of target cells. For example, in addition to inducing granule exocytosis, cross-linking of FcγRIIIA on NK cells induces transcriptional upregulation of FAS ligands (FAS-L), thereby enabling NK cells to become effectors that can kill target cells expressing FAS receptors.[25] This may be relevant in the context of ADCC, as the killing by macrophages of antibody-coated mesanglial cells and vascular smooth muscle cells via ADCC can be inhibited by anti-FAS-L or anti-CD16 antagonistic antibodies.[26]

The ROS/ROI Pathway

The role of the reactive oxygen species/reactive oxygen intermediates (ROS/ROI) pathway in ADCC remains controversial. It is well known that ROS are produced by phagocytic cells during the "oxidative" or "metabolic" burst that occurs in response to antigen opsonization. This burst is characterized by an increase in oxygen consumption by the cell and the subsequent release of ROS such as hydrogen peroxide, superoxide, and other free radicals that can damage the integrity of opsonized antigens and can thus confer protection against intracellular bacteria, viruses, or parasites. It is unclear, however, whether ROS or the oxidative burst are involved during target cell lysis via ADCC. Early experiments indicated that hypoxia and metabolic burst inhibitors (such as cation chelators) reduced the ability of monocytes to kill antibody-sensitized erythrocytes, suggesting a role for the metabolic burst in ADCC.[27] However, these data were at odds with two observations: (1) Monocytes from patients with chronic granulomatous disease (CGD) (i.e., patients who have a genetic impairment in mounting a metabolic burst) had normal levels of ADCC; and (2) the addition of ROS scavengers (such as superoxide dismutase) did not inhibit the ADCC reaction. Similarly, experiments with granulocytes confirmed that ROS scavengers did not inhibit granulocyte-mediated ADCC and that granulocytes from CGD patients had an even greater capacity to kill compared to granulocytes from normal donors.[28] In contrast, data from a third study indicated that both mononuclear (PBMC) and polymorphonuclear (PMN) cells from CGD patients had significantly reduced levels of ADCC against T cells.[29] These discrepancies may be best explained by the fact that the CGD phenotype is not caused by a unique mutation; instead, it is the result of a genetically heterogeneous group of immunodeficiencies rendering cells from CGD patients differentially affected in their capacity to perform ROS-dependent ADCC.

In a recent report, Horner et al.[6] argued that the ADCC activity of PMN is neither ROS mediated nor perforin dependent but is instead related to trogocytosis, the ability of effector cells and target cells to exchange membrane lipids during the ADCC reaction *in vitro*. They showed that membrane lipid exchange (assessed visually by microscopy) correlated with target cell apoptosis and target cell lysis. Recently, an *in vivo* role of trogocytosis in ADCC has also been proposed using a mouse model.[30] Future experiments may elucidate whether trogocytosis is a novel mechanism of ADCC or merely a consequence of the known mechanisms described earlier. In any case, the trogocytosis and ROS data summarized here illustrate how ADCC killing mechanisms for PMN and monocytes may differ substantially from the predominant perforin/granzyme pathway described for NK cells. Consistent with the notion that effector cell populations may act by different mechanisms, antibody fucosylation has been found to differentially impact ADCC mediated by NK and PMN effectors.[31]

ADCC Assays in Relation to Killing Mechanisms

Final considerations over the killing mechanisms involved in ADCC are the variety, the significance, and the limitations of available ADCC assays (Table 1.2). Historically, while the original ADCC assays were target cell-based and involved assessing the lysis of target cells by measuring the release of chromium-51 or other radioisotopes,[32] subsequent assays were effector cell based and consisted of measuring the release of esterases[33] and perforin[34] into the cell medium or into the adjacent cell microenvironment (as a surrogate marker of degranulation). The advent of flow cytometry has also facilitated the development of numerous assays that can measure target cell viability or effector cell degranulation.[35–38] A broader variety of new-generation ADCC assays, however, may be required to clarify the role of the Fas/Fas-L pathway, the ROS/ROI oxidative burst pathway and a possible trogocytosis pathway in ADCC mediated by both NK and non-NK cells.

ADCC IN MONOCLONAL ANTIBODY THERAPY OF CANCER

Monoclonal antibodies are well-established cancer therapies due to their specificity, versatility, and clinical efficacy. In addition to their direct anti-tumor effects through targeting of

TABLE 1.2 Examples of Methods Used to Measure ADCC Activity *In Vitro*

Category	Method	Concept	Major Equipment Required	Refs.
Target cell-based	Chromium release assay (CRA)	Target cells are labeled with chromium[51] (Cr^{51}). Antibody and effector cells are added. Incubation ensues to allow ADCC to occur. Cr^{51} release is measured as a surrogate marker of killing and target cell lysis. Variations include labeling targets with other radioisotopes such as tritium (H^3) or iodine.[125]	Scintillation counter	Timonen and Saksela[32]
	Viability dye flow-based assays	Target cells are labeled with a cell membrane dye. Antibody and effector cells are added. Incubation ensues to allow ADCC to occur. A viability dye is added at the end of the reaction. Cells are fixed and flow cytometry is used to measure the percentage of non-viable cells that retain the membrane dye and lose the viability dye. Variations include the rapid fluorometric ADCC (RFADCC) assay, in which target cells are dually labeled with a membrane dye and a viability dye at the beginning of the ADCC reaction.	Flow cytometer	Jacobs and Pipho,[35] Lee-MacAry et al.,[36] Gomez-Roman et al.,[37] Wilkinson et al.[121]
	Apoptosis-based assays	These assays focus on the Fas/Fas-L pathway and employ a combination of flow-cytometry and microscopy methods to assess the apoptotic state of target cells.	Electron microscope, flow cytometer	Boyle[26]
	ADCC-GranToxiLux (ADCC-GLT) assay	Target cells are labeled with a fluorogenic peptide substrate containing a sequence recognized by granzyme B. Targets are incubated with antibody and effectors and ADCC is allowed to occur. Granzyme B is delivered from effectors into the target cells and hydrolysis of the fluorogenic peptide substrate occurs. Hydrolysis of the substrate within target cells is quantitated by flow cytometry as a surrogate marker of granzyme B diffusion.	Flow cytometer	Pollara et al.[38]
	Lactate dehydrogenase release assay	Target cells are incubated with antibody and effector cells. ADCC is allowed to occur. The release of lactate dehydrogenase (LDH) is measured as a surrogate marker of killing and target cell lysis. LDH released from dead cells is used to produce a red dye	Microplate reader	Seidel et al.[122]
	Electrical impedance assay	Adherent target cells are incubated with antibody and effector cells. ADCC is allowed to occur, leading to detachment of target cells from microplate wells and resulting in a change in electrical impedance. Impedance can be measured over time yielding kinetic or time course data of the ADCC reaction.	xCELLigence™ system	Yamashita-Kashima et al.[123]

(*Continued*)

TABLE 1.2 (Continued)

Category	Method	Concept	Major Equipment Required	Refs.
Effector cell-based	Esterase release assay	Target cells are incubated with antibody and effector cells. ADCC is allowed to occur. Upon degranulation, effectors release granules containing esterases (mainly granzyme A) that can cleave the substrate *N*-α-benzyloxycarbonyl-L-lysine thiobenzyl ester (BLT). Aliquots from the ADCC culture supernatant are incubated with the BLT substrate, and esterase activity is measured by colorimetry as a surrogate marker of effector cell activity.	Microplate reader	Kato et al.[33]
	Perforin deposition assays	Effectors, antibody, and targets are mixed and ADCC is allowed to occur. Cells are fixed and stained with gold-conjugated, perforin-specific monoclonal antibodies. Perforin deposition at the effector–target cell synapse is monitored by microscopy.	Electron microscope	Ortaldo et al.[34]
	Whole blood intracellular cytokine staining (ICS) assay	Whole blood is incubated with peptide antigens in the presence of brefeldin A and monensin for 6 hours. ADCC is allowed to occur. At the end of the incubation, cells are stained with monoclonal antibodies against NK cells, granzyme B, and the CD107, a surface degranulation marker. The number of CD107-positive NK cells is measured as a surrogate marker of degranulation. Cells that have lost intracellular granzyme B expression can also be quantified.	Flow cytometer	Chung et al.[124]

tumor antigens, monoclonal antibodies can, as described above, engage immune effector mechanisms such as antibody-dependent cell-mediated cytotoxicity (ADCC). Pivotal *in vivo* studies established the role of activating and inhibitory Fc receptors (FcRs) expressed on immune effector cells in mouse models of monoclonal antibody cancer therapy. A multitude of *in vitro* preclinical studies have confirmed that ADCC and other FcR-dependent effector mechanisms are relevant for the anti-tumor effects of therapeutic monoclonal antibodies. In clinical trials, FcR polymorphisms have been associated with monoclonal antibody affinity and clinical efficacy, supporting ADCC as a putative mechanism of action. Translational studies have attempted to verify immune effector mechanisms in patients responding to monoclonal antibody therapy. Aside from ADCC, monoclonal antibodies have also been used to target receptors on immune effector cells—independent of FcRs—in an effort to enhance responses against tumors.

Versatility of Monoclonal Antibodies as Platforms for Cancer Therapy

The desire for targeted therapy in cancer has spurred the development of monoclonal antibody therapies that recognize tumor antigens. The structure of monoclonal antibodies has provided a versatile platform with which to

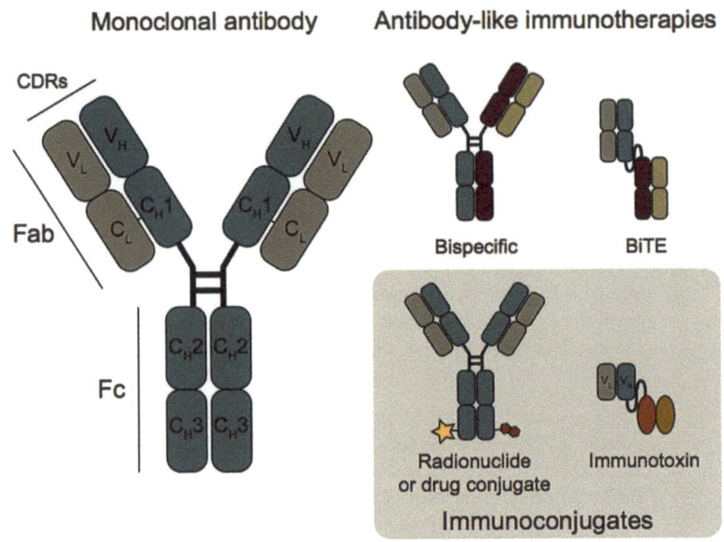

FIGURE 1.4 **The structure of monoclonal antibody and antibody-like therapies.** Most monoclonal antibody (mAb)-based cancer therapies are IgG isotype structures with three main regions: (1) Two fragment antigen-binding (Fab) "arms," which contain complementarity-determining regions (CDRs) that recognize specific antigens; and (2) the crystallizable fragment (Fc) region, which can promote immune effector mechanisms. IgG mAbs also contain structural domains known as heavy and light chains. Each Fab portion contains a variable light (V_L) and variable heavy (V_H) chain and constant light (C_L) and heavy (C_H1) chain. The Fc portion contains the rest of the heavy chains (C_H2 and C_H3). Modifications to the Fab regions involve enhancing affinity to antigens or using portions of the Fabs to generate other antibody-like molecules (i.e., using V_L and V_H chains in immunotoxins). Fc modifications modulate immune effector function and have included (1) *replacement*, to reduce intrinsic immunogenicity through chimerism (e.g., mouse variable regions with human Fc regions) or "humanization" (e.g., mouse CDRs with otherwise human antibody sequence); (2) *amino acid substitutions*, to enhance Fc receptor (FcR) specificity and affinity to engage immune effectors (e.g., reduced inhibitory FcR affinity and enhanced activating FcR affinity) and modify neonatal FcR (FcRn) engagement to change serum stability; and (3) *conjugation*, to deliver therapeutic payloads to targeted sites (i.e., immunoconjugates). Examples of mAb structure and various mAb-like molecules including bispecifics, BiTEs, and immunoconjugates are depicted. *Figure reproduced with permission from Louis M. Weiner, Joseph C. Murray, Casey W. Shuptrine, Antibody-Based Immunotherapy of Cancer, Cell, Volume 148, Issue 6, 16 March 2012, pp. 1081–1084, ISSN 0092-8674, 10.1016/j.cell.2012.02.034.*

develop targeted therapies (Figure 1.4). Many therapeutic monoclonal antibodies have targeted cell surface-expressed antigens found on tumor cells, due to their relative accessibility and specificity (Table 1.3). Rituximab, the first U.S. Food and Drug Administration (FDA)-approved monoclonal antibody therapy for cancer, targets CD20 expressed on B-cell non-Hodgkin lymphoma (NHL).[39] Rituximab engagement of CD20 induced antiproliferative and apoptotic activity against NHL cell lines *in vitro*. Trastuzumab was the first monoclonal antibody therapy approved for a solid tumor, targeting HER2/ErbB2-positive breast cancer.[40] Cetuximab is an anti-EGFR/ErbB1 antibody for metastatic colorectal and head and neck cancers.[41–43] The antigen-binding activities of trastuzumab and cetuximab perturb oncogenic growth factor receptor signaling of their respective ErbB family members, reducing the proliferation and viability of tumor cells.

The Fc region of monoclonal antibodies has served as a foundation for modifying antibody activity without impinging upon antigen specificity found in the Fab regions. Early attempts were aimed at enhancing the pharmacokinetic and pharmacodynamic properties of monoclonal antibodies derived from

TABLE 1.3 Approved Antibody-Based Cancer Immunotherapies

Name	Antigen	Format	Isotype and Subtype[a]	Indication(s)
Tumor Antigen-Targeted Antibodies[b]				
Rituximab	CD20	Chimeric	IgG_1	Non-Hodgkin lymphoma
^{131}I-tositumomab	CD20	Humanized conjugate	Murine IgG_2	Relapsed and/or refractory lymphoma
Ofatumumab	CD20	Human	IgG_1	Chronic lymphocytic leukemia
^{90}Y-Ibritumomab tiuxetan	CD20	Mouse conjugate	Murine IgG_1	Relapsed and/or refractory lymphoma
Alemtuzumab	CD52	Humanized	IgG_1	Chronic lymphocytic leukemia
Brentuximab vedotin	CD30	Chimeric	IgG_1	Hodgkin lymphoma and anaplastic large cell lymphoma
Trastuzumab	HER2	Humanized	IgG_1	Breast and gastric cancers
Cetuximab	EGFR	Chimeric	IgG_1	Colorectal and head and neck cancers
Panitumumab	EGFR	Human	IgG_2	Metastatic colorectal cancer
Bevacizumab	VEGF-A	Humanized	IgG_1	Metastatic colorectal, non-small cell lung, glioblastoma, and kidney cancers
Immune Effector Antigen-Targeted Antibodies				
Ipilimumab	CTLA-4	Human	IgG_1	Metastatic melanoma

[a]*Human isotype and subtype, unless otherwise specified.*
[b]*Gemtuzumab ozogamicin (Mylotarg™) was withdrawn from the market in June, 2010.*
Table reproduced with permission from Louis M. Weiner, Joseph C. Murray, Casey W. Shuptrine, Antibody-Based Immunotherapy of Cancer, Cell, Volume 148, Issue 6, 16 March 2012, pp. 1081–1084, ISSN 0092-8674, 10.1016/j.cell.2012.02.034.

non-human mammals. Chimeric antibodies reduced unwanted antigenicity through recombination, mainly in the Fc, with human regions. Rituximab was the first chimeric antibody approved by the FDA for its clinical efficacy, and this human IgG_1 Fc demonstrated effective complement-dependent cytotoxicity (CDC) and ADCC *in vitro*.[39] Cetuximab is an anti-EGFR chimeric IgG_1 antibody with similar capacity to induce ADCC.[44,45] The incorporation of a human Fc into these antibodies, while allowing for superior pharmacological properties, also allowed for enhanced engagement of immune effector mechanisms.

Following on the success of chimeric antibodies, humanized antibodies were designed to replace the majority of a non-human-derived antibody—aside from the critical complementarity-determining regions (CDRs) that impart antigen specificity—with human polypeptide sequences.[46] Trastuzumab represents a recombinant humanized antibody that has retained its capacity for ADCC.[40] "Fully human" antibodies are now developed via phage display or genetically modified mice and can be produced in mammalian cell systems. Panitumumab, a fully human anti-EGFR antibody approved for use in colorectal cancer, differs from cetuximab in that it targets a distinct epitope and contains an IgG_2 isotype, which lessens its potency in conventional ADCC assays that employ natural killer (NK) cells as effectors. However, panitumumab has the capacity to induce ADCC by innate immune cells of the myeloid lineage preferentially.[47] By incorporating specific human Fc regions, therapeutic monoclonal antibodies now can be engineered with fine-tuned Fc-mediated effector mechanisms.

Evidence for ADCC in Cancer Therapy

The seminal work of Clynes and Ravetch established the role of inhibitory and activating FcR in modifying response to monoclonal antibody therapy in mouse models of cancer.[48] Their studies—along with others utilizing FcR-associated γ-chain (FcRγ) knockout or signaling-deficient mice—defined a role of FcR-mediated immune effector activity, such as ADCC, in monoclonal antibody therapy.[49]

In mouse models of monoclonal antibody therapy, various FcRs and innate immune effectors—most commonly of myeloid lineage—have demonstrated the capacity for FcR-mediated anti-tumor activity, including ADCC.[50] However, identifying immune effectors in the act of ADCC has been challenging *in vivo*. In a Tn antigen-positive mouse breast cancer (TA3Ha) intraperitoneal xenograft model, ADCC immune synapses were visualized *ex vivo* between macrophage and tumor cells in peritoneal fluid.[51] Combining conjugated antibodies with high-resolution intravital imaging of immune effectors and tumor cells may reveal more about the *in vivo* dynamics of ADCC in mouse models.

In antibody therapy in humans, there is evidence that multiple innate immune effectors, including macrophage, granulocytes, and NK cells, play a role in ADCC.[52] However, NK cells—and specifically those expressing the activating FcR *FCGR3A*—have been shown to be the predominant effector cell capable of eliciting ADCC.[53] *FCGR3A* polymorphisms can independently predict responses to rituximab in patients with non-Hodgkin lymphoma.[54,55] Specifically, high-affinity *FCGR3A* polymorphisms resulting in homozygous valine versus phenylalanine at residue 158 (V/V158 vs. F/F158) correlated with significantly better objective responses (90% vs. 67%) at one year.[54] These findings suggest that FcR-mediated activity affects the clinical efficacy of monoclonal antibody therapy. Beyond hematological malignancies, FcR polymorphisms have been shown to predict response to antibody therapy in solid tumors. FcR polymorphisms predict responses to trastuzumab in breast cancer.[56] Similar correlations have been found with cetuximab in metastatic colorectal cancer.[57,58] Despite some negative retrospective analyses, the correlation of FcR polymorphisms with therapeutic responses represents the strongest clinical evidence for ADCC.

In the clinical application of antibody therapies, *in vivo* assessment of ADCC has been especially challenging. Even where a tumor microenvironment could be deemed relatively accessible, such as in rituximab-treated lymphoma, ADCC has yet to be observed directly; however, rituximab therapy has been shown to induce activation of peripheral blood NK cells in patients with high-affinity FcR polymorphisms.[59] In histological assessment of solid tumors, NK cells are apparent but few in number and rarely assessed for FCGR3A expression.[52,60] It is conceivable that NK cells in peripheral blood may inhibit metastatic disease via ADCC, but translational evidence is lacking.

ADCC IN INFECTIOUS DISEASE: A CORRELATE OF PROTECTION?

A protective role of ADCC against infectious disease has been postulated in numerous studies (Table 1.4). In many of these, significant associations have been observed between the *in vitro* ADCC activity of serum antibodies and *in vivo* protection from infection or disease progression in animals or humans. These strong associations have generated both enthusiasm and skepticism among immunologists. On the

TABLE 1.4 Examples of ADCC Being Implicated in Protection vs. Infectious Diseases

Pathogen	Disease or Pathology	Model	Relevant Observations	Refs.
Herpes simplex virus type 2 (HSV-2)	Death	Mice	Passive transfer of non-neutralizing monoclonal antibodies with *in vitro* ADCC activity protects complement-deficient mice against lethal challenge.	Balachandran et al.[62]
	Genital herpes	Humans	Limited induction of antibodies with ADCC activity may be related to the poor efficacy of an HSV-2 vaccine containing recombinant glycoproteins B and D.	Kohl et al.[125]
Influenza virus	Flu	Humans	Antibody with *in vitro* ADCC activity against influenza-virus-infected cells is detectable in sera of children after natural infection and after immunization with live attenuated or inactivated influenza vaccines.	Hashimoto et al.[126]
		Mice	Vaccine-elicited M2-specific antibodies are able to bind to influenza-virus-infected cells *in vitro* but fail to protect against a high-dose challenge *in vivo.*	Jegerlehner et al.[127]
Sendai virus	Pneumonia	Mice	Passive transfer of non-neutralizing monoclonal antibodies with no complement-mediated lysis activity protected mice against pneumonia via an Fc-dependent mechanism.	Mochizuki et al.[128]
African swine fever virus (ASFV)	Fever, viremia, and death	Pigs	Passive transfer ASFV-specific antibodies with *in vitro* ADCC activity confers protection of pigs against challenge.	Wardley et al.[129]
Chlamydia trachomatis	Secondary genital chlamydial infection	Mice	Peritoneal exudate macrophages and anti-chlamydial antibodies with *in vitro* ADCC activity control secondary genital infection.	Moore et al.[130]
Schistosoma japonicum	Schistosomiasis	Mice	An intramuscular cDNA vaccine induces antibodies with ADCC activity *in vitro* and is efficient against cercariae.	Zhou et al.[131]
Human immunodeficiency virus (HIV)	AIDS	Humans	*In vitro* ADCC activity correlates with prognostic predictors of HIV infection.	Ahmad et al.[63]
		Humans	*In vitro* ADCC activity correlates with lower viral loads *in vivo.*	Forthal et al.[64]
		Humans	A higher frequency and magnitude of *in vitro* ADCC responses is observed in serum among recipients of a prime-boost HIV vaccine compared to placebo recipients.	Karnasuta et al.[75]
		Humans	*In vitro* ADCC activity is detectable in the sera of HIV controllers (i.e., HIV-infected individuals in whom viral replication is undetectable in spite of receiving no antiretroviral treatment) and is significantly higher than in viremic individuals.	Lambotte et al.[69]

(*Continued*)

TABLE 1.4 (Continued)

Pathogen	Disease or Pathology	Model	Relevant Observations	Refs.
Simian immunodeficiency virus (SIV)	AIDS	Rhesus macaques	*In vitro* ADCC activity is associated with delayed disease progression in a small group of macaques ($n = 3$).	Banks et al.[65]
		Rhesus macaques	Vaccine-elicited antibodies mediate ADCC activity correlating with protection against a rectal SIV challenge.	Gomez-Roman et al.[66]
		Rhesus macaques	Vaccine-elicited antibodies mediate ADCC activity at high titers correlating with reduced acute viremia after a rectal SIV challenge.	Hidajat et al.[67]
		Rhesus macaques	The magnitude of *in vitro* ADCC responses is inversely associated with viral load in animals with moderate to high levels of viral replication.	Sun et al.[71]
		Rhesus macaques	ADCC titers correlate with the number of exposures required for infection in a repeated low-dose SIV rectal challenge.	Xiao et al.[72]
Genetically engineered simian–human immunodeficiency virus (SHIV)	High levels of acute viral load after infection; CD4T cell depletion	Rhesus macaques	Passive transfer of b12, an HIV neutralizing antibody, confers protection against challenge with SHIV. When the *in vitro* Fc-receptor binding activity of the antibody is obliterated, it loses some *in vivo* protective properties.	Hessell et al.[77]
		Rhesus macaques	Vaccine-elicited antibodies with ADCC activity are observed in macaques with reduced chronic viremia following an intravenous SHIV challenge.	Florese et al.[68]
		Rhesus macaques	Vaccine-elicited antibodies mediate ADCC activity correlating with reduced acute and chronic viremia following an intravenous SHIV challenge.	Xiao et al.[70]
		Rhesus macaques	A non-fucosylated variant of b12 (NFb12) has a higher affinity to FcγRIIIA and is more effective than its wild-type counterpart in mediating *in vitro* ADCC. However, no significant differences in protection are observed *in vivo* when macaques are infused with b12 or NFb12 prior to a repeated low-dose vaginal challenge with SHIV.	Moldt et al.[78]

one hand, ADCC enthusiasts, including vaccine experts from the World Health Organization,[61] consider ADCC a possible mechanism of protection worth exploring in the context of vaccine research and development. On the other hand, ADCC skeptics argue that the strong associations with protection establish neither causality nor a definitive, clear, unequivocal role of ADCC in protection. Here we present evidence supporting both views.

Studies of Herpes Simplex Virus

Among the studies listed in Table 1.4, the herpes simplex virus (HSV) studies are a notable exception supporting ADCC enthusiasts.[62] Soon after the advent of monoclonal antibody technology, several monoclonal antibodies against HSV-2 glycoproteins were derived in mice. These antibodies were characterized *in vitro* for their ability to neutralize the virus, for their ability to kill virus-infected cells via ADCC and for their ability to kill virus-infected cells via CDC. Although none of the antibodies had neutralizing activity, some had dual ADCC and CDC activity, and a few had strong ADCC activity and very low CDC activity only, thus providing a good opportunity to study the protective role of ADCC by infusing them into mice and then challenging with live virus. To further rule out any interference of CDC in these studies, complement-deficient mice were used in these experiments, thereby providing a "clean" system in which any observed protection could be attributed exclusively to ADCC and not to CDC or to neutralization. Infusion of monoclonal antibodies with high ADCC activity (*in vitro* ADCC titers greater than 1:3000) protected mice against a lethal HSV-2 challenge (70% survival or greater), while infusion of monoclonal antibodies with intermediate ADCC activity (*in vitro* ADCC titers of 1:1000) resulted in reduced protection (35 to 55% survival). Infusion of monoclonal antibodies with low ADCC activity (*in vitro* ADCC titers of 1:30) conferred no protection upon challenge (0% survival), providing a direct link between *in vivo* protection from infectious disease and high ADCC titers observed *in vitro*.

Studies of Human and Simian Immunodeficiency Virus

The remaining examples outlined in Table 1.4 do not provide the clear-cut evidence or the "neutralization and complement-free" clean systems so elegantly designed in the HSV-2 studies described above. This lack of clean, "ADCC-only" experimental systems confounds our ability to differentiate the impact of the multiple effector mechanisms by which antibodies may provide protection. For example, much enthusiasm has been generated lately because several associations have been observed between antiviral ADCC activity in serum and protection from AIDS in humans and in rhesus macaques.[63–72] It has been speculated that ADCC could play a role in protection by intercepting the "eclipse" phase of human or simian immunodeficiency virus (HIV/SIV) infections—that is, the narrow window of opportunity shortly after mucosal transmission, during which HIV/SIV can be found only in mucosal cells but not in systemic compartments.[73] It is conceivable that, shortly after mucosal exposure to the virus, ADCC may prevent acquisition by killing small, discrete foci of virus-infected cells before the infection spreads to systemic compartments. This notion has been revisited recently in light of data that are being analyzed from the RV144 Phase III HIV vaccine trial. In this trial, the rate of HIV infection among volunteers receiving an HIV vaccine was 31.2% lower than the rate of HIV infection among volunteers who received the placebo.[74] The hypothesis that protection may have been due to ADCC was soon raised, primarily based on earlier findings reporting that sera from vaccinees had had binding antibodies that possessed ADCC activity but lacked broadly neutralizing antibodies or potent T cell responses.[75,76]

Ongoing Debate and a Possible Consensus

Skeptics may argue that the above associations do not warrant causality. Toward this end, monoclonal antibodies can be manipulated to alter their neutralizing, CDC, and ADCC activities *in vitro* prior to their use in challenge studies *in vivo*. This elegant strategy has been used to establish that the Fc receptor-binding capacity, but not the complement-binding capacity of b12, an HIV-neutralizing antibody, is important in mediating protection against a chimeric simian–human immunodeficiency virus (SHIV) challenge in macaques.[77] Contrastingly, recent evidence has also shown that a non-fucosylated variant of this antibody (NFb12) had greater *in vitro* ADCC activity against HIV-infected cells compared to its wild-type counterpart (b12), but did not confer greater protection against a vaginal SHIV challenge.[78] Yet, a host of similar experiments in other disease models in which monoclonal antibodies have been engineered to possess differential ADCC activity have likewise provided support for a protective role of ADCC.[79,80] While ADCC on its own may be unlikely to be protective against HIV infection or other infectious diseases, it is possible that induction of ADCC may potentiate protection conferred by the other potential immune correlates, such as CTLs and neutralizing antibodies. As investigation into the possible causal relationship of antibody–FcgR interactions and protection continues, the role of ADCC relative to other effector functions remains challenging to resolve.

RATIONAL MODIFICATION OF ADCC ACTIVITY

As described above, attempts to modify the *in vivo* activity of monoclonal antibodies have focused on enhancing selective Fc- and FcR-mediated responses. The differential glycosylation of specific amino acid residues in the Fc has been shown to modify Fc-mediated CDC and Fc–FcR-mediated ADCC.[81] Therefore, glycoengineering of monoclonal antibodies is an important consideration in antibody development.[82] Mutations introduced into IgG_1 Fc regions have been shown to modulate C1q binding, which could modify CDC activity.[83] Non-fucosylated rituximab and trastuzumab antibodies have enhanced FcR binding and ADCC versus their fucosylated equivalents.[84,85]

Besides glycoengineering techniques, mutagenesis has revealed ways to modify Fc–FcR interactions at the amino acid level. Assessment of human IgG_1 residues that affect binding to activating or inhibitory FcR—including the activating FcγRIIIa (FCGR3A), commonly associated with ADCC—provided insight into the structure-function relationship of Fc–FcR interactions.[86] Based on these findings, genetic modification of Fc residues has increased FCGR3A binding and ADCC, with antibody variants that have overcome the reduced clinical efficacy correlated with low-affinity *FCGR3A* polymorphisms.[87] Inhibitory FcγRIIb (FCGR2B)—expressed primarily on innate immune effectors besides NK cells—has been shown to decrease monoclonal antibody therapy efficacy in mouse models.[48] However, as binding to the FcγR family is shared in the hinge region of the Fc domain, it has proved challenging to engineer preferentially enhanced FCGR3A and reduced FCGR2B binding.[87,88] Fc engagement with the neonatal FcR (FcRn) has been shown to modify the pharmacokinetic profile of therapeutic monoclonal antibodies.[89] IgG_1 Fc variants with enhanced affinity to FcRn have demonstrated greater serum stability.[90]

Afucosylated monoclonal antibodies designed with reduced CDC activity, increased FCGR3A affinity, and enhanced FcRn-mediated serum retention could yield potent therapeutic antibodies with maximal capacity for ADCC. Accordingly, such Fc-optimized monoclonal antibodies are being translated into the clinic. Obinutuzumab, a glycol-engineered anti-CD20 antibody with reduced CDC and enhanced ADCC and direct apoptosis, is being tested in Phase III clinical trials in combination with chemotherapeutic agents, after demonstrating Phase I/II efficacy as a monotherapy.[91] Several antibodies optimized for FcR affinity are in preclinical or Phase I studies, including an anti-CD20 antibody, AME-133v, that contains two amino acid changes that enhance FcR binding and ADCC.[92] Rational engineering of monoclonal antibodies is expected to translate into significantly enhanced anti-tumor activity and clinical efficacy.

Beyond the antibody engineering discussed here, the modular domains of antibodies—including Fv, Fab, and Fc domains—have been recombined into a multitude of antibody-like therapies. These therapies include bispecific (including bispecific T-cell engagers [BiTEs]) and trispecific (e.g., TrioMabs) antibodies with various non FcR-mediated anti-tumor effects (Figure 1.5). Most of these therapies target non-FcR mediated anti-tumor mechanisms, although some novel approaches have attempted to engage FcR and tumor antigens directly.[93] Reviews of these and other antibody-derived therapies are available elsewhere.[94–96]

In contrast to the spectrum of tools available for manipulating monoclonal antibodies, less is known about whether or how vaccination strategies may differ in their capacity to elicit antibodies with variable ADCC activity, whether by tuning IgG subclass composition or by altering Fc glycosylation. However, these represent promising avenues of investigation, and the glycosylation state of IgG_1 secreted from B cells *ex vivo* has been shown to be modulated by B cell stimuli such as CpG, retinoic acid, or IL-21.[97] Experiments in mice have shown that repeated immunizations with ovalbumin (OVA) elicit OVA-specific IgG with a higher fucose content compared to the less-fucosylated OVA-specific IgG elicited by a single priming and a single boosting immunization.[98] This finding would suggest that repeated boosts during vaccination against infectious diseases may bias humoral immunity toward the production of fucosylated IgG versions. Based on the known effect of fucosylation on ADCC activity, the implications of this bias in the context of ADCC ought to be investigated. "More" vaccine may not necessarily translate into the induction of "better" functional antibodies in the case of ADCC.

ENHANCING THE LINK BETWEEN ADCC AND ADAPTIVE IMMUNITY

A common goal of immunotherapies is the induction of a persistent host immune response. Immunological persistence is acquired through adaptive immune responses that yield antigen-specific memory. Initiation of ADCC by therapeutic antibodies does not depend on preexisting host adaptive immunity, requiring only FcR engagement on innate immune effector cells. However, FcR-mediated effector mechanisms by therapeutic monoclonal antibodies could themselves enable adaptive immunity—and their associated memory responses—against tumors (Figure 1.5).

In mouse models of monoclonal antibody therapy, antigens within apoptotic tumor cells can be cross-presented by antigen-presenting cells (APCs) to induce adaptive T cell responses.[99] Later studies confirmed that effective T-cell responses following antibody therapy were dependent on FcRs and dendritic cells, which are APCs.[100] Whether this process depends on an immunogenic tumor cell death due to ADCC or antibody-dependent cell-mediated phagocytosis (ADCP) remains to be elucidated. Intriguingly, it is plausible that immune effector activity is irrelevant. Activating or inhibitory FcR cross-linking of agonistic antibodies against death receptor 5 (DR5) alone has been shown to induce apoptosis in tumor cells, without FcR-mediated immune effector activity.[101] Independent of mechanism, the evidence supporting a critical link between therapeutic monoclonal antibody therapy, tumor cell death, ADCC, and induction of adaptive immunity continues to grow.[102] Although it has been demonstrated that monoclonal antibody and FcR interactions are required for induction of adaptive immunity,

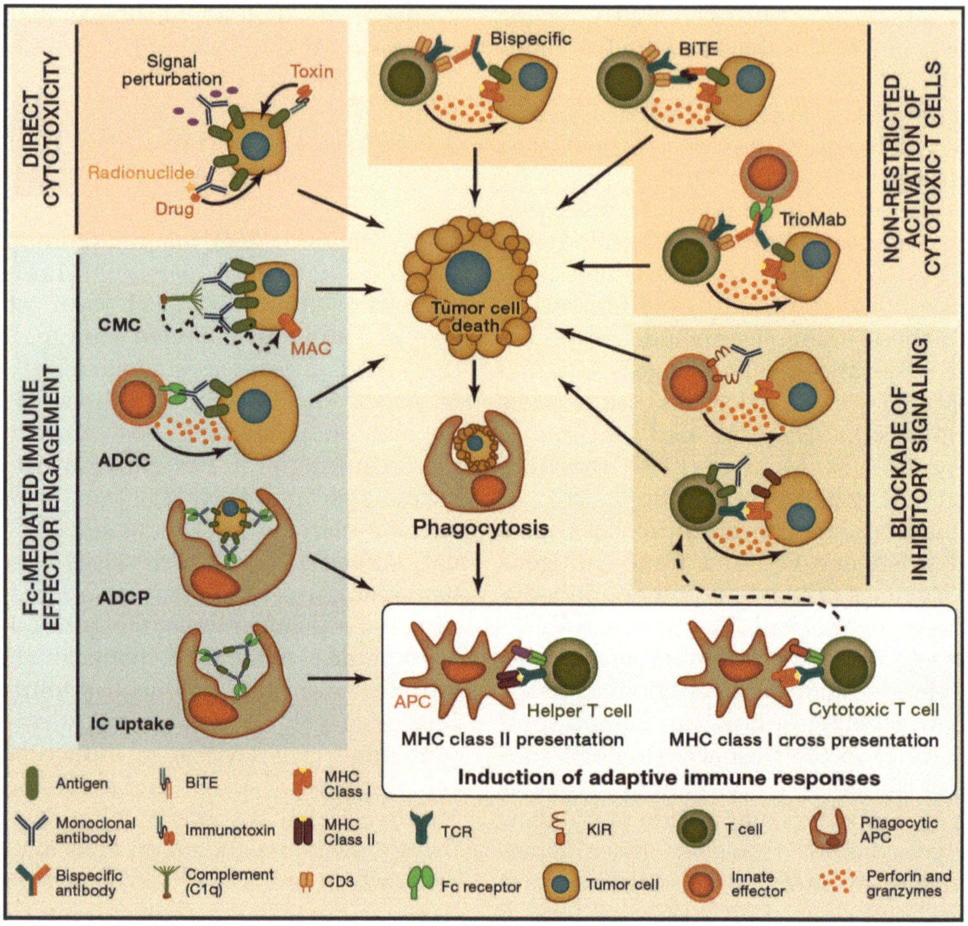

FIGURE 1.5 **Mechanisms of action of antibody immunotherapy in cancer.** Mechanisms of action of antibodies in cancer therapy are diverse and represent the versatility of antibody-based approaches. Here, four different strategies are depicted. (Upper left) Direct cytotoxicity, in which mAbs can induce direct cytotoxicity in tumor cells by perturbing oncogenic signaling pathways or where immunoconjugates can carry cytotoxic agents to targeted cells. (Lower left) FcR-mediated immune effector engagement, in which the Fc portion of mAbs can engage immune effector cells including soluble complement-mediated cytotoxicity (CMC, through the membrane attack complex, MAC) as well as NK cells, macrophages, and dendritic cells through FcRs, allowing for antibody-dependent cellular cytotoxicity (ADCC), antibody-dependent cellular phagocytosis (ADCP), and immune complex (IC) uptake. (Upper right) Non-restricted activation of cytotoxic T cells, in which tumor-infiltrating cytotoxic T lymphocytes (CTLs) can be activated against tumor cells—independent of T cell receptor (TCR) specificity—by engaging co-receptors on the T cells and tumor antigens. (Lower right) Blockade of inhibitory signaling, in which cytotoxic lymphocytes, including NK cells and CTLs, express inhibitory receptors for various ligands that may be expressed by tumor cells. Antagonistic antibodies that target these inhibitory receptors can block ligand–receptor interactions so that targeted cytotoxicity can ensue. These four strategies enhance tumor cell death, which can promote phagocytosis of tumor cell antigens, and induction of adaptive immune responses (bottom right) in two ways: MHC class I cross presentation and priming of cytotoxic T cells and MHC class II presentation and priming of helper T cells. These adaptive immune responses can lead to enhanced—and possibly persistent—anti-tumor immunity. *Figure reproduced with permission from Louis M. Weiner, Joseph C. Murray, Casey W. Shuptrine, Antibody-Based Immunotherapy of Cancer, Cell, Volume 148, Issue 6, 16 March 2012, pp. 1081–1084, ISSN 0092-8674, 10.1016/j.cell.2012.02.034.*

comprehensive understanding of the underlying mechanisms remains elusive. Nonetheless, several antibody- and FcR-based therapeutic approaches are being assessed in which enhanced antibody-induced target cell death may promote induction of adaptive immunity.

Several preclinical studies have demonstrated enhanced anti-tumor activity by targeting immune cell receptors in concert with tumor-antigen targeting or FcR engagement. Besides FcRs, several families of activating or inhibitory cell surface receptors are expressed on innate immune effectors—such as macrophage and NK cells—that recognize ligands expressed on virally infected or transformed cells.[103,104] Antibody blockade of CD47-SIRPA interactions has enhanced rituximab-mediated ADCP, although not ADCC, in mouse models of non-Hodgkin lymphoma.[105] Antibody cross-linking of a costimulatory NK cell receptor, CD137 (4-1BB), has increased rituximab-mediated ADCC in mouse and human xenograft models of B cell lymphoma.[106] In both studies, enhancement of the FcR-dependent mechanisms led to increased anti-tumor effect. Therefore, combinatorial antibody strategies, which enable selective and enhanced FcR-mediated activities, could further the clinical utility of tumor-antigen targeting approaches.

Monoclonal antibodies have also been conjugated with therapeutic payloads, including radionuclides, chemotherapeutics, and toxins bound often to their Fc regions, in an effort to turn systemically toxic payloads into targeted therapies. Radioimmunotherapies (RITs) represent a class of these immunoconjugates where a monoclonal antibody is conjugated with radionuclides. Two RITs targeting CD20—^{90}Y-ibritumomab tiuxetan and ^{131}I-tositumomab—were approved by the FDA for treatment of relapsed and/or rituximab-refractory lymphomas.[107,108] RITs targeting solid malignancies are being developed.[109] Brentuximab vedotin, the only antibody–drug conjugate (ADC) approved by the FDA, is used to treat anaplastic large cell and Hodgkin lymphoma.[110] It contains a potent anti-mitotic chemotherapeutic conjugated to a chimeric anti-CD30 monoclonal antibody. The Phase III success of trastuzumab emtansine (T-DM1), where trastuzumab is conjugated with a microtubule inhibitor, even in trastuzumab-refractory breast cancer has reinforced the clinical utility of ADCs beyond their unconjugated counterparts.[111] T-DM1 has also been shown to retain its capacity to induce ADCC *in vitro*, suggesting that its FcR-mediated immune effects are intact independent of conjugation.[112] Although antibody-based immunotoxins incorporating catalytic toxins have yet to gain FDA approval as cancer therapies, one has shown distinct promise in Phase II trials: BL22, an anti-CD22 Fv conjugated with recombinant *Pseudomonas* exotoxin.[113] As BL22 lacks an Fc domain, it is unlikely to engage in FcR-dependent effector mechanisms such as ADCC. Nonetheless, it remains to be seen whether Fc–FcR interactions are linked to clinical efficacy of antibody-conjugated therapies, as tumor targeting of toxic agents has been the predominant focus of immunoconjugate development.

Human NK cells also express inhibitory killer immunoglobulin-like receptors (KIRs) that recognize host human leukocyte antigen (HLA) ligands in order to inhibit deleterious cytotoxic attacks against themselves. Combinatorial therapeutic strategies that cross-link activating FcRs on NK cells to induce ADCC while blocking inhibitory receptor interactions may enhance targeted potency and clinical efficacy.[114] This strategy for blocking inhibitory immune receptors is not restricted to those expressed on NK cells (Figure 1.5). The success of ipilimumab, a monoclonal antibody targeting the inhibitory CTLA4 receptor on T cells, has demonstrated safety, feasibility, and efficacy in metastatic melanoma.[115,116] Blockade of inhibitory KIRs by an anti-KIR antibody, IPH2101, has demonstrated safety in Phase 1 clinical trials for acute myelogenous leukemia and relapsed/refractory multiple myeloma.[117,118] While the combination of inhibitory KIR blockade and activating FcR engagement has not been tested in the clinic, these clinical studies provide sufficient justification for such an approach.

PERSPECTIVES: FUTURE DIRECTIONS

Key questions remain to be answered and may provide fertile areas for future studies:

- How does Fc receptor expression and ADCC activity compare in mucosal tissue or sites of solid tumors versus peripheral blood? Can γδT cells, a subset of which express Fc receptors and are rather abundant in the mucosa, mediate ADCC? What is the role of non-NK cells, including PMN, in ADCC-mediated activity *in vivo*? What are the mechanistic differences between different effector cell populations, and can these be exploited?
- How does expression of modulatory receptors, such as MPR and PAF-R on target cells, or KIR and other regulatory receptors on effectors affect killing via ADCC?
- How can a causal link between ADCC and *in vivo* efficacy be demonstrated?
- How can vaccine regimens be manipulated to bias the humoral response toward the production of IgG with potentiated ADCC activity?
- How can therapeutic antibodies and ADCC be utilized to link innate immune activation with persistent adaptive immune responses?

Antibodies represent the correlate of protection for most vaccines, and monoclonal antibodies have transformed cancer therapy and represent the nexus of both targeted and immune-activating therapies. The ability of antibodies to target tumors, infected cells, or free pathogens while simultaneously engaging Fc- and FcR-dependent effector activity, and specifically ADCC, has allowed for potent activity. The versatility of antibodies as engineered therapeutic platforms has increased their clinical utility, while their unique capacity to induce adaptive immune responses remains an exciting translational avenue. Building upon their specificity and versatility, combinations of monoclonal antibody therapies may further enhance targeted effects to yield significant increases in clinical efficacy. Likewise, the correlations between binding antibodies with ADCC activity and protection observed in the setting of vaccination have also pointed toward an important role of ADCC *in vivo*. Because the first ADCC-optimized monoclonal has been approved for use in Japan, with many more currently being evaluated in efficacy studies,[119] and with tantalizing associations from major vaccine efficacy studies,[76] our understanding of the *in vivo* importance of this mode of antibody action will continue to evolve.

Acknowledgments

The authors thank Marjorie Robert-Guroff, Pascal Hérion, and Kristoffer Jarlov Jensen for critical reading and useful discussions during the writing stages of this chapter.

References

1. Möeller E. Contact-induced cytotoxicity by lymphoid cells containing foreign isoantigens. *Science* 1965;**147**(3660):873–9.
2. MacLennan IC, Loewi G, Harding B. The role of immunoglobulins in lymphocyte-mediated cell damage, *in vitro*. I. Comparison of the effects of target cell specific antibody and normal serum factors on cellular damage by immune and non-immune lymphocytes. *Immunology* 1970;**18**(3):397–404.
3. Pudifin DJ, Harding B, MacLennan IC. The differential effect of gamma irradiation on the sensitizing and effector stages of antibody dependent lymphocyte mediated cytotoxicity. *Immunology* 1971;**21**(5):853–60.
4. Wallace PK, Howell AL, Fanger MW. Role of Fc gamma receptors in cancer and infectious disease. *J Leukocyte Biol* 1994;**55**(6):816–26.
5. Tudor D, Bomsel M. The broadly neutralizing HIV-1 IgG 2F5 elicits gp41-specific antibody-dependent cell

cytotoxicity in a FcgammaRI-dependent manner. *Aids* 2011;**25**(6):751–9.

6. Horner H, Frank C, Dechant C, et al. Intimate cell conjugate formation and exchange of membrane lipids precede apoptosis induction in target cells during antibody-dependent, granulocyte-mediated cytotoxicity. *J Immunol* 2007;**179**(1):337–45.
7. Shen R, Richter HE, Clements RH, et al. Macrophages in vaginal but not intestinal mucosa are monocyte-like and permissive to human immunodeficiency virus type 1 infection. *J Virol* 2009;**83**(7):3258–67.
8. Kato K, Fridman WH, Arata Y, Sautes-Fridman C. A conformational change in the Fc precludes the binding of two Fcgamma receptor molecules to one IgG. *Immunol Today* 2000;**21**(7):310–2.
9. Shields RL, Lai J, Keck R, et al. Lack of fucose on human IgG1 N-linked oligosaccharide improves binding to human Fcgamma RIII and antibody-dependent cellular toxicity. *J Biol Chem* 2002;**277**(30):26733–40.
10. Ferrara C, Grau S, Jager C, et al. Unique carbohydrate–carbohydrate interactions are required for high affinity binding between FcgammaRIII and antibodies lacking core fucose. *Proc Natl Acad Sci USA* 2011;**108**(31):12669–74.
11. Liao F, Shin HS, Rhee SG. Cross-linking of Fc gamma RIIIA on natural killer cells results in tyrosine phosphorylation of PLC-gamma 1 and PLC-gamma 2. *J Immunol* 1993;**150**(7):2668–74.
12. Saxena RK, Saxena QB, Adler WH. Identity of effector cells participating in the reverse antibody-dependent cell-mediated cytotoxicity. *Immunology* 1982;**46**(2):459–64.
13. Leibson PJ. Signal transduction during natural killer cell activation: inside the mind of a killer. *Immunity* 1997;**6**(6):655–61.
14. Sanchez-Mejorada G, Rosales C. Signal transduction by immunoglobulin Fc receptors. *J Leukocyte Biol* 1998;**63**(5):521–33.
15. Zompi S, Colucci F. Anatomy of a murder—signal transduction pathways leading to activation of natural killer cells. *Immunol Lett* 2005;**97**(1):31–9.
16. Procopio AD, Paolini R, Vecchio I, Frati L, Santoni A. GTP-binding proteins transduce signals generated via human FC gamma receptor IIIA (CD16). *J Immunol* 1991;**146**(10):3550–6.
17. Ortiz-Stern A, Rosales C. Cross-talk between Fc receptors and integrins. *Immunol Lett* 2003;**90**(2–3):137–43.
18. Karsten CM, Pandey MK, Figge J, et al. Anti-inflammatory activity of IgG1 mediated by Fc galactosylation and association of FcgammaRIIB and dectin-1. *Nat Med* 2012;**18**(9):1401–6.
19. Galandrini R, Tassi I, Mattia G, et al. SH2-containing inositol phosphatase (SHIP-1) transiently translocates to raft domains and modulates CD16-mediated cytotoxicity in human NK cells. *Blood* 2002;**100**(13):4581–9.
20. Lichtfuss GF, Meehan AC, Cheng WJ, et al. HIV inhibits early signal transduction events triggered by CD16 cross-linking on NK cells, which are important for antibody-dependent cellular cytotoxicity. *J Leukocyte Biol* 2011;**89**(1):149–58.
21. Wood SM, Meeths M, Chiang SC, et al. Different NK cell-activating receptors preferentially recruit Rab27a or Munc13-4 to perforin-containing granules for cytotoxicity. *Blood* 2009;**114**(19):4117–27.
22. Trapani JA, Smyth MJ. Functional significance of the perforin/granzyme cell death pathway. *Nat Rev Immunol* 2002;**2**(10):735–47.
23. Smyth MJ, Kelly JM, Sutton VR, et al. Unlocking the secrets of cytotoxic granule proteins. *J Leukocyte Biol* 2001;**70**(1):18–29.
24. Berthou C, Bourge JF, Zhang Y, et al. Interferon-gamma-induced membrane PAF-receptor expression confers tumor cell susceptibility to NK perforin-dependent lysis. *Blood* 2000;**95**(7):2329–36.
25. Eischen CM, Schilling JD, Lynch DH, Krammer PH, Leibson PJ. Fc receptor-induced expression of Fas ligand on activated NK cells facilitates cell-mediated cytotoxicity and subsequent autocrine NK cell apoptosis. *J Immunol* 1996;**156**(8):2693–9.
26. Boyle JJ. Human macrophages kill human mesangial cells by Fas-L-induced apoptosis when triggered by antibody via CD16. *Clin Exp Immunol* 2004;**137**(3):529–37.
27. Koller CA, LoBuglio AF. Monocyte-mediated antibody-dependent cell-mediated cytotoxicity: the role of the metabolic burst. *Blood* 1981;**58**(2):293–9.
28. Bruchelt G, Handgretinger R, Fierlbeck G, et al. Lysis of neuroblastoma cells by the ADCC-reaction: granulocytes of patients with chronic granulomatous disease are more effective than those of healthy donors. *Immunol Lett* 1989;**22**(3):217–20.
29. Golub RM, Descamps-Latscha B. Role of oxygen-dependent mechanisms in monoclonal antibody-induced lysis of normal T cells by phagocytes. I. Human phagocytes. *Ann Inst Pasteur Immunol* 1985;**136D**(1):3–18.
30. Boross P, Jansen JH, Pastula A, van der Poel CE, Leusen JH. Both activating and inhibitory Fc gamma receptors mediate rituximab-induced trogocytosis of CD20 in mice. *Immunol Lett* 2012;**143**(1):44–52.
31. Peipp M, Lammerts van Bueren JJ, Schneider-Merck T, et al. Antibody fucosylation differentially impacts cytotoxicity mediated by NK and PMN effector cells. *Blood* 2008;**112**(6):2390–9.
32. Timonen T, Saksela E. A simplified isotope release assay for cell-mediated cytotoxicity against anchorage dependent target cells. *J Immunol Meth* 1977;**18**(1–2):123–32.
33. Kato K, Agatsuma T, Tanabe T, Masuko T, Hashimoto Y. Release of esterase from murine

lymphokine-activated killer cells in antibody-dependent cellular cytotoxic reaction. *Jpn J Cancer Res (Gann)* 1991;**82**(2):206–12.
34. Ortaldo JR, Winkler-Pickett RT, Nagashima K, Yagita H, Okumura K. Direct evidence for release of pore-forming protein during NK cellular lysis. *J Leukocyte Biol* 1992;**52**(5):483–8.
35. Jacobs DB, Pipho C. Use of propidium iodide staining and flow cytometry to measure anti-mediated cytotoxicity: resolution of complement-sensitive and resistant target cells. *J Immunol Meth* 1983;**62**(1):101–8.
36. Lee-MacAry AE, Ross EL, Davies D, et al. Development of a novel flow cytometric cell-mediated cytotoxicity assay using the fluorophores PKH-26 and TO-PRO-3 iodide. *J Immunol Meth* 2001;**252**(1–2):83–92.
37. Gomez-Roman VR, Florese RH, Patterson LJ, et al. A simplified method for the rapid fluorometric assessment of antibody-dependent cell-mediated cytotoxicity. *J Immunol Meth* 2006;**308**(1–2):53–67.
38. Pollara J, Hart L, Brewer F, et al. High-throughput quantitative analysis of HIV-1 and SIV-specific ADCC-mediating antibody responses. *Cytometry A J Int Soc Analyt Cytol* 2011;**79**(8):603–12.
39. Maloney DG, Grillo-Lopez AJ, Bodkin DJ, et al. IDEC-C2B8: results of a phase I multiple-dose trial in patients with relapsed non-Hodgkin's lymphoma. *J Clin Oncol* 1997;**15**(10):3266–74.
40. Baselga J, Tripathy D, Mendelsohn J, et al. Phase II study of weekly intravenous recombinant humanized anti-p185HER2 monoclonal antibody in patients with HER2/neu-overexpressing metastatic breast cancer. *J Clin Oncol* 1996;**14**(3):737–44.
41. Cunningham D, Humblet Y, Siena S, et al. Cetuximab monotherapy and cetuximab plus irinotecan in irinotecan-refractory metastatic colorectal cancer. *New Engl J Med* 2004;**351**(4):337–45.
42. Bonner JA, Harari PM, Giralt J, et al. Radiotherapy plus cetuximab for squamous-cell carcinoma of the head and neck. *New Engl J Med* 2006;**354**(6):567–78.
43. Vermorken JB, Trigo J, Hitt R, et al. Open-label, uncontrolled, multicenter phase II study to evaluate the efficacy and toxicity of cetuximab as a single agent in patients with recurrent and/or metastatic squamous cell carcinoma of the head and neck who failed to respond to platinum-based therapy. *J Clin Oncol* 2007;**25**(16):2171–7.
44. Fan Z, Masui H, Altas I, Mendelsohn J. Blockade of epidermal growth factor receptor function by bivalent and monovalent fragments of 225 anti-epidermal growth factor receptor monoclonal antibodies. *Cancer Res* 1993;**53**(18):4322–8.
45. Kurai J, Chikumi H, Hashimoto K, et al. Antibody-dependent cellular cytotoxicity mediated by cetuximab against lung cancer cell lines. *Clin Cancer Res* 2007;**13**(5):1552–61.
46. Riechmann L, Clark M, Waldmann H, Winter G. Reshaping human antibodies for therapy. *Nature* 1988;**332**(6162):323–7.
47. Schneider-Merck T, Lammerts van Bueren JJ, Berger S, et al. Human IgG2 antibodies against epidermal growth factor receptor effectively trigger antibody-dependent cellular cytotoxicity but, in contrast to IgG1, only by cells of myeloid lineage. *J Immunol* 2010;**184**(1):512–20.
48. Clynes RA, Towers TL, Presta LG, Ravetch JV. Inhibitory Fc receptors modulate *in vivo* cytotoxicity against tumor targets. *Nat Med* 2000;**6**(4):443–6.
49. de Haij S, Jansen JH, Boross P, et al. *In vivo* cytotoxicity of type I CD20 antibodies critically depends on Fc receptor ITAM signaling. *Cancer Res* 2010;**70**(8):3209–17.
50. Minard-Colin V, Xiu Y, Poe JC, et al. Lymphoma depletion during CD20 immunotherapy in mice is mediated by macrophage FcgammaRI, FcgammaRIII, and FcgammaRIV. *Blood* 2008;**112**(4):1205–13.
51. Hubert P, Heitzmann A, Viel S, et al. Antibody-dependent cell cytotoxicity synapses form in mice during tumor-specific antibody immunotherapy. *Cancer Res* 2011;**71**(15):5134–43.
52. Gennari R, Menard S, Fagnoni F, et al. Pilot study of the mechanism of action of preoperative trastuzumab in patients with primary operable breast tumors overexpressing HER2. *Clin Cancer Res* 2004;**10**(17):5650–5.
53. Dall'Ozzo S, Tartas S, Paintaud G, et al. Rituximab-dependent cytotoxicity by natural killer cells: influence of FCGR3A polymorphism on the concentration-effect relationship. *Cancer Res* 2004;**64**(13):4664–9.
54. Cartron G, Dacheux L, Salles G, et al. Therapeutic activity of humanized anti-CD20 monoclonal antibody and polymorphism in IgG Fc receptor FcgammaRIIIa gene. *Blood* 2002;**99**(3):754–8.
55. Weng WK, Levy R. Two immunoglobulin G fragment C receptor polymorphisms independently predict response to rituximab in patients with follicular lymphoma. *J Clin Oncol* 2003;**21**(21):3940–7.
56. Musolino A, Naldi N, Bortesi B, et al. Immunoglobulin G fragment C receptor polymorphisms and clinical efficacy of trastuzumab-based therapy in patients with HER-2/neu-positive metastatic breast cancer. *J Clin Oncol* 2008;**26**(11):1789–96.
57. Zhang W, Gordon M, Schultheis AM, et al. FCGR2A and FCGR3A polymorphisms associated with clinical outcome of epidermal growth factor receptor expressing metastatic colorectal cancer patients treated with single-agent cetuximab. *J Clin Oncol* 2007;**25**(24):3712–8.
58. Bibeau F, Lopez-Crapez E, Di Fiore F, et al. Impact of Fc{gamma}RIIa-Fc{gamma}RIIIa polymorphisms and KRAS mutations on the clinical outcome of patients with metastatic colorectal cancer treated with cetuximab plus irinotecan. *J Clin Oncol* 2009;**27**(7):1122–9.

59. Veeramani S, Wang SY, Dahle C, et al. Rituximab infusion induces NK activation in lymphoma patients with the high-affinity CD16 polymorphism. *Blood* 2011;**118**(12):3347–9.
60. Arnould L, Gelly M, Penault-Llorca F, et al. Trastuzumab-based treatment of HER2-positive breast cancer: an antibody-dependent cellular cytotoxicity mechanism? *Brit J Cancer* 2006;**94**(2):259–67.
61. Assaad F, Bektimirov T, Ennis F, et al. Immune responses to viral antigens in man and their relevance to vaccine development: memorandum from a WHO meeting. *Bull WHO* 1983;**61**(6):935–40.
62. Balachandran N, Bacchetti S, Rawls WE. Protection against lethal challenge of BALB/c mice by passive transfer of monoclonal antibodies to five glycoproteins of herpes simplex virus type 2. *Infect Immun* 1982;**37**(3):1132–7.
63. Ahmad R, Sindhu ST, Toma E, et al. Evidence for a correlation between antibody-dependent cellular cytotoxicity-mediating anti-HIV-1 antibodies and prognostic predictors of HIV infection. *J Clin Immunol* 2001;**21**(3):227–33.
64. Forthal DN, Landucci G, Keenan B. Relationship between antibody-dependent cellular cytotoxicity, plasma HIV type 1 RNA, and CD4+ lymphocyte count. *AIDS Res Hum Retroviruses* 2001;**17**(6):553–61.
65. Banks ND, Kinsey N, Clements J, Hildreth JE. Sustained antibody-dependent cell-mediated cytotoxicity (ADCC) in SIV-infected macaques correlates with delayed progression to AIDS. *AIDS Res Hum Retroviruses* 2002;**18**(16):1197–205.
66. Gomez-Roman VR, Patterson LJ, Venzon D, et al. Vaccine-elicited antibodies mediate antibody-dependent cellular cytotoxicity correlated with significantly reduced acute viremia in rhesus macaques challenged with SIVmac251. *J Immunol* 2005;**174**(4):2185–9.
67. Hidajat R, Xiao P, Zhou Q, et al. Correlation of vaccine-elicited systemic and mucosal nonneutralizing antibody activities with reduced acute viremia following intrarectal simian immunodeficiency virus SIVmac251 challenge of rhesus macaques. *J Virol* 2009;**83**(2):791–801.
68. Florese RH, Demberg T, Xiao P, et al. Contribution of nonneutralizing vaccine-elicited antibody activities to improved protective efficacy in rhesus macaques immunized with Tat/Env compared with multigenic vaccines. *J Immunol* 2009;**182**(6):3718–27.
69. Lambotte O, Ferrari G, Moog C, et al. Heterogeneous neutralizing antibody and antibody-dependent cell cytotoxicity responses in HIV-1 elite controllers. *Aids* 2009;**23**(8):897–906.
70. Xiao P, Zhao J, Patterson LJ, et al. Multiple vaccine-elicited nonneutralizing antienvelope antibody activities contribute to protective efficacy by reducing both acute and chronic viremia following simian/human immunodeficiency virus SHIV89.6P challenge in rhesus macaques. *J Virol* 2010;**84**(14):7161–73.
71. Sun Y, Asmal M, Lane S, et al. Antibody-dependent cell-mediated cytotoxicity in simian immunodeficiency virus-infected rhesus monkeys. *J Virol* 2011;**85**(14):6906–12.
72. Xiao P, Patterson LJ, Kuate S, et al. Replicating adenovirus-simian immunodeficiency virus (SIV) recombinant priming and envelope protein boosting elicits localized, mucosal IgA immunity in rhesus macaques correlated with delayed acquisition following a repeated low-dose rectal SIV(mac251) challenge. *J Virol* 2012;**86**(8):4644–57.
73. Haase AT. Targeting early infection to prevent HIV-1 mucosal transmission. *Nature* 2010;**464**(7286):217–23.
74. Rerks-Ngarm S, Pitisuttithum P, Nitayaphan S, et al. Vaccination with ALVAC and AIDSVAX to prevent HIV-1 infection in Thailand. *New Engl J Med* 2009;**361**(23):2209–20.
75. Karnasuta C, Paris RM, Cox JH, et al. Antibody-dependent cell-mediated cytotoxic responses in participants enrolled in a phase I/II ALVAC-HIV/AIDSVAX B/E prime-boost HIV-1 vaccine trial in Thailand. *Vaccine* 2005;**23**(19):2522–9.
76. Haynes BF, Gilbert PB, McElrath MJ, et al. Immune-correlates analysis of an HIV-1 vaccine efficacy trial. *New Engl J Med* 2012;**366**(14):1275–86.
77. Hessell AJ, Hangartner L, Hunter M, et al. Fc receptor but not complement binding is important in antibody protection against HIV. *Nature* 2007;**449**(7158):101–4.
78. Moldt B, Shibata-Koyama M, Rakasz EG, et al. A nonfucosylated variant of the anti-HIV-1 monoclonal antibody b12 has enhanced FcgammaRIIIa-mediated antiviral activity *in vitro* but does not improve protection against mucosal SHIV challenge in macaques. *J Virol* 2012;**86**(11):6189–96.
79. Zalevsky J, Leung IW, Karki S, et al. The impact of Fc engineering on an anti-CD19 antibody: increased Fcgamma receptor affinity enhances B-cell clearing in nonhuman primates. *Blood* 2009;**113**(16):3735–43.
80. Junttila TT, Parsons K, Olsson C, et al. Superior *in vivo* efficacy of afucosylated trastuzumab in the treatment of HER2-amplified breast cancer. *Cancer Res* 2010;**70**(11):4481–9.
81. Jefferis R. Glycosylation as a strategy to improve antibody-based therapeutics. *Nat Rev Drug Disc* 2009;**8**(3):226–34.
82. Jiang XR, Song A, Bergelson S, et al. Advances in the assessment and control of the effector functions of therapeutic antibodies. *Nat Rev Drug Disc* 2011;**10**(2):101–11.
83. Idusogie EE, Wong PY, Presta LG, et al. Engineered antibodies with increased activity to recruit complement. *J Immunol* 2001;**166**(4):2571–5.

84. Iida S, Misaka H, Inoue M, et al. Nonfucosylated therapeutic IgG1 antibody can evade the inhibitory effect of serum immunoglobulin G on antibody-dependent cellular cytotoxicity through its high binding to FcgammaRIIIa. *Clin Cancer Res* 2006;**12**(9):2879–87.
85. Suzuki E, Niwa R, Saji S, et al. A nonfucosylated anti-HER2 antibody augments antibody-dependent cellular cytotoxicity in breast cancer patients. *Clin Cancer Res* 2007;**13**(6):1875–82.
86. Shields RL, Namenuk AK, Hong K, et al. High resolution mapping of the binding site on human IgG1 for Fc gamma RI, Fc gamma RII, Fc gamma RIII, and FcRn and design of IgG1 variants with improved binding to the Fc gamma R. *J Biol Chem* 2001;**276**(9):6591–604.
87. Lazar GA, Dang W, Karki S, et al. Engineered antibody Fc variants with enhanced effector function. *Proc Natl Acad Sci USA* 2006;**103**(11):4005–10.
88. Radaev S, Sun P. Recognition of immunoglobulins by Fcgamma receptors. *Molec Immunol* 2002;**38**(14):1073–83.
89. Suzuki T, Ishii-Watabe A, Tada M, et al. Importance of neonatal FcR in regulating the serum half-life of therapeutic proteins containing the Fc domain of human IgG1: a comparative study of the affinity of monoclonal antibodies and Fc-fusion proteins to human neonatal FcR. *J Immunol* 2010;**184**(4):1968–76.
90. Yeung YA, Leabman MK, Marvin JS, et al. Engineering human IgG1 affinity to human neonatal Fc receptor: impact of affinity improvement on pharmacokinetics in primates. *J Immunol* 2009;**182**(12):7663–71.
91. Sehn LH, Assouline SE, Stewart DA, et al. A phase 1 study of obinutuzumab induction followed by 2 years of maintenance in patients with relapsed CD20-positive B-cell malignancies. *Blood* 2012;**119**(22):5118–25.
92. Forero-Torres A, de Vos S, Pohlman BL, et al. Results of a phase 1 study of AME-133v (LY2469298), an Fc-engineered humanized monoclonal anti-CD20 antibody, in FcgammaRIIIa-genotyped patients with previously treated follicular lymphoma. *Clin Cancer Res* 2012;**18**(5):1395–403.
93. Shahied LS, Tang Y, Alpaugh RK, Somer R, Greenspon D, Weiner LM. Bispecific minibodies targeting HER2/neu and CD16 exhibit improved tumor lysis when placed in a divalent tumor antigen binding format. *J Biol Chem* 2004;**279**(52):53907–14.
94. Nelson AL, Reichert JM. Development trends for therapeutic antibody fragments. *Nat Biotechnol* 2009;**27**(4):331–7.
95. Hudson PJ, Souriau C. Engineered antibodies. *Nat Med* 2003;**9**(1):129–34.
96. Beck A, Wurch T, Bailly C, Corvaia N. Strategies and challenges for the next generation of therapeutic antibodies. *Nat Rev Immunol* 2010;**10**(5):345–52.
97. Wang J, Balog CI, Stavenhagen K, et al. Fc-glycosylation of IgG1 is modulated by B-cell stimuli. *Molec Cell Proteomics* 2011;**10**(5) M110 004655.
98. Guo N, Liu Y, Masuda Y, et al. Repeated immunization induces the increase in fucose content on antigen-specific IgG N-linked oligosaccharides. *Clin Biochem* 2005;**38**(2):149–53.
99. Dhodapkar KM, Krasovsky J, Williamson B, Dhodapkar MV. Antitumor monoclonal antibodies enhance cross-presentation of cellular antigens and the generation of myeloma-specific killer T cells by dendritic cells. *J Exp Med* 2002;**195**(1):125–33.
100. Harbers SO, Crocker A, Catalano G, et al. Antibody-enhanced cross-presentation of self antigen breaks T cell tolerance. *J Clin Invest* 2007;**117**(5):1361–9.
101. Wilson NS, Yang B, Yang A, et al. An Fcgamma receptor-dependent mechanism drives antibody-mediated target-receptor signaling in cancer cells. *Cancer Cell* 2011;**19**(1):101–13.
102. Yang X, Zhang X, Mortenson ED, Radkevich-Brown O, Wang Y, Fu YX. Cetuximab-mediated tumor regression depends on innate and adaptive immune responses. *Molec Ther* 2013;**21**(1):91–100.
103. Taylor PR, Martinez-Pomares L, Stacey M, Lin HH, Brown GD, Gordon S. Macrophage receptors and immune recognition. *Annu Rev Immunol* 2005;**23**:901–44.
104. Lanier LL. Up on the tightrope: natural killer cell activation and inhibition. *Nat Immunol* 2008;**9**(5):495–502.
105. Chao MP, Alizadeh AA, Tang C, et al. Anti-CD47 antibody synergizes with rituximab to promote phagocytosis and eradicate non-Hodgkin lymphoma. *Cell* 2010;**142**(5):699–713.
106. Kohrt HE, Houot R, Goldstein MJ, et al. CD137 stimulation enhances the antilymphoma activity of anti-CD20 antibodies. *Blood* 2011;**117**(8):2423–32.
107. Kaminski MS, Zelenetz AD, Press OW, et al. Pivotal study of iodine I 131 tositumomab for chemotherapy-refractory low-grade or transformed low-grade B-cell non-Hodgkin's lymphomas. *J Clin Oncol* 2001;**19**(19):3918–28.
108. Witzig TE, Gordon LI, Cabanillas F, et al. Randomized controlled trial of yttrium-90-labeled ibritumomab tiuxetan radioimmunotherapy versus rituximab immunotherapy for patients with relapsed or refractory low-grade, follicular, or transformed B-cell non-Hodgkin's lymphoma. *J Clin Oncol* 2002;**20**(10):2453–63.
109. Steiner M, Neri D. Antibody-radionuclide conjugates for cancer therapy: historical considerations and new trends. *Clin Cancer Res* 2011;**17**(20):6406–16.
110. Younes A, Bartlett NL, Leonard JP, et al. Brentuximab vedotin (SGN-35) for relapsed CD30-positive lymphomas. *New Engl J Med* 2010;**363**(19):1812–21.

111. Verma S, Miles D, Gianni L, et al. Trastuzumab emtansine for HER2-positive advanced breast cancer. *New Engl J Med* 2012;**367**(19):1783–91.
112. Junttila TT, Li G, Parsons K, Phillips GL, Sliwkowski MX. Trastuzumab-DM1 (T-DM1) retains all the mechanisms of action of trastuzumab and efficiently inhibits growth of lapatinib insensitive breast cancer. *Breast Cancer Res Treat* 2011;**128**(2):347–56.
113. Kreitman RJ, Stetler-Stevenson M, Margulies I, et al. Phase II trial of recombinant immunotoxin RFB4(dsFv)-PE38 (BL22) in patients with hairy cell leukemia. *J Clin Oncol* 2009;**27**(18):2983–90.
114. Binyamin L, Alpaugh RK, Hughes TL, Lutz CT, Campbell KS, Weiner LM. Blocking NK cell inhibitory self-recognition promotes antibody-dependent cellular cytotoxicity in a model of anti-lymphoma therapy. *J Immunol* 2008;**180**(9):6392–401.
115. Wolchok JD, Yang AS, Weber JS. Immune regulatory antibodies: are they the next advance? *Cancer J* 2010;**16**(4):311–7.
116. Lipson EJ, Drake CG. Ipilimumab: an anti-CTLA-4 antibody for metastatic melanoma. *Clin Cancer Res* 2011;**17**(22):6958–62.
117. Benson Jr DM, Hofmeister CC, Padmanabhan S, et al. A phase 1 trial of the anti-KIR antibody IPH2101 in patients with relapsed/refractory multiple myeloma. *Blood* 2012;**120**(22):4324–33.
118. Vey N, Bourhis JH, Boissel N, et al. A phase 1 trial of the anti-inhibitory KIR mAb IPH2101 for AML in complete remission. *Blood* 2012;**120**(22):4317–23.
119. Beck A, Reichert JM. Marketing approval of mogamulizumab: a triumph for glyco-engineering. *mAbs* 2012;**4**(4):419–25.
120. Chen Z, Freedman MS. Correlation of specialized CD16(+) gammadelta T cells with disease course and severity in multiple sclerosis. *J Neuroimmunol* 2008;**194**(1–2):147–52.
121. Wilkinson RW, Lee-MacAry AE, Davies D, Snary D, Ross EL. Antibody-dependent cell-mediated cytotoxicity: a flow cytometry-based assay using fluorophores. *J Immunol Meth* 2001;**258**(1–2):183–91.
122. Seidel MG, Freissmuth M, Pehamberger H, Micksche M. Stimulation of natural killer activity in peripheral blood lymphocytes of healthy donors and melanoma patients *in vitro*: synergism between interleukin (IL)-12 and IL-15 or IL-12 and IL-2. *Naunyn Schmiedebergs Arch Pharmacol* 1998;**358**(3):382–9.
123. Yamashita-Kashima Y, Iijima S, Yorozu K, et al. Pertuzumab in combination with trastuzumab shows significantly enhanced antitumor activity in HER2-positive human gastric cancer xenograft models. *Clin Cancer Res* 2011;**17**(15):5060–70.
124. Chung AW, Rollman E, Center RJ, Kent SJ, Stratov I. Rapid degranulation of NK cells following activation by HIV-specific antibodies. *J Immunol* 2009;**182**(2):1202–10.
125. Kohl S, Charlebois ED, Sigouroudinia M, et al. Limited antibody-dependent cellular cytotoxicity antibody response induced by a herpes simplex virus type 2 subunit vaccine. *J Infect Dis* 2000;**181**(1):335–9.
126. Hashimoto G, Wright PF, Karzon DT. Antibody-dependent cell-mediated cytotoxicity against influenza virus-infected cells. *J Infect Dis* 1983;**148**(5):785–94.
127. Jegerlehner A, Schmitz N, Storni T, Bachmann MF. Influenza A vaccine based on the extracellular domain of M2: weak protection mediated via antibody-dependent NK cell activity. *J Immunol* 2004;**172**(9):5598–605.
128. Mochizuki Y, de Ming T, Hayashi T, Itoh M, Hotta H, Homma M. Protection of mice against Sendai virus pneumonia by non-neutralizing anti-F monoclonal antibodies. *Microbiol Immunol* 1990;**34**(2):171–83.
129. Wardley RC, Norley SG, Wilkinson PJ, Williams S. The role of antibody in protection against African swine fever virus. *Vet Immunol Immunopathol* 1985;**9**(3):201–12.
130. Moore T, Ananaba GA, Bolier J, et al. Fc receptor regulation of protective immunity against *Chlamydia trachomatis*. *Immunology* 2002;**105**(2):213–21.
131. Zhou S, Liu S, Song G, Xu Y, Sun W. Protective immunity induced by the full-length cDNA encoding paramyosin of Chinese *Schistosoma japonicum*. *Vaccine* 2000;**18**(27):3196–204.

CHAPTER

2

Antibody-Dependent Cellular Phagocytosis and Its Impact on Pathogen Control

*Stefan S. Weber and Annette Oxenius**

Institute of Microbiology, ETH Zürich, Zürich, Switzerland

INTRODUCTION

Humoral immunity relies on the induction of antigen-specific B cells and resulting production and secretion of antibodies specific for the antigen. Effector functions of antibodies include neutralization of toxins and viruses as well as complement activation, but also functions that require the interaction of antibodies with Fcγ receptors (FcγRs) on cells, thus initiating intracellular signal transduction by protein phosphorylation cascades. By means of these signaling pathways, activating signals by FcRs can lead to a large variety of effector responses in innate immune effector cells such as oxidative burst, cytokine release, degranulation of mast cells, antibody-dependent cellular cytotoxicity (ADCC), and antibody-dependent cellular phagocytosis (ADCP).[1]

By ingesting and in particular by digesting microbial threats, phagocytic cells act as a first line of defense of the innate immune system. They are widely dispersed throughout the body and prevalent in various tissues that may serve as potential entry sites for microbes. Interestingly, phagocyte activity can be enhanced by cytokines such as IFN-γ, but also by opsonizing agents such as complement and antibodies, thus linking innate and adaptive immunity. Phagocytic cells of the immune system such as monocytes, macrophages, neutrophils, and dendritic cells (DCs) express FcRs in order to efficiently take up antibody-opsonized particles. This allows not only direct clearance of microbes from the system but also modulation of cellular immunity—for example, by enhancing the presentation of antigens to T cells.

* Corresponding Author

PHAGOCYTIC CELLS AND THEIR Fcγ RECEPTORS

Various Receptors for IgG

Four different classes of FcγRs have been identified in mammals, namely the high-affinity receptor FcγRI (CD64) and the low-to-medium affinity receptors FcγRII (CD32), FcγRIII (CD16) and FcγRIV. All bind the different IgG subclasses with varying affinity and specificity. Only high-affinity receptors bind monomeric IgG and thus are usually saturated with serum IgG, whereas low- to medium-affinity receptors preferentially bind antibody in the form of immune complexes. The human set of FcγRs is comprised of FcγRI, IIA, IIB, IIC, IIIA, and IIIB, while mice have a less complex repertoire of FcγRI, IIB, III, and IV (reviewed in Nimmerjahn and Ravetch[2]). Both, human and murine FcγRI and IIB share sequence and functional homology. FcγRIIA is found only in primates but is considered to be most closely related to murine FcγRIII, while the human FcγRIIIA is thought to be an ortholog of the murine FcγRIV. In addition to being a receptor for IgG, FcγRIV was shown to bind IgE immune complexes.[3] Mice have FcγRs homologous to neither the human FcγRIIC nor to FcγRIIIB, the latter of which has no signaling capacity, functions as a decoy receptor, and is mainly expressed on neutrophils.[2,4]

FcγRs can be functionally divided into inhibitory receptors (FcγRIIB), which transmit signals via immunoreceptor tyrosine-based inhibitory motifs (ITIMs), and activating FcγRs (all others) signaling through immunoreceptor tyrosine-based activation motifs (ITAMs). ITAMs either are directly encoded on the intracellular domain of the FcγR (human FcγRs IIA and IIC), or, more commonly, the FcγRs need to associate with the common γ-chain that harbors the ITAM sequence to transmit an activating signal.[5,6] Many cell types express both activating and inhibitory FcRs, and the simultaneous engagement sets a threshold for innate immune effector cell activation and ensures a balanced immune response.[7]

Differential Expression of Fcγ Receptors on Phagocytic Cells

FcγRs are expressed on most myeloid cells, including neutrophils, eosinophils, basophils, mast cells, NK cells, monocytes, macrophages, and DCs. Lymphocytes generally do not express FcγRs with the exception of B cells, which exclusively express the inhibitory FcγRIIB. Here we will focus on FcγR expression on phagocytic cells of the immune system.

Freshly isolated human blood monocytes express mainly two FcγRs, namely FcγRI and FcγRIIA.[8] Monocytes are phagocytic cells that circulate in the bloodstream and migrate into organs to mature into tissue-specific macrophages such as red pulp macrophages in the spleen, Kupffer cells in the liver, microglia in the central nervous system, or alveolar macrophages in the lung. Human and murine macrophages express all types of activating FcγRs and the inhibitory FcγRIIB,[1,2,9] although FcγRI might be the most abundantly expressed isoform as has been shown for alveolar macrophages in humans and rats.[10,11] The presence of FcγRIIB on macrophages is of importance, as these cells can trigger a strong proinflammatory response that needs to be tightly controlled. Murine monocytes can be divided into classical inflammatory and non-classical resident cells. While the classical monocytes only express FcγRs I, III, and IIB, resident monocytes express in addition high levels of FcγRIV.[9]

Neutrophils are innate immune cells that are rapidly attracted to sites of inflammation where they contribute to the clearance of the source of inflammation such as an infection. Murine blood neutrophils express the low-affinity FcγRs III, IV, and IIB, though at lower densities compared to the other cell types.[9] Human neutrophils express the low-affinity FcγRIIA and are, with the exception of human basophils, the only cell type that expresses the GPI-anchored FcγRIIIB.[4,12] The simultaneous engagement of FcγRs IIA and IIIB on neutrophils results in a synergistic enhancement of phagocytosis of immune complexes.[13] Engagement of FcγRIIIB was shown to stimulate the influx of extracellular calcium into human neutrophils, which is required for optimal phagocytosis.[14] Moreover, neutrophils express FcγRI upon interferon-γ (IFN-γ) stimulation. While this induced FcγR is unable to mediate phagocytosis, it nonetheless contributes to an efficient calcium rise.[15,16] Interestingly, the surface expression of FcγRIIA is reduced upon cross-linking of the receptor by immune complexes in a mechanism involving internalization, ubiquitylation by E3 ubiquitin ligase c-Cbl, and subsequent targeting to the proteasome.[17] This results in downregulation of FcγRIIA signaling and the phagocytic capacity of neutrophils, a mechanism that is of importance in the absence of inhibitory FcγRIIB. Recently, the MHC class I related neonatal FcR (FcRn) was shown to relocate from specific granules of neutrophils to nascent phagosomes, thereby facilitating IgG-mediated bacterial phagocytosis.[18] Interestingly, FcRn does not bind IgG at physiologic pH (7.4) but has high affinity to IgG at the lower pH (≤6.5) found in endocytic compartments.

DCs are professional antigen-presenting cells (APCs) that are important in priming T-cell responses. They express all activating FcγRs as well as the inhibitory FcγRIIB. It has been shown that DCs are able to prime stronger immune responses if antigen is taken up by FcγR-mediated phagocytosis. Moreover, peptides of antigens internalized by DCs via FcγR-mediated phagocytosis are not only presented on MHC class II but are also cross-presented on MHC class I, allowing the priming of CD4 as well as CD8 T-cell responses.[19,20]

The expression of FcRs by cells is not static, but rather regulated by the cytokine milieu. For instance, the transcription of the *fcγRI* gene is induced by IFN-γ, but not by type I IFN.[21] As discussed above, human neutrophils express FcγRI after activation with IFN-γ.[15] Remarkably, mouse microglia were also shown to upregulate the expression of FcγRI upon treatment with IFN-γ, while treatment with IL-4 and IL-13 increased the expression of the inhibitory receptor FcγRIIB.[22] These responses reflect the activation state of the cells in pro- or antiinflammatory environments, respectively, and allow the phagocytes to react in the appropriate manner. Consequently, in the presence of IFN-γ, FcγR-mediated phagocytosis of *Staphylococcus aureus* was more efficient, while treatment of the phagocytes with IL-4 and IL-13 resulted in reduced uptake.[22] In contrast, maturation of DCs results in moderate downregulation of FcγR expression but does not inhibit subsequent capture, processing and presentation of an antigen.[23]

Fcγ RECEPTOR-MEDIATED PHAGOCYTOSIS BY PHAGOCYTES

Phagocytosis is the active uptake and endocytosis of a particle larger than 0.5 μm into a cell. Though professional phagocytic cells are able to ingest all kinds of particles, the presence of opsonizing factors such as complement or antibodies provides additional ligand–receptor interaction sites and thus significantly contributes to the enhancement of phagocytosis. Furthermore, receptor ligation by the opsonized particle activates the phagocyte and triggers phagocytosis (see below). For the efficient capture of IgG-opsonized particles, phagocytes continuously probe their environment by extending membrane protrusions in an actin-dependent manner, comparable to the sampling of the fluid milieu by DCs.[24] This mechanism is of specific importance when the phagocyte is confronted with scarcely opsonized or highly motile targets. Moreover, the density of IgG opsonizing the particle correlates with the magnitude of early FcγR signals and thus results in an "all or none" response of FcγR-mediated phagocytosis, depending on whether or not threshold levels of downstream secondary signaling molecules are reached.[25] Genetically engineered antibodies with additional Fcγ domains in tandem repeats can be used to increase binding avidity to FcγRs and thus to enhance antibody-mediated cellular phagocytosis.[26]

Signaling by Activating FcγRs

The clustering and cross-linking of FcγRs by immune complexes results in a coordinated signal transduction that initiates FcγR-mediated phagocytosis (reviewed in Garcia-Garcia and Rosales[27] and Swanson and Hoppe[28]). The signaling cascade is initiated by phosphorylation of tyrosine residues in the ITAM sequences on FcγRs or associated proteins through Src family kinases such as Lyn, Hck, and Fgr.[8,29] Interestingly, the phosphorylation of ITAM motifs feeds back and facilitates the clustering of activated receptors that is required for efficient particle binding and subsequent phagocytosis.[30] More important, the phosphorylation of signal-transducing cytoplasmic tails of FcRs also leads to the recruitment and activation of spleen tyrosine kinase (Syk) and phosphoinositide-3 kinase (PI3K), followed by the activation of various downstream targets.[31,32] These include the Ras–Raf–MAP kinase (Erk) pathway, c-Jun N-terminal kinases (JNK), and phospholipase C-γ (PLCγ).[33–35] Though PI3K and Erk are required for efficient phagocytosis in professional phagocytes, poorly phagocytic cells such as monocytes do not require these kinases for phagocytosis.[36,37] PI3K phosphorylates phosphatidylinositol 4,5-bisphosphate (PtdIns(4,5)P_2) to produce PtdIns(3,4,5)P_3, by which Tec kinase and Bruton's tyrosine kinase (BTK) are recruited to the membrane and engaged in activation and signaling through MAC-1 (CD11b), Rac, and Rho.[38,39]

Moreover, PI3Ks and PtdIns(3,4,5)P_3 are involved in the activation of the small GTPases Rac1, Cdc42 and Arf6 that are involved in actin remodeling necessary for membrane extension and engulfment of particles.[40–44] In contrast, PLC hydrolyses PtdIns(4,5)P_2 to create diacylglycerol (DAG) and soluble second messenger inositol 1,4,5-trisphosphate (InsP_3), which activates the InsP_3 receptor on the endoplasmic reticulum (ER), ultimately leading to calcium release.[45] Simultaneously, the membrane-anchored DAG engages protein kinase C-α (PKCα), which initiates downstream signaling pathways leading to actin polymerization and remodeling, resulting in phagocytosis and activation of the NADPH oxidase complex.[46–48] Indeed, cross-linking of FcγRI on human monocytic cell lines using monoclonal antibodies leads to NADPH oxidase activation and superoxide anion (O_2^-) production[49] directly correlated with the quantity of antibody bound to FcγRs (i.e., the sum of activated receptors).[50]

In contrast to complement receptor-mediated phagocytosis that was shown to be mediated through Rho, cross-linking of FcγRIIA specifically results in the activation of Cdc42, which in turn activates the Cdc42–Rac–Rho cascade in phagocytic cell lines.[51,52] Because Rac is an important regulatory component of the NADPH oxidase complex, FcγR-mediated uptake results in oxidative burst and thus an inflammatory response, whereas complement-mediated phagocytosis does not. Nevertheless, Rac was more recently shown to be involved in complement-mediated phagocytosis in primary macrophages from murine bone marrow.[53] Interestingly, the assembly of the NADPH oxidase complex in response to immune complex binding on mouse neutrophils happens on a tubulovesicular compartment that subsequently fuses to the emerging phagosome.[54]

Regulation of FcR Signals

The inhibitory FcγRIIB is a single-chain receptor that contains an ITIM motif in its cytoplasmic tail.[2] FcγRIIB engagement acts as a negative regulator of immune complex-triggered activation as it counteracts effector cell functions triggered through activating receptors. Analogous to cross-linking of activating FcγRs, engagement of FcγRIIB results in activation of Src-family kinases that in this situation phosphorylate tyrosine residues of the ITIM.[55] This generates docking sites for the phosphatase SHIP which in turn hydrolyses PtdIns(3,4,5)P_3 to PtdIns(3,4)P_2.[56] Through the depletion of PtdIns(3,4,5)P_3 by SHIP, docking sites for BTK and Tec are no longer produced by PI3K, thus recruitment of these protein kinases to the membrane and the signaling cascade initiated through ITAM motifs is terminated.[57] Being the only FcR expressed in B cells, its inhibitory signaling is implicated in maintenance of the humoral tolerance in the immune system.[58] Negative regulation of FcγR-mediated phagocytosis is also accomplished through inactivation of PI3K by protein kinase C-δ (PKCδ), thus limiting the recruitment of Akt/protein kinase B (PKB) to the membrane.[59]

Phagosome Maturation

After FcγR-mediated phagocytosis of a particle, the phagosome matures into a phagolysosome, in which its contents are subsequently degraded.[60] Besides recruitment of and fusion with lysosomes, phagosome maturation also includes the activation of NADPH oxidase (see above) that is recruited to PtdIns3*P* on endosomes, resulting in production of reactive oxygen species (ROS) and oxidative burst.[61–63] Interestingly, endosomes containing IgG-coated beads targeted to FcγRIIA mature significantly faster into phagolysosomes, as compared to endosomes containing uncoated control beads.[64] However, this process does not involve signaling via the ITAM motif, but rather via a leucine–threonine–leucine sequence in the cytoplasmic tail of FcγRIIA that induces the calcium signaling required for phagolysosomal fusion.[65,66]

The functional consequences of FcγR-mediated ingestion differ between macrophages and DCs. Macrophages utilize phagocytosis to kill ingested microbes, while DCs acquire antigen for efficient presentation to T cells on MHC class II molecules. Thus, DCs fail to mobilize calcium[67] and do not generate reactive oxygen intermediates.[68] Moreover, DCs are resistant to leukotriene LTB4, a proinflammatory lipid mediator that is produced in response to FcγR engagement and potently contributes to antimicrobial functions in alveolar macrophages.[69] LTB4 increases FcγR-mediated phagocytosis by enhancing the activation of Erk, PI3K, and PKCα in alveolar macrophages.[70,71] Interestingly, FcγRI redistributes to lipid rafts with the LTB4 receptor after immune complex engagement, allowing enhanced antimicrobial signaling.[11]

ROLE OF FcγR-MEDIATED PHAGOCYTOSIS FOR PATHOGEN UPTAKE, CELLULAR LOCALIZATION, AND PATHOGEN CONTROL

Bacteria

Pathogenic bacteria have evolved different strategies to evade recognition and killing by their host's immune system. Extracellular bacteria (e.g., *Yersinia*) avoid being taken up by phagocytes that patrol the tissues to clear microbial threats. In contrast, intracellular bacteria such as *Legionella* or *Salmonella* enter cells and establish an immune-privileged site so as to be protected from humoral or cell-mediated immunity. Nevertheless, in many cases the immune system is still able to detect pathogenic threats and reacts appropriately by raising a potent immune response that not only clears the intruders but also forms immunological memory. In a secondary infection, cell-mediated as well as humoral immunity can result in more efficient clearance of the bacteria—for example, by enhanced ADCP. In this section, we will discuss phagocytosis of bacterial pathogens in the presence of an opsonizing antibody and the resulting downstream effects of ADCP. We will also elaborate on bacteria evasion strategies.

Avoiding Uptake into Phagocytes

Among the clinically relevant *Yersinia* species is the causative agent of plague (*Y. pestis*) as well as an enterocolitis-causing microorganism (*Y. enterocolitica*), which have evolved mechanisms to interfere with (FcR-mediated) phagocytosis. By injecting type III secretion system (T3SS) effectors such as *Yersinia* outer protein H (YopH), YopT, and YopO, *Y. enterocolitica* was shown to resist phagocytic uptake by macrophages and PMNs, even under antibody-opsonizing conditions.[72] This antiphagocytic activity of the T3SS might be critical for the resistance to killing by neutrophils or activated macrophages. The effector YopO was shown to interfere with FcγR signaling by specifically preventing the activation of Rac, thus blocking FcγR-mediated phagocytosis,[73] while several other *Yersinia* effector proteins interfere with Rho GTPases involved in actin mobilization and phagocytosis.[74] Though its role for opsonic phagocytosis was not evaluated formally, FcγR-mediated phagocytosis might also be hampered by the *Yersinia* effector YopJ, which inhibits the activation of Erk by blocking phosphorylation.[75]

Establishing an Intracellular Niche

In contrast to extracellular bacteria that avoid being taken up into phagocytes, intracellular bacteria either are able to invade nonphagocytic cells by utilizing virulence factors (*Salmonella*, *Chlamydia*) or are readily taken up by phagocytic cells but use various strategies to avoid intracellular degradation. Either bacteria escape from the phagosome to escape the hostile lysosomal environment (*Francisella*, *Listeria*) or they modulate phagosome maturation to avoid acidification (*Legionella*, *Mycobacteria*). A last class of bacteria has evolved to thrive within the low pH in phagolysosomes (*Coxiella*).

Because these intracellular bacteria are well hidden and thus not accessible to humoral immunity, protection against intracellular pathogens was long thought to be mediated by innate and adaptive cellular immunity. Nevertheless, recent advances in research on humoral components of the immune system revealed that antibodies can have notable activity in protection against intracellular pathogens via various mechanisms.[76,77]

Francisella tularensis is the highly virulent causative agent of tularemia in humans and other mammals. As few as 10 colony-forming units of aerosolized bacteria can cause disease and death in exposed individuals. Immune serum containing IgG was shown to protect from a lethal challenge in a murine infection model in an indirect manner. Though phagocytosis of bacteria in the presence of opsonizing antibody was much more efficient, subsequent intracellular killing of the pathogens was shown to depend on parallel cellular activation by IFN-γ, probably of T or NK cell source.[78–80] Thus, the humoral and cell-mediated branches of immunity need to interact *in vivo* to provide sufficient resistance against *F. tularensis*. Nevertheless, recent *in vitro* studies with bone marrow-derived macrophages showed that FcγR-dependent phagocytosis results in restricted phagosomal escape and intracellular growth of *F. tularensis* in an NADPH oxidase-dependent manner.[81]

Obligate intracellular bacteria of the *Chlamydia* genus can infect and multiply within mucosal epithelial cells, thus causing clinical infections of the genital tract or granular conjunctivitis also called trachoma. Knock-out mice defective in FcγRI, FcγRII, and FcγRIII clear primary infections as efficiently as wild-type animals but are more susceptible to a secondary infection. This phenotype was shown to be due to less efficient priming of T_H1 cells in the absence of antibodies or FcRs, as FcR-mediated uptake of antibody-opsonized *Ch. trachomatis* into APCs such as macrophages and DCs resulted in enhanced antigen presentation and pathogen killing.[82–84]

Likewise, *Salmonella enterica* serovar Typhimurium escapes from antigen presentation by avoiding lysosomal degradation in DCs; however, targeting of the bacteria to FcγRIII via opsonizing IgG leads to enhanced antigen presentation and thus to a robust activation of *Salmonella*-specific T cells.[85,86] Nevertheless, the enhanced internalization of IgG-coated *Salmonella* is dependent on neither FcγRs nor downstream signaling such as PI3K and actin activation, but results in rapid targeting of lysosomal compartments.[87] The molecular mechanism of FcγR-independent internalization of IgG-opsonized *Salmonella* in DCs remains to be discovered.

Legionella and *Mycobacteria* are intracellular pathogens that are associated with the pulmonary infections Legionnaires' disease and tuberculosis, respectively. Antibodies are able to confer protection against *Legionella pneumophila* by enhanced uptake and targeting of internalized bacteria for lysosomal degradation in alveolar macrophages in an FcγR-dependent mechanism.[88] Likewise, internalization of *Mycobacterium bovis* BCG was also enhanced in the presence of immune serum, and the bacteria were targeted to lysosomal compartments in cells activated via FcRs.[88–90] Moreover, inhibitory effects on mycobacterial growth in phagocytes as well as proliferation and IFN-γ production of mycobacterium-specific T cells were enhanced in presence of BCG-induced specific antibodies, the latter possibly resulting from enhanced antigen presentation.[89]

Passive immunization by serum transfer from vaccinated animals revealed that antibodies are able to confer protective immunity against the bacteria *Coxiella burnetii*, which causes Q fever.[91,92] These are obligate intracellular organisms dwelling in phagolysosome-like compartments in DCs without inducing cell maturation or activation. Yet, *in vitro* infections of DCs in the presence of immune serum containing *Coxiella*-specific antibodies resulted in DC maturation and inflammatory cytokine production in an FcR-dependent manner.[93] However, antibody-mediated protection via an FcR-mediated mechanism could not be confirmed *in vivo*.[93]

Evasion Strategy of Bacteria: Proteolytic Degradation of Antibodies

Streptococcus pyogenes, the organism associated with necrotizing fasciitis, secretes enzymes that abolish the interaction of antibodies with FcRs. One of these enzymes, the endoglycosidase of *Streptococcus* (EndoS), can remove glycan moieties from antibodies, thus inducing conformational changes in the Fc part structure such that FcR binding is no longer possible.[94,95] In contrast, the endoproteases streptopain (SpeB) and immunoglobulin-degrading enzyme of *Streptococcus* (IdeS) cleave antibodies in their hinge region to produce $F(ab)_2$ and Fc fragments, also terminating signal-inducing antibody–FcR interactions, thereby inhibiting phagocytosis.[94–97] To achieve the proteolytic degradation of an opsonizing antibody, *Francisella tularensis* interacts with the host serine protease plasmin, resulting in proximal antibody cleavage, leading to reduced phagocytosis into macrophages and poor induction of protective proinflammatory cytokines.[98]

Hence, proteolytic cleavage of antibodies in the hinge region may function as an important immune evasion mechanism employed by pathogenic bacteria to render antibodies incapable of linking antigen to FcRs on immune effector cells.[99] Nevertheless, by the induction of anti-hinge autoantibodies against cleaved antibodies, FcR effector functions can be restored and might counteract the immune evasion.[100]

Remarkably, FcγRs can also be used by pathogenic bacteria to invade host cells in the absence of IgG. The outer membrane protein A (OmpA) of the meningitis-causing *Escherichia coli* strain K1 interacts with the FcγRI α-chain as a receptor, which is necessary for cell invasion and disease onset.[101] The resulting signaling cascade is different from common FcγR signaling, as recruitment of the common γ-chain is prevented.

Viruses

A classical role of antibodies in mediating control of viral infections is via neutralizing activity.[102,103] Neutralization activity can be mediated at multiple stages of infection, ranging from preventing viral attachment and/or fusion with target cells to blocking the uncoating of the virus to inhibiting viral assembly and release.[104] Recently, a further mechanism of antibody-mediated interference with viral replication of non-enveloped viruses was reported, namely that capsid-bound antibodies can bind to the cytoplasmic Fc-binding protein TRIM21 and thereby target cytosolic viruses for proteasomal degradation.[105]

Antibody-mediated neutralization is generally achieved by antibodies masking target cell receptor binding sites or inhibiting conformational changes in viral spike proteins generally required for the fusion process between the viral lipid envelope and cellular plasma membrane.[104] In consequence, such antibodies can inhibit *de novo* infection of target cells by free virus particles or interfere with cell-to-cell transmission of a virus. Because neutralizing antibodies act directly on viral particles, they are autonomous and do not require accessory cells or molecules to operate. However, there are a number of additional mechanisms by which antibodies (including neutralizing and non-neutralizing antibodies) regulate viral infection processes and thereby contribute to control (or enhancement) of viral infections *in vivo*. These further mechanisms generally rely on additional effector cells or effector molecules and include complement-mediated lysis of opsonized viral particles or opsonized infected target cells, antibody-dependent cellular cytotoxicity by FcR-bearing effector cells such as NK cells, and FcR-mediated phagocytosis of opsonized virus particles or of virus-containing immune complexes into FcR-bearing target cells. The focus of this section will be on the consequences of FcR-mediated phagocytosis of opsonized virus particles or of virus-containing immune complexes by FcR-bearing phagocytes on viral infection and replication.

Targeting of Viruses to FcRs

Viral infection of target cells in the absence of virus-specific antibodies is in general dependent on the interaction between viral spike proteins and corresponding receptors on target cells, thereby conferring a specific tropism of individual viruses to their target cells. Antibody-opsonized virus particles, however, may gain access to additional FcR-expressing target cells. Uptake of opsonized virus particles into FcR-bearing phagocytes via FcR-dependent phagocytosis may have different outcomes for the infection process and for the ensuing spread and control of the virus infection. While very little is known about the exact intracellular fate of opsonized virus particles and how this relates to their infectivity in phagocytes, most available data indicate that FcR-mediated uptake into phagocytes does not interfere with intracellular viral replication. However, in situations when opsonizing antibodies have direct neutralizing effects on the fusion or uncoating process of the virus, and when this property is maintained under acidic conditions as present in late phagosomes/lysosomes,[106–108] FcR-mediated uptake of opsonized viruses might restrict replication within phagocytes. In cases where the infected phagocyte does not support the requirements of a specific viral life cycle, FcR-mediated uptake of opsonized viruses may also lead to enhanced control of viral replication.

Antibody-Dependent Enhancement of Infection

Directly opposed to this scenario, namely that FcR-mediated uptake might restrict viral replication, antibody-dependent enhancement of infection (ADE) has been well documented for a number of viruses.[109] Two components of ADE have been described, a "cell-extrinsic" mechanism by which FcR-mediated uptake increases the number of infected cells or increases the cell tropism of a given virus to include FcR-bearing phagocytes, and a "cell-intrinsic" mechanism by which FcR triggering of phagocytes by opsonized virus particles modulates innate immune responses; for instance via production of IL-10 which consequently induces a shift toward a Th2 response profile.[109]

The number of viruses for which ADE has been described is large and includes most prominently dengue virus,[110–115] HIV,[116–119] γ-herpes virus,[68,120] influenza virus,[121–125] murine cytomegalovirus (MCMV),[126] foot and mouth disease virus,[127,128] measles virus,[129] coxsackievirus,[130] Ross river virus,[131] and aleutian mink disease parvovirus.[132] In particular, for dengue virus, influenza, and HIV, it is known that neutralizing antibodies at suboptimal concentrations or non-neutralizing antibodies can promote infection of FcR-bearing phagocytes with little or no inhibitory effect on intracellular replication. However, this enhancement of viral replication is likely to vary among phagocytes, as immature DCs were shown not to exhibit enhanced infection in case of opsonized dengue virus.[112] Furthermore, enhanced infection of FcR-positive target cells with opsonized dengue virus was shown to be mediated predominantly by the FcγRII pathway,[113] suggesting that antibody subclass may play a role in directing opsonized virus to specific FcγR-positive cell types.

Suboptimal concentrations of dengue-specific antibodies are prevalent in cases of cross-reactive or heterotypic antibodies induced by different serotypes or in cases of HIV infection by continuous intra-individual or inter-individual selection of viral variants that exhibit reduced sensitivity to neutralizing activity. While suboptimal concentrations of dengue-specific antibodies promote binding to and infection of human monocytes, high concentrations of antibodies, favoring the formation of immune complexes, hinder binding to monocytes, thereby interfering with infection.[110] In contrast, immune complexes of HIV and specific antibodies were shown to exhibit enhanced infection of monocytes and macrophages via FcRs and complement receptors.[116,117] Cytomegalovirus (CMV)- or Herpes simplex virus (HSV)-induced upregulation of FcR expression was proposed to generate new target cells for CD4-independent HIV infection.[117] In opposition to the large body of evidence that opsonized dengue or HIV can get access to FcR-positive phagocytes and thereby enlarge the target cell spectrum of these viruses, there are also reports indicating a suppressive function of FcR-mediated uptake with respect to the replication capacity of these viruses. HIV-specific non-neutralizing antibodies were shown to protect against acquiring HIV infection in combination with FcR polymorphisms in a gp120 vaccination trial (Vax004 trial).[129,133,134] Furthermore, inhibition of replication of opsonized HIV was reported in human macrophages and was attributed to FcRI engagement,[135] and might be caused by a post-entry restriction of replication, likely inhibition of proviral integration.[136]

Also in case of influenza virus infection, there are contradicting reports on the enhancing or suppressing function of FcR-mediated uptake with respect to viral restriction. In a cell-intrinsic manner it was reported for non-hematopoietic cells that some antibodies may achieve FcRn-dependent intracellular neutralization of influenza virus (i.e., antibodies that exhibit neutralizing activity even at low pH), thereby possibly inhibiting fusion in endosomes.[137] Furthermore, dimeric flu-specific IgA antibodies protected against intracellular flu replication in FcγR-positive cells.[138,139] However, other reports have indicated that, in particular, cross-serotype-specific antibodies (i.e., non-neutralizing antibodies[121,122]) or subneutralizing concentrations of flu-specific antibodies promoted infection of FcR-positive target cells.[123–125] It was suggested that neutralization versus enhanced infection capacity of individual flu-specific antibodies might critically depend on the fine specificity of those.[123] However, *in vivo*, alveolar macrophages were found to critically contribute to control of influenza virus infection via phagocytosis of opsonized virus particles[140] and to eliminate influenza-infected cells in an FcR-dependent mechanism in the presence of M2-specific antibodies.[141]

Besides the effects of FcR-mediated uptake of opsonized viruses on infection and replication described above, there are additional downstream effects of this process that have been shown to modulate ensuing innate and adaptive immune responses. Most prominently, FcR triggering on activated macrophages by immune complexes results in production of IL-10,[142] which exerts various immunosuppressive effects on innate and adaptive immune cells and might thereby contribute to increased severity of disease, as suggested for dengue virus infection.[143] Opposed to this immunosuppressive role for immune complexes, it was also reported that antibody-coated adenovirus was more efficiently internalized by macrophages and targeted to phagolysosomes, which led to more pronounced induction of intracellular innate immune pathways.[144]

FcR-Mediated Uptake of Parasites and Fungi

In the context of intracellular parasites, most knowledge about the role of FcR-mediated uptake with respect to intracellular localization and replication exists for *Leishmania* and *Toxoplasma gondii*. Opsonized *Leishmania* are more efficiently phagocytized via FcRs in macrophages[145] and thereafter replicate in the parasitophorous vacuole.[146] In some reports, however, it was shown that phagocytosis of opsonized *Leishmania* via FcRs promotes parasite killing, whereas complement-mediated phagocytosis leads to parasite survival,[147] and triggering of FcRs in macrophages prior to infection induces a parasiticidal state via induction of reactive oxygen species.[148]

Leishmania-Specific Antibodies Can Shift the Balance between Th1 and Th2 Responses

In vivo, during infection, it was shown for *Leishmania major*[149,150] and *Leishmania mexicana*[151,152] that opsonized parasites trigger the secretion of anti-inflammatory cytokines in an FcR-dependent manner that impairs parasite killing by activated macrophages. Thus, host IgG essentially acts as a virulence factor by subverting a Th1-based inflammatory reaction toward an antiinflammatory Th2-based environment. This is in contrast to a report that highlighted a protective role of antibodies and FcRs in *Leishmania major* infection: Only IgG opsonized parasites were efficiently taken up by DCs *in vivo* via FcRs (FcγRI and FcγRIII) which was required for induction of protective parasite-specific T-cell responses.[153]

Toxoplasma is Targeted to Lysosomes in the Presence of Specific Antibody

Toxoplasma gondii enters host cells via an active mechanism involving actin-driven parasite movement into the cell, eventually establishing a vacuole in which *T. gondii* replicates. This vacuole resists fusion with lysosomes and thereby escapes acidification of its replicative niche.[154] In contrast, opsonized *T. gondii* is targeted to lysosomal compartments in an FcR-dependent manner,[154,155] parasite replication is halted and parasites are killed.[156,157] However, in human monocytes, opsonization of *T. gondii* had little effect on intracellular replication, and opsonized parasites did not localize in lysosomal compartments.[158] These different outcomes might be explained by an active means of parasite penetration in monocytes that persists even when parasites were opsonized. Consistent with these *in vitro* studies, B cell-deficient mice were highly susceptible to *T. gondii* infection, indicating the importance of antibodies in conferring resistance to this parasite *in vivo*.[159] It is conceivable that antibodies activate macrophages via FcRs *in vivo* such that they no longer support intracellular replication of *T. gondii*.

Antibody-Mediated Phagocytosis of Invasive Fungi

In the case of invasive fungal infections, the role of antibodies and FcR-mediated effector functions is less well studied. Nonetheless, there is evidence that antibodies can confer protection during infection with *Cryptococcus neoformans* and *Candida albicans*. In *C. albicans* infection, polymorphonuclear leukocytes exhibited enhanced phagocytosis and killing of *C. albicans* upon engagement of either FcγRI (CD64) or FcαRI (CD89).[160] A number of protective B-cell antigens have been described for *C. albicans*[161] whose efficacy might be compromised by binding of antibodies directed against other *C. albicans* epitopes that mask or even block their protective effect.[162,163] Furthermore, there are indications that specific subclasses of *C. albicans*-specific antibodies differ with respect to their protective capacity.[164] This issue of different protective capacities of specific IgG subclasses has been more clearly elaborated in the context of infection with *Cryptococcus neoformans*, where a non-protective murine IgG3 antibody could be converted into a protective one by fusing its variable region to murine IgG1.[165,166] Opsonization of *C. neoformans* with this IgG1 antibody resulted in augmented phagocytosis and led to the arrest of fungal growth in macrophages *in vitro*,[167,168] and passive transfer to protected mice in a strictly FcR-dependent manner.[168] As this *in vivo* protective effect was dependent on the presence of activating FcRs, and since opsonization halted fungal growth in macrophages *in vitro*, it is likely that antibody–FcR-mediated lysosomal targeting contributes to antibody-mediated protection against fungal pathogens.

CONCLUDING REMARKS

Phagocytes of the innate immune system are pivotal for the elimination and the degradation of cellular debris originating from apoptotic cells or tissue renewal. Moreover, phagocytic cells are also of importance for killing potentially harmful microbial invaders, such as bacteria, viruses, parasites, or fungi, but they can also participate in the destruction of tumors. The presence of opsonizing agents such as complement or antibody can increase the efficiency of phagocytosis, thus linking adaptive and innate immunity.

FcγR polymorphisms in the human population have been described and associated with autoimmune and infectious diseases. A higher binding efficiency of antibodies to FcγRs may trigger detrimental inflammatory responses, while reduced binding can result in inefficient immune complex clearance, which may hamper the containment of bacterial infections (reviewed in van Sorge et al.[169]). Thus, FcγR allelic polymorphisms may contribute to susceptibility to infectious diseases.

In this chapter, we highlighted antibody-dependent cellular phagocytosis and its impact on a variety of pathogens belonging to different domains of life (Figure 2.1). In the presence of an opsonizing antibody, bacteria, but also eukaryotic parasites, can be targeted to lysosomal killing and degradation of the pathogen. Subsequently, their degradation may also result in enhanced antigen presentation and thus promote an efficient priming of T cells. Interestingly, for several intracellular pathogens, the lysosomal targeting following FcγR-mediated phagocytosis is dominant over pathogen strategies to avoid lysosomal fusion in order to establish an intracellular replicative

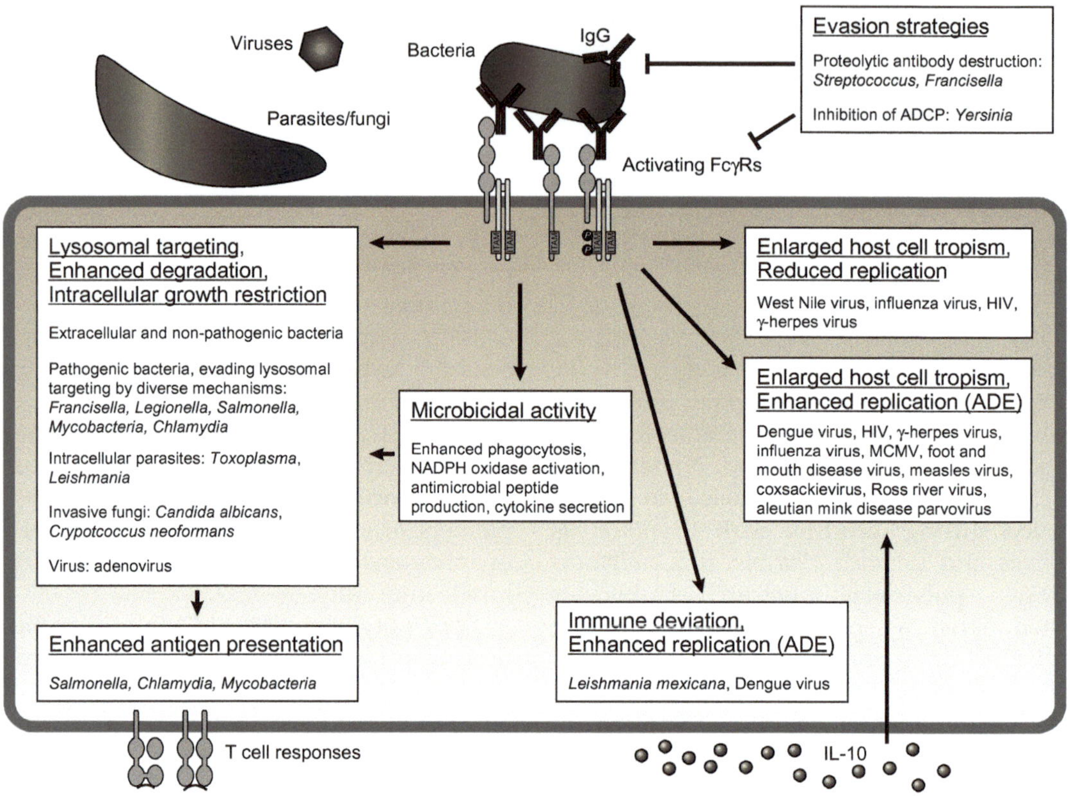

FIGURE 2.1 **Role of FcR-mediated phagocytosis in phagocytes for pathogen uptake, cellular localization, and pathogen control.** Activation of FcRs by antibody opsonized pathogens can lead to a large variety of effector responses in innate immune cells including enhanced phagocytosis, production of ROS and antimicrobial peptides, secretion of cytokines, and lysosomal targeting of the pathogen. Intracellular degradation in lysosomal compartments of different pathogenic organisms results in enhanced antigen presentation to prime efficient T-cell responses. Opsonized viruses gain the capability to enter host cells bearing FcRs resulting in either reduced or enhanced intracellular replication. Several bacteria have evolved to restrict ADCP, either by the proteolytic degradation of antibodies or by interfering with FcR signaling.

niche. Thus, antibodies can protect against intracellular bacteria, a finding that allows new strategies for vaccine design that were formerly underestimated.

Viruses, in contrast, can gain a broader host cell spectrum when opsonized by specific antibodies, particularly in the case of non- or poorly neutralizing antibodies. As such, antibodies may enable the infection of FcR-bearing host cells that lack virus-specific receptors and function as an adjuvant for infection in this situation.

From an evolutionary point of view, it is interesting to speculate why the immune system developed a mechanism that promotes viral infection of FcR-expressing target cells. It is conceivable that this is a trade-off situation, as antibody-mediated phagocytosis by FcRs is key for protection against a multitude of bacterial, protozoan, and fungal pathogens. However, the immune system has evolved other means to control viral infections such as cytotoxic T cells that specifically recognize and kill virus-infected cells.

A challenge for the future will be to translate the current and still accumulating knowledge on FcγR-mediated effector functions such as phagocytosis to optimize prophylactic and therapeutic approaches against microbial pathogens. As the various FcγRs not only have different affinities for IgG subclasses but also exert different effector functions, it will be important to be able to shape immune responses—and in particular antibody responses—in a targeted manner.

References

1. Ravetch JV, Nimmerjahn F. Fc Receptors and their role in immune regulation and inflammation. In: Paul WE, editor. *Fundamental Immunology*. 6th ed. Philadelphia PA: Lippincott Williams & Wilkins; 2008. p. 684–707.
2. Nimmerjahn F, Ravetch JV. Fcγ receptors as regulators of immune responses. *Nat Rev Immunol* 2008;**8**(1):34–47.
3. Mancardi DA, Iannascoli B, Hoos S, England P, Daeron M, Bruhns P. FcγRIV is a mouse IgE receptor that resembles macrophage FcεRI in humans and promotes IgE-induced lung inflammation. *J Clin Invest* 2008;**118**(11):3738–50.
4. Li M, Wirthmueller U, Ravetch JV. Reconstitution of human FcγRIII cell type specificity in transgenic mice. *J Exp Med* 1996;**183**(3):1259–63.
5. Bonnerot C, Amigorena S, Choquet D, Pavlovich R, Choukroun V, Fridman WH. Role of associated γ-chain in tyrosine kinase activation via murine FcγRIII. *EMBO J* 1992;**11**(7):2747–57.
6. Indik ZK, Hunter S, Huang MM, Pan XQ, Chien P, Kelly C, et al. The high affinity Fcγ receptor (CD64) induces phagocytosis in the absence of its cytoplasmic domain: the γ subunit of Fcγ RIIIA imparts phagocytic function to Fcγ RI. *Exp Hematol* 1994;**22**(7):599–606.
7. Nimmerjahn F, Ravetch JV. Fcγ receptors: old friends and new family members. *Immunity* 2006;**24**(1):19–28.
8. Pan XQ, Darby C, Indik ZK, Schreiber AD. Activation of three classes of nonreceptor tyrosine kinases following Fcγ receptor crosslinking in human monocytes. *Clin Immunol* 1999;**90**(1):55–64.
9. Biburger M, Aschermann S, Schwab I, Lux A, Albert H, Danzer H, et al. Monocyte subsets responsible for immunoglobulin G-dependent effector functions *in vivo*. *Immunity* 2011;**35**(6):932–44.
10. Berger M, Norvell TM, Tosi MF, Emancipator SN, Konstan MW, Schreiber JR. Tissue-specific Fcγ and complement receptor expression by alveolar macrophages determines relative importance of IgG and complement in promoting phagocytosis of *Pseudomonas aeruginosa*. *Pediatr Res* 1994;**35**(1):68–77.
11. Serezani CH, Aronoff DM, Sitrin RG, Peters-Golden M. FcγRI ligation leads to a complex with BLT1 in lipid rafts that enhances rat lung macrophage antimicrobial functions. *Blood* 2009;**114**(15):3316–24.
12. Meknache N, Jonsson F, Laurent J, Guinnepain MT, Daeron M. Human basophils express the glycosylphosphatidylinositol-anchored low-affinity IgG receptor FcγRIIIB (CD16B). *J Immunol* 2009; **182**(4):2542–50.
13. Edberg JC, Kimberly RP. Modulation of Fcγ and complement receptor function by the glycosyl-phosphatidylinositol-anchored form of FcγRIII. *J Immunol* 1994;**152**(12):5826–35.
14. Marois L, Pare G, Vaillancourt M, Rollet-Labelle E, Naccache PH. FcγRIIIb triggers raft-dependent calcium influx in IgG-mediated responses in human neutrophils. *J Biol Chem* 2011;**286**(5):3509–19.
15. Petroni KC, Shen L, Guyre PM. Modulation of human polymorphonuclear leukocyte IgG Fc receptors and Fc receptor-mediated functions by IFN-γ and glucocorticoids. *J Immunol* 1988;**140**(10):3467–72.
16. Rivas-Fuentes S, Garcia-Garcia E, Nieto-Castaneda G, Rosales C. Fcγ receptors exhibit different phagocytosis potential in human neutrophils. *Cell Immunol* 2010;**263**(1):114–21.
17. Marois L, Vaillancourt M, Marois S, Proulx S, Pare G, Rollet-Labelle E, et al. The ubiquitin ligase c-Cbl down-regulates FcγRIIa activation in human neutrophils. *J Immunol* 2009;**182**(4):2374–84.
18. Vidarsson G, Stemerding AM, Stapleton NM, Spliethoff SE, Janssen H, Rebers FE, et al. FcRn: an IgG receptor on phagocytes with a novel role in phagocytosis. *Blood* 2006;**108**(10):3573–9.
19. Regnault A, Lankar D, Lacabanne V, Rodriguez A, Thery C, Rescigno M, et al. Fcγ receptor-mediated induction of dendritic cell maturation and major histocompatibility complex class I-restricted antigen presentation after immune complex internalization. *J Exp Med* 1999;**189**(2):371–80.
20. Rafiq K, Bergtold A, Clynes R. Immune complex-mediated antigen presentation induces tumor immunity. *J Clin Invest* 2002;**110**(1):71–9.
21. Pearse RN, Feinman R, Ravetch JV. Characterization of the promoter of the human gene encoding the high-affinity IgG receptor: transcriptional induction by γ-interferon is mediated through common DNA response elements. *Proc Nat Acad Sci USA* 1991;**88**(24):11305–9.
22. Quan Y, Möller T, Weinstein JR. Regulation of Fcγ receptors and immunoglobulin G-mediated

phagocytosis in mouse microglia. *Neurosci Lett* 2009;**464**(1):29–33.

23. Platt CD, Ma JK, Chalouni C, Ebersold M, Bou-Reslan H, Carano RA, et al. Mature dendritic cells use endocytic receptors to capture and present antigens. *Proc Nat Acad Sci USA* 2010;**107**(9):4287–92.
24. Flannagan RS, Harrison RE, Yip CM, Jaqaman K, Grinstein S. Dynamic macrophage "probing" is required for the efficient capture of phagocytic targets. *J Cell Biol* 2010;**191**(6):1205–18.
25. Zhang Y, Hoppe AD, Swanson JA. Coordination of Fc receptor signaling regulates cellular commitment to phagocytosis. *Proc Nat Acad Sci USA* 2010;**107**(45):19332–7.
26. Nagashima H, Ootsubo M, Fukazawa M, Motoi S, Konakahara S, Masuho Y. Enhanced antibody-dependent cellular phagocytosis by chimeric monoclonal antibodies with tandemly repeated Fc domains. *J Biosci Bioeng* 2011;**111**(4):391–6.
27. Garcia-Garcia E, Rosales C. Signal transduction during Fc receptor-mediated phagocytosis. *J Leukocyte Biol* 2002;**72**(6):1092–108.
28. Swanson JA, Hoppe AD. The coordination of signaling during Fc receptor-mediated phagocytosis. *J Leukocyte Biol* 2004;**76**(6):1093–103.
29. Wang AV, Scholl PR, Geha RS. Physical and functional association of the high affinity immunoglobulin G receptor (FcγRI) with the kinases Hck and Lyn. *J Exp Med* 1994;**180**(3):1165–70.
30. Sobota A, Strzelecka-Kiliszek A, Gladkowska E, Yoshida K, Mrozinska K, Kwiatkowska K. Binding of IgG-opsonized particles to FcγR is an active stage of phagocytosis that involves receptor clustering and phosphorylation. *J Immunol* 2005;**175**(7):4450–7.
31. Crowley MT, Costello PS, Fitzer-Attas CJ, Turner M, Meng F, Lowell C, et al. A critical role for Syk in signal transduction and phagocytosis mediated by Fcγ receptors on macrophages. *J Exp Med* 1997;**186**(7):1027–39.
32. Cooney DS, Phee H, Jacob A, Coggeshall KM. Signal transduction by human-restricted FcγRIIa involves three distinct cytoplasmic kinase families leading to phagocytosis. *J Immunol* 2001;**167**(2):844–54.
33. Rose DM, Winston BW, Chan ED, Riches DW, Gerwins P, Johnson GL, et al. Fcγ receptor cross-linking activates p42, p38, and JNK/SAPK mitogen-activated protein kinases in murine macrophages: role for $p42^{MAPK}$ in Fc gamma receptor-stimulated TNF-α synthesis. *J Immunol* 1997;**158**(7):3433–8.
34. Kiener PA, Rankin BM, Burkhardt AL, Schieven GL, Gilliland LK, Rowley RB, et al. Cross-linking of Fcγ receptor I (FcγRI) and receptor II (FcγRII) on monocytic cells activates a signal transduction pathway common to both Fc receptors that involves the stimulation of p72 Syk protein tyrosine kinase. *J Biol Chem* 1993;**268**(32):24442–8.
35. Darby C, Geahlen RL, Schreiber AD. Stimulation of macrophage FcγRIIIA activates the receptor-associated protein tyrosine kinase Syk and induces phosphorylation of multiple proteins including p95Vav and p62/GAP-associated protein. *J Immunol* 1994;**152**(11):5429–37.
36. Araki N, Johnson MT, Swanson JA. A role for phosphoinositide 3-kinase in the completion of macropinocytosis and phagocytosis by macrophages. *J Cell Biol* 1996;**135**(5):1249–60.
37. Garcia-Garcia E, Rosales R, Rosales C. Phosphatidylinositol 3-kinase and extracellular signal-regulated kinase are recruited for Fc receptor-mediated phagocytosis during monocyte-to-macrophage differentiation. *J Leukocyte Biol* 2002;**72**(1): 107–14.
38. Saito K, Scharenberg AM, Kinet JP. Interaction between the Btk PH domain and phosphatidylinositol-3,4,5-trisphosphate directly regulates Btk. *J Biol Chem* 2001;**276**(19):16201–6.
39. Jongstra-Bilen J, Puig Cano A, Hasija M, Xiao H, Smith CI, Cybulsky MI. Dual functions of Bruton's tyrosine kinase and Tec kinase during Fcγ receptor-induced signaling and phagocytosis. *J Immunol* 2008;**181**(1):288–98.
40. Massol P, Montcourrier P, Guillemot JC, Chavrier P. Fc receptor-mediated phagocytosis requires CDC42 and Rac1. *EMBO J* 1998;**17**(21):6219–29.
41. Castellano F, Montcourrier P, Chavrier P. Membrane recruitment of Rac1 triggers phagocytosis. *J Cell Sci* 2000;**113**(Pt 17):2955–61.
42. Castellano F, Montcourrier P, Guillemot JC, Gouin E, Machesky L, Cossart P, et al. Inducible recruitment of Cdc42 or WASP to a cell-surface receptor triggers actin polymerization and filopodium formation. *Curr Biol* 1999;**9**(7):351–60.
43. Zhang Q, Cox D, Tseng CC, Donaldson JG, Greenberg S. A requirement for ARF6 in Fcγ receptor-mediated phagocytosis in macrophages. *J Biol Chem* 1998;**273**(32):19977–81.
44. Venkateswarlu K, Cullen PJ. Signalling via ADP-ribosylation factor 6 lies downstream of phosphatidylinositide 3-kinase. *Biochem J* 2000;**345**(Pt 3):719–24.
45. Liao F, Shin HS, Rhee SG. Tyrosine phosphorylation of phospholipase C-γ 1 induced by cross-linking of the high-affinity or low-affinity Fc receptor for IgG in U937 cells. *Proc Nat Acad Sci USA* 1992;**89**(8):3659–63.
46. Zheleznyak A, Brown EJ. Immunoglobulin-mediated phagocytosis by human monocytes requires

protein kinase C activation. Evidence for protein kinase C translocation to phagosomes. *J Biol Chem* 1992;**267**(17):12042–8.

47. Breton A, Descoteaux A. Protein kinase C-α participates in FcγR-mediated phagocytosis in macrophages. *Biochem Biophys Res Commun* 2000;**276**(2):472–6.
48. Larsen EC, DiGennaro JA, Saito N, Mehta S, Loegering DJ, Mazurkiewicz JE, et al. Differential requirement for classic and novel PKC isoforms in respiratory burst and phagocytosis in RAW 264.7 cells. *J Immunol* 2000;**165**(5):2809–17.
49. Anderson CL, Guyre PM, Whitin JC, Ryan DH, Looney RJ, Fanger MW. Monoclonal antibodies to Fc receptors for IgG on human mononuclear phagocytes. Antibody characterization and induction of superoxide production in a monocyte cell line. *J Biol Chem* 1986;**261**(27):12856–64.
50. Pfefferkorn LC, Fanger MW. Cross-linking of the high affinity Fc receptor for human immunoglobulin G1 triggers transient activation of NADPH oxidase activity. Continuous oxidase activation requires continuous *de novo* receptor cross-linking. *J Biol Chem* 1989;**264**(24):14112–20.
51. Nobes CD, Hall A. Rho, rac, and cdc42 GTPases regulate the assembly of multimolecular focal complexes associated with actin stress fibers, lamellipodia, and filopodia. *Cell* 1995;**81**(1):53–62.
52. Caron E, Hall A. Identification of two distinct mechanisms of phagocytosis controlled by different Rho GTPases. *Science* 1998;**282**(5394):1717–21.
53. Hall AB, Gakidis MA, Glogauer M, Wilsbacher JL, Gao S, Swat W, et al. Requirements for Vav guanine nucleotide exchange factors and Rho GTPases in FcγR- and complement-mediated phagocytosis. *Immunity* 2006;**24**(3):305–16.
54. Anderson KE, Chessa TA, Davidson K, Henderson RB, Walker S, Tolmachova T, et al. PtdIns3P and Rac direct the assembly of the NADPH oxidase on a novel, pre-phagosomal compartment during FcR-mediated phagocytosis in primary mouse neutrophils. *Blood* 2010;**116**(23):4978–89.
55. Muta T, Kurosaki T, Misulovin Z, Sanchez M, Nussenzweig MC, Ravetch JVA. 13-amino-acid motif in the cytoplasmic domain of FcγRIIB modulates B-cell receptor signalling. *Nature* 1994;**368**(6466):70–3.
56. Ono M, Bolland S, Tempst P, Ravetch JV. Role of the inositol phosphatase SHIP in negative regulation of the immune system by the receptor FcγRIIB. *Nature* 1996;**383**(6597):263–6.
57. Bolland S, Pearse RN, Kurosaki T, Ravetch JV. SHIP modulates immune receptor responses by regulating membrane association of Btk. *Immunity* 1998;**8**(4):509–16.
58. Baerenwaldt A, Lux A, Danzer H, Spriewald BM, Ullrich E, Heidkamp G, et al. Fcγ receptor IIB (FcγRIIB) maintains humoral tolerance in the human immune system *in vivo*. *Proc Nat Acad Sci USA* 2011;**108**(46):18772–7.
59. Hazeki K, Inoue K, Nigorikawa K, Hazeki O. Negative regulation of class IA phosphoinositide 3-kinase by protein kinase Cδ limits Fcγ receptor-mediated phagocytosis in macrophages. *J Biochem* 2009;**145**(1):87–94.
60. Kinchen JM, Ravichandran KS. Phagosome maturation: going through the acid test. *Nat Rev Mol Cell Biol* 2008;**9**(10):781–95.
61. Ellson CD, Anderson KE, Morgan G, Chilvers ER, Lipp P, Stephens LR, et al. Phosphatidylinositol 3-phosphate is generated in phagosomal membranes. *Curr Biol* 2001;**11**(20):1631–5.
62. Vieira OV, Botelho RJ, Rameh L, Brachmann SM, Matsuo T, Davidson HW, et al. Distinct roles of class I and class III phosphatidylinositol 3-kinases in phagosome formation and maturation. *J Cell Biol* 2001;**155**(1):19–25.
63. Ueyama T, Nakakita J, Nakamura T, Kobayashi T, Son J, Sakuma M, et al. Cooperation of $p40^{phox}$ with $p47^{phox}$ for Nox2-based NADPH oxidase activation during Fcg receptor (FcγR)-mediated phagocytosis: mechanism for acquisition of $p40^{phox}$ phosphatidylinositol 3-phosphate (PI(3)P) binding. *J Biol Chem* 2011;**286**(47):40693–705.
64. Trivedi V, Zhang SC, Castoreno AB, Stockinger W, Shieh EC, Vyas JM, et al. Immunoglobulin G signaling activates lysosome/phagosome docking. *Proc Nat Acad Sci USA* 2006;**103**(48):18226–31.
65. Worth RG, Mayo-Bond L, Kim MK, van de Winkel JG, Todd III RF, Petty HR, et al. The cytoplasmic domain of FcγRIIA (CD32) participates in phagolysosome formation. *Blood* 2001;**98**(12):3429–34.
66. Worth RG, Kim MK, Kindzelskii AL, Petty HR, Schreiber AD. Signal sequence within FcγRIIA controls calcium wave propagation patterns: apparent role in phagolysosome fusion. *Proc Nat Acad Sci USA* 2003;**100**(8):4533–8.
67. Shibaki A, Ohkawara A, Cooper KD. Differential extracellular signaling via FcγR and FMLP in functionally distinct antigen-presenting cell subsets: ultraviolet-induced epidermal macrophages versus Langerhans cells. *J Invest Dermatol* 1995;**105**(3):383–7.
68. Fanger NA, Voigtlaender D, Liu C, Swink S, Wardwell K, Fisher J, et al. Characterization of expression, cytokine regulation, and effector function of the high affinity IgG receptor FcγRI (CD64) expressed on human blood dendritic cells. *J Immunol* 1997;**158**(7):3090–8.

69. Canetti C, Aronoff DM, Choe M, Flamand N, Wettlaufer S, Toews GB, et al. Differential regulation by leukotrienes and calcium of Fcγ receptor-induced phagocytosis and Syk activation in dendritic cells versus macrophages. *J Leukocyte Biol* 2006;**79**(6):1234–41.
70. Mancuso P, Peters-Golden M. Modulation of alveolar macrophage phagocytosis by leukotrienes is Fc receptor-mediated and protein kinase C-dependent. *Am J Respir Cell Mol Biol* 2000;**23**(6):727–33.
71. Campos MR, Serezani CH, Peters-Golden M, Jancar S. Differential kinase requirement for enhancement of FcγR-mediated phagocytosis in alveolar macrophages by leukotriene B4 vs. D4. *Mol Immunol* 2009;**46**(6):1204–11.
72. Grosdent N, Maridonneau-Parini I, Sory MP, Cornelis GR. Role of Yops and adhesins in resistance of *Yersinia enterocolitica* to phagocytosis. *Infect Immun* 2002;**70**(8):4165–76.
73. Groves E, Rittinger K, Amstutz M, Berry S, Holden DW, Cornelis GR, et al. Sequestering of Rac by the *Yersinia* effector YopO blocks Fcγ receptor-mediated phagocytosis. *J Biol Chem* 2010;**285**(6):4087–98.
74. Fallman M, Gustavsson A. Cellular mechanisms of bacterial internalization counteracted by *Yersinia*. *Int Rev Cytol* 2005;**246**:135–88.
75. Mukherjee S, Keitany G, Li Y, Wang Y, Ball HL, Goldsmith EJ, et al. *Yersinia* YopJ acetylates and inhibits kinase activation by blocking phosphorylation. *Science* 2006;**312**(5777):1211–4.
76. Casadevall A, Pirofski LA. A reappraisal of humoral immunity based on mechanisms of antibody-mediated protection against intracellular pathogens. *Adv Immunol* 2006;**91**:1–44.
77. Joller N, Weber SS, Oxenius A. Antibody-Fc receptor interactions in protection against intracellular pathogens. *Eur J Immunol* 2011;**41**(4):889–97.
78. Rhinehart-Jones TR, Fortier AH, Elkins KL. Transfer of immunity against lethal murine Francisella infection by specific antibody depends on host γ interferon and T cells. *Infect Immun* 1994;**62**(8):3129–37.
79. Balagopal A, MacFarlane AS, Mohapatra N, Soni S, Gunn JS, Schlesinger LS. Characterization of the receptor–ligand pathways important for entry and survival of *Francisella tularensis* in human macrophages. *Infect Immun* 2006;**74**(9):5114–25.
80. Kirimanjeswara GS, Golden JM, Bakshi CS, Metzger DW. Prophylactic and therapeutic use of antibodies for protection against respiratory infection with *Francisella tularensis*. *J Immunol* 2007;**179**(1):532–9.
81. Geier H, Celli J. Phagocytic receptors dictate phagosomal escape and intracellular proliferation of *Francisella tularensis*. *Infect Immun* 2011;**79**(6):2204–14.
82. Yang X, Brunham RC. Gene knockout B cell-deficient mice demonstrate that B cells play an important role in the initiation of T cell responses to *Chlamydia trachomatis* (mouse pneumonitis) lung infection. *J Immunol* 1998;**161**(3):1439–46.
83. Moore T, Ananaba GA, Bolier J, Bowers S, Belay T, Eko FO, et al. Fc receptor regulation of protective immunity against *Chlamydia trachomatis*. *Immunology* 2002;**105**(2):213–21.
84. Moore T, Ekworomadu CO, Eko FO, MacMillan L, Ramey K, Ananaba GA, et al. Fc receptor-mediated antibody regulation of T cell immunity against intracellular pathogens. *J Infect Dis* 2003;**188**(4):617–24.
85. Tobar JA, Gonzalez PA, Kalergis AM. Salmonella escape from antigen presentation can be overcome by targeting bacteria to Fcγ receptors on dendritic cells. *J Immunol* 2004;**173**(6):4058–65.
86. Herrada AA, Contreras FJ, Tobar JA, Pacheco R, Kalergis AM. Immune complex-induced enhancement of bacterial antigen presentation requires Fcγ receptor III expression on dendritic cells. *Proc Nat Acad Sci USA* 2007;**104**(33):13402–7.
87. Riquelme SA, Bueno SM, Kalergis AM. IgG keeps virulent *Salmonella* from evading dendritic cell uptake. *Immunology* 2012;**136**(3):291–305.
88. Joller N, Weber SS, Müller AJ, Spörri R, Selchow P, Sander P, et al. Antibodies protect against intracellular bacteria by Fc receptor-mediated lysosomal targeting. *Proc Nat Acad Sci USA* 2010;**107**(47):20441–6.
89. de Valliere S, Abate G, Blazevic A, Heuertz RM, Hoft DF. Enhancement of innate and cell-mediated immunity by antimycobacterial antibodies. *Infect Immun* 2005;**73**(10):6711–20.
90. Armstrong JA, Hart PD. Phagosome-lysosome interactions in cultured macrophages infected with virulent tubercle bacilli. Reversal of the usual nonfusion pattern and observations on bacterial survival. *J Exp Med* 1975;**142**(1):1–16.
91. Humphres RC, Hinrichs DJ. Role of antibody in *Coxiella burnetii* infection. *Infect Immun* 1981;**31**(2):641–5.
92. Zhang G, Russell-Lodrigue KE, Andoh M, Zhang Y, Hendrix LR, Samuel JE. Mechanisms of vaccine-induced protective immunity against *Coxiella burnetii* infection in BALB/c mice. *J Immunol* 2007;**179**(12):8372–80.
93. Shannon JG, Cockrell DC, Takahashi K, Stahl GL, Heinzen RA. Antibody-mediated immunity to the obligate intracellular bacterial pathogen *Coxiella burnetii* is Fc receptor- and complement-independent. *BMC Immunol* 2009;**10**:26.
94. Collin M, Olsen A. EndoS, a novel secreted protein from *Streptococcus pyogenes* with endoglycosidase activity on human IgG. *EMBO J* 2001;**20**(12):3046–55.
95. Collin M, Svensson MD, Sjoholm AG, Jensenius JC, Sjobring U, Olsen A. EndoS and SpeB from

Streptococcus pyogenes inhibit immunoglobulin-mediated opsonophagocytosis. *Infect Immun* 2002;**70**(12):6646–51.

96. Vincents B, von Pawel-Rammingen U, Bjorck L, Abrahamson M. Enzymatic characterization of the streptococcal endopeptidase, IdeS, reveals that it is a cysteine protease with strict specificity for IgG cleavage due to exosite binding. *Biochemistry* 2004;**43**(49):15540–9.
97. von Pawel-Rammingen U, Johansson BP, Bjorck L. IdeS, a novel streptococcal cysteine proteinase with unique specificity for immunoglobulin G. *EMBO J* 2002;**21**(7):1607–15.
98. Crane DD, Warner SL, Bosio CM. A novel role for plasmin-mediated degradation of opsonizing antibody in the evasion of host immunity by virulent, but not attenuated, *Francisella tularensis*. *J Immunol* 2009;**183**(7):4593–600.
99. Brezski RJ, Jordan RE. Cleavage of IgGs by proteases associated with invasive diseases: an evasion tactic against host immunity? *MAbs* 2010;**2**(3):212–20.
100. Brezski RJ, Luongo JL, Petrone D, Ryan MH, Zhong D, Tam SH, et al. Human anti-IgG1 hinge autoantibodies reconstitute the effector functions of proteolytically inactivated IgGs. *J Immunol* 2008;**181**(5):3183–92.
101. Mittal R, Sukumaran SK, Selvaraj SK, Wooster DG, Babu MM, Schreiber AD, et al. Fcγ receptor I α-chain (CD64) expression in macrophages is critical for the onset of meningitis by *Escherichia coli* K1. *PLoS Pathog* 2010;**6**(11):e1001203.
102. Burton DR. Antibodies, viruses and vaccines. *Nat Rev Immunol* 2002;**2**(9):706–13.
103. Hangartner L, Zinkernagel RM, Hengartner H. Antiviral antibody responses: the two extremes of a wide spectrum. *Nat Rev Immunol* 2006;**6**(3):231–43.
104. Reading SA, Dimmock NJ. Neutralization of animal virus infectivity by antibody. *Arch Virol* 2007;**152**(6):1047–59.
105. Mallery DL, McEwan WA, Bidgood SR, Towers GJ, Johnson CM, James LC. Antibodies mediate intracellular immunity through tripartite motif-containing 21 (TRIM21). *Proc Nat Acad Sci USA* 2010;**107**(46):19985–90.
106. Thompson BS, Moesker B, Smit JM, Wilschut J, Diamond MS, Fremont DH. A therapeutic antibody against West Nile virus neutralizes infection by blocking fusion within endosomes. *PLoS Pathog* 2009;**5**(5):e1000453.
107. Imai M, Sugimoto K, Okazaki K, Kida H. Fusion of influenza virus with the endosomal membrane is inhibited by monoclonal antibodies to defined epitopes on the hemagglutinin. *Virus Res* 1998;**53**(2):129–39.
108. Glauser DL, Kratz AS, Gillet L, Stevenson PG. A mechanistic basis for potent, glycoprotein B-directed γ-herpesvirus neutralization. *J Gen Virol* 2011;**92** (Pt 9):2020–33.
109. Halstead SB, Mahalingam S, Marovich MA, Ubol S, Mosser DM. Intrinsic antibody-dependent enhancement of microbial infection in macrophages: disease regulation by immune complexes. *Lancet Infect Dis* 2010;**10**(10):712–22.
110. Sun P, Bauza K, Pal S, Liang Z, Wu SJ, Beckett C, et al. Infection and activation of human peripheral blood monocytes by dengue viruses through the mechanism of antibody-dependent enhancement. *Virology* 2011;**421**(2):245–52.
111. Dejnirattisai W, Jumnainsong A, Onsirisakul N, Fitton P, Vasanawathana S, Limpitikul W, et al. Cross-reacting antibodies enhance dengue virus infection in humans. *Science* 2010;**328**(5979):745–8.
112. Boonnak K, Dambach KM, Donofrio GC, Tassaneetrithep B, Marovich MA. Cell type specificity and host genetic polymorphisms influence antibody-dependent enhancement of dengue virus infection. *J Virol* 2011;**85**(4):1671–83.
113. Huang KJ, Yang YC, Lin YS, Huang JH, Liu HS, Yeh TM, et al. The dual-specific binding of dengue virus and target cells for the antibody-dependent enhancement of dengue virus infection. *J Immunol* 2006;**176**(5):2825–32.
114. Halstead SB, Venkateshan CN, Gentry MK, Larsen LK. Heterogeneity of infection enhancement of dengue 2 strains by monoclonal antibodies. *J Immunol* 1984;**132**(3):1529–32.
115. Halstead SB. Neutralization and antibody-dependent enhancement of dengue viruses. *Adv Virus Res* 2003;**60**:421–67.
116. Fust G. Enhancing antibodies in HIV infection. *Parasitology* 1997;**115**(Suppl):S127–40.
117. McKeating JA, Griffiths PD, Weiss RA. HIV susceptibility conferred to human fibroblasts by cytomegalovirus-induced Fc receptor. *Nature* 1990;**343**(6259):659–61.
118. Takeda A, Tuazon CU, Ennis FA. Antibody-enhanced infection by HIV-1 via Fc receptor-mediated entry. *Science* 1988;**242**(4878):580–3.
119. Robinson Jr WE, Montefiori DC, Gillespie DH, Mitchell WM. Complement-mediated, antibody-dependent enhancement of HIV-1 infection *in vitro* is characterized by increased protein and RNA syntheses and infectious virus release. *J Acquir Immune Defic Syndr* 1989;**2**(1):33–42.
120. Rosa GT, Gillet L, Smith CM, de Lima BD, Stevenson PG. IgG fc receptors provide an alternative infection route for murine γ-herpesvirus-68. *PLoS One* 2007;**2**(6):e560.

121. Tamura M, Webster RG, Ennis FA. Subtype cross-reactive, infection-enhancing antibody responses to influenza A viruses. *J Virol* 1994;**68**(6):3499–504.
122. Gotoff R, Tamura M, Janus J, Thompson J, Wright P, Ennis FA. Primary influenza A virus infection induces cross-reactive antibodies that enhance uptake of virus into Fc receptor-bearing cells. *J Infect Dis* 1994;**169**(1):200–3.
123. Tamura M, Webster RG, Ennis FA. Neutralization and infection-enhancement epitopes of influenza A virus hemagglutinin. *J Immunol* 1993;**151**(3):1731–8.
124. Ochiai H, Kurokawa M, Matsui S, Yamamoto T, Kuroki Y, Kishimoto C, et al. Infection enhancement of influenza A NWS virus in primary murine macrophages by anti-hemagglutinin monoclonal antibody. *J Med Virol* 1992;**36**(3):217–21.
125. Tamura M, Webster RG, Ennis FA. Antibodies to HA and NA augment uptake of influenza A viruses into cells via Fc receptor entry. *Virology* 1991;**182**(1):211–9.
126. Inada T, Chong KT, Mims CA. Enhancing antibodies, macrophages and virulence in mouse cytomegalovirus infection. *J Gen Virol* 1985;**66**(Pt 4):871–8.
127. Baxt B, Mason PW. Foot-and-mouth disease virus undergoes restricted replication in macrophage cell cultures following Fc receptor-mediated adsorption. *Virology* 1995;**207**(2):503–9.
128. Mason PW, Baxt B, Brown F, Harber J, Murdin A, Wimmer E. Antibody-complexed foot-and-mouth disease virus, but not poliovirus, can infect normally insusceptible cells via the Fc receptor. *Virology* 1993;**192**(2):568–77.
129. Iankov ID, Pandey M, Harvey M, Griesmann GE, Federspiel MJ, Russell SJ. Immunoglobulin G antibody-mediated enhancement of measles virus infection can bypass the protective antiviral immune response. *J Virol* 2006;**80**(17):8530–40.
130. Kishimoto C, Kurokawa M, Ochiai H. Antibody-mediated immune enhancement in coxsackievirus B3 myocarditis. *J Mol Cell Cardiol* 2002;**34**(9):1227–38.
131. Mahalingam S, Lidbury BA. Suppression of lipopolysaccharide-induced antiviral transcription factor (STAT-1 and NF-κB) complexes by antibody-dependent enhancement of macrophage infection by Ross River virus. *Proc Nat Acad Sci USA* 2002;**99**(21):13819–24.
132. Bloom ME, Best SM, Hayes SF, Wells RD, Wolfinbarger JB, McKenna R, et al. Identification of aleutian mink disease parvovirus capsid sequences mediating antibody-dependent enhancement of infection, virus neutralization, and immune complex formation. *J Virol* 2001;**75**(22):11116–27.
133. McMichael AJ, Haynes BF. Lessons learned from HIV-1 vaccine trials: new priorities and directions. *Nat Immunol* 2012;**13**(5):423–7.
134. Forthal DN, Gilbert PB, Landucci G, Phan T. Recombinant gp120 vaccine-induced antibodies inhibit clinical strains of HIV-1 in the presence of Fc receptor-bearing effector cells and correlate inversely with HIV infection rate. *J Immunol* 2007;**178**(10):6596–603.
135. Holl V, Hemmerter S, Burrer R, Schmidt S, Bohbot A, Aubertin AM, et al. Involvement of FcγRI (CD64) in the mechanism of HIV-1 inhibition by polyclonal IgG purified from infected patients in cultured monocyte-derived macrophages. *J Immunol* 2004;**173**(10):6274–83.
136. Perez-Bercoff D, David A, Sudry H, Barre-Sinoussi F, Pancino G. Fcγ receptor-mediated suppression of human immunodeficiency virus type 1 replication in primary human macrophages. *J Virol* 2003;**77**(7):4081–94.
137. Bai Y, Ye L, Tesar DB, Song H, Zhao D, Bjorkman PJ, et al. Intracellular neutralization of viral infection in polarized epithelial cells by neonatal Fc receptor (FcRn)-mediated IgG transport. *Proc Nat Acad Sci USA* 2011;**108**(45):18406–11.
138. Mazanec MB, Coudret CL, Fletcher DR. Intracellular neutralization of influenza virus by immunoglobulin A anti-hemagglutinin monoclonal antibodies. *J Virol* 1995;**69**(2):1339–43.
139. Mazanec MB, Kaetzel CS, Lamm ME, Fletcher D, Peterra J, Nedrud JG. Intracellular neutralization of Sendai and influenza viruses by IgA monoclonal antibodies. *Adv Exp Med Biol* 1995;**371A**:651–4.
140. Huber VC, Lynch JM, Bucher DJ, Le J, Metzger DW. Fc receptor-mediated phagocytosis makes a significant contribution to clearance of influenza virus infections. *J Immunol* 2001;**166**(12):7381–8.
141. El Bakkouri K, Descamps F, De Filette M, Smet A, Festjens E, Birkett A, et al. Universal vaccine based on ectodomain of matrix protein 2 of influenza A: Fc receptors and alveolar macrophages mediate protection. *J Immunol* 2011;**186**(2):1022–31.
142. Sutterwala FS, Noel GJ, Salgame P, Mosser DM. Reversal of proinflammatory responses by ligating the macrophage Fcγ receptor type I. *J Exp Med* 1998;**188**(1):217–22.
143. Green S, Vaughn DW, Kalayanarooj S, Nimmannitya S, Suntayakorn S, Nisalak A, et al. Elevated plasma interleukin-10 levels in acute dengue correlate with disease severity. *J Med Virol* 1999;**59**(3):329–34.
144. Zaiss AK, Vilaysane A, Cotter MJ, Clark SA, Meijndert HC, Colarusso P, et al. Antiviral antibodies target adenovirus to phagolysosomes and amplify the innate immune response. *J Immunol* 2009;**182**(11):7058–68.
145. Guy RA, Belosevic M. Comparison of receptors required for entry of *Leishmania major* amastigotes into macrophages. *Infect Immun* 1993;**61**(4):1553–8.

146. Peters C, Aebischer T, Stierhof YD, Fuchs M, Overath P. The role of macrophage receptors in adhesion and uptake of Leishmania mexicana amastigotes. *J Cell Sci* 1995;**108**(Pt 12):3715–24.
147. Mosser DM. Receptors on phagocytic cells involved in microbial recognition. *Immunol Ser* 1994;**60**:99–114.
148. Dasgupta D, Chakraborty P, Basu MK. Ligation of Fc receptor of macrophages stimulates protein kinase C and anti-leishmanial activity. *Mol Cell Biochem* 2000;**209**(1–2):1–8.
149. Padigel UM, Farrell JP. Control of infection with Leishmania major in susceptible BALB/c mice lacking the common γ-chain for FcR is associated with reduced production of IL-10 and TGF-β by parasitized cells. *J Immunol* 2005;**174**(10):6340–5.
150. Kane MM, Mosser DM. The role of IL-10 in promoting disease progression in leishmaniasis. *J Immunol* 2001;**166**(2):1141–7.
151. Buxbaum LU. A detrimental role for IgG and FcγR in *Leishmania mexicana* infection. *Immunol Res* 2008;**42**(1–3):197–209.
152. Thomas BN, Buxbaum LU. FcγRIII mediates immunoglobulin G-induced interleukin-10 and is required for chronic *Leishmania mexicana* lesions. *Infect Immun* 2008;**76**(2):623–31.
153. Woelbing F, Kostka SL, Moelle K, Belkaid Y, Sunderkoetter C, Verbeek S, et al. Uptake of *Leishmania major* by dendritic cells is mediated by Fcγ receptors and facilitates acquisition of protective immunity. *J Exp Med* 2006;**203**(1):177–88.
154. Sibley LD, Weidner E, Krahenbuhl JL. Phagosome acidification blocked by intracellular *Toxoplasma gondii*. *Nature* 1985;**315**(6018):416–9.
155. Joiner KA, Fuhrman SA, Miettinen HM, Kasper LH, Mellman I. *Toxoplasma gondii*: fusion competence of parasitophorous vacuoles in Fc receptor-transfected fibroblasts. *Science* 1990;**249**(4969):641–6.
156. Anderson Jr SE, Bautista SC, Remington JS. Specific antibody-dependent killing of *Toxoplasma gondii* by normal macrophages. *Clin Exp Immunol* 1976;**26**(3):375–80.
157. Erbe DV, Pfefferkorn ER, Fanger MW. Functions of the various IgG Fc receptors in mediating killing of *Toxoplasma gondii*. *J Immunol* 1991;**146**(9):3145–51.
158. Fadul CE, Channon JY, Kasper LH. Survival of immunoglobulin G-opsonized *Toxoplasma gondii* in nonadherent human monocytes. *Infect Immun* 1995;**63**(11):4290–4.
159. Kang H, Remington JS, Suzuki Y. Decreased resistance of B cell-deficient mice to infection with *Toxoplasma gondii* despite unimpaired expression of IFN-γ, TNF-α, and inducible nitric oxide synthase. *J Immunol* 2000;**164**(5):2629–34.
160. van Spriel AB, van den Herik-Oudijk IE, van Sorge NM, Vile HA, van Strijp JA, van de Winkel JG. Effective phagocytosis and killing of *Candida albicans* via targeting FcγRI (CD64) or FcαRI (CD89) on neutrophils. *J Infect Dis* 1999;**179**(3):661–9.
161. Cutler JE, Deepe Jr GS, Klein BS. Advances in combating fungal diseases: vaccines on the threshold. *Nat Rev Microbiol* 2007;**5**(1):13–28.
162. Bromuro C, Torosantucci A, Chiani P, Conti S, Polonelli L, Cassone A. Interplay between protective and inhibitory antibodies dictates the outcome of experimentally disseminated candidiasis in recipients of a *Candida albicans* vaccine. *Infect Immun* 2002;**70**(10):5462–70.
163. Torosantucci A, Chiani P, Bromuro C, De Bernardis F, Palma AS, Liu Y, et al. Protection by anti-β-glucan antibodies is associated with restricted β-1,3 glucan binding specificity and inhibition of fungal growth and adherence. *PLoS One* 2009;**4**(4):e5392.
164. Hu Y, Farah CS, Ashman RB. Isolates of *Candida albicans* that differ in virulence for mice elicit strain-specific antibody-mediated protective responses. *Microbes Infect* 2006;**8**(3):612–20.
165. Yuan R, Casadevall A, Spira G, Scharff MD. Isotype switching from IgG3 to IgG1 converts a nonprotective murine antibody to *Cryptococcus neoformans* into a protective antibody. *J Immunol* 1995;**154**(4):1810–6.
166. Yuan RR, Casadevall A, Oh J, Scharff MD. T cells cooperate with passive antibody to modify *Cryptococcus neoformans* infection in mice. *Proc Nat Acad Sci USA* 1997;**94**(6):2483–8.
167. Mukherjee S, Lee SC, Casadevall A. Antibodies to *Cryptococcus neoformans* glucuronoxylomannan enhance antifungal activity of murine macrophages. *Infect Immun* 1995;**63**(2):573–9.
168. Yuan R, Clynes R, Oh J, Ravetch JV, Scharff MD. Antibody-mediated modulation of *Cryptococcus neoformans* infection is dependent on distinct Fc receptor functions and IgG subclasses. *J Exp Med* 1998;**187**(4):641–8.
169. van Sorge NM, van der Pol WL, van de Winkel JG. FcγR polymorphisms: implications for function, disease susceptibility and immunotherapy. *Tissue Antigens* 2003;**61**(3):189–202.

CHAPTER

3

Interactions Between the Complement System and Fcγ Receptors

Margaret A. Lindorfer[a], *Jörg Köhl*[b] *and Ronald P. Taylor*[a,*]

[a]Department of Biochemistry and Molecular Genetics, University of Virginia School of Medicine, Charlottesville, Virginia, [b]Institute for Systemic Inflammation Research, University of Lübeck, Lübeck, Germany; Division of Cellular and Molecular Immunology, Cincinnati Children's Hospital and University, Cincinnati, Ohio

PRELIMINARY COMMENTS

The sequences of activation of the three complement pathways are very well understood in molecular detail.[1–7] After converging at C3 activation, all three pathways share the terminal pathway of complement activation, formation of the membrane attack complex (MAC). The MAC has been demonstrated to be quite efficient at lysing and destroying sheep erythrocytes as well as a wide variety of selected cellular targets. However, with respect to actual defense against infection, it appears that the generation of nascent activated C3b, which can covalently tag infectious agents to allow for recognition by cognate receptors on effector cells, constitutes a more important role for complement in host defense.[8–10] For example, it is well known that individuals with defects in the terminal pathway of complement, or patients who receive eculizumab anti-C5 mAb therapy, are susceptible to *Neisseria* infection, but they are otherwise, to a great extent, immunologically intact.[5,6,11,12] However, a lack of functional C3 is associated with an increased risk of a number of pyrogenic bacterial infections.[6,12] An immune response, provoked by infection or vaccination, leads to the generation of IgG antibodies; deposition of C3b on immune IgG-sensitized infectious agents represents the classic pattern by which complement participates in neutralizing and clearing such targets based on their subsequent recognition by receptors specific for both complement fragments (C3b/iC3b; CR1, and CR3 and CR4 respectively) and for bound IgG (Fcγ receptors).[5,13] Moreover, emerging evidence demonstrates that several U.S. Food and Drug Administration (FDA)-approved anti-tumor mAbs make use of complement as well as Fcγ receptors to eliminate targeted cells.[14–21] Therefore, many investigations have focused on developing a detailed understanding of the mechanisms by which C3b opsonization can synergize with Fcγ receptor functions in immune defense.[8,22,23] More recently,

* Corresponding Author

the cross-talk between C5a and Fcγ receptors, which plays a role in both immune defense as well as in mechanisms of inflammation in autoimmune diseases, has been the subject of intense investigation.[24–28] The principal emphasis in this chapter will center on the most important and key findings in these two areas of research. The schematics in Figure 3.1 highlight the steps and

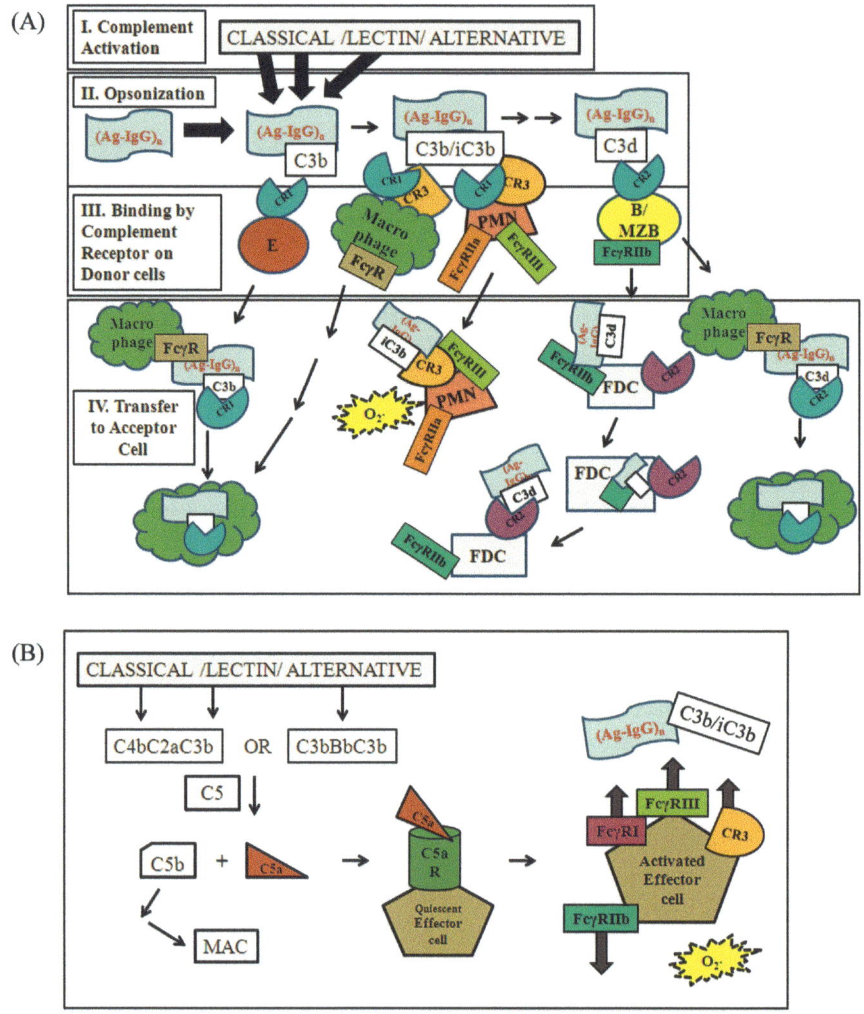

FIGURE 3.1 **(A) Simplified schematic of the major points of interaction between the complement system and Fcγ receptors, all of which converge at the C3b opsonization step.** I. *Complement Activation.* The classical pathway, followed by amplification mediated by the alternative pathway, is principally responsible for C3b opsonization of immune complexes $(Ag–IgG)_n$. However, as noted, the alternative pathway can be directly activated by certain immune complexes. The lectin pathway is directly activated after binding of mannan binding lectin or of ficollins to certain bacteria, and if IgG were also bound these immune complexes could be subjected to the reactions shown. II. *Opsonization.* Although not explicitly shown, numerous C3b fragments covalently tag the immune complexes, thus allowing the complexes to bind to the low avidity

molecules in the complement activation pathways that are most relevant for our presentation, and Table 3.1 summarizes many of the key reports that are discussed. More detailed descriptions of the complement cascade may be found in several excellent recent reviews.[1–7]

COMPLEMENT FRAGMENT C3b MEDIATES BINDING OF IgG IMMUNE COMPLEXES TO PRIMATE ERYTHROCYTES: IMMUNE ADHERENCE

Historical Perspective

The immune adherence phenomenon, whereby C3b-opsonized substrates are bound to primate erythrocytes, was first described by Nelson 60 years ago.[29,30] This phenomenon remains one of the most instructive and important manifestations of the synergy between the complement system and the interaction of IgG antibodies with their receptors. It is interesting to note that neither complement receptors nor Fcγ receptors had been characterized when Nelson first described immune adherence. However, his prescient findings and analyses, as well as the investigations of Robineaux, performed in part in collaboration with Nelson, provided phenomenological descriptions of the interplay among bacteria, specific antibodies, complement, primate erythrocytes, and white cells.[31] Their observations led to the development of paradigms for understanding these complex systems that still apply today.

Nelson reported that in the presence of serum complement, antibody-opsonized bacteria are first bound to human erythrocytes, and, *once bound to the erythrocytes*, the bacteria are then transferred to and internalized and killed by leukocytes;[29,30] however, under these conditions, the erythrocytes appear to emerge from this reaction undamaged. The details of this transfer process have now been dissected and are

complement receptors on the cells. Due to the action of Factor I, C3b is rapidly degraded to iC3b, and then to C3d. The immune complexed "antigens" that have been documented to be processed by one or more of these pathways include soluble proteins, dsDNA, viruses (including HIV) bacteria, erythrocytes, and tumor cells. III. and IV. *Binding to donor cells and transfer to acceptor cells. Erythrocytes*, the immune adherence reaction—C3b-opsonized immune complexes bind to clusters of CR1 on primate erythrocytes. The complexes are recognized by Fcγ receptors on monocyte/macrophages and then transferred to these acceptor cells, in a concerted reaction that includes transfer of CR1. The complexes are then phagocytosed. *Macrophages and neutrophils*—Substrates opsonized with C3b/iC3b (as well as with IgG) can bind directly to cells via both Fcγ receptors and via complement receptors. C3b-IgG (and likely iC3b-IgG) can function as a "superopsonin" and chelate CR1 (and likely CR3) along with Fcγ receptors on monocytes/macrophages or on neutrophils (PMN), thus promoting greatly enhanced phagocytosis. Synergy and direct interaction between CR3 and FcγRIII on neutrophils leads to cooperative uptake of substrates opsonized at the iC3b stage. These complexes can be phagocytosed, and in addition co-stimulation of both CR3 and FcγRIII leads to neutrophil activation associated with a respiratory burst (release of O_2^-/H_2O_2) and release of other inflammatory mediators including β-glucuronidase and lysozyme. *B cells*. C3d-opsonized immune complexes bound to B-cell CR2 can be taken up by and transferred to macrophages in a process that analogously follows the immune adherence reaction pathway. The complexes, along with CR2, are internalized by the acceptor macrophages. Alternatively, after these complexes bind to marginal zone B cells via CR2, they are taken up by and transferred to FDC. In this latter reaction, the immune complexes, along with CR2, are removed from the marginal zone B cell and, after internalization, are recycled and held on the cell surface by CR2 of the FDC. This is accomplished through the recycling action of FcγIIb on the FDC. **(B) Downstream, the classical and alternative pathway C5 convertases generate C5a and C5b, which can mediate tissue damage.** The MAC is subsequently assembled from C5b and C6–C9. C5a binds to C5aR on effector cells, including mast cells, monocytes, macrophages, and neutrophils. The net effect is to drive the quiescent effector cell into an inflammatory poise, based in large part on upregulation of activating Fcγ receptors and upregulation of CR3. Levels of the inhibitory receptor FcγRIIb are also decreased. Under these conditions, the activated effector cell will interact with the IgG/C3b(iC3b)-opsonized immune complexes and promote inflammation. This inflammatory response can include phagocytosis as well as the release of inflammatory mediators (e.g., O_2^-, hydrolytic enzymes, cytokines, chemokines).

TABLE 3.1 Examples of Interactions Between the Complement System and Fcγ Receptors

Interactions	Description	Implications in Human Disease	Selected References
Immune adherence CR1–C3b–IgG–FcγR	C3b-opsonized immune complexes bound to primate erythrocytes via CR1 are taken up by effector cells due to recognition by Fcγ receptors.	+, Removal of opsonized inflammatory and infectious agents –, Enhancement of HIV infection	Nelson[29,30] Robineaux and Pinet[31] Fearon[44] Lindorfer et al.[34]
Antigen trafficking by non-cognate B cells CR2–C3d–IgG–FcγR	C3d-opsonized immune complexes bound to marginal zone B cells via CR2 are delivered to and displayed on the surface of FDC.	+, Enhanced immune response –, FDC are a reservoir for HIV	Brown et al.[73] Humphrey et al.[76] Lindorfer et al.[67] Cyster et al.[74] Carroll et al.[75]
C3b and IgG synergize to increase immunologic recognition of targets	Opsonization of substrates with C3b and IgG substantially enhances *in vivo* clearance and *in vitro* phagocytosis mediated by effector cells.	+, More efficient removal of opsonized inflammatory and infectious agents; C3b–IgG as a superopsonin –, Possibly increased infectivity of HIV	Frank et al.[23] da Silveira et al.[102] Ehlenberger and Nussenzweig[22] Stoiber et al.[84]
FcγRIII and CR3 communicate	Stimulus or blockade of one receptor affects the function/downstream cell biology associated with the other; the receptors co-cap and also cooperate in targeting opsonized cancer cells.	+, Enhanced activity of complement-fixing mAbs in cancer immunotherapy	Brown et al.[104] Zhou and Brown[106] Leusen et al.[113] Di Gaetano et al.[14]
The C5a/C5aR axis regulates FcγR expression	C5a, induced by immune complex-mediated complement activation, reduces the threshold for FcγR-mediated cell activation by increasing the A/I ratio—that is, upregulation of activating FcγR (A) and dowregulation of of inhibitory receptor FcγRIIb (I).	+, Enhanced removal of inflammatory agents –, Potent mediator of inflammation in SLE, RA	Frank et al.[140] Gerard et al.[125] Schmidt and Gessner[25] Heller et al.[127] Godau et al.[130]
FcγRIIB with Dectin-1 to block C5aR-mediated effector functions	Galactosylated IgG_1 immune complexes bind to FcγRIIb and Dectin-1, resulting in a Syk- and SHIP-dependent inhibition of C5aR signaling in neutrophils and macrophages.	+, Inhibitory feedback loop to prevent excessive C5aR activation; protect from C5a-mediated inflammation in autoimmune diseases –, Possibly decreased defense against bacterial infections	Karsten et al.[28]

(Continued)

TABLE 3.1 (Continued)

Interactions	Description	Implications in Human Disease	Selected References
Complement and immune complex processing in SLE	Complement activation mediated by immune complexes produces C5a; as expected, FcγRI is upregulated, but FcγRII and FcγRIII are downregulated/partially exhausted, likely due to chronic phagocytosis of immune complexes.	+, New therapeutic targets may be identified	Fries et al.[139] Salmon et al.[141] Kavai and Szegedi[138] Ahuja et al.[148]
Essential role of the alternative pathway of complement and FcγR in murine models of antibody-induced arthritis	Clinical disease mediated by IgG immune complexes deposited on collagen requires complement activation and C5aR activity; disease is increased by MAC generation. A positive feedback loop due to complement may enhance IgG deposition.		Ji et al.[128] Banda et al.[152]

understood in molecular detail. IgG antibodies first bind to the bacteria and activate the classical pathway of complement, thus promoting covalent deposition of large numbers of C3 activation fragments (C3b) on the bound IgG and on the bacterial surface. The affinity of the erythrocyte complement receptor (CR1) for its cognate ligand, C3b, is low;[32–34] however, the large number of C3b molecules covalently fixed to the bacterium/IgG complex allow for multivalent binding of the opsonized bacteria to *clusters* of CR1 on the erythrocyte, thus immobilizing the bacteria.[34] Subsequently, uptake and phagocytosis of the erythrocyte-bound IgG-opsonized bacteria by acceptor leukocytes "was markedly enhanced compared to controls in which B-Ab-C [bacterium opsonized with antibody and complement] was floating free in the plasma."[30]

Nelson extended his studies to a monkey model,[30] and it is now well established that only primate erythrocytes express CR1 and are capable of binding C3b-opsonized IgG immune complexes and then transferring these complexes to acceptor cells for phagocytosis and destruction.[34,35] The immune complexes that have been examined have been constructed with a wide range of substrate antigens, including bacteria, viruses, double-stranded DNA, and proteins. The processing of the immune complexes is *trans* in the sense that the immune complexed substrate is opsonized with complement and adhered to one cell (the erythrocyte), and this allows for uptake followed by phagocytosis and degradation of the substrate by another cell, the leukocyte. Based on the monkey models, the immune complexes are taken up by Kupffer cells in the liver and other fixed macrophages in the spleen.[34,35] Finberg and colleagues have recently replicated this system in mice.[36] They generated transgenic mice whose erythrocytes express human CR1; immune complexes opsonized with mouse C3b were processed by the transgenic murine erythrocytes closely following the immune adherence reaction pathway described by Nelson.

Nelson also demonstrated that the erythrocytes survive the transfer step in the immune adherence reaction. Phase contrast microscopy experiments revealed that the leukocyte appeared to "scour" the erythrocyte surface in order to remove bound bacteria. There was a transient deformity of the erythrocyte during its interaction with the leukocyte; however, after the bacteria were removed, the erythrocyte appeared to regain its normal shape.[30] Obviously, these early studies could not have elucidated the *mechanism of transfer* of these particulate immune complexes, but the experiments set the stage for investigating and understanding more complex systems and mechanisms, including animal models and clinical studies.

Modern Times and Mechanisms: CR1 is Removed from Erythrocytes

Based on a voluminous literature on immune complex clearance,[34,37,38] it is now established that transfer of the bacteria (or other opsonized substrates) from erythrocytes to acceptor cells (monocytes/macrophages) is mediated principally by Fcγ receptors on the acceptor cells that recognize IgG bound to the bacteria. As noted, activation of complement leads to opsonization of a substrate with multiple copies of C3b, thus promoting its binding to CR1 clusters and immobilization on the erythrocyte surface. This IgG-rich immobilized substrate is a particularly inviting target for multivalent chelation by several Fcγ receptors on a leukocyte, and this chelation is followed by removal of the substrate from the erythrocyte, which leads to phagocytosis and degradation of the substrate by the acceptor cell. However, the important underlying question is exactly *how* does the leukocyte *remove* the immune complex from the erythrocyte without promoting substantial damage to the erythrocyte? Based on basic tenets of complement, it is possible that factor I-mediated degradation of C3b to iC3b on erythrocyte-bound immune complexes would cause release of the immune complexes, thus leading to solution-phase transfer of iC3b-opsonized complexes to acceptor cells.[38–40] However, observations in a chimpanzee model argued against this mechanism.[34,41,42] *In vitro* experiments demonstrated that factor I-mediated release does not take place in the serum of the chimpanzee. In addition, C3b-opsonized IgG anti-dsDNA/dsDNA immune complex substrates bound to chimpanzee erythrocytes are rapidly cleared from the circulation without any apparent damage to the erythrocytes.[34,41] That is, this *rapid* transfer in the chimpanzee model appears to preclude a mechanism that makes use of factor I. Also, the close contact ("scouring") between the erythrocyte and leukocyte reported by Nelson would suggest that at least for some period of time there is direct interaction between the cells, rather than simply release of the immune complexes into solution.

To address the question of the transfer mechanism in more detail, we first focus on the *site of attachment* of the C3b-opsonized immune complexes to the erythrocyte, CR1. This receptor is a type I transmembrane glycoprotein that spans the membrane once and has a small intracytoplasmic portion; it was first described by Fearon in 1979 and 1980.[43,44] Soon thereafter, several reports emerged that demonstrated *substantial reductions* in the levels of erythrocyte CR1 associated with numerous diseases characterized by complement activation and immune complex processing.[45–49] It was hypothesized that after the CR1-associated IgG-containing immune complexes are recognized and chelated by Fc receptors on the acceptor cell, they would then be transferred to the acceptor cell in a concerted reaction in which the CR1 molecules associated with the immune complexes would *also* be removed from the erythrocytes and taken up and internalized by the phagocytic cell.[34,48] CR1 is known to be quite sensitive to proteases,[50–52] and it is possible that one or more proteases are secreted by the acceptor cells and then CR1 is proteolyzed close to the plasma membrane, thus allowing release of the bound immune complexes.

Reductions in erythrocyte CR1 have been documented in patients with systemic lupus erythematosus (SLE), rheumatoid arthritis (RA), and AIDS.[47–49,53,54] Moreover, both *in vitro* and animal models have been used to examine this phenomenon, and they all lead to the same conclusion: IgG-containing immune complexes bound to primate erythrocytes via CR1 are taken up by acceptor cells that express Fcγ receptors, and all or almost all of immune complex-associated CR1 is taken up as well.[34] It appears that the rate of clearance/transfer may be simply related to the number of IgG bound per immune complex, with immune complexes containing multiple IgG being cleared much more quickly, because there would be more effective interaction with and engagement of Fcγ receptors on the acceptor cells.

In some of these model systems, the immune complexes were constructed and bound to CR1 *in the absence of complement*, based on using high-affinity mAbs to CR1 as surrogates for multiple molecules of C3b.[34] For example Taylor et al.[34,55–57] examined the clearance of bispecific mAb complexes (heteropolymers, anti-CR1 cross-linked with an irrelevant mouse IgG) in a monkey model. These model immune complexes bind to erythrocyte CR1 and are cleared in about one day, coincident with loss of CR1. To confirm the key role of Fcγ receptors, they also demonstrated that immune complexes constructed with $F(ab)_2$ antibody fragments were not taken up by acceptor cells, and that the transfer reaction can be blocked *in vitro* by high concentrations of intact IgG due to blockade of Fcγ receptors. The transfer reaction could be a form of trogocytosis. Trogocytosis is now recognized as a general reaction in which receptors (e.g. Fcγ receptors) on an acceptor cell can pinch off and remove cognate ligands (e.g., immune complexes) and associated plasma membrane from another cell.[58–60] Thus, small portions of the erythrocyte membrane associated with CR1 and the immune complexes could also be taken up by clusters of Fcγ receptors on the macrophage. For example, Zimring[61] has reported that in models of autoimmune anemia, antibodies bound to certain erythrocyte antigens can be removed from the erythrocytes, along with the cognate antigens, by Fcγ receptors on macrophages ("antigen loss") without otherwise damaging the erythrocytes. Beum et al.[62,63] have reported that CD20 IgG mAbs bound to B cells, along with the CD20 antigen, can be almost quantitatively removed and internalized by monocytes due to interaction with their Fcγ receptors. At the present time it is not clear if trogocytosis or CR1 cleavage or both mechanisms are utilized when immune complexes bound to erythrocytes via CR1 are removed from the erythrocyte and then internalized by acceptor cells. Definitive studies that do or do not demonstrate a cytoplasmic stump of CR1 on post-transfer erythrocytes could resolve this issue; however, as noted previously, studies of the immune adherence reaction provide a valuable lesson for understanding other systems. That is, substrates/ligands presented on a donor cell to receptors on an acceptor cell can be removed from the donor cell with minimal damage to the donor.

The report of Wilson et al.[64] in 1985 can now be understood in light of these considerations. They evaluated the erythrocytes of an SLE patient who had IgG autoantibodies specific for CR1. High titers of the anti-CR1 antibodies correlated with severe reductions in the levels of erythrocyte CR1, and the reductions were not due to simple blockade of epitopes on CR1. The most likely explanation for these findings is that the autoantibodies had bound to erythrocyte CR1 and were processed as immune complexes, thus leading to loss of CR1 as well.

COMPLEMENT FRAGMENT C3d MEDIATES BINDING OF SUBSTRATES TO CR2 ON B CELLS: ANTIGEN TRAFFICKING AND ITS SIGNIFICANCE IN HIV DISEASE

Similarities and Differences between CR1 and CR2

CR1 and CR2 are both type I transmembrane glycoproteins, and each is composed almost entirely of similar repeating structural subunits, the short consensus repeat found in many complement control proteins.[33] CR2 is located most abundantly on B cells and follicular dendritic cells and is specific for C3d, the final breakdown product of C3b.[33,65–68] The affinity of CR2 for C3d is modest, but B cells are able to bind immune complexed substrates containing multiple copies of C3d through multivalent chelation, in a manner similar to that described for the binding of C3b-opsonized immune complexes by clusters of CR1 on primate erythrocytes.[65–67] An obvious and interesting question is whether there is a comparable process of immunological significance in which immune complexes bound to B cells via CR2 can be transferred to acceptor cells. Indeed, several *in vitro* and animal models, in mice and in monkeys, have all demonstrated that prototype IgG-containing immune complex substrates bound to B-cell CR2 can be removed from the B cells and transferred to and internalized by acceptor cells. This transfer reaction also leads to loss of CR2 from the B cells and requires Fcγ receptors on the acceptor cells.[67,69,70] This process is obviously quite similar to the final transfer step of the immune adherence reaction. In some of these studies, this process was replicated, both *in vitro* and *in vivo*, based on making use of high-affinity IgG mAbs specific for human (and monkey) or mouse CR2. In analogy to the studies with CR1, these mAbs serve as surrogates for multiple molecules of C3d. In the presence of acceptor cells, binding of these mAbs to B-cell CR2 promotes removal of the mAb and CR2 from the B cell, followed by internalization of both the mAb *and CR2* by the acceptor cell.[67,69,70] The extracellular portion of CR2 is indeed removed from the B cells, but a fraction of its intracellular domain remains within the B cell, suggesting that this transfer reaction may be mediated in part by *proteolysis* of CR2. Although most (but not all) B cells recirculate, only a small fraction of the B cells are in the circulation at any time; instead, they are found within the lymphatic system.[71,72] Therefore, it is perhaps not surprising that the principal compartment for the processing of IC bound to B cells is the lymphatic system, and in fact the animal model studies clearly demonstrated that substrates bound to B cells via CR2 are localized to the spleen, and not to the liver.[69,70,73–75]

The Shuttle Mechanism: CR2 and Antigen Presentation

B cells can transport complement (C3d)-opsonized immune complexes in the bloodstream, and B cells also have access to the lymphatic system. Thus, in principle, a B cell can transfer C3d-opsonized immune complexes between these compartments. Alternatively, marginal-zone B cells, which do not recirculate and are located at the interface between the blood and the white pulp of the spleen, are very well situated to capture circulating C3d-opsonized immune complexes. As first described by Brown et al.[73] and then in more detail by Humphrey et al.,[76] marginal zone B cells in the spleen can bind and transport C3d-opsonized antigen-IgG-containing immune complexes to the follicle, and this allows for transfer to and display of the intact antigen *on the surface* of follicular dendritic cells (FDCs). This reaction plays a major role in the normal immune response.[70,75,77,78] After transfer, the FDC-associated antigen can then be recognized and bound by cognate B cells in the follicle, ultimately initiating a strong immune response. Several model systems have been developed and studied to gain insight into the mechanisms associated with the transport of C3d-opsonized immune complexes bound to CR2 on marginal zone B cells. In a comprehensive series of papers, Cyster et al.[74,78,79] have elucidated many of the key details. They have demonstrated that, due to competing chemotactic factors (sphingosine-1-phosphate/CXCL13) and transitory and differential expression of sphingosine phosphate receptors, marginal-zone B cells actually "shuttle" between the marginal zone and the B-cell follicle. Thus, these cells, which are sessile and remain in the spleen,[76] are uniquely suited to provide "an efficient mechanism for systemic antigen capture and delivery to follicular dendritic cells."[74,78] Transfer of the C3d-opsonized immune complexes from marginal zone B cells to FDCs follows a pathway that is in part similar to that delineated for the erythrocyte-based immune adherence reaction. However, as will be discussed below, one major difference must be explained: Although the reaction leads to analogous loss of CR2 from the marginal-zone B cell, the released immune complex substrates are apparently not permanently internalized and degraded by acceptor cells but instead are found bound to CR2 on the surface of FDCs.

CR1, CR2, and AIDS

It is well established that HIV can activate complement and capture C3 fragments; this reaction is considerably more effective for HIV/anti-HIV IgG immune complexes.[80–85] HIV-containing immune complexes can bind to erythrocyte CR1 *in vitro*, and HIV has also been found to be associated with erythrocytes in the circulation of AIDS patients.[83,86] Moreover, as noted above, substantial reductions in erythrocyte CR1 have been reported in patients with AIDS, strongly suggesting that at least some of these erythrocyte CR1-bound IgG-containing immune complexes can be chelated by Fc receptors on fixed cells and then taken up by macrophages in the liver and spleen. Whether in a given patient this processing leads to the destruction of HIV or serves as a mechanism to infect the acceptor macrophages likely depends upon several factors, including the concentration and nature of the anti-HIV antibodies as well as the complement titer of the patient.[80,82,84,85,87]

There is considerable evidence, however, indicating that a substantial fraction of these HIV immune complexes experience a different fate. As opposed to the other immune complex substrates bound to erythrocyte CR1 mentioned earlier, a fraction of the HIV-containing immune complexes *are released* into the bloodstream as C3d–HIV–IgG immune complexes, due to factor I-mediated decay of C3b to iC3b and then to C3d.[88] These C3d-opsonized substrates then bind to B cells via CR2 and can, in principle, be removed by trogocytosis of the B cells *by other cells* that express receptors for one or more constituents of these B cell-bound substrates. These include CD4 (specific for gp120), Fcγ receptors (specific for IgG), or CR2 (specific for C3d). There is evidence that these immune complexes can indeed be subjected to several different processing reactions.

Moir et al.[89] have reported that T cells can become infected with HIV when they are allowed to react with B cells that have bound HIV immune complexes on their surface. In this case, it is CD4 on the T cells that interacts with the HIV immune complex. In order for the HIV to infect the T cells *it must be released from the B cells* and internalized by the acceptor T cells, and it is likely that the transfer process is accomplished via trogocytosis and/or proteolysis of CR2.

Alternatively, due to recognition by Fcγ receptors, the C3d–HIV–IgG immune complexes can be stripped off the B cells and internalized by macrophages. The question of whether this leads to degradation and destruction of HIV or infection of the macrophage remains complex and may depend upon the concentration and avidity of the IgG antibodies associated with HIV.[80,84,87] However, both of these transfer processes should also lead to loss of CR2 from the B cell, and several studies have documented that reduced levels of B-cell CR2 are associated with AIDS.[89,90] It is also noteworthy that several reports have indicated that solution phase immune complexes containing IgG and HIV can indeed infect monocyte/macrophages. Infection can also be mediated if the immune complexes are opsonized with complement, thus indicating that entry of the HIV into cells can be promoted by Fcγ receptors, or by receptors most specific for iC3b, CR3, or CR4.[87,91–93]

Immune complexes such as C3d–HIV–IgG can first bind to marginal-zone B cells and then be transferred to FDCs in the spleen and lymph nodes (see previous section). This is a very important reaction, because it is now established that C3d-opsonized HIV bound to FDCs makes up the vast majority of the infectious and long-lasting extracellular HIV reservoir in AIDS.[81,84,90,94] Most of this HIV is apparently bound to CR2 on the FDCs, because it can be released either by treatment with an anti-CR2 mAb that blocks its C3d binding site or by treatment with a mAb specific for C3d that blocks its binding to CR2.[81,94] The *mechanism* of transfer of HIV immune complexes from marginal zone B cells to FDCs is most likely to follow the immune complex-processing pathway first described by Brown et al.[73] and Humphrey et al.[76] FDCs have two important receptors that participate in the reaction, CR2 and FcγRIIb. Based on the observation that CR2 on B cells is substantially reduced in AIDS, during the transfer process CR2 will likely be removed from the B cells in order to promote release of the bound IC. Once again, trogocytosis and/or CR2 proteolysis are the most reasonable candidate mechanisms, but both of these reactions lead to *internalization* of the IC by the acceptor cells. The key question is how can CR2 be cut and the immune complexes transferred to the *surface* of the FDC?

A Clue to a Mechanism: Lessons Learned from Dendritic Cells

Clynes and colleagues[95] examined immune complex processing by dendritic cells and concluded that FcγRIIb is the likely key mediator of transfer of the complexes to the cell surface. In their model, activating Fcγ receptors on the dendritic cells were either blocked or genetically ablated, and they reported that FcγRIIb promoted internalization of the immune complexes, but the immune complexes were processed outside the lysosomal pathway and then returned/recycled to the cell surface. FDCs do not express activating Fcγ receptors and thus, by analogy, FcγRIIb on the FDC should be able to remove CR2 from the marginal-zone B cells and promote release of the cell-bound C3d-opsonized IgG-containing immune complexes. The intact immune complex would be internalized and then recycle to the surface of the FDC and bind to CR2 of the FDC (expressed at high copy number). The FDC would be able to display the IgG–antigen C3d immune complex (or HIV–IgG–C3d immune complex) on its surface for an extended period of time.[84,90] This mechanism follows a pathway that is part of the normal protective immune response by which marginal zone B cells can transfer other immune complexes to FDC, thus allowing long-term display of antigens on their surface.

COOPERATION/SYNERGY BETWEEN Fcγ RECEPTORS AND COMPLEMENT RECEPTORS ON EFFECTOR CELLS

In Vivo Studies of the Clearance of Opsonized Erythrocytes

The investigations of the handling of immune complexes bound to erythrocyte CR1 or to B-cell CR2 can be clearly classified as *trans* because the interactions are between cells. The immune complexes are bound to the carrier erythrocyte or B cells via complement receptors and are then removed and transferred to acceptor cells based on recognition of the bound IgG by Fcγ receptors on the acceptor cells. Alternatively, complement and Fcγ receptors can also synergize on the same effector cell, based on enhanced recognition and phagocytosis of substrates that are opsonized with both IgG and with C3b or iC3b fragments.

The most compelling early evidence for synergy between complement receptors and

Fcγ receptors emerged from the classic animal model studies of autoimmune hemolytic anemia reported by Frank and colleagues.[96–100] They found that guinea pig erythrocytes opsonized with polyclonal rabbit IgM anti-erythrocyte antibodies could capture complement C3 fragments and were temporarily sequestered in the liver, presumably by CR1 and CR3 on Kupffer cells;[101] however, a substantial fraction of the erythrocytes was later released back into the bloodstream, most likely due to conversion of C3b/iC3b to C3d. This finding indicates that the C3b/iC3b-opsonized erythrocytes could indeed adhere to macrophages in the liver, but that phagocytosis was inefficient. The investigators went on to demonstrate that erythrocytes opsonized with low levels of polyclonal rabbit IgG anti-erythrocyte antibodies (too low to induce significant complement activation) were removed from the circulation, principally by the splenic macrophages. This finding emphasizes that receptors specific for IgG, especially in the spleen, are much more effective than complement receptors in promoting phagocytosis. Use of higher doses of antibody, however, led to increasing levels of opsonization with IgG; therefore, complement activation and C3b deposition on the erythrocytes was increased. Under these conditions, clearance to the liver was favored. The most reasonable explanation is that the C3b fragments deposited on the cells would promote adherence to CR1 and CR3 on the surface of Kupffer cells in the liver. Thus, based on the observations of Nelson, these adhered cells would then be subject to more efficient phagocytosis. This synergy was clearly evident when the clearance experiment was repeated in C4-deficient guinea pigs, which have no functional classical pathway of complement activation.[99] Atkinson and Frank reported that erythrocytes opsonized with large amounts of IgG were cleared to the liver (58%) and the spleen (42%) in wild-type animals; however, in C4-deficient animals, clearance of the opsonized erythrocytes to the spleen increased (49%), but clearance to the liver decreased substantially (29%). Moreover, these findings, combined with this group's earlier work, strongly suggest that, in these models, complement plays no role in clearance to the spleen.

Decades later, Izui and colleagues[102] investigated the relative contributions of complement and Fcγ receptors in promoting clearance of targeted erythrocytes in very well-characterized mouse models. They compared different doses of mouse mAb IgG isotype switch variants of a high-affinity anti-erythrocyte mAb with respect to their ability to promote anemia in either wild-type mice or in engineered mice in which either C3 or Fcγ receptors or both were ablated. At a 50-μg dose, the IgG_{2a} variant, which binds with high affinity to Fcγ receptors, promoted erythrocyte clearance independent of complement. However, in analogy to the reports by Frank's group, at high antibody doses (200 μg) the mAb promoted C3b deposition on the erythrocytes, and the hematocrit (Ht) was reduced from 45 to 10%, providing clear evidence for synergy between Fcγ receptors and complement in promoting erythrocyte clearance. Elimination of the contribution of either complement (C3 knockout mice) or Fcγ receptors only partially reduced erythrocyte clearance (Ht of 21% and 28%, respectively), thus emphasizing the synergistic effect. Both Fcγ receptors and complement had to be eliminated in order to restore a full hematocrit in mAb-treated mice. These results also demonstrated that at the high mAb input in the Fcγ knockout mice, complement-mediated clearance to the liver does occur (final Ht of 28%). Finally, the investigators reported similar experiments with the IgG_{2b} anti-erythrocyte isotype, which binds weakly to Fcγ receptors. Dose–response experiments revealed that C3b opsonization was necessary to enhance and synergize with the otherwise relatively weak Fcγ receptor-mediated clearance.

In Vitro Evidence for Synergy between Fcγ Receptors and Complement Receptors

Animal model studies of synergy between Fcγ receptor biology and complement biology were complemented (no pun intended!) by an important early contribution by Ehlenberger and Nussenzweig.[22] They reported that opsonization of sheep erythrocytes with small amounts of C3b dramatically increased phagocytosis of IgG-opsonized cells by neutrophils or monocytes. The C3b was deposited on the erythrocytes by using rabbit IgM antibodies followed by isolated complement components, up to the C3b stage. Rabbit IgG was then independently bound to these C3b-opsonized cells or to naïve cells. Their findings, based on careful quantitative analyses, indicated that phagocytosis mediated by either neutrophils or monocytes was quite modest unless large amounts of IgG were bound to the sheep erythrocytes. In contrast, opsonization of the sheep erythrocytes with even large amounts of C3b did not promote any phagocytosis. The synergistic effect of C3b opsonization on phagocytosis was correlated with its ability to induce rosette formation. In quantitative terms, 1000 molecules of C3b bound to the erythrocyte could promote rosette formation (cell-to-cell contact) with neutrophils, presumably mediated by both CR1 and possibly CR3, but there was no phagocytosis; however, if the C3b-coated erythrocytes were also opsonized with 2000 molecules of IgG, this gave considerably more neutrophil-mediated phagocytosis than if erythrocytes were only opsonized with as many as 60,000 molecules of IgG. These studies were confirmed and the immunological significance extended by Newman and Johnston, who also investigated how opsonized substrates could trigger bactericidal responses of neutrophils.[103] They reported that erythrocytes opsonized with C3b formed rosettes with neutrophils, but this did not cause the neutrophils to release O_2^- or to degranulate and release β-glucuronidase or lysozyme. Reaction of neutrophils with IgG-opsonized erythrocytes did promote some activation and release of these inflammatory agents; however, clear evidence for synergy was demonstrated, based on increased release of the inflammatory mediators, when sheep erythrocytes opsonized with both C3b and IgG were allowed to react with the neutrophils.

Interaction between FcγRIII and CR3

Research into additional mechanisms of synergy has focused on the observation of direct interaction or communication between FcγRIII and CR3. Several independent investigations have demonstrated that FcγRIII appears to be a ligand for CR3, and in the case of neutrophils, in which FcγRIII is anchored to the membrane via glycosylphosphatidylinositol, its interaction with CR3 likely provides a means of signaling. Brown's group has found that $F(ab)_2$ mAbs that target CR3 on human monocytes and neutrophils can inhibit their rosetting with and phagocytosis of IgG-opsonized substrates.[104] Based in part on the results of cross-competition binding experiments with aggregated IgG, they concluded that an immobile subset (~50%) of CR3 is directly associated with FcγRIII. Zhou et al.[105] conducted capping experiments on human neutrophils that focused on CR3 and FcγRIII. They found that when specific agents were used to induce capping of one of these receptors, a substantial fraction of the other receptor was also localized to the cap. In a separate study by Zhou and Brown,[106] synergy between the two receptors with respect to neutrophil activation was most simply demonstrated based on experiments in which the cells were plated on a surface coated with an anti-FcγRIII mAb (as a model for aggregated IgG) and with either iC3b or with an anti-CR3 mAb (a surrogate for iC3b). If the surface was coated with ligands for both receptors, a profound respiratory burst was generated; however, if only one of the receptors was stimulated (the ligand for only one receptor was on the plate), there was little, if any, respiratory burst. The findings in this paper are indeed similar to and in agreement with the earlier report of Newman and Johnston,[103] who used opsonized sheep erythrocytes to stimulate the neutrophils. In terms of the immunological significance, the results strongly suggest that substrates/bacteria that are opsonized with IgG *and have activated complement* will provoke a vigorous and synergistic cytotoxic response by neutrophils and that macrophage-mediated phagocytosis will also be substantially enhanced.

Bouhal et al. reported on a direct interaction between CR3 and FcγRIII with particular relevance to AIDS.[107] As stated earlier, HIV can activate complement and become opsonized with C3 activation fragments in the absence of antibodies. The C3b/iC3b-opsonized HIV can then enter and infect monocyte/macrophages based on chelation of complement receptors CR1 or CR3. In the present study, the investigators noted that the soluble form of FcγRIII is a natural ligand for CR3, and they found that blocking mAbs specific for CR3, or for soluble FcγRIII, could substantially block infection of monocytes/macrophages by serum-opsonized HIV. They also reported that levels of soluble FcγRIII are reduced in HIV disease, and the extent of reduction appeared to correlate with disease severity, suggesting a possible protective role of soluble FcγRIII. Although the mechanism responsible for the reduction in FcγRIII remains to be delineated, the investigators recognized that soluble FcγRIII may have therapeutic applications in AIDS.

C3b–IgG as a Superopsonin

In view of the close interaction between FcγRIII and CR3, it would seem quite reasonable that one could develop or identify a natural ligand that can effectively engage both receptors. Frank and colleagues[8,23] suggested that C3b covalently bound to IgG could function as a "superopsonin." When IgG-opsonized antigens/substrates activate complement, the nascent C3b that is generated can form covalent bonds with either the substrates or with the bound IgG. These substrates include soluble proteins, double-stranded DNA, bacteria, viruses, and cancer cells targeted by immunotherapeutic mAbs.[18,34,38] There do not appear to be any established rules that govern how much of the substrate versus the IgG is covalently labeled with the C3b, except that the substrate must have available acceptor sites (hydroxyl or amino groups) to form ester or amide bonds with the nascent C3b. Frank and colleagues developed a preparative procedure, based on activating C3 with trypsin in the presence of purified anti-sheep erythrocyte IgG, to generate purified C3b–IgG. They found that these complexes were far more effective in promoting phagocytosis of sensitized sheep erythrocytes by neutrophils compared to sensitization with IgG alone. They replicated earlier findings that *random placement* of C3b on the erythrocyte would enhance phagocytosis when the erythrocytes were also opsonized with IgG. However, their quantitative results clearly demonstrated that the C3b–IgG heterodimers *were far more effective* at promoting phagocytosis than was observed when the C3b and IgG were bound independently to the erythrocytes. In other words, the covalent C3b–IgG complex did appear to function as a superopsonin. Although the investigators attributed these effects as due to chelation of Fcγ receptors and CR1 (specific for C3b), it is certainly possible that FcγRIII and CR3 (more specific for iC3b) were engaged as well. In addition, *in vivo* C3b is rapidly decayed to iC3b,[108] and so it is quite likely that the iC3b–IgG heterocomplex will also act as a superopsonin.

Interaction between FcγR and Complement: Cancer Models

There is good evidence that FcγRIII effector functions are compromised in the absence of CR3 (Mac-1, CD11b/CD18). For example, patients with leukocyte adhesion deficiency lack β-2 integrins and have defects in FcγRIII-mediated cytotoxic functions.[109] In a syngeneic melanoma challenge model, van Spriel et al.[110] compared the efficacy of mAb TA99 (anti-gp75) in wild-type mice to Mac-1-knockout mice (lacking CR3). The protective action of mAb TA99, which killed targeted melanoma cells by promoting antibody-dependent cell-mediated cytotoxicity (ADCC) mediated by FcγRIII on effector cells, was reduced considerably in the Mac-1-knockout mice, even though the neutrophils of these mice appeared to have intact chemotactic function and antibody binding was preserved. Thus, the phenotype of the Mac-1 knockout mice appears to be manifested as a defect in Fcγ-mediated cytotoxicity. The downstream signaling mechanisms by which FcγRIII and CR3 interact are the subject of active investigations.[10]

The Taylor laboratory has reported that binding of CD20 mAbs rituximab (RTX) or ofatumumab (OFA) to B cells, and to primary chronic lymphocytic leukemia cells in particular, is accompanied by substantial complement activation and a very high level of C3b deposition, both *in vitro* and *in vivo*.[18,21,111] Moreover, there is a very good evidence for considerable co-localization of the deposited C3b with the bound human IgG mAbs.[18,111,112] This does not prove that the C3b formed a covalent bond with the CD20 mAb, but, based on the high degree of co-localization, it would certainly be anticipated that these opsonized cells would indeed be rapidly cleared to the liver based on the synergistic action of complement receptors (presumably CR1 and CR3) with Fcγ receptors, which would follow the patterns reported by the groups of Frank and Izui.

Di Gaetano et al.[14] found that complement activation was required for therapeutic activity of RTX in a syngeneic mouse model in which C57Bl/6 mice were challenged with EL4 cells that had been transfected with human CD20. Injection of RTX was quite effective at suppressing tumor growth, even when the tumors were allowed to grow for three days before RTX treatment; the therapeutic activity of RTX was lost in C1q-knockout mice, providing clear and unambiguous evidence for the key role of complement.

Additional evidence for such synergy was recently reported by Leusen's group.[113] They made use of the same syngeneic mouse model to evaluate cytotoxic effector mechanisms mediated by CD20 mAbs against varying doses of CD20-expresssing EL4 cells that were injected into the peritoneal cavities of mice. The mice received CD20 mAb therapy or PBS control at 18 hours, and 24 hours later the number of live tumor cells in the peritoneum was measured. At low tumor challenge burdens, complement was required to kill injected cells in mice that received either RTX or OFA; tumor killing was blocked if the mAb-treated mice were injected with cobra venom factor to compromise complement activity. On the other hand, effective mAb-mediated protection against the low tumor challenges was observed in both wild-type mice and in mice in which FcγR were either ablated or compromised in function by abrogation of their normal downstream signaling activities. However, at high tumor burdens, comparable experiments indicated that both complement and functional Fcγ receptors, as well as functional CR3 were required to promote CD20 mAb-mediated protection. The fact that no partial, statistically significant protection was observed when either Fcγ receptor functions or complement was compromised suggests that these separate mAb-mediated effector cell mechanisms function in a synergistic fashion. The investigators provided additional evidence based on *in vitro* assays of macrophage-mediated killing. In the presence of serum complement, macrophage-mediated killing of the EL4–CD20 cells that were opsonized by RTX or OFA was enhanced substantially. Moreover, when the macrophages were not included in the assay, complement-mediated killing alone was negligible. The investigators recognized that the most reasonable and likely explanation for this finding is that the deposited C3b fragments enhanced ADCC mediated by Fcγ receptors, in cooperation with both CR3 and CR4. The results of these investigations, as well as a previous report by these authors,[20] provide very powerful evidence that type I CD20 mAbs absolutely require effector functions to kill targeted cells in these mouse models; there is simply no reliable evidence that apoptosis is a valid mechanism of cytotoxicity of the mAb-opsonized target cells.[21,114] At the higher tumor burdens, the dose of mAb was adequate to saturate all CD20 sites, but more live tumor cells were observed after 24 hours. Thus, their work strongly suggests that even at high mAb doses the cytotoxic effector mechanisms mediated by mAbs can be saturated or exhausted at high tumor burdens, in agreement with the results of several clinical investigations of CD20 mAbs.[18,19,21,114]

In view of the reports of Di Gaetano, Leusen, and van Spriel and their colleagues, it would seem quite reasonable that part of the effect of complement seen in these cancer models is based on recruitment of CR3-positive effector cells to promote killing of tumor cells opsonized with mAbs and then covalently tagged with C3b/iC3b. As discussed in the next section, a role for C5a in upregulating Fcγ receptors would also likely contribute to tumor cell killing in these models.

Tomlinson's group has developed a novel approach to cancer therapy that makes explicit use of both complement and Fcγ receptors, and they have generated provocative first-order proof-of-concept evidence based on *in vitro* studies and mouse models.[115,116] They have constructed chimeric molecules in which the C3d binding domain of either human or mouse CR2 (respectively specific for human or mouse C3d) is linked to an Fcγ domain (either human IgG_1 or mouse IgG_{2a}) that is capable of fixing complement and binding to Fcγ receptors. The hypothesis is that cancer cells that are first targeted by complement-fixing mAbs in the presence of serum complement will be tagged with fragments of iC3b and C3d, and these tagged cells will therefore be susceptible to secondary attack by the chimeric constructs. This will lead to placement of additional Fcγ regions (human IgG_1 or mouse IgG_{2a}) on the cells, which should promote increased tumor cell killing by effector mechanisms. They demonstrated that binding of the CR2–Fc constructs to iC3b/C3d fragments on tumor cells that had been opsonized with specific mAbs caused increased C3b deposition, complement-mediated cytotoxicity, and ADCC mediated by effector cells. These constructs increased the therapeutic efficacy of complement-fixing mAbs in several murine cancer models. Translation of this paradigm to the clinic would likely be focused on FDA-approved mAbs that have been demonstrated to make use of complement in their therapeutic mechanisms, which would include OFA, RTX, and alemtuzumab.[15–18,21,111]

CROSS-TALK BETWEEN THE C5a RECEPTOR AND FcγR ON EFFECTOR CELLS

How Important is the MAC?

In view of the ability of the MAC of complement to lyse cells, it would seem reasonable to examine its role in inflammatory and autoimmune diseases, and in particular to ask what is the role of the MAC in the pathophysiology of tissue injury in such human diseases? On one hand, in paroxysmal nocturnal hemoglobinuria (PNH), the action of the MAC plays a primary and direct role in inducing cell destruction/tissue injury. In PNH, due to an acquired defect in the assembly of glycosylphosphatidylinositol-linked membrane proteins, a variable fraction of an individual's erythrocytes lack or have considerably reduced levels of complement control proteins CD55 and CD59, and these cells are quite vulnerable to alternative pathway-mediated deposition of C3b and then attack by the MAC.[11,117] As noted by Walport[118] in a comprehensive review, it was also thought that the MAC itself promoted tissue damage in autoimmune diseases, based on clinical investigations and animal models that correlated complement activation with tissue damage;[11] however, the issue is far more complex. As is discussed below, animal models based on the reverse Arthus reaction have been particularly useful in elucidating mechanisms of tissue damage mediated by immune complexes.[119] In these models, purified antibodies specific for an antigen (e.g., ovalbumin or bovine serum albumin) are injected into the target tissue (e.g., skin or lung) and the antigen is injected intravenously, thus allowing the formation of inflammatory immune complexes in the targeted site.

The elegant pioneering work of Ravetch and associates,[120–124] based on studies with knockout mice in which either Fcγ receptors or C3 were ablated, clearly demonstrated that tissue damage associated with immune complex diseases was almost exclusively induced by effector cells that expressed functional Fcγ receptors. Their findings, in several mouse models, including the reverse Arthus reaction and SLE, indicated that the effector cells recognized the IgG immune complex and generated a variety of inflammatory agents, all of which promoted local tissue destruction. One of the major implications of this work would be that the major tissue damage in most human diseases associated with immune complexes *is not directly induced by the MAC*. By inference, one might also conclude that *complement* does not play a role in the immunopathology of diseases associated with immune complexes.

The Importance of C5a

Reports from several groups, however, have now established that complement does play a key role in tissue damage in immune complex disease, and the mediators of damage are upstream of the MAC and are at the level of C5a. Gerard and coworkers[125] first reported that genetic deletion of the C5a receptor on effector cells led to substantial decreases in both inflammation and tissue damage in three different tissue-specific mouse models of the reverse Arthus reaction. Similarly, the Köhl laboratory showed that pharmacological targeting of the C5a receptor attenuated neutrophilic inflammation in skin, lung, and peritoneum in the reverse Arthus reaction.[126] Further, in a model of immune complex peritonitis, they showed for the first time that C5a receptor and activating Fcγ receptor signaling act in concert to promote the inflammatory response in immune complex disease.[127] Along the same lines, lessons learned from the K/BxN mouse model for arthritis have also been quite instructive.[128] In this model, mice develop antibodies specific for glucose-6-phosphate isomerase (GPI) and they have a severe arthritis, due to localization of GPI–anti-GPI immune complexes to the joints. The anti-GPI antibodies are indeed directly causative because transfer of serum or of purified IgG from these mice induces arthritis in recipients. This serum transfer model allowed identification of key mediators of arthritis, based on transfer of the pathogenic antibodies to a variety of genetically engineered recipient mice in which specific effector functions were missing. The results of these studies revealed that inflammation and tissue destruction are mediated by and require activation of the alternative pathway of complement, although the mechanism by which the immune complexes activate the alternative pathway has not been clearly delineated. In addition, tissue damage requires functional Fcγ receptors (disease is abrogated in γ-knockout mice) and requires both C5 and normal expression of the C5a receptor on effector cells.

The complement connection was firmly established by the comprehensive work of the Gessner and Köhl laboratories.[25,126,127,129–132] They described a critical role of C5a and the C5a receptor in mouse models of immune complex associated inflammation. These investigators examined several classic models of immune complex disease, and they were able to establish highly reproducible and general trends that described the mechanisms of tissue injury. Cooperation between the complement system and Fcγ receptors was most evident based on the key and virtually indispensable role of C5a and on the binding of C5a to the C5a receptor on effector cells which include neutrophils, mast cells, and macrophages. In numerous models they demonstrated that C5a played an important chemotactic role in attracting leukocytes to sites of inflammation. In addition, their experiments revealed a second role for C5a, that of promoting an inflammatory phenotype in monocyte/macrophages by upregulating activating receptors (FcγRI and FcγRIII) while downregulating the inhibitor receptor FcγRIIb. The C5a receptor is G-protein coupled, and chelation of this receptor by C5a leads to downstream signaling mediated though phosphatidyl-inositol 3-kinase-γ.[133–135] Moreover, the activating/inhibitor receptor ratio on effector cells is controlled at the transcriptional level. Binding of C5a to C5aR ultimately leads to transcriptional upregulation of activating Fcγ receptors FcγRI and III, the common γ-chain and simultaneous downregulation of inhibitory receptor FcγIIb.[131,132]

In a mouse model of lethal autoimmune hemolytic anemia, Gessner and colleagues[131] demonstrated that compared to wild-type mice, mice in which either Fcγ receptors or the C5a receptor were ablated were resistant to lethal infusion of 300 μg of an anti-erythrocyte IgG_{2a} (complement-fixing) mAb. As noted by Atkinson,[13] the fact that C3-knockout mice were still sensitive to the mAb infusion could not rule out a role for complement, because of cross-talk between the complement system, in particular C5a, and Fcγ receptors. Binding of immune-complexed IgG (in this case, IgG-opsonized erythrocytes) to macrophages induced direct synthesis of C5, followed by its cleavage to C5a. This reaction clearly defines a feed-forward model of inflammation, because the C5a can further increase the ratio of activating to inhibitory receptors on the macrophages, thus enhancing clearance of the IgG-opsonized erythrocytes. In close concordance with these findings, Huber-Lang et al.[136] examined lung tissue injury in a reverse Arthus mouse model and also reported that, due to immune complex deposition, C5 could be locally produced in C3 knockout mice and that cleavage of the secreted C5 to active C5a was apparently mediated by thrombin. The net effect is that substantial lung injury can be induced by immune complexes in the absence of C3 because of local production of C5 (presumably by macrophages) and its cleavage to C5a. Indeed, these investigators also found that anti-C5a antibodies reduced lung damage in the C3 knockout mice.

As stated above, complement activation, and in particular the generation of C5a, stimulates the cytotoxic action of effector cells in part by promoting rapid increases in the number of activating Fcγ receptors expressed on their surface. In view of the synergistic interactions documented for the CR3–FcγRIII pair, it is not surprising that C5a can also upregulate CR3, in a biologically meaningful context. Mollnes's group reported that addition of *Escherichia coli* to whole human blood (anti-coagulated with lepirudin) promoted complement activation; they noted that both IgG and IgM antibodies specific for *E. coli* were present in the serum of the blood donors, but apparently complement activation was mediated most effectively by the alternative pathway. They found that CR3 was upregulated on granulocytes, and based on use of blocking antibodies and specific antagonists, they were able to demonstrate that the upregulation of CR3 was mediated by C5a. Thus, it is reasonable to anticipate that an *in vivo* stimulus or danger signal that generates C5a would induce parallel increases in CR3 and activating Fcγ receptors that synergize in the elimination of C3 fragment/IgG-opsonized substrates.[137]

More recently, the Köhl laboratory found that the cross-talk between C5a receptor and Fcγ receptors is even more complex. In several *in vitro* and *in vivo* experiments, they showed that IgG_1 immune complexes can suppress C5aR-mediated effector functions by an FcγRIIb and Dectin-1-dependent pathway.[28] Importantly, this effect depends on Fc–glycan galactosylation of the IgG_1 molecules. Only highly galactosylated IgG_1 immune complexes have the ability to link FcγRIIb and the C-type lectin receptor Dectin-1, which is the prerequisite for induction of the signaling pathway that suppresses C5a-mediated effector functions. The importance of this inhibitory feedback loop between IgG_1–FcγRIIb–Dectin-1 and the C5aR was observed in an experimental model of epidermolysis bullosa acquisita, an autoimmune skin-blistering disease. Administration of highly galactosylated IgG_1 immune complexes significantly suppressed development of inflammatory skin lesions, whereas low galactosylated IgG immune complexes had no protective effect. Thus, complement and Fcγ receptors are intertwined by a complex regulatory network that is likely to affect not only the inflammatory response in autoimmunity but also in allergy, cancer, and infection.

Immune Complexes, C5a, and SLE

In diseases such as SLE, chronic generation of immune complexes followed by complement activation will have consequences that will impact on Fcγ receptors.[138] On one hand, the production of C5a would be expected to promote increases in Fcγ receptors on effector cells, including monocyte/macrophages. In 1984, Frank's group first reported that monocyte Fcγ receptors are increased in SLE, and soon thereafter they demonstrated that C5a indeed induced rapid upregulation of monocyte Fcγ receptor activity based on rosetting assays with IgG-opsonized sheep erythrocytes.[139,140] On the other hand, *processing* of immune complexes by these cells involves phagocytosis/internalization, and this can lead to internalization of the Fcγ receptors and exhaustion of effector function. In fact, both Salmon et al.[141] and Fries et al.[139] reported what at the time (1984) appeared to be a contradiction: Both groups found that Fcγ receptors on monocytes appeared to be *increased* in SLE, and the increases tended to correlate with disease activity (more immune complexes). However, assays of Fcγ receptor *functions* gave opposite results. That is, *in vivo* clearance of IgG-opsonized erythrocytes was reduced in SLE patients with active disease, and similarly *in vitro* phagocytosis of IgG-opsonized erythrocytes was decreased in the same patients who appeared to have increased numbers of Fcγ receptors. As first noted by Kavai, resolution of these apparent contradictions had to await the identification and characterization of the different classes of Fcγ receptors that are expressed on effector cells.[138] There is now very good evidence that FcγRIIa and FcγRIII play the most important roles in immune complex processing and phagocytosis, and during normal immune complex processing these receptors can be internalized and degraded and possibly released into the bloodstream in their soluble forms as well.[138,142–145] FcγRI plays less of a role in immune complex processing, and in addition it is rapidly recycled to the cell surface when it does internalize certain substrates.[146,147] Thus, in SLE, simple IgG binding activity by monocytes would be increased due to C5a-mediated upregulation of activating FcγRI, but more complex functional activity (phagocytosis, clearance of IgG-opsonized erythrocytes) would be reduced due to chronic immune complex processing and attendant internalization of FcγRIIa and FcγRIII.

Quite recently these findings have been validated to some extent in mouse models of SLE. Shlomchik and colleagues[148] noted the decreased efficacy of RTX-mediated clearance of B cells in SLE and suggested that the effect could be related to defects in Fcγ receptor-mediated processing; they reported that elimination of human CD20+ B cells by CD20 mAbs was markedly impaired in several SLE mouse models. Moreover, they were able to show that transfer of either serum or purified IgG from the SLE mice (MRL.Fas^{lpr}) to wild-type mice also transferred resistance to CD20 mAb-mediated B-cell depletion. Complement activation is quite pronounced in SLE mice, and it would be interesting to determine their profile of Fcγ receptor expression on monocyte/macrophages. That is, due to generation of C5a, upregulation of FcγRI but downregulation of FcγRIIb would be predicted; however, FcγRIII would be downregulated due to chronic immune complex processing.

New Animal Models Continue to Demonstrate Synergy

Tsuboi et al.[27] revisited the K/BxN mouse serum-transfer arthritis model and demonstrated that there also appears to be cross-talk between FcγRIIa and C5aR. Mice that had the murine γ-chain knocked out were engineered to express the human FcγRIIa on their neutrophils in order to specifically examine the role of this receptor in the K/BxN serum transfer model. Expression of the human FcγRIIa receptor alone on neutrophils was sufficient to restore arthritis in the γ-knockout mice. They also found that treatment of these hFcγRIIa^{+} γ-knockout mice with either cobra venom factor, to deplete complement, or with C5a receptor antagonists substantially attenuated arthritis in the serum transfer model. This result reinforces the key role of the C5a/C5a receptor in upregulating Fcγ receptor-mediated cytotoxicity. However, in this case, the investigators were able to eliminate, as a mechanism, changes in the ratio of activating to inhibitory receptors on the cells. Instead, they found, based on *in vitro* experiments, that chelation of C5a by the C5a receptor on the neutrophils could dramatically increase both phagocytosis of IgG-opsonized sheep erythrocytes and production of reactive oxygen species upon cross-linking of FcγRIIa. The authors recognized that these findings suggest a level of control in FcγR-expressing cells that is downstream of simple IgG binding, and it is likely that additional studies will be instructive as to the details of mechanism.

Banda and colleagues[149–152] have recently evaluated mechanisms of tissue damage in a mouse model in which intraperitoneal injection of a cocktail of collagen-specific mAbs (followed three days later by an LPS injection) induced severe inflammatory arthritis in less than two weeks. The underlying mechanisms were explored in some detail by determining clinical disease activity in a variety of genetically engineered and otherwise matched C57BL/6 mice. They reported that, in common with the observations in several other already cited animal models and inflammatory diseases associated with immune complexes, activation of the alternative pathway of complement was required in order to mediate tissue damage. Moreover, based on numerous gene-targeting investigations, they found that when complement was activated, the single most important downstream mediator of inflammation appeared to be the C5aR on effector cells. That is, complement activation was needed to generate C5a, and it was the interaction of the C5a-activated effector cells with immune complexes associated with collagen in the joints that led to tissue damage. Although the investigators did not explicitly examine the role of Fcγ receptors in their model, based on several similar mouse models it would indeed be expected that disease activity would be abrogated in FcγR knockout mice.[121–124,128] The investigations also revealed cross-talk between the lectin pathway and the alternative pathway. They found that mannose-binding lectin-associated serine protease-1 (MASP-1) plays an essential role in disease activity because it is required to generate *active* factor D from its zymogen precursor pro-factor D. That is, mice lacking MASP-1/3 have a phenotype quite similar to that of mice lacking factor D, thus precluding activation of the alternative pathway and therefore severely suppressing disease activity, even in the presence of the injected arthritis-promoting antibodies. Finally, deposition of C3 fragments and IgG in the joints was reduced in mice deficient in C6 as well as in mice lacking either the C3a receptor or C5a receptor. These results suggested that perhaps the high level of inflammation mediated by full functioning of these receptors, as well inflammation mediated by the terminal pathway of complement, may additionally increase tissue damage by a feedback loop that amplifies upstream pathology associated with complement activation and IgG deposition.

CONCLUDING REMARKS

Of Mice and Men: An Important Caveat

There must be an implicit and cautionary note in the interpretation and possible over-generalization of the results in murine disease models (e.g., specific knockouts, use of neutralizing mAbs). It will be important, wherever possible, to test for clear and unambiguous validation of murine models in human diseases. Ultimately the (sometimes unstated) goal of this research is to use the results of these investigations to develop new and more effective therapies for human diseases such as SLE, RA, or cancer. Several of the key demonstrations of synergy between the complement system and Fcγ receptors that we have cited were made in human systems. Nelson's observations of immune adherence were made based on measurements in a human system, and he and several other investigators extended this work to monkey models.[29,30,34,35] Although Frank and colleagues first examined patterns of erythrocyte clearance in animal models, they were able to translate their approach to investigations of mononuclear phagocytic system function by studying the clearance of IgG-opsonized erythrocytes in humans.[96–98,139] Frank's group also reported that human C5a rapidly increased expression of FcγR on human neutrophils and monocytes long before it was even recognized that multiple different classes of Fcγ receptors existed.[140] Mollnes' group found, in a human whole blood model, that C5a could also upregulate CR3, a partner of FcγRIII.[137] The work of Ehlenberger and Nussenzweig, which documented cooperation between C3b and IgG in promoting enhanced phagocytosis, was also based on studies with human effector cells.[22] The approach of the Tomlinson group, which envisions use of CR2-Fc chimeric molecules to enhance mAb-based cancer immunotherapy, is noteworthy. They have developed appropriate reagents to allow for parallel testing of their paradigm in both murine models and in human systems.[115,116]

Lessons Learned and Future Directions

The clear demonstrations of synergy between Fcγ receptor functions and the complement system add to our understanding of immunologic defense. Indeed, a danger signal or threat that alerts one of the systems leads to cross-communication with the other, thus conspiring to rapidly up-regulate appropriate effector mechanisms in both systems that can then cooperate in eliminating the threat. This synergy gives approximately equal credit to both systems, as well as to the investigators who may have focused their work in only one of these areas of research.[13] It is also not at all surprising that inappropriate signals (autoantibodies, immune complexes deposited in tissue) will promote activation and cooperation of the complement system and Fcγ receptor functions in mediating tissue pathology. Perhaps the greatest challenge for workers in these fields is to use the lessons learned from this research to devise specific therapeutic approaches in human disease that appropriately regulate these two powerful effector systems. That is, interventions should concentrate on augmenting and enhancing inflammation and cytotxoicity in infectious diseases and in cancer. However, in autoimmune diseases, efforts should be focused in the opposite direction.

ABBREVIATIONS

ADCC, antibody-dependent cell-mediated cytoxicity; C3, complement component 3; C3b, iC3b, C3d, fragments of C3; C5aR, CD88, the C5a receptor; CR1, CD35, complement receptor 1, specific for C3b; CR2, CD21, complement receptor 2, specific for C3d; CR3, CD11b/CD18, complement receptor 3, specific for iC3b; CR4, CD11c/CD18, specific for iC3b; FDC, follicular dendritic cell; GPI, glucose-6-phosphate isomerase; MAC, membrane attack complex; OFA, ofatumumab; PNH, paroxysmal nocturnal hemoglobinuria; RTX, rituximab; SLE, systemic lupus erythematosus.

References

1. Walport MJ. Complement. *N Engl J Med* 2001;**344**:1058–66.
2. Degn SE, Thiel S, Jensenius JC. New perspectives on mannan-binding lectin-mediated complement activation. *Immunobiology* 2007;**212**:301–11.
3. Gros P, Milder FJ, Janssen BJ. Complement driven by conformational changes. *Nat Rev Immunol* 2008;**8**:48–58.
4. Ricklin D, Hajishengallis G, Yang K, Lambris JD. Complement: a key system for immune surveillance and homeostasis. *Nat Immunol* 2010;**11**:785–97.
5. Wagner E, Frank MM. Therapeutic potential of complement modulation. *Nat Rev Drug Disc* 2010;**9**:43–56.
6. Dunkelberger JR, Song WC. Complement and its role in innate and adaptive immune responses. *Cell Res* 2010;**20**:34–50.
7. Ehrnthaller C, Ignatius A, Gebhard F, Huber-Lang M. New insights of an old defense system: structure, function, and clinical relevance of the complement system. *Mol Med* 2011;**17**:317–29.
8. Fries LF, Siwik SA, Malbran A, Frank MM. Phagocytosis of target particles bearing C3b-IgG covalent complexes by human monocytes and polymorphonuclear leukocytes. *Immunology* 1987;**62**:45–51.
9. Brown EJ, Joiner KA, Cole RM, Berger M. Localization of complement component 3 on *Streptococcus pneumoniae*: anti-capsular antibody causes complement deposition on the pneumococcal capsule. *Infect Immun* 1983;**39**:403–9.
10. Huang ZY, Hunter S, Chien P, et al. Interaction of two phagocytic host defense systems: Fcγ receptors and complement receptor 3. *J Biol Chem* 2011;**286**:160–8.
11. Parker C. Eculizumab for paroxysmal nocturnal haemoglobinuria. *Lancet* 2009;**373**:759–67.
12. Botto M, Kirschfink M, Macor P, et al. Complement in human diseases: lessons from complement deficiencies. *Mol Immunol* 2009;**46**:2774–83.
13. Atkinson JP. C5a and Fcγ receptors: a mutual admiration society. *J Clin Invest* 2006;**116**:304–6.
14. Di Gaetano N, Cittera E, Nota R, et al. Complement activation determines the therapeutic activity of Rituximab *in vivo*. *J Immunol* 2003;**171**:1581–7.
15. Manches O, Lui G, Chaperot L, et al. *In vitro* mechanisms of action of rituximab on primary non-Hodgkin's lymphomas. *Blood* 2003;**101**:949–54.
16. Zent CS, Chen JB, Kurten RC, et al. Alemtuzumab (CAMPATH 1H) does not kill chronic lymphocytic leukemia cells in serum free medium. *Leuk Res* 2004;**28**:495–507.
17. Teeling JL, French RR, Cragg MS, et al. Characterization of new human CD20 monoclonal antibodies with potent cytolytic activity against non-Hodgkin's lymphomas. *Blood* 2004;**104**:1793–800.
18. Kennedy AD, Beum PV, Solga MD, et al. Rituximab infusion promotes rapid complement depletion and acute CD20 loss in chronic lymphocytic leukemia. *J Immunol* 2004;**172**:3280–8.
19. Berdeja JG, Hess A, Lucas DM, et al. Systemic interleukin-2 and adoptive transfer of lymphokine-activated killer cells improves antibody-dependent cellular cytotoxicity in patients with relapsed B-cell lymphoma treated with rituximab. *Clin Cancer Res* 2007;**13**:2392–9.
20. de Haij S, Jansen JHM, Boross P, et al. *In vivo* cytotoxicity of type I CD20 antibodies critically depends on Fc receptor ITAM signaling. *Cancer Res* 2010;**70**:3209–17.
21. Beurskens FJ, Lindorfer MA, Farooqui M, et al. Exhaustion of cytotoxic effector systems may limit monoclonal antibody-based immunotherapy in cancer patients. *J Immunol* 2012;**188**:3532–41.
22. Ehlenberger AG, Nussenzweig V. The role of membrane receptors for C3b and C3d in phagocytosis. *J Exp Med* 1977;**145**:357–70.
23. Frank MM, Basta M, Fries LF. The effects of intravenous immune globulin on complement-dependent immune damage of cells and tissues. *Clin Immunol Immunopathol* 1992;**62**:S82–6.

24. Solomon S, Kassahn D, Illges H. The role of the complement and the FcγR system in the pathogenesis of arthritis. *Arthritis Res* 2005;**7**:129–35.
25. Schmidt RE, Gessner JE. Fc receptors and their interaction with complement in autoimmunity. *Immunol Lett* 2005;**100**:56–67.
26. Holers VM. The spectrum of complement alternative pathway-mediated diseases. *Immunol Rev* 2008;**223**:300–16.
27. Tsuboi N, Ernandez T, Li X, et al. Regulation of human neutrophil Fcγ receptor IIa by C5a receptor promotes inflammatory arthritis in mice. *Arthritis Rheum* 2011;**63**:467–78.
28. Karsten CM, Pandey MK, Figge J, et al. Galactosylated IgG_1 links FcγRIIB and Dectin-1 to block complement-mediated inflammation. *Nat Med* 2012;**18**:1401–6.
29. Nelson RA. The immune-adherence phenomenon. An immunologically specific reaction between microorganisms and erythrocytes leading to enhanced phagocytosis. *Science* 1953;**118**:733–7.
30. Nelson RA. The immune-adherence phenomenon. A hypothetical role of erythrocytes in defense against bacteria and viruses. *Proc Royal Soc Med* 1955;**49**:55–8.
31. Robineaux R, Pinet J. An *in vitro* study of some mechanisms of antigen uptake by cells. In: Woldstenholme GEW, editor. *Ciba foundation symposium on cellular aspects of immunity*. Boston, MA: Little, Brown; 1960. p. 5–43.
32. Arnaout MA, Melamed J, Tack BF, Colten HR. Characterization of the human complement (C3b) receptor with a fluid phase C3b dimer. *J Immunol* 1981;**127**:1348–54.
33. Ahearn JM, Fearon DT. Structure and function of the complement receptors, CR1 (CD35) and CR2 (CD21). *Adv Immunol* 1989;**46**:183–217.
34. Lindorfer MA, Hahn CS, Foley PL, Taylor RP. Heteropolymer-mediated clearance of immune complexes via erythrocyte CR1: mechanisms and applications. *Immunol Rev* 2001;**183**:10–24.
35. Cornacoff JB, Hebert LA, Smead WL, et al. Primate erythrocyte-immune complex-clearing mechanism. *J Clin Invest* 1983;**71**:236–47.
36. Li J, Wang JP, Ghiran I, et al. Complement receptor 1 expression on mouse erythrocytes mediates clearance of *Streptococcus pneumoniae* by immune adherence. *Infect Immun* 2010;**78**:3129–35.
37. Hebert LA, Cosio FG. The erythrocyte–immune complex–glomerulonephritis connection in man. *Kidney Int* 1987;**31**:877–85.
38. Schifferli JA, Taylor RP. Physiological and pathological aspects of circulating immune complexes. *Kidney Int* 1989;**35**:993–1003.
39. Medof ME, Iida K, Mold C, Nussenzweig V. Unique role of the complement receptor CR1 in the degradation of C3b associated with immune complexes. *J Exp Med* 1982;**156**:1739–54.
40. Nielsen CH, Matthiesen SH, Lyng I, Leslie RG. The role of complement receptor type 1 (CR1, CD35) in determining the cellular distribution of opsonized immune complexes between whole blood cells: kinetic analysis of the buffering capacity of erythrocytes. *Immunology* 1997;**90**:129–37.
41. Kimberly RP, Edberg JC, Merriam LT, et al. *In vivo* handling of soluble complement fixing Ab/dsDNA immune complexes in chimpanzees. *J Clin Invest* 1989;**84**:962–70.
42. Edberg JC, Kimberly RP, Taylor RP. Functional characterization of non-human primate erythrocyte immune adherence receptors: implications for the uptake of immune complexes by the cells of the mononuclear phagocytic system. *Eur J Immunol* 1992;**22**:1333–9.
43. Fearon DT. Regulation of the amplification C3 convertase of human complement by an inhibitory protein isolated from human erythrocyte membrane. *Proc Natl Acad Sci USA* 1979;**76**:5867–71.
44. Fearon DT. Identification of the membrane glycoprotein that is the C3b receptor of the human erythrocyte, polymorphonuclear leukocyte, B lymphocyte, and monocyte. *J Exp Med* 1980;**152**:20–30.
45. Miyakawa Y, Yamada A, Kosaka K, et al. Defective immune-adherence (C3b) receptor on erythrocytes from patients with systemic lupus erythematosus. *Lancet* 1981;**2**:493–7.
46. Iida K, Mornaghi R, Nussenzweig V. Complement receptor (CR1) deficiency in erythrocytes from patients with systemic lupus erythematosus. *J Exp Med* 1982;**155**:1427–38.
47. Taylor RP, Horgan C, Buschbacher R, et al. Decreased complement mediated binding of antibody/3H-dsDNA immune complexes to the red blood cells of patients with systemic lupus erythematosus, rheumatoid arthritis, and hematologic malignancies. *Arthritis Rheum* 1983;**26**:736–44.
48. Ross GD, Yount WJ, Walport MJ, et al. Disease-associated loss of erythrocyte complement receptors (CR1, C3b receptors) in patients with systemic lupus erythematosus and other diseases involving autoantibodies and/or complement activation. *J Immunol* 1985;**135**:2005–14.
49. Tausk FA, McCutchan A, Spechko P, Schreiber RD, Gigli I. Altered erythrocyte C3b receptor expression, immune complexes, and complement activation in homosexual men: varying risk groups for acquired immune deficiency syndrome. *J Clin Invest* 1986;**78**:977–82.
50. Ripoche J, Sim RB. Loss of complement receptor type 1 (CR1) on ageing of erythrocytes: studies of proteolytic release of the receptor. *Biochem J* 1986;**235**:815–21.

51. Pascual M, Danielsson C, Steiger G, Schifferli JA. Proteolytic cleavage of CR1 on human erythrocytes *in vivo*: evidence for enhanced cleavage in AIDS. *Eur J Immunol* 1994;**24**:702–8.
52. Sadallah S, Hess C, Miot S, et al. Elastase and metalloproteinase activities regulate soluble complement receptor 1 release. *Eur J Immunol* 1999;**29**:3754–61.
53. Jouvin MH, Rozenbaum W, Russo R, Kazatchkine MD. Decreased expression of the C3b/C4b complement receptor (CR1) in AIDS and AIDS-related syndromes correlates with clinical subpopulations of patients with HIV infection. *AIDS* 1987;**1**:89–94.
54. Currie MS, Vala M, Pisetsky DS, et al. Correlation between erythrocyte CR1 reduction and other blood proteinase markers in patients with malignant and inflammatory disorders. *Blood* 1990;**75**:1699–704.
55. Taylor RP, Sutherland WM, Martin EN, et al. Bispecific monoclonal antibody complexes bound to primate erythrocyte CR1 facilitate virus clearance in a monkey model. *J Immunol* 1997;**158**:842–50.
56. Taylor RP, Martin EN, Reinagel ML, et al. Bispecific monoclonal antibody complexes facilitate erythrocyte binding and liver clearance of a prototype particulate pathogen in a monkey model. *J Immunol* 1997;**159**:4035–44.
57. Craig ML, Reinagel ML, Martin EN, et al. Infusion of bispecific monoclonal antibody complexes into monkeys provides immunologic protection against later challenge with a model pathogen. *Clin Immunol* 1999;**92**:170–80.
58. Joly E, Hudrisier D. What is trogocytosis and what is its purpose?. *Nat Immunol* 2003;**4**:815.
59. Hudrisier D, Aucher A, Puaux AL, Bordier C, Joly E. Capture of target cell membrane components via trogocytosis is triggered by a selected set of surface molecules on T or B cells. *J Immunol* 2007;**178**:3637–47.
60. Daubeuf S, Lindorfer MA, Taylor RP, Joly E, Hudrisier D. The direction of plasma membrane exchange between lymphocytes and accessory cells by trogocytosis is influenced by the nature of the accessory cell. *J Immunol* 2010;**184**:1897–908.
61. Zimring JC, Cadwell CM, Spitalnik SL. Antigen loss from antibody-coated red blood cells. *Transfusion Med Rev* 2009;**23**:189–204.
62. Beum PV, Kennedy AD, Williams ME, Lindorfer MA, Taylor RP. The shaving reaction: rituximab/CD20 complexes are removed from mantle cell lymphoma and chronic lymphocytic leukemia cells by THP-1 monocytes. *J Immunol* 2006;**176**:2600–9.
63. Beum PV, Peek EM, Lindorfer MA, et al. Loss of CD20 and bound CD20 antibody from opsonized B cells occurs more rapidly because of trogocytosis mediated by Fc receptor-expressing effector cells than direct internalization by the B cells. *J Immunol* 2011;**187**:3438–47.
64. Wilson JG, Jack RM, Wong WW, Schur PH, Fearon DT. Autoantibody to the C3b/C4b receptor and absence of this receptor from erythrocytes of a patient with systemic lupus erythematosus. *J Clin Invest* 1985;**76**:182–90.
65. Dempsey PW, Allison ME, Akkaraju S, Goodnow CC, Fearon DT. C3d of complement as a molecular adjuvant: bridging innate and acquired immunity. *Science* 1996;**271**:348–50.
66. Henson SE, Smith D, Boackle SA, Holers VM, Karp DR. Generation of recombinant human C3dg tetramers for the analysis of CD21 binding and function. *J Immunol Methods* 2001;**258**:97–109.
67. Lindorfer MA, Jinivizian HB, Foley PL, et al. The B cell complement receptor 2 transfer reaction. *J Immunol* 2003;**170**:3671–8.
68. Holers VM, Kulik L. Complement receptor 2, natural antibodies and innate immunity: inter-relationships in B cell selection and activation. *Mol Immunol* 2007;**44**:64–72.
69. Whipple EC, Shanahan RS, Ditto AH, Taylor RP, Lindorfer MA. Analyses of the *in vivo* trafficking of stoichiometric doses of an anti-complement receptor 1/2 monoclonal antibody infused intravenously in mice. *J Immunol* 2004;**173**:2297–306.
70. Whipple EC, Ditto AH, Shanahan RS, et al. Low doses of antigen coupled to anti-CR2 mAbs induce rapid and enduring IgG immune responses in mice and in cynomolgus monkeys. *Mol Immunol* 2007;**44**:377–88.
71. Westermann J, Pabst R. Lymphocyte subsets in the blood: a diagnostic window on the lymphoid system. *Immunol Today* 1990;**11**:406–10.
72. Yazawa N, Hamaguchi Y, Poe JC, Tedder TF. Immunotherapy using unconjugated CD19 monoclonal antibodies in animal models for B lymphocyte malignancies and autoimmune disease. *Proc Natl Acad Sci USA* 2005;**102**:15178–83.
73. Brown JC, Harris G, Papamichail M, Sljivic VS, Holborow EJ. The localization of aggregated human γ-globulin in the spleens of normal mice. *Immunology* 1973;**24**:955–68.
74. Cinamon G, Zachariah MA, Lam OM, Foss Jr FW, Cyster JG. Follicular shuttling of marginal zone B cells facilitates antigen transport. *Nat Immunol* 2008;**9**:54–62.
75. Gonzalez SF, Degn SE, Pitcher LA, et al. Trafficking of B cell antigen in lymph nodes. *Ann Rev Immunol* 2011;**29**:215–33.
76. Humphrey JH, Grennan D, Sundaram V. The origin of follicular dendritic cells in the mouse and the mechanism of trapping of immune complexes on them. *Eur J Immunol* 1984;**14**:859–64.
77. Heyman B. Regulation of antibody responses via antibodies, complement, and Fc receptors. *Ann Rev Immunol* 2000;**18**:709–37.

78. Cyster JG. B cell follicles and antigen encounters of the third kind. *Nat Immunol* 2010;**11**:989–96.
79. Phan TG, Grigorova I, Okada T, Cyster JG. Subcapsular encounter and complement-dependent transport of immune complexes by lymph node B cells. *Nat Immunol* 2007;**8**:992–1000.
80. Montefiori DC. Role of complement and Fc receptors in the pathogenesis of HIV-1 infection. *Springer Sem Immunopathol* 1997;**18**:371–90.
81. Kacani L, Prodinger WM, Sprinzl GM, et al. Detachment of human immunodeficiency virus type 1 from germinal centers by blocking complement receptor type 2. *J Virol* 2000;**74**:7997–8002.
82. Subbramanian RA, Xu J, Toma E, et al. Comparison of human immunodeficiency virus (HIV)-specific infection-enhancing and -inhibiting antibodies in AIDS patients. *J Clin Microbiol* 2002;**40**:2141–6.
83. Horakova E, Gasser O, Sadallah S, et al. Complement mediates the binding of HIV to erythrocytes. *J Immunol* 2004;**173**:4236–41.
84. Huber G, Banki Z, Lengauer S, Stoiber H. Emerging role for complement in HIV infection. *Curr Opin HIV AIDS* 2011;**6**:419–26.
85. Willey S, Aasa-Chapman MM, O'Farrell S, et al. Extensive complement-dependent enhancement of HIV-1 by autologous non-neutralising antibodies at early stages of infection. *Retrovirology* 2011;**8**:16.
86. Hess C, Klimkait T, Schlapbach L, et al. Association of a pool of HIV-1 with erthrocytes *in vivo*: cohort study. *Lancet* 2002;**359**:2230–4.
87. Stoiber H. Complement, Fc receptors and antibodies: a Trojan horse in HIV infection?. *Curr Opin HIV AIDS* 2009;**4**:394–9.
88. Banki Z, Wilflingseder D, Ammann CG, et al. Factor I-mediated processing of complement fragments on HIV immune complexes targets HIV to CR2-expressing B cells and facilitates B cell-mediated transmission of opsonized HIV to T cells. *J Immunol* 2006;**177**:3469–76.
89. Moir S, Malaspina A, Li Y, et al. B cells of HIV-1-infected patients bind virions through CD21–complement interactions and transmit infectious virus to activated T cells. *J Exp Med* 2000;**192**:637–46.
90. Ho J, Moir S, Kulik L, et al. Role for CD21 in the establishment of an extracellular HIV reservoir in lymphoid tissues. *J Immunol* 2007;**178**:6968–74.
91. Thieblemont N, Haeffner-Cavaillon N, Ledur A, et al. CR1 (CD35) and CR3 (CD11b/CD18) mediate infection of human monocytes and monocytic cell lines with complement-opsonized HIV independently of CD4. *Clin Exp Immunol* 1993;**92**:106–13.
92. Bajtay Z, Speth C, Erdei A, Dierich MP. Productive HIV-1 infection of dendritic cells via complement receptor type 3 (CR3, CD11b/CD18). *J Immunol* 2004;**173**:4775–8.
93. Bouhlal H, Chomont N, Requena M, et al. Opsonization of HIV with complement enhances infection of dendritic cells and viral transfer to CD4 T cells in a CR3 and DC-SIGN-dependent manner. *J Immunol* 2007;**178**:1086–95.
94. Joling P, Bakker LJ, Van Strijp JAG, et al. Binding of human immunodeficiency virus type-1 to follicular dendritic cells *in vitro* is complement dependent. *J Immunol* 1993;**150**:1065–73.
95. Bergtold A, Desai DD, Gavhane A, Clynes R. Cell surface recycling of internalized antigen permits dendritic cell priming of B cells. *Immunity* 2005;**23**:503–14.
96. Schreiber AD, Frank MM. Role of antibody and complement in the immune clearance and destruction of erythrocytes. I. *In vivo* effects of IgG and IgM complement fixing sites. *J Clin Invest* 1972;**51**:575–82.
97. Schreiber AD, Frank MM. Role of antibody and complement in the immune clearance and destruction of erythrocytes. II. Molecular nature of IgG and IgM complement-fixing sites and effects of their interaction with serum. *J Clin Invest* 1972;**51**:583–9.
98. Atkinson JP, Frank MM. Studies on the *in vivo* effects of antibody. Interaction of IgM antibody and complement in the immune clearance and destruction of erythrocytes in man. *J Clin Invest* 1974;**54**:339–48.
99. Atkinson JP, Frank MM. Complement-independent clearance of IgG-sensitized erythrocytes: inhibition by cortisone. *Blood* 1974;**44**:629–37.
100. Atkinson JP, Schreiber AD, Frank MM. Effects of corticosteroids and splenectomy on the immune clearance and destruction of erythrocytes. *J Clin Invest* 1973;**52**:1509–17.
101. Hinglais N, Kazatchkine MD, Mandet C, Appay M, Bariety J. Human liver Kupffer cells express CR1, CR3, and CR4 complement receptor antigens. *Lab Invest* 1989;**61**:509–14.
102. da Silveira SA, Kikuchi S, Fossati-Jimack L, et al. Complement activation selectively potentiates the pathogenicity of the IgG2b and IgG3 isotypes of a high affinity anti-erythrocyte autoantibody. *J Exp Med* 2002;**195**:665–72.
103. Newman SL, Johnson Jr. RB. Role of binding through C3b and IgG in polymorphonuclear neutrophil function: studies with trypsin-generated C3b. *J Immunol* 1979;**123**:1839–46.
104. Brown EJ, Bohnsack JF, Gresham HD. Mechanism of inhibition of immunoglobulin G-mediated phagocytosis by monoclonal antibodies that recognize the Mac-1 antigen. *J Clin Invest* 1988;**81**:365–75.
105. Zhou M, Todd RF, van de Winkel JGJ, Petty HR. Cocapping of the leukoadhesin molecules complement receptor type 3 and lymphocyte function-associated antigen-1 with Fcγ Receptor III on human neutrophils. *J Immunol* 1993;**150**:3030–41.

106. Zhou MJ, Brown EJ. CR3 (Mac-1, alpha M beta 2, CD11b/CD18) and FcγRIII cooperate in generation of a neutrophil respiratory burst: requirement for FcγRIII and tyrosine phosphorylation. *J Cell Biol* 1994;**125**:1407–16.
107. Bouhlal H, Galon J, Kazatchkine M, et al. Soluble CD16 inhibits CR3(CD11b/CD18)-mediated infection of monocytes/macrophages by opsonized primary R5 HIV-1. *J Immunol* 2000;**166**:3377–83.
108. Ross GD, Vetvicka V, Yan J, Xia Y, Vetvickova J. Therapeutic intervention with complement and β-glucan in cancer. *Immunopharmacology* 1999;**42**:61–74.
109. van Spriel AB, Leusen JHW, van Egmond M, et al. Mac-1 (CD11b/CD18) is essential for Fc receptor mediated neutrophil cytotoxicity and immunologic synapse formation. *Blood* 2001;**97**:2478–86.
110. van Spriel AB, van Ojik HH, Bakker A, Jansen MJH, van de Winkel JGJ. Mac-1 (CD11b/CD18) is crucial for effective Fc receptor-mediated immunity to melanoma. *Blood* 2003;**101**:253–8.
111. Beum PV, Lindorfer MA, Beurskens F, et al. Complement activation on B lymphocytes opsonized with rituximab or ofatumumab produces substantial changes in membrane structure preceding cell lysis. *J Immunol* 2008;**181**:822–32.
112. Beum PV, Lindorfer MA, Hall BE, et al. Quantitative analysis of protein co-localization on B cells opsonized with rituximab and complement using the ImageStream multispectral imaging flow cytometer. *J Immunol Methods* 2006;**317**:90–9.
113. Boross P, Jansen JHM, de Haij S, et al. The *in vivo* mechanism of action of CD20 monoclonal antibodies depends on local tumor burden. *Haematologica* 2011;**96**:1822–30.
114. Lindorfer MA, Wiestner A, Zent CS, Taylor RP. Monoclonal antibody (mAb)-based cancer therapy: is it time to reevaluate dosing strategies? *OncoImmunology* 2012.
115. Imai M, Ohta R, Varela JC, Song H, Tomlinson S. Enhancement of antibody-dependent mechanisms of tumor cell lysis by a targeted activator of complement. *Canc Res* 2007;**67**:9535–41.
116. Elvington M, Huan Y, Morgan BP, et al. A targeted complement-dependent strategy to improve the outcome of mAb therapy, and characterization in a murine model of metastatic cancer. *Blood* 2012.
117. Parker CJ. The pathophysiology of paroxysmal nocturnal hemoglobinuria. *Exp Hematol* 2007;**35**:523–33.
118. Walport MJ. Complement and systemic lupus erythematosus. *Arthritis Res* 2002;**4**:S279–93.
119. Köhl J, Gessner JE. On the role of complement and Fcγ-receptors in the Arthus reaction. *Mol Immunol* 1999;**36**:893–903.
120. Sylvestre DL, Ravetch JV. Fc receptors initiate the Arthus reaction: redefining the inflammatory cascade. *Science* 1994;**265**:1095–8.
121. Clynes R, Dumitru C, Ravetch JV. Uncoupling of immune complex formation and kidney damage in autoimmune glomerulonephritis. *Science* 1998;**279**:1052–4.
122. Clynes R, Maizes JS, Guinamard R, et al. Modulation of immune complex-induced inflammation *in vivo* by the coordinate expression of activation and inhibitory Fc receptors. *J Exp Med* 1999;**189**:179–85.
123. Nimmerjahn F, Ravetch JV. Fc-receptors as regulators of immunity. *Adv Immunol* 2007;**96**:179–203.
124. Ravetch J. *In vivo* veritas: the surprising roles of Fc receptors in immunity. *Nat Immunol* 2010;**11**:183–5.
125. Hopken UE, Lu B, Gerard NP, Gerard C. Inpaired inflammatory responses in the reverse Arthus reaction through genetic deletion of the C5a receptor. *J Exp Med* 1997;**186**:749–56.
126. Heller T, Hennecke M, Baumann U, et al. Selection of a C5a receptor antagonist from phage libraries attenuating the inflammatory resonse in immune complex disease and ischemia/reperfusion injury. *J Immunol* 1999;**163**:985–94.
127. Heller T, Gessner JE, Schmidt RE, et al. Cutting edge: Fc receptor type I for IgG macrophages and complement mediate the inflammatory response in immune complex peritonitis. *J Immunol* 1999;**162**:5657–61.
128. Ji H, Ohmura K, Mahmood U, et al. Arthritis critically dependent on innate immune system players. *Immunity* 2002;**16**:157–68.
129. Baumann U, Chouchakova N, Gewecke B, et al. Distinct tissue site-specific requirements of mast cells and complement components C3/C5a receptor in IgG immune complex-induced injury of skin and lung. *J Immunol* 2001;**167**:1022–7.
130. Godau J, Heller T, Hawlisch H, et al. C5a initiates the inflammatory cascade in immune complex peritonitis. *J Immunol* 2004;**173**:3437–45.
131. Kumar V, Ali SR, Konrad S, et al. Cell-derived anaphylatoxins as key mediators of antibody-dependent type II autoimmunity in mice. *J Clin Invest* 2006;**116**:512–20.
132. Shushakova N, Skokowa J, Schulman J, et al. C5a anaphylatoxin is a major regulator of activating versus inhibitory FcγRs in immune complex-induced lung disease. *J Clin Invest* 2002;**110**:1823–30.
133. Konrad S, Engling L, Schmidt RE, Gessner JE. Characterization of the murine IgG Fc receptor III and IIB gene promoters. A single two-nucleotide difference determines their inverse responsiveness to C5a. *J Biol Chem* 2007;**282**:37906–12.
134. Konrad S, Ali SR, Wiege K, et al. Phosphoinositide 3-kinases γ and δ, linkers of coordinate C5a receptor-Fcγ

receptor activation and immune complex-induced inflammation. *J Biol Chem* 2008;**283**:33296–303.

135. Skokowa J, Ali SR, Felda O, et al. Macrophages induce the inflammatory response in the pulmonary Arthus reaction through G-αi2 activation that controls C5aR and Fc receptor cooperation. *J Immunol* 2005;**174**:3041–50.
136. Huber-Lang M, Sarma JV, Zetoune FS, et al. Generation of C5a in the absence of C3: a new complement activation pathway. *Nat Med* 2006;**12**:682–7.
137. Brekke OL, Christiansen D, Fure H, Fung M, Mollnes TE. The role of complement C3 opsonization, C5a receptor, and CD14 in *E.coli*-induced up-regulation of granulocyte and monocyte CD11b/CD18 (CR3), phagocytosis, and oxidative burst in human whole blood. *J Leuk Biol* 2007;**81**:1404–13.
138. Kavai M, Szegedi G. Immune complex clearance by monocytes and macrophages in systemic lupus erythematosus. *Autoimmun Rev* 2007;**6**:497–502.
139. Fries LF, Mullins WW, Cho KR, Plotz PH, Frank MM. Monocyte receptors for the Fc portion of IgG are increased in systemic lupus erythematosus. *J Immunol* 1984;**132**:695–700.
140. Yancey KB, O'Shea J, Chused T, et al. Human C5a modulates monocyte Fc and C3 receptor expression. *J Immunol* 1985;**135**:465–70.
141. Salmon JE, Kimberly RP, Gibofsky A, Fotina M. Defective mononuclear phagocyte function in systemic lupus erythematosus: dissociation of Fc receptor–ligand binding and internalization. *J Immunol* 1984;**133**:2525–31.
142. Zhang CY, Booth JW. Divergent intracellular sorting of FcγRIIA and FcγRIIB2. *J Biol Chem* 2010;**285**:34250–528.
143. Ukkonen P, Lewis V, Marsh M, Helenius A, Mellman I. Transport of macrophage Fc receptors and Fc receptor-bound ligands to lysosomes. *J Exp Med* 1986;**163**:952–71.
144. Taylor RP, Lindorfer MA. Drug insight: the mechanism of action of rituximab in autoimmune disease—the immune complex decoy hypothesis. *Nat Clin Pract Rheum* 2007;**3**:86–95.
145. Bowles JA, Weiner GJ. CD16 polymorphisms and NK activation induced by monoclonal antibody-coated target cells. *J Immunol Methods* 2005;**304**:88–99.
146. Davis W, Harrison PT, Hutchinson MJ, Allen JM. Two distinct regions of FcγRI initiate separate signalling pathways involved in endocytosis and phagocytosis. *EMBO J* 1995;**14**:432–41.
147. Lovdal T, Andersen E, Brech ABT. Fc receptor mediated endocytosis of small soluble immunoglobulin G immune complexes in Kupffer and endothelial cells from rat liver. *J Cell Sci* 2000;**113**:3255–66.
148. Ahuja A, Teichmann LL, Wang H, et al. An acquired defect in IgG-dependent phagocytosis explains the impairment in antibody-mediated cellular depletion in lupus. *J Immunol* 2011;**187**:3888–94.
149. Banda NK, Thurmann JM, Kraus D, et al. Alternative complement pathway activation is essential for inflammation and joint destruction in the passive transfer model of collagen-induced arthritis. *J Immunol* 2006;**177**:1904–12.
150. Banda NK, Takahashi K, Wood AK, Holers VM, Arend WP. Pathogenic complement activation in collagen antibody-induced arthritis in mice requires amplification by the alternative pathway. *J Immunol* 2007;**179**:4101–9.
151. Banda N, Takahashi M, Levitt B, et al. Essential role of complement mannose-binding lectin-associated serine proteases-1/3 in the murine collagen antibody-induced model of inflammatory arthritis. *J Immunol* 2010;**185**:5598–606.
152. Banda NK, Hyatt S, Antonioli AH, et al. Role of C3a receptors, C5a receptors, and complement protein C6 deficiency in collagen antibody-induced arthritis. *J Immunol* 2012;**188**:1469–78.

CHAPTER

4

Natural Killer Cells

Andreas Diefenbach

Department of Medical Microbiology and Hygiene (IMMH), University of Freiburg, Freiburg, Germany

Natural killer (NK) cells are a bone marrow-derived lymphocyte subset of the innate immune system that expresses Fc receptors.[1] NK cells are granular lymphocytes that play important roles in immunity against viruses and in the immune surveillance of tumors.[1] While NK cells were for a long time considered the only relevant innate lymphocyte subset in adults, additional innate lymphocyte lineages have been identified recently.[2,3] These new innate lymphocyte subsets and NK cells are now lumped together as innate lymphoid cells (ILCs).[2] Three distinct groups of ILCs have currently been identified.[2] Group 1 ILCs are characterized by the production of interferon (IFN)-γ and the expression of the transcription factor T-bet.[2] NK cells fulfill these criteria[1,4–6] and are considered to be one ILC1 subset. In addition, various groups have described ILC subsets that co-express T-bet and RORγt and produce IFN-γ.[7–10] It is debated whether these are ILC1s or rather part of the RORγt-expressing ILC3s (see below).[11] Group 2 ILCs are IL-5- and IL-13-producing innate lymphocytes.[12,13] ILC2s express high levels of the transcription factor Gata-3, which is also required for their lineage specification and maintenance.[14,15] In addition, mice lacking the retinoic acid-related orphan receptor alpha (RORα) are deficient for ILC2s,[16,17] and it has been proposed that RORα may be a transcriptional target of Gata-3.[18] Group 3 ILCs continuously express and developmentally depend on the transcription factor RORγt.[19,20] ILC3s produce "type 17" cytokines, such as IL-17A, IL-17F, and IL-22.[21–25] In addition, subsets of ILC3s have lymphoid tissue-inducing (LTi) function;[19,20,26–29] therefore, mice lacking ILC3s do not have lymph nodes and Peyer's patches.[19,28] In addition, ILC3s are also required for the generation of postnatally forming intestinal lymphoid follicles (i.e., cryptopatches and isolated lymphoid follicles).[29–31] Insights into the biology of ILCs have generated quite some interest because of the striking analogies in the transcriptional and functional programs of ILC and Th cell effector fates.

While ILC2s and ILC3s share similarities with Th2 and Th17 cells, respectively, NK cells resemble in various aspects cytotoxic $CD8^+$ T cells. NK cells require IL-15 for their differentiation or maintenance,[32,33] whereas ILC2s and ILC3s are independent of IL-15 but instead require IL-7R signaling for their maintenance.[22,34–36] This is similar to the CD4 and CD8 that show differential dependence on these cytokines for homeostatic maintenance.[37] In addition to being a potent innate source of IFN-γ, NK cells hold cytoplasmic granula that contain perforin and granzymes mediating cell-mediated cytotoxicity.[1] NK cells express various types of immunoreceptors that all are designed to sense pathological changes of self cells. In contrast to myeloid cells, NK cells have limited phagocytic activity and do not directly interact with pathogen components via pattern recognition receptors such as Toll-like receptors. NK cells also differ from lymphocytes of the adaptive immune system (i.e., T and B cells), because they do not express one major immune recognition receptor generated by recombination of receptor elements. Instead, NK cells express an arsenal of inhibitory and activating germline-encoded immunoreceptors that interact with ligands expressed by self cells.[38–40] The balance of inhibitory and activating input to an NK cell determines its activation state. This chapter focuses on NK cells and highlights how the activity of NK cells is regulated by inhibitory and activating input. NK cells express the stimulatory, low-affinity Fc receptor FcγRIIIa or CD16, which will be discussed as one pathway to activate NK cells. Finally, the spotlight will be put on recent work that has identified previously unappreciated, adaptive features of NK cells.

INHIBITORY RECEPTOR MODULES INFORM A USEFUL AND SELF-TOLERANT NK CELL REPERTOIRE

Most inhibitory receptors expressed by human and mouse NK cells recognize, either directly or indirectly, class I MHC molecules, keeping NK cells tolerant of normal self cells, as all nucleated cells express high levels of class I MHC molecules. Viral infection and tumor transformation are often accompanied by the downregulation of class I MHC molecules, possibly to evade recognition by CD8 T cells. The proposal that NK cells recognize target cells with low-level class I MHC expression was informed by data that NK cells would preferentially target infected or transformed cells[41] or transplanted cells with an incomplete complement of host class I MHC as observed in "hybrid resistance."[42–44] However, no causal link was made between low-level class I MHC expression and arousal of NK cell reactivity until a direct comparison of NK cell-mediated rejection of a class I MHC-expressing lymphoma and its class I MHC-deficient mutant variant was performed.[45] This study proposed that NK cells have an immune recognition apparatus that can sense loss of class I MHC.[45] This study and others[46,47] led to the initial proposal that NK cells target self cells that have downregulated class I MHC molecules, the "missing self hypothesis."[45,48] Interestingly, in the initial report showing that NK cells target class I MHC-negative tumor variants, it was proposed that NK cells may express inhibitory receptors specific for class I MHC.[45]

Some years later, inhibitory NK cell receptors with specificity for mouse and human class I MHC were identified. The inhibitory receptors expressed by human and mouse NK cells are quite diverse, suggesting that these receptors emerged after the separation of human and rodent ancestors. In humans, a group of killer cell immunoglobulin-like receptors (KIRs) with a long cytoplasmic domain containing immunoreceptor tyrosine-based inhibitory motifs (ITIMs) directly bind to HLA molecules.[49,50] KIR molecules are type I transmembrane, Ig-superfamily proteins and are subdivided into those with two and three extracellular immunoglobulin-like domains, KIR2DL and KIR3DL, respectively. KIR2DL1 interacts with group 2 HLA-C alleles, whereas KIR2DL2 and KIR2DL3 interact with group 1 HLA-C. The KIRs containing three Ig domains, KIR3DL1 and KIR3DL2, bind to HLA-B or HLA-A alleles, respectively. Mouse class I-specific inhibitory receptors belong to the Ly49 family of type II, lectin-like transmembrane proteins. Ly49 family proteins can interact with class I MHC alleles (H2-D, H2-K, and H2-L molecules).[51–53]

The inhibitory CD94/NKG2A receptor is conserved between humans and mice.[54–58] CD94/NKG2A does not directly bind to class I MHC molecules but rather uses an indirect mode to survey class I MHC expression. The heterodimeric CD94/NKG2A complex binds to the non-classical class I MHC-like molecules HLA-E in humans[59,60] and Qa-1^b (also known as H2-T23) in mice.[61] CD94/NKG2A only bind to HLA-E or Qa-1^b molecules if they are loaded with a self peptide derived from the leader sequence of classical class I MHC molecules.[62] Exchange of the self peptide in the context of an infection leads to loss of CD94/NKG2A binding and reduced inhibitory input to NK cells.

Both KIR and HLA genes are polymorphic, and the gene content of loci encoding KIR and HLA varies on the population level which may suggest pathogen-driven selection.[63,64] Indeed, recent data have provided compelling evidence that certain HLA–KIR haplotype combinations correlate with improved resistance to chronic viral infections such as hepatitis C and HIV.[65,66] It is now recognized that individuals homozygous for group 1 HLA-C and KIR2DL3 alleles are largely protected against such persistent infections. KIR2DL2 also binds to group 1 HLA-C alleles, albeit with higher affinity resulting in a stronger inhibitory signal.[67] Consequently, stronger activating signals are required for NK cell stimulation in individuals homozygous or heterozygous for KIR2DL2, which correlated with reduced protection against HCV.[65] Another important clinical application came from the discovery that KIR alloreactivity in stem cell transplantation increases the graft-*versus*-leukemia effect while decreasing unwanted graft-*versus*-host disease.[68,69] Thus, harnessing the power of NK cells by exploiting the polymorphic inhibitory receptor/ligand systems has become a constituent of clinical therapies.

Interestingly, individual NK cells do not express a full complement of KIR and Ly49 molecules but rather show variegation of expression.[70] This leads to the formation of an NK cell repertoire in which individual NK cells have distinct specificities based on their expression of inhibitory class I MHC-specific receptors. Variegation is believed to come into play through stochastic upregulation of inhibitory receptors, a process that is shaped when a productive interaction between an inhibitory receptor and a cognate class I MHC molecule occurs.[70–74] A further level of complexity is generated by the interaction of inhibitory receptors with class I MHC molecules expressed within the plane of the same cells (referred to as *cis* interactions).[75]

It is striking that, despite their diverse genetic material, human and mouse inhibitory NK cell receptors have a similar mode of action. As mentioned above, inhibitory receptors contain one or two ITIMs with the consensus sequence I/V*x*Y*xx*L/V (with *x* representing any amino acid). Inhibitory, ITIM-based signaling is not specific to NK cells and is a conserved theme in biology.[76] Crosslinking of inhibitory receptors results in the phosphorylation of the tyrosine residue of the ITIM by activated Src family kinases (e.g., Lck).[77,78] Phosphorylated ITIMs serve as docking sites for the protein tyrosine phosphatase SH2 domain-containing tyrosine phosphatase (SHP)-1.[57,77–82] Overexpression of a dominant-negative mutant of SHP-1 in NK cells reverses the inhibitory effect of KIR-mediated inhibitory signaling on both natural killer and antibody-dependent cell-mediated cytotoxicity (ADCC).[77,78] Our mechanistic understanding of how inhibitory signaling negatively regulates activating signals is far from complete. It is believed that SHP-1 dephosphorylates proximal tyrosine kinases, thereby restraining NK cell activation. In the case of FcR-mediated ADCC, co-ligation of KIR or CD94/NKG2A leads to reduced tyrosine phosphorylation of CD3ζ, FcRγ, ZAP-70, Syk, and PLC-γ, resulting in the inhibition of inositol phosphate release and calcium mobilization.[77,83] The exact molecular targets of SHP-1 associated with inhibitory NK cell receptors remain to be investigated.[84]

Interestingly, expression of self class I MHC-specific inhibitory receptors and their ligands is required to retain functional NK cells. This was initially supported by data showing that NK cells developing in mice lacking ligands for inhibitory NK cell receptors (i.e., β_2 microglobulin-deficient mice) do not display NK cell-mediated autoimmunity but rather have a hyporesponsive NK cell pool.[47,85,86] This was then extended by the observation, in normal mice, of a subpopulation of NK cells that do not express inhibitory receptors for self class I MHC.[87] Similar to NK cells of class I MHC-deficient mice, this subset was hyporesponsive when triggered by class I MHC-deficient target cells.[87] Another report showed that interaction of NK cell-expressed inhibitory receptors with its cognate MHC renders NK cells functional, a process requiring ITIM signaling in NK cells[88] and referred to as licensing or education of NK cells.[88,89] However, there are also data incompatible with the idea that interaction between inhibitory NK receptors and cognate class I MHC provide an "on" switch for NK cells. In an alternative model, NK cell education is a process in which a developing NK cell is already functional and integrates both inhibitory and activating signals. If the activating signal cannot be balanced by an inhibitory signal, these potentially autoreactive NK cells are rendered hyporesponsive (i.e., "disarming model").[89] It is currently unclear which of the models to explain NK cell education is correct, and it also remains to be seen where this process occurs and which cell types supply the cognate class I MHC.

It was initially believed that NK cell education is an "on/off" process that occurs during a distinct stage of NK cell differentiation at which a useful and self-tolerant NK cell repertoire is formed. However, it is now becoming apparent that NK cell education is a tunable rather than an "on/off" process.[90–93] In addition, mature NK cells may be reprogrammed, which is an important aspect for therapeutic approaches using anti-KIR antibodies.[94–96]

ACTIVATING IMMUNORECEPTORS MEDIATE NK CELL RECOGNITION OF TUMORS AND INFECTED CELLS

Missing-self recognition was the first model to explain how NK cells may recognize target cells. However, it has become clear that loss of inhibitory input is not sufficient for NK cell-mediated attack of target cells and that cognate interaction between activating receptors and their ligands on target cells is a prerequisite for NK cell activation. This became apparent from data investigating the formation of the NK cell/target cell synapse that supported the idea that stimulatory receptor/ligand interactions are required to polarize NK cells for the efficient and directed attack of the target cell.[97–103] Interestingly, activating receptors are quite conserved between mice and humans and, in contrast to the variegated expression of inhibitory receptors, are often expressed by virtually all NK cells. All known activating receptors do not display signaling motifs in their cytoplasmic domains but rather need to associate with signaling adapter molecules that mediate downstream signaling. Adapter proteins have very short extracellular domains that do not contribute to ligand binding. On the basis of the signaling pathways engaged by these adapter molecules, ITAM-containing and non-ITAM adapter proteins can be distinguished. One example of an ITAM-containing activating receptor is the low-affinity FcγRIIIa (CD16), which is expressed by most NK cells. The best studied non-ITAM-containing receptor complex is the NKG2D receptor complex. These receptor systems are discussed in more detail below.

Fc Receptor-Mediated Recognition of Immunoglobulin-Coated Target Cells by NK Cells

When it was determined that NK cells are a separate lymphocyte subset,[104–107] it became clear that the majority of NK cells express immunoglobulin-binding Fc receptors and can mediate ADCC (i.e., the ability of NK cells to kill antibody-coated target cells).[108–110] Once monoclonal antibodies against Fc receptors became available, it was shown that preincubation of NK cells with such FcR-specific antibodies abrogated ADCC.[111–113] NK cells mainly express FcγRIIIa (CD16), a low-affinity receptor for IgG.[114,115] For signaling, human CD16 associates with the ITAM-containing CD3ζ and FcRγ adapter proteins, whereas in mice CD16 only associates with FcRγ.[116–121] Analysis of mice genetically lacking the FcRγ adapter revealed a loss of ADCC mediated by NK cells.[122,123] ADCC is best triggered by antibodies of the IgG_{2a} and IgG_{2b} isotypes followed by IgG_1.[124]

In humans, two functionally distinct NK cell subsets can be discriminated based on the expression levels of the cell surface marker CD56 and CD16.[125] $CD56^{dim}$ NK cells co-express CD16 and are highly cytolytic including ADCC. In contrast, $CD56^{high}$ NK cells are $CD16^-$ and are relatively poor killer cells (no ADCC) but they produce large amounts of cytokines such as IFN-γ, TNF, and GM-CSF.[126] While $CD56^{high}$ $CD16^-$ NK cells are only a small fraction of NK cells in the peripheral blood, they are the major NK cell subset in secondary lymphoid organs.[127–129] It is currently believed that $CD56^{high}$ $CD16^-$ NK cells are immature NK cells that develop into mature $CD56^{dim}$ $CD16^+$ NK cells.[130,131] In mice, CD16 is already expressed by immature NK cells, and CD16 upregulation preceded the expression of NKG2D but was absent from earlier NK cell precursors (stage 1 to 3).[132]

Recently a hierarchy of NK cell receptors was established based on their propensities to fully stimulate NK cell function by themselves or in synergy with other NK cell receptors.[133] If insect cells were used as target cells for human resting NK cells, ICAM-1 expression on insect cells was sufficient to induce granule polarization but not for degranulation of NK cells.[101] Coating of ICAM-1-negative insect cells with IgG molecules led to the degranulation of resting NK cells without any obvious polarization. Such direct triggering of degranulation was characteristic of CD16-mediated signaling because engagement of the activating 2B4 receptor by its ligand CD48 expressed on insect cells resulted in only weak polarization but no degranulation.[101] IgG-coated insect cells expressing ICAM-1 were efficiently killed by NK cells because combinatorial engagement of CD16 and LFA-1 (the receptor for ICAM-1) led to polarization and degranulation of resting NK cells. The exceptional potency of the CD16 receptor to trigger cytotoxicity of resting NK cells was confirmed in redirected lysis assays.[134] While CD16 crosslinking alone led to NK cell-mediated cytotoxicity, other NK cell receptors (e.g., NKp46, NKG2D, 2B4, DNAM-1, CD2) were unable to do so. Resting NK cells could only be triggered for cytokine production by combinatorial triggering of various activating receptors, a scenario resembling at least some target cells that often express multiple ligands for various NK cell receptors.[39]

Recognition of Induced Self Molecules by NK Cells

It is now clear that NK cell activation requires cognate interaction of activating NK cell receptors with their ligands expressed on offending cells. This has been best documented for the NKG2D receptor/ligand system that is introduced here. The *Nkg2d* gene encodes a C-type lectin-like receptor that is located within a *Nkg2* gene cluster within the NK gene complex (mouse chromosome 6 or human chromosome 12), which also contains the genes for *Nkg2a*, *Nkg2c*, and *Nkg2e*.[56,135,136]

Although structurally related, NKG2D does not share much sequence homology with the other NKG2 proteins and does not associate with CD94, whereas NKG2A, NKG2C, and NKG2E do. In contrast, NKG2D forms homodimers and associates with the adaptor protein DNAX-associated protein of 10 kDa (DAP10).[137–139] DAP10 does not contain an ITAM motif but does contain a phosphatidylinositol (PI)3-kinase binding site. DAP10-mediated signaling activates PI3-kinase, Vav1, Rho family GTPases, and phospholipase C, resulting in Syk-independent activation of NK cells.[140,141] Full activation of human NK cells after NKG2D triggering requires the formation of a complex of DAP10 with the p85 subunit of PI3-kinase, Grb2, and Vav1.[142]

Data from mice genetically lacking the *Dap10* gene showed normal expression of NKG2D on activated NK cells, suggesting that NKG2D associates with an alternative adapter protein.[143] Interestingly, in mice, two alternative transcripts of the *Nkg2d* gene were found that differ in the length of the cytoplasmic C-terminus of the protein: NKG2D-short (S)[136,144] and NKG2D-long (L).[135,144] While NKG2D-L can only associate with DAP10, NKG2D-S can pair with both DAP10 and an ITAM-containing adapter protein called KARAP[144,145] or DAP12.[144,146] Domain-swapping experiments revealed that the long cytoplasmic tail of NKG2D repels KARAP/DAP12.[147] Like the other ITAM-containing adapter molecules, DAP12 leads to Syk-dependent activation of NK cells.[146] Expression of NKG2D-S is regulated in NK cells, allowing the signaling quality to be tuned downstream of the NKG2D receptor.[143,144] DAP12-deficient NK cells could not be triggered for IFN-γ production, whereas NK cell-mediated cytotoxicity against certain target cell lines was preserved.[141,144,148] Interestingly, in activated CD8$^+$ T cells NKG2D associates with DAP10 only, because DAP12 is not expressed by T cells.[144] Triggering of the NKG2D/DAP10 complex does not lead to T cell activation but can enhance T cell function in the context of T cell receptor triggering.[149–151] Ectopic expression of DAP12 in T cells allowed for direct, TCR-independent activation of T cells by triggering of the NKG2D receptor only.[144] These data show that regulated association of NKG2D with DAP10 and DAP12 can initiate two distinct signaling pathways that control the discrete functional profiles of lymphocytes.

Although activating NK cell receptors were identified, beginning in the 1980s,[152,153] their specificity remained obscure. NKG2D was the first activating receptor involved in natural cytotoxicity for which ligands have been identified. The human NKG2D receptor binds to two non-classical class I MHC molecules, MICA and MICB (MHC class I chain-related genes A and B), that are encoded within the MHC locus.[154–156] MICA and MICB were previously identified as stress-inducible ligands expressed by intestinal epithelial cells and recognized by Vδ1$^+$ γδ TCR-expressing T cells.[157,158] Consecutive studies revealed that MICA and MICB serve as ligands for both Vδ1$^+$ γδ TCRs and NKG2D.[159] In mice, no MICA or MICB orthologs could be identified because the syntenic region of the mouse MHC locus is very different in structure and gene content, and it is possible that no functional orthologs of the MIC genes exist in this region.[160,161]

Instead, studies in mice have identified a second group of NKG2D ligands. These belong to a multigene family encoded on mouse chromosome 10 and the syntenic human locus located on human chromosome 6. In mice, nine distinct genes have been identified: retinoic acid early inducible (Rae)1α–ε, H60a–c, and mouse ULBP-like transcript (MULT) 1.[162–166] A similar group of genes variably referred to as *ULBP (UL16 binding proteins)* or *RAET1* genes has been identified in humans.[167–170] Structural analysis of the various NKG2D ligands has revealed that they strikingly resemble class I MHC molecules, although the sequence homology to class I MHC is rather limited.[171,172] The existence of a large group of NKG2D ligands is striking. Although the various ligands have different affinities for the NKG2D receptor, distinct functions have not been observed;[173,174] therefore, it appears likely that the diversification of the NKG2D ligands was driven by the co-evolution with viruses because large DNA viruses such as mouse cytomegalovirus (MCMV) encode various proteins that serve to downregulate the expression of NKG2D ligands in infected cells.[175–177]

Analysis of expression of NKG2D ligands revealed that they are not expressed, or only at low levels, in healthy normal tissues;[157,162,163] however, transformed cells and infected cells express high levels of NKG2D ligands, making them targets for NK cells.[151,178,179] This scenario led to the formulation of a model in which NK cells recognize self ligands, the expression of which is upregulated on transformed or infected cells (i.e., recognition of induced self ligands).[161,180–182] Indeed, target cells ectopically expressing NKG2D ligands were efficiently killed by NK cells.[156,162,163] Data from mice genetically lacking NKG2D provided evidence that the NKG2D receptor/ligand system may be an important sentinel system to survey nascent tumors.[183]

The finding that NKG2D ligands are upregulated by stressed cells raised the important question of how these events are regulated on a molecular level. We do not have a complete picture yet of the molecular events leading to NKG2D ligand expression by stressed cells. For the MICA and MICB ligands, heat shock promoters have been implicated.[157,184] Studies in mice revealed an additional pathway for upregulation of the Rae1 family of ligands following DNA damage.[185] Indeed, several forms of DNA damage led to an ATM/ATR-dependent upregulation of murine NKG2D ligands.[186,187] As the DNA damage response cascade has been involved in tumor transformation and viral infection, this may indeed be a central pathway leading to induced expression of NKG2D ligands by tumor cells.[186,187] Another clue to how NKG2D ligands may be regulated came from studies investigating the contribution of senescence to fibrotic and cirrhotic processes in the liver.[188] In mice treated to develop liver fibrosis, senescent cells accumulate in livers. Senescent cells expressed increased levels of NKG2D ligands, and depletion of NK cells led to aggravated liver fibrosis.[188] Thus, NK cells may not only be required to prevent virus infection or tumor development but may also be involved in maintaining organ homeostasis by eliminating pro-fibrotic cells. This important avenue of research will reveal insights into previously unappreciated roles of NK cells.

Although many tumor cells express NKG2D ligands, various mechanisms have been identified that lead to the downregulation of NKG2D ligands on advanced tumors. First, shedding of NKG2D ligands has been observed leading to effective escape from immune-mediated recognition of tumors.[189–193] Second, epigenetic regulation of NKG2D ligand expression in late-stage tumors involving histone deacetylases has been reported.[194–197] Remodeling of chromatin at the NKG2D ligand loci by reduced acetylation of histone residues may lead to reduced transcription of NKG2D ligands and escape from immune-mediated control of tumor progression.

Collectively, the NKG2D receptor/ligand system is currently the best explored paradigm of how NK cells recognize target cells. Research into this and other stimulatory NK cell receptors has revealed important insights into the co-evolution of the innate immune system and viruses. It has also provided a rationale for therapeutic interventions based on harnessing the power of NK cells for the immunotherapy of tumors and viral infections.

ADAPTIVE FEATURES OF NK CELLS

Natural killer cells are considered part of the innate immune system because they can rapidly respond to infections and because of their expression of germline-encoded immune recognition receptors. Recent research has, however, provided evidence that NK cells already show some features of the adaptive immune system in that they require interactions with the myeloid lineage for potent effector function (a process referred to as "priming") and previously activated NK cells are better effector cells upon rechallenge (a process resembling "immunological memory").

NK Cell Priming

For a long time, NK cells were considered to follow a cell-autonomous activation program when their activating receptors are triggered by their cognate ligands expressed by offending cells. However, this view seems dated because freshly isolated NK cells from human peripheral blood and from mice are remarkably poor killers of various well-recognized NK target cells.[134,198] In addition, naïve NK cells were found to demonstrate only very low-level expression of the cytotoxic proteins granzyme B and perforin.[198,199] These findings lend support to a model in which NK cells require "priming" of effector functions, a process that involves interaction with cells of the myeloid lineage. This view first received support by a study showing that NK cell-mediated rejection of a mesothelioma tumor cell line in mice required the presence of dendritic cells (DCs).[200] In addition, NK cells co-cultured with either a DC line or with stimulated bone marrow-derived DCs displayed potent cytotoxicity against target cells, whereas control NK cells were very inefficient in killing.[200] These data effectively challenged the view that NK cells can cell-autonomously mediate potent effector functions once confronted with a target cell.

Additional evidence came from *in vivo* studies in mice infected with MCMV.[201] $CD8\alpha\alpha^+$ DCs were required for expansion of the $Ly49H^+$ subset of NK cells in C57BL/6 mice. Ly49H is an activating immunoreceptor that binds to an MCMV-encoded ligand (m157) required for virus control in the C57BL/6 strain of mice.[202,203] In addition, this study revealed bidirectional interaction between NK cells and DCs because NK cell-depleted mice could not retain DCs in the spleen.[201] NK cell activation in co-cultures with syngeneic, stimulated splenic DCs was also observed in the human system.[204] In addition, NK cells that are normally excluded from lymph nodes are recruited in a CCR7-independent and CXCR3-dependent manner, where they can interact with DCs and induce Th1-type of immunity.[205] These previous studies relied on *in vitro* stimulation of NK cells with various types of DCs, subcutaneous injections of DCs, or antibody-mediated depletion of DC subsets not entirely specific to DCs. When mice became available that allow for the specific ablation of DCs,[206,207] it was shown that NK cell-mediated immunity to viruses, bacteria, and parasites required the presence of DCs.[198,207–210]

What are the molecular signals provided by DCs that prime NK cell function? The conventional view has been that the various cytokines provided by DCs initiate distinct functional programs of NK cells.[204] Type I IFNs were believed to directly trigger cytotoxic function by NK cells, whereas IL-12 induces IFN-γ expression. In addition, IL-15 is required for NK cell expansion and survival. However, IL-12-deficient mice could still produce significant amounts of IFN-γ, whereas mice lacking the type I IFN receptor (*Ifnar*$^{-/-}$ mice) were unable to mount NK cell cytotoxicity or cytokine production.[198] In addition, NK cells lacking the IFNAR could still be activated relatively well, suggesting that the relevant type I IFN signaling occurs in another cell type.[198,211] This was recently supported by tissue-specific targeting of the IFNAR showing that selective deficiency of IFNAR on NK cells still allowed for potent NK cell activation and immunity to MCMV.[212] Indeed, various lines of evidence have suggested that DCs can be stimulated by type I IFNs that activate antiproliferative, antiviral, and lymphocyte-activating gene networks in DCs.[212] Of the lymphocyte-activating genes, *trans*-presentation of IL-15 on its high-affinity IL-15Rα chain is potently enhanced by type I IFN-stimulated DCs.[213] IL-15 *trans*-presented by IL-15Rα$^+$ DCs has been identified as the central priming signal provided by DCs to NK cells.[198,212,214,215] Indeed, IL-15 is a potent signal inducing translation of perforin and granzyme from pre-existing mRNA pools in naïve NK cells.[199] Thus, NK cell recognition of target cells requires previous priming by DCs. Recently, this concept was extended by data showing that other myeloid cell subsets (e.g., neutrophils and inflammatory macrophages) may also contribute to NK cell activation.[216–218]

Collectively, these data lend support to a model in which NK cells do not follow a cell-autonomous activation program but rather require previous interaction with cells of the myeloid lineage that allows acquisition of effector molecules arming NK cells for interaction with target cells.

NK Cell Memory

The formation of antigen-specific, long-lived memory cells emerging after the initial antigen encounter is considered to be a quality of adaptive lymphocytes expressing recombining, antigen-specific receptors (i.e., B and T cells). However, recent data have provided some evidence that, under certain conditions, NK cells may exhibit a memory of previous activation. One line of research has investigated NK cell responses in the context of MCMV infection. A number of inbred mouse strains (e.g., C57BL/6) are resistant to MCMV infection, whereas others (e.g., BALB/c) are susceptible.[219] Depletion of NK cells[219] or perforin deficiency[220] in resistant mice leads to the loss of virus control. Extensive genetic mapping studies have indicated that a single autosomal dominant locus, termed *Cmv1*, controls both survival and spleen viral titers.[219,221–223] The *Cmv1* locus maps to the NK gene complex on mouse chromosome 6 and contains the various genes encoding Ly49 receptors.[224] Interestingly, one activating Ly49 receptor, Ly49H, is required for resistance to MCMV infection in C57BL/6 mice because blocking of the receptor leads to the loss of virus control.[224] This was confirmed in a genetic study showing that the *Cmv1* locus of congenic mice susceptible to MCMV infection lacks the *Ly49h* (*Klra8*) gene.[225] Significantly, the Ly49H receptor recognizes a MCMV-encoded cell surface protein called m157.[202,203] Ectopic expression of m157 on cell lines that are normally poor NK cell targets resulted in effective recognition by NK cells that was dependent on cognate interaction between Ly49H on NK cells and m157 on target cells.[202] Importantly, some of the susceptible mouse strains lacking the *Ly49h* gene encoded related inhibitory receptors recognizing m157, suggesting that m157 may be a virus-encoded gene that has developed to evade immune recognition by NK cells.[202]

The immune response in C57BL/6 mice to MCMV is peculiar in that it is dominated by the cognate interaction between one activating receptor (Ly49H) with a virus-encoded ligand (m157). This is an unusual scenario because NK cell responses are often driven by various stimulatory receptors and their ligands, making the MCMV system almost T cell like. Ly49H associates with the adaptor protein KARAP or DAP12, and mice lacking DAP12 lack cell surface expression of Ly49H.[226,227] Similar to what has been found for antigen-specific T cells, adoptive transfer of NK cells into mice lacking DAP12 expression led to an expansion of Ly49H$^+$ NK cells that proliferated in response to the virus-encoded ligand for the Ly49H receptor.[228] Expansion of these "MCMV-specific" NK cells was followed by a contraction phase; after contraction, these MCMV-experienced NK cells had a distinct cell surface phenotype and, upon restimulation, produced higher levels of IFN-γ compared to naïve NK cells. Lower numbers of MCMV-experienced

NK cells were required to protect newborn mice against MCMV infection when compared to "naïve," MCMV-inexperienced NK cells.[228] Interestingly, IL-12 signaling in NK cells was important for the generation of a memory-like phenotype in NK cells.[229] This is supported by findings that NK cells stimulated with IL-12 *in vitro* have similar phenotypic and functional characteristics as MCMV-experienced NK cells[230] and have higher antitumor activity when transferred into mice with established tumors.[231] Recently, evidence was provided that human NK cells expanded in individuals infected with Puumula hantavirus, and NK cell frequency was enhanced over a time frame of more than 6 months.[232] The increase in NK cell numbers was most pronounced in NKG2C$^+$ NK cells, and elevated levels of its cognate ligand (HLA-E) were observed on hantavirus-infected endothelial cells.

Another line of evidence for the memory-like qualities of NK cells came from studies of hapten-specific contact hypersensitivity (CHS) reactions in mice lacking all B and T cells (i.e., *Rag2*$^{-/-}$ mice). The CHS response is considered a classical example of an antigen-specific, adaptive memory response. During the sensitization phase, epithelial surfaces (e.g., skin) are exposed to an organic or inorganic compound that chemically modifies proteins. These "haptenated" proteins are recognized as "non-self" and induce T and B cell responses. Upon rechallenge, typically at a previously unexposed site, a local recall response occurs that was widely believed to involve recruitment of memory B and T cells. Recently, it was shown that Rag-deficient mice that lack all B and T cells but have normal numbers of innate lymphocytes (NK cells and ILCs) show an intact cutaneous CHS response that is dependent on the presence of NK cells.[233] While *Rag2*$^{-/-}$*Il2rg*$^{-/-}$ mice, which lack all lymphocytes (including NK cells and ILC), do not develop CHS, transfer of hepatic Thy1$^+$ (CD90$^+$) NK cells into such alymphoid mice has been shown to restore CHS responses.[233] In consecutive studies, liver NK cells were shown to also provide antigen-specific recall reactions to virus-like particles containing VSV, influenza, or HIV-1 antigens.[234] NK cell memory of haptens and viruses required expression of the chemokine receptor CXCR6. CXCR6 was needed for persistence of antigen-experienced NK cells but was not involved in antigen recognition.[234] Collectively, these data indicate that NK cells show traits of adaptive lymphocytes such as expansion to stimulation and an antigen-experienced status allowing for rapid and more effective recall responses.

References

1. Trinchieri G. Biology of natural killer cells. *Adv Immunol* 1989;**47**(187):187–376.
2. Spits H, Artis D, Colonna M, Diefenbach A, Di Santo JP, Eberl G, et al. Innate lymphoid cells: a proposal for uniform nomenclature. *Nat Rev Immunol* 2013;**13**(2):145–9.
3. Spits H, Cupedo T. Innate lymphoid cells: emerging insights in development, lineage relationships, and function. *Annu Rev Immunol* 2012;**30**:647–75.
4. Gordon SM, Chaix J, Rupp LJ, Wu J, Madera S, Sun JC, et al. The transcription factors T-bet and Eomes control key checkpoints of natural killer cell maturation. *Immunity* 2012;**36**(1):55–67.
5. Townsend MJ, Weinmann AS, Matsuda JL, Salomon R, Farnham PJ, Biron CA, et al. T-bet regulates the terminal maturation and homeostasis of NK and Valpha14i NKT cells. *Immunity* 2004;**20**(4):477–94.
6. Klose CS, Hoyler T, Kiss EA, Tanriver Y, Diefenbach A. Transcriptional control of innate lymphocyte fate decisions. *Curr Opin Immunol* 2012;**24**(3):290–6.
7. Klose CS, Kiss EA, Schwierzeck V, Ebert K, Hoyler T, d'Hargues Y, et al. A T-bet gradient controls the fate and function of CCR6−RORγt+ innate lymphoid cells. *Nature* 2013;**494**(7436):261–5.
8. Bernink JH, Peters CP, Munneke M, Te Velde AA, Meijer SL, Weijer K, et al. Human type 1 innate lymphoid cells accumulate in inflamed mucosal tissues. *Nat Immunol* 2013;**14**:221–9.
9. Rankin LC, Groom JR, Chopin M, Herold MJ, Walker JA, Mielke LA, et al. The transcription factor T-bet is essential for the development of NKp46(+) innate lymphocytes via the Notch pathway. *Nat Immunol* 2013;**14**(4):389–95.

10. Sciume G, Hirahara K, Takahashi H, Laurence A, Villarino AV, Singleton KL, et al. Distinct requirements for T-bet in gut innate lymphoid cells. *J Exp Med* 2012;**209**(13):2331–8.
11. Leavy O. Innate-like lymphocytes: will the real ILC1 please stand up?. *Nat Rev Immunol* 2013;**13**(2):67.
12. Moro K, Yamada T, Tanabe M, Takeuchi T, Ikawa T, Kawamoto H, et al. Innate production of T(H)2 cytokines by adipose tissue-associated c-Kit(+)Sca-1(+) lymphoid cells. *Nature* 2010;**463**(7280):540–4.
13. Neill DR, Wong SH, Bellosi A, Flynn RJ, Daly M, Langford TK, et al. Nuocytes represent a new innate effector leukocyte that mediates type-2 immunity. *Nature* 2010;**464**(7293):1367–70.
14. Hoyler T, Klose CS, Souabni A, Turqueti-Neves A, Pfeifer D, Rawlins EL, et al. The transcription factor GATA3 controls cell fate and maintenance of type 2 innate lymphoid cells. *Immunity* 2012;**37**(4):634–48.
15. Mjosberg J, Bernink J, Golebski K, Karrich JJ, Peters CP, Blom B, et al. The transcription factor GATA3 is essential for the function of human type 2 innate lymphoid cells. *Immunity* 2012;**37**(4):649–59.
16. Wong SH, Walker JA, Jolin HE, Drynan LF, Hams E, Camelo A, et al. Transcription factor RORα is critical for nuocyte development. *Nat Immunol* 2012;**13**:229–36.
17. Halim TY, MacLaren A, Romanish MT, Gold MJ, McNagny KM, Takei F. Retinoic-acid-receptor-related orphan nuclear receptor alpha is required for natural helper cell development and allergic inflammation. *Immunity* 2012;**37**(3):463–74.
18. Vosshenrich CA, Di Santo JP. Developmental programming of natural killer and innate lymphoid cells. *Curr Opin Immunol* 2013;**25**(2):130–8.
19. Sun Z, Unutmaz D, Zou YR, Sunshine MJ, Pierani A, Brenner-Morton S, et al. Requirement for RORγ in thymocyte survival and lymphoid organ development. *Science* 2000;**288**(5475):2369–73.
20. Eberl G, Marmon S, Sunshine MJ, Rennert PD, Choi Y, Littman DR. An essential function for the nuclear receptor RORγ(t) in the generation of fetal lymphoid tissue inducer cells. *Nat Immunol* 2004;**5**(1):64–73.
21. Cupedo T, Crellin NK, Papazian N, Rombouts EJ, Weijer K, Grogan JL, et al. Human fetal lymphoid tissue-inducer cells are interleukin 17-producing precursors to RORC+ CD127+ natural killer-like cells. *Nat Immunol* 2009;**10**(1):66–74.
22. Sanos SL, Bui VL, Mortha A, Oberle K, Heners C, Johner C, et al. RORγt and commensal microflora are required for the differentiation of mucosal interleukin 22-producing NKp46+ cells. *Nat Immunol* 2009;**10**(1):83–91.
23. Cella M, Fuchs A, Vermi W, Facchetti F, Otero K, Lennerz JK, et al. A human natural killer cell subset provides an innate source of IL-22 for mucosal immunity. *Nature* 2009;**457**(7230):722–5.
24. Luci C, Reynders A, Ivanov II, Cognet C, Chiche L, Chasson L, et al. Influence of the transcription factor RORγt on the development of NKp46+ cell populations in gut and skin. *Nat Immunol* 2009;**10**(1):75–82.
25. Satoh-Takayama N, Vosshenrich CA, Lesjean-Pottier S, Sawa S, Lochner M, Rattis F, et al. Microbial flora drives interleukin 22 production in intestinal NKp46+ cells that provide innate mucosal immune defense. *Immunity* 2008;**29**(6):958–70.
26. Mebius RE, Rennert P, Weissman IL. Developing lymph nodes collect CD4 + CD3– LTbeta+ cells that can differentiate to APC, NK cells, and follicular cells but not T or B cells. *Immunity* 1997;**7**(4):493–504.
27. Yoshida H, Honda K, Shinkura R, Adachi S, Nishikawa S, Maki K, et al. IL-7 receptor alpha+ CD3(–) cells in the embryonic intestine induces the organizing center of Peyer's patches. *Int Immunol* 1999;**11**(5):643–55.
28. Kurebayashi S, Ueda E, Sakaue M, Patel DD, Medvedev A, Zhang F, et al. Retinoid-related orphan receptor gamma (RORgamma) is essential for lymphoid organogenesis and controls apoptosis during thymopoiesis. *Proc Natl Acad Sci USA* 2000;**97**(18):10132–7.
29. Kiss EA, Vonarbourg C, Kopfmann S, Hobeika E, Finke D, Esser C, et al. Natural aryl hydrocarbon receptor ligands control organogenesis of intestinal lymphoid follicles. *Science* 2011;**334**(6062):1561–5.
30. Eberl G, Littman DR. Thymic origin of intestinal alphabeta T cells revealed by fate mapping of RORgammat+ cells. *Science* 2004;**305**(5681):248–51.
31. Bouskra D, Brezillon C, Berard M, Werts C, Varona R, Boneca IG, et al. Lymphoid tissue genesis induced by commensals through NOD1 regulates intestinal homeostasis. *Nature* 2008;**456**(7221):507–10.
32. Kennedy MK, Glaccum M, Brown SN, Butz EA, Viney JL, Embers M, et al. Reversible defects in natural killer and memory CD8 T cell lineages in interleukin 15-deficient mice. *J Exp Med* 2000;**191**(5):771–80.
33. Lodolce JP, Boone DL, Chai S, Swain RE, Dassopoulos T, Trettin S, et al. IL-15 receptor maintains lymphoid homeostasis by supporting lymphocyte homing and proliferation. *Immunity* 1998;**9**(5):669–76.
34. Satoh-Takayama N, Lesjean-Pottier S, Vieira P, Sawa S, Eberl G, Vosshenrich CA, et al. IL-7 and IL-15 independently program the differentiation of intestinal CD3–NKp46+ cell subsets from Id2-dependent precursors. *J Exp Med* 2010;**207**(2):273–80.
35. Vonarbourg C, Mortha A, Bui VL, Hernandez PP, Kiss EA, Hoyler T, et al. Regulated expression of nuclear receptor RORγt confers distinct functional fates to

NK cell receptor-expressing RORγt(+) innate lymphocytes. *Immunity* 2010;**33**(5):736–51.
36. Vonarbourg C, Diefenbach A. Multifaceted roles of interleukin-7 signaling for the development and function of innate lymphoid cells. *Sem Immunol* 2012;**24**(3):165–74.
37. Boyman O, Purton JF, Surh CD, Sprent J. Cytokines and T-cell homeostasis. *Curr Opin Immunol* 2007;**19**(3):320–6.
38. Lanier LL. NK cell recognition. *Annu Rev Immunol.* 2005;**23**:225–74.
39. Moretta L, Bottino C, Vitale M, Pende D, Cantoni C, Mingari M, et al. Activating receptors and coreceptors involved in human natural killer cell-mediated cytolysis. *Annu Rev Immunol* 2001;**19**:197–223.
40. Lanier LL. NK cell receptors. *Annu Rev Immunol.* 1998;**16**(2):359–93.
41. Stern P, Gidlund M, Orn A, Wigzell H. Natural killer cells mediate lysis of embryonal carcinoma cells lacking MHC. *Nature* 1980;**285**(5763):341–2.
42. Cudkowicz G, Bennett M. Peculiar immunobiology of bone marrow allografts. II. Rejection of parental grafts by resistant F_1 hybrid mice. *J Exp Med* 1971;**134**:1513–28.
43. Kiessling R, Petranyi G, Klein G, Wigzell H. Genetic variation of *in vitro* cytolytic activity and *in vivo* rejection potential of non-immunized semi-syngeneic mice against a mouse lymphoma line. *Int J Cancer* 1975;**15**(6):933–40.
44. Kiessling R, Hochman PS, Haller O, Shearer GM, Wigzell H, Cudkowicz G. Evidence for a similar or common mechanism for natural killer cell activity and resistance to hemopoietic grafts. *Eur J Immunol* 1977;**7**(9):655–63.
45. Karre K, Ljunggren HG, Piontek G, Kiessling R. Selective rejection of H-2-deficient lymphoma variants suggests alternative immune defense strategy. *Nature* 1986;**319**:675–8.
46. Bix M, Liao N-S, Zijlstra M, Loring J, Jaenisch R, Raulet D. Rejection of class I MHC-deficient hemopoietic cells by irradiated MHC-matched mice. *Nature* 1991;**349**:329–31.
47. Liao N, Bix M, Zijlstra M, Jaenisch R, Raulet D. MHC class I deficiency: susceptibility to natural killer (NK) cells and impaired NK activity. *Science* 1991;**253**:199–202.
48. Karre K. NK cells, MHC class I molecules and the missing self. *Scand J Immunol* 2002;**55**(3):221–8.
49. Colonna M, Samaridis J. Cloning of immunoglobulin-superfamily members associated with HLA-C and HLA-B recognition by human natural killer cells. *Science* 1995;**268**(5209):405–8.
50. Wagtmann N, Rajagopalan S, Winter CC, Peruzzi M, Long EO. Killer cell inhibitory receptors specific for HLA-C and HLA-B identified by direct binding and by functional transfer. *Immunity* 1995;**3**(6):801–9.
51. Karlhofer FM, Ribaudo RK, Yokoyama WM. MHC class I alloantigen specificity of Ly-49$^+$ IL-2 activated natural killer cells. *Nature* 1992;**358**:66–70.
52. Hanke T, Takizawa H, McMahon CW, Busch DH, Pamer EG, Miller JD, et al. Direct assessment of MHC class I binding by seven Ly49 inhibitory NK cell receptors. *Immunity* 1999;**11**:67–77.
53. Natarajan K, Boyd LF, Schuck P, Yokoyama WM, Eliat D, Margulies DH. Interaction of the NK cell inhibitory receptor Ly49A with H-2Dd: identification of a site distinct from the TCR site. *Immunity* 1999;**11**(5):591–601.
54. Brooks AG, Posch PE, Scorzelli CJ, Borrego F, Coligan JE. NKG2A complexed with CD94 defines a novel inhibitory natural killer cell receptor. *J Exp Med* 1997;**185**(4):795–800.
55. Phillips JH, Chang C, Mattson J, Gumperz JE, Parham P, Lanier LL. CD94 and a novel associated protein (94AP) form a NK receptor involved in the recognition of HLA-A, HLA-B and HLA-C allotypes. *Immunity* 1996;**5**(2):163–72.
56. Houchins JP, Yabe T, McSherry C, Bach FH. DNA sequence analysis of NKG2, a family of related cDNA clones encoding type II integral membrane proteins on human natural killer cells. *J Exp Med* 1991;**173**(4):1017–20.
57. Houchins JP, Lanier LL, Niemi EC, Phillips JH, Ryan JC. Natural killer cell cytolytic activity is inhibited by NKG2-A and activated by NKG2-C. *J Immunol* 1997;**158**(8):3603–9.
58. Carretero M, Cantoni C, Bellon T, Bottino C, Biassoni R, Rodriguez A, et al. The CD94 and NKG2-A C-type lectins covalently assemble to form a natural killer cell inhibitory receptor for HLA class I molecules. *Eur J Immunol* 1997;**27**(2):563–7.
59. Braud VM, Allan DSJ, O'Callaghan CA, Soderstrom K, D'Andrea A, Ogg GS, et al. HLA-E binds to natural killer cell receptors CD94/NKG2A, B, and C. *Nature* 1998;**391**:795–9.
60. Lee N, Llano M, Carretero M, Ishitani A, Navarro F, Lopez-Botet M, et al. HLA-E is a major ligand for the natural killer inhibitory receptor CD94/NKG2A. *Proc Natl Acad Sci USA* 1998;**95**(9):5199–204.
61. Vance RE, Kraft JR, Altman JD, Jensen PE, Raulet DH. Mouse CD94/NKG2A is a natural killer cell receptor for the nonclassical MHC class I molecule Qa-1^b. *J Exp Med* 1998;**188**:1841–8.
62. Kraft JR, Vance RE, Pohl J, Martin AM, Raulet DH, Jensen PE. Analysis of Qa-1(b) peptide binding specificity and the capacity of CD94/NKG2A to discriminate between Qa-1–peptide complexes. *J Exp Med* 2000;**192**(5):613–24.

63. Valiante NM, Lienert K, Shilling HG, Smits BJ, Parham P. Killer cell receptors: keeping pace with MHC class I evolution. *Immunol Rev* 1997;**155**:155–64.
64. Khakoo SI, Rajalingam R, Shum BP, Weidenbach K, Flodin L, Muir DG, et al. Rapid evolution of NK cell receptor systems demonstrated by comparison of chimpanzees and humans. *Immunity* 2000;**12**(6):687–98.
65. Khakoo SI, Thio CL, Martin MP, Brooks CR, Gao X, Astemborski J, et al. HLA and NK cell inhibitory receptor genes in resolving hepatitis C virus infection. *Science* 2004;**305**(5685):872–4.
66. Alter G, Heckerman D, Schneidewind A, Fadda L, Kadie CM, Carlson JM, et al. HIV-1 adaptation to NK-cell-mediated immune pressure. *Nature* 2011;**476**(7358):96–100.
67. Winter CC, Gumperz JE, Parham P, Long EO, Wagtmann N. Direct binding and functional transfer of NK cell inhibitory receptors reveal novel patterns of HLA-C allotype recognition. *J Immunol* 1998;**161**(2):571–7.
68. Ruggeri L, Capanni M, Urbani E, Perruccio K, Shlomchik WD, Tosti A, et al. Effectiveness of donor natural killer cell alloreactivity in mismatched hematopoietic transplants. *Science* 2002;**295**(5562):2097–100.
69. Cooley S, Trachtenberg E, Bergemann TL, Saeteurn K, Klein J, Le CT, et al. Donors with group B KIR haplotypes improve relapse-free survival after unrelated hematopoietic cell transplantation for acute myelogenous leukemia. *Blood* 2009;**113**(3):726–32.
70. Raulet DH, Vance RE, McMahon CW. Regulation of the natural killer cell receptor repertoire. *Annu Rev Immunol* 2001;**19**:291–330.
71. Held W, Raulet DH. Ly49A transgenic mice provide evidence for a major histocompatibility complex-dependent education process in NK cell development. *J Exp Med* 1997;**185**:2079–88.
72. Held W, Roland J, Raulet DH. Allelic exclusion of Ly49 family genes encoding class I-MHC-specific receptors on NK cells. *Nature* 1995;**376**:355–8.
73. Tanamachi DM, Hanke T, Takizawa H, Jamieson AM, Raulet DH. Expression of natural killer cell receptor alleles at different Ly49 loci occurs independently and is regulated by major histocompatibility complex class I molecules. *J Exp Med* 2001;**193**(3):307–15.
74. Uhrberg M, Valiente N, Shum B, Shilling H, Lienert-Weidenbach K, Corliss B, et al. Human diversity in killer cell inhibitory receptor genes. *Immunity* 1997;**7**(6):753–63.
75. Doucey MA, Scarpellino L, Zimmer J, Guillaume P, Luescher IF, Bron C, et al. Cis association of Ly49A with MHC class I restricts natural killer cell inhibition. *Nat Immunol* 2004;**5**(3):328–36.
76. Boehm T. Quality control in self/nonself discrimination. *Cell* 2006;**125**(5):845–58.
77. Binstadt BA, Brumbaugh KM, Dick CJ, Scharenberg AM, Williams BL, Colonna M, et al. Sequential involvement of Lck and SHP-1 with MHC-recognizing receptors on NK cells inhibits FcR-initiated tyrosine kinase activation. *Immunity* 1996;**5**(6):629–38.
78. Burshtyn D, Scharenberg A, Wagtmann N, Rajagopalan S, Peruzzi M, Kinet J-P, et al. Recruitment of tyrosine phosphatase HCP by the NK cell inhibitory receptor. *Immunity* 1996;**4**:77–85.
79. Campbell KS, Dessing M, Lopez-Botet M, Cella M, Colonna M. Tyrosine phosphorylation of a human killer inhibitory receptor recruits protein tyrosine phosphatase 1C. *J Exp Med* 1996;**184**(1):93–100.
80. Olcese L, Lang P, Vely F, Cambiaggi A, Marguet D, Blery M, et al. Human and mouse killer-cell inhibitory receptors recruit Ptp1c and Ptp1d protein tyrosine phosphatases. *J Immunol* 1996;**156**:4531–4.
81. Fry AM, Lanier LL, Weiss A. Phosphotyrosines in the killer cell inhibitory receptor motif of NKB1 are required for negative signaling and for association with protein tyrosine phosphatase 1C. *J Exp Med* 1996;**184**(1):295–300.
82. Nakamura MC, Niemi EC, Fisher MJ, Shultz LD, Seaman WE, Ryan JC. Mouse Ly-49A interrupts early signaling events in natural killer cell cytotoxicity and functionally associates with the SHP-1 tyrosine phosphatase. *J Exp Med* 1997;**185**(4):673–84.
83. Kaufman DS, Schoon RA, Robertson MJ, Leibson PJ. Inhibition of selective signaling events in natural killer cells recognizing major histocompatibility complex class I. *Proc Natl Acad Sci USA* 1995;**92**(14):6484–8.
84. Leibson PJ. Signal transduction during natural killer cell activation: inside the mind of a killer. *Immunity* 1997;**6**:655–61.
85. Dorfman JR, Raulet DH. Acquisition of Ly49 receptor expression by developing natural killer cells. *J Exp Med* 1998;**187**(4):609–18.
86. Dorfman JR, Zerrahn J, Coles MC, Raulet DH. The basis for self-tolerance of natural killer cells in β_2m^- and TAP-1^- mice. *J Immunol* 1997;**159**:5219–25.
87. Fernandez NC, Treiner E, Vance RE, Jamieson AM, Lemieux S, Raulet DH. A subset of natural killer cells achieves self-tolerance without expressing inhibitory receptors specific for self-MHC molecules. *Blood* 2005;**105**(11):4416–23.
88. Kim S, Poursine-Laurent J, Truscott SM, Lybarger L, Song YJ, Yang L, et al. Licensing of natural killer cells by host major histocompatibility complex class I molecules. *Nature* 2005;**436**(7051):709–13.
89. Raulet DH, Vance RE. Self-tolerance of natural killer cells. *Nat Rev Immunol* 2006;**6**(7):520–31.

90. Johansson S, Johansson M, Rosmaraki E, Vahlne G, Mehr R, Salmon-Divon M, et al. Natural killer cell education in mice with single or multiple major histocompatibility complex class I molecules. *J Exp Med* 2005;**201**(7):1145–55.
91. Joncker NT, Fernandez NC, Treiner E, Vivier E, Raulet DH. NK cell responsiveness is tuned commensurate with the number of inhibitory receptors for self-MHC class I: the rheostat model. *J Immunol* 2009;**182**(8):4572–80.
92. Brodin P, Lakshmikanth T, Johansson S, Karre K, Hoglund P. The strength of inhibitory input during education quantitatively tunes the functional responsiveness of individual natural killer cells. *Blood* 2009;**113**(11):2434–41.
93. Brodin P, Karre K, Hoglund P. NK cell education: not an on-off switch but a tunable rheostat. *Trends Immunol* 2009;**30**(4):143–9.
94. Sola C, Andre P, Lemmers C, Fuseri N, Bonnafous C, Blery M, et al. Genetic and antibody-mediated reprogramming of natural killer cell missing-self recognition *in vivo*. *Proc Natl Acad Sci USA* 2009;**106**(31):12879–84.
95. Joncker NT, Shifrin N, Delebecque F, Raulet DH. Mature natural killer cells reset their responsiveness when exposed to an altered MHC environment. *J Exp Med* 2010;**207**(10):2065–72.
96. Elliott JM, Wahle JA, Yokoyama WM. MHC class I-deficient natural killer cells acquire a licensed phenotype after transfer into an MHC class I-sufficient environment. *J Exp Med* 2010;**207**(10):2073–9.
97. Davis DM. Assembly of the immunological synapse for T cells and NK cells. *Trends Immunol* 2002;**23**(7):356–63.
98. Davis DM, Chiu I, Fassett M, Cohen GB, Mandelboim O, Strominger JL. The human natural killer cell immune synapse. *Proc Natl Acad Sci USA* 1999;**96**(26):15062–7.
99. Lou Z, Jevremovic D, Billadeau DD, Leibson PJ. A balance between positive and negative signals in cytotoxic lymphocytes regulates the polarization of lipid rafts during the development of cell-mediated killing. *J Exp Med* 2000;**191**(2):347–54.
100. Orange JS, Harris KE, Andzelm MM, Valter MM, Geha RS, Strominger JL. The mature activating natural killer cell immunologic synapse is formed in distinct stages. *Proc Natl Acad Sci USA* 2003;**100**(24):14151–6.
101. Bryceson YT, March ME, Barber DF, Ljunggren HG, Long EO. Cytolytic granule polarization and degranulation controlled by different receptors in resting NK cells. *J Exp Med* 2005;**202**(7):1001–12.
102. Brilot F, Strowig T, Roberts SM, Arrey F, Munz C. NK cell survival mediated through the regulatory synapse with human DCs requires IL-15Rα. *J Clin Invest* 2007;**117**(11):3316–29.
103. Barreira da Silva R, Munz C. Natural killer cell activation by dendritic cells: balancing inhibitory and activating signals. *CMLS* 2011;**68**(21):3505–18.
104. Herberman RB, Nunn ME, Lavrin DH. Natural cytotoxic reactivity of mouse lymphoid cells against syngeneic and allogeneic tumors. I. Distribution of reactivity and specificity. *Int J Cancer* 1975;**16**(2):216–29.
105. Herberman RB, Nunn ME, Holden HT, Lavrin DH. Natural cytotoxic reactivity of mouse lymphoid cells against syngeneic and allogeneic tumors. II. Characterization of effector cells. *Int J Cancer* 1975;**16**(2):230–9.
106. Kiessling R, Klein E, Wigzell H. "Natural" killer cells in the mouse. I. Cytotoxic cells with specificity for mouse Moloney leukemia cells. Specificity and distribution according to genotype. *Eur J Immunol* 1975;**5**:112–7.
107. Kiessling R, Klein E, Pross H, Wigzell H. "Natural" killer cells in the mouse. II. Cytotoxic cells with specificity for mouse Moloney leukemia cells. Characteristic of the killer cell. *Eur J Immunol* 1975;**5**:117–21.
108. Peter HH, Pavie-Fischer J, Fridman WH, Aubert C, Cesarini JP, Roubin R, et al. Cell-mediated cytotoxicity *in vitro* of human lymphocytes against a tissue culture melanoma cell line (igr3). *J Immunol* 1975;**115**(2):539–48.
109. West WH, Cannon GB, Kay HD, Bonnard GD, Herberman RB. Natural cytotoxic reactivity of human lymphocytes against a myeloid cell line: characterization of effector cells. *J Immunol* 1977;**118**(1):355–61.
110. Herberman RB, Bartram S, Haskill JS, Nunn M, Holden HT, West WH. Fc receptors on mouse effector cells mediating natural cytotoxicity against tumor cells. *J Immunol* 1977;**119**(1):322–6.
111. Perussia B, Acuto O, Terhorst C, Faust J, Lazarus R, Fanning V, et al. Human natural killer cells analyzed by B73.1, a monoclonal antibody blocking Fc receptor functions. II. Studies of B73.1 antibody–antigen interaction on the lymphocyte membrane. *J Immunol* 1983;**130**(5):2142–8.
112. Perussia B, Trinchieri G. Antibody 3G8, specific for the human neutrophil Fc receptor, reacts with natural killer cells. *J Immunol* 1984;**132**(3):1410–5.
113. Perussia B, Trinchieri G, Jackson A, Warner NL, Faust J, Rumpold H, et al. The Fc receptor for IgG on human natural killer cells: phenotypic, functional, and comparative studies with monoclonal antibodies. *J Immunol* 1984;**133**(1):180–9.
114. Perussia B, Tutt MM, Qiu WQ, Kuziel WA, Tucker PW, Trinchieri G, et al. Murine natural killer

cells express functional Fc gamma receptor II encoded by the Fc gamma R alpha gene. *J Exp Med* 1989;**170**(1):73–86.

115. Lanier LL, Le AM, Phillips JH, Warner NL, Babcock GF. Subpopulations of human natural killer cells defined by expression of the Leu-7 (HNK-1) and Leu-11 (NK-15) antigens. *J Immunol* 1983;**131**(4):1789–96.

116. Lanier LL, Yu G, Phillips JH. Co-association of CD3 zeta with a receptor (CD16) for IgG Fc on human natural killer cells. *Nature* 1989;**342**(6251):803–5.

117. Ra C, Jouvin MH, Blank U, Kinet JP. A macrophage Fc gamma receptor and the mast cell receptor for IgE share an identical subunit. *Nature* 1989;**341**(6244):752–4.

118. Hibbs ML, Selvaraj P, Carpen O, Springer TA, Kuster H, Jouvin MH, et al. Mechanisms for regulating expression of membrane isoforms of Fc gamma RIII (CD16). *Science* 1989;**246**(4937):1608–11.

119. Anderson P, Caligiuri M, O'Brien C, Manley T, Ritz J, Schlossman SF. Fc gamma receptor type III (CD16) is included in the zeta NK receptor complex expressed by human natural killer cells. *Proc Natl Acad Sci USA* 1990;**87**(6):2274–8.

120. Kurosaki T, Gander I, Ravetch JV. A subunit common to an IgG Fc receptor and the T-cell receptor mediates assembly through different interactions. *Proc Natl Acad Sci USA* 1991;**88**(9):3837–41.

121. Wirthmueller U, Kurosaki T, Murakami MS, Ravetch JV. Signal transduction by Fc gamma RIII (CD16) is mediated through the gamma chain. *J Exp Med* 1992;**175**(5):1381–90.

122. Takai T, Li M, Sylvestre D, Clynes R, Ravetch J. FcR γ chain deletion results in pleiotrophic effector cell defects. *Cell* 1994;**76**:519–29.

123. Zhang M, Zhang Z, Garmestani K, Goldman CK, Ravetch JV, Brechbiel MW, et al. Activating Fc receptors are required for antitumor efficacy of the antibodies directed toward CD25 in a murine model of adult T-cell leukemia. *Cancer Res* 2004;**64**(16):5825–9.

124. Kipps TJ, Parham P, Punt J, Herzenberg LA. Importance of immunoglobulin isotype in human antibody-dependent, cell-mediated cytotoxicity directed by murine monoclonal antibodies. *J Exp Med* 1985;**161**(1):1–17.

125. Lanier LL, Le AM, Civin CI, Loken MR, Phillips JH. The relationship of CD16 (Leu-11) and Leu-19 (NKH-1) antigen expression on human peripheral blood NK cells and cytotoxic T lymphocytes. *J Immunol* 1986;**136**(12):4480–6.

126. Vitale M, Della Chiesa M, Carlomagno S, Romagnani C, Thiel A, Moretta L, et al. The small subset of $CD56^{bright}$CD16– natural killer cells is selectively responsible for both cell proliferation and interferon-gamma production upon interaction with dendritic cells. *Eur J Immunol* 2004;**34**(6):1715–22.

127. Caligiuri MA, Zmuidzinas A, Manley TJ, Levine H, Smith KA, Ritz J. Functional consequences of interleukin 2 receptor expression on resting human lymphocytes. Identification of a novel natural killer cell subset with high affinity receptors. *J Exp Med* 1990;**171**(5):1509–26.

128. Fehniger TA, Cooper MA, Nuovo GJ, Cella M, Facchetti F, Colonna M, et al. $CD56^{bright}$ natural killer cells are present in human lymph nodes and are activated by T cell-derived IL-2: a potential new link between adaptive and innate immunity. *Blood* 2003;**101**(8):3052–7.

129. Jacobs R, Hintzen G, Kemper A, Beul K, Kempf S, Behrens G, et al. $CD56^{bright}$ cells differ in their KIR repertoire and cytotoxic features from $CD56^{dim}$ NK cells. *Eur J Immunol* 2001;**31**(10):3121–7.

130. Romagnani C, Juelke K, Falco M, Morandi B, D'Agostino A, Costa R, et al. $CD56^{bright}$CD16– killer Ig-like receptor-NK cells display longer telomeres and acquire features of $CD56^{dim}$ NK cells upon activation. *J Immunol* 2007;**178**(8):4947–55.

131. Caligiuri MA. Human natural killer cells. *Blood* 2008;**112**(3):461–9.

132. Narni-Mancinelli E, Chaix J, Fenis A, Kerdiles YM, Yessaad N, Reynders A, et al. Fate mapping analysis of lymphoid cells expressing the NKp46 cell surface receptor. *Proc Natl Acad Sci USA* 2011;**108**(45):18324–9.

133. Bryceson YT, March ME, Ljunggren HG, Long EO. Activation, coactivation, and costimulation of resting human natural killer cells. *Immunol Rev.* 2006;**214**:73–91.

134. Bryceson YT, March ME, Ljunggren HG, Long EO. Synergy among receptors on resting NK cells for the activation of natural cytotoxicity and cytokine secretion. *Blood* 2006;**107**(1):159–66.

135. Ho EL, Heusel JW, Brown MG, Matsumoto K, Scalzo AA, Yokoyama WM. Murine Nkg2d and Cd94 are clustered within the natural killer complex and are expressed independently in natural killer cells. *Proc Natl Acad Sci USA* 1998;**95**:6320–5.

136. Vance RE, Tanamachi DM, Hanke T, Raulet DH. Cloning of a mouse homolog of CD94 extends the family of C-type lectins on murine natural killer cells. *Eur J Immunol* 1997;**27**:3236–41.

137. Wu J, Song Y, Bakker AB, Bauer S, Spies T, Lanier LL, et al. An activating immunoreceptor complex formed by NKG2D and DAP10. *Science* 1999;**285**(5428):730–2.

138. Chang C, Dietrich J, Harpur AG, Lindquist JA, Haude A, et al. KAP10, a Novel Transmembrane Adapter Protein Genetically Linked to DAP12 but with Unique Signaling Properties. *J Immunol* 1999;**163**(9):4652–4.

139. Garrity D, Call ME, Feng J, Wucherpfennig KW. The activating NKG2D receptor assembles in the membrane with two signaling dimers into a hexameric structure. *Proc Natl Acad Sci USA* 2005;**102**(21):7641–6.
140. Billadeau DD, Upshaw JL, Schoon RA, Dick CJ, Leibson PJ. NKG2D-DAP10 triggers human NK cell-mediated killing via a Syk-independent regulatory pathway. *Nat Immunol* 2003;**4**(6):557–64.
141. Zompi S, Hamerman JA, Ogasawara K, Schweighoffer E, Tybulewicz VL, Santo JP, et al. NKG2D triggers cytotoxicity in mouse NK cells lacking DAP12 or Syk family kinases. *Nat Immunol* 2003;**4**(6):565–72.
142. Upshaw JL, Arneson LN, Schoon RA, Dick CJ, Billadeau DD, Leibson PJ. NKG2D-mediated signaling requires a DAP10-bound Grb2–Vav1 intermediate and phosphatidylinositol-3-kinase in human natural killer cells. *Nat Immunol* 2006;**7**(5):524–32.
143. Gilfillan S, Ho EL, Cella M, Yokoyama WM, Colonna M. NKG2D recruits two distinct adapters to trigger natural killer cell activation and costimulation. *Nat Immunol* 2002;**3**(12):1150–5.
144. Diefenbach A, Tomasello E, Lucas M, Jamieson AM, Hsia JK, Vivier E, et al. Selective associations with signaling molecules determines stimulatory versus costimulatory activity of NKG2D. *Nat Immunol* 2002;**3**(12):1142–9.
145. Tomasello E, Olcese L, Vély F, Geourgeon C, Bléry M, Moqrich A, et al. Gene structure, expression pattern, and biological activity of mouse killer cell activating receptor-associated protein (KARAP)/DAP-12. *J Biol Chem* 1998;**273**(51):34115–9.
146. Lanier LL, Corliss BC, Wu J, Leong C, Phillips JH. Immunoreceptor DAP12 bearing a tyrosine-based activation motif is involved in activating NK cells. *Nature* 1998;**391**(6668):703–7.
147. Rosen DB, Araki M, Hamerman JA, Chen T, Yamamura T, Lanier LL. A Structural basis for the association of DAP12 with mouse, but not human, NKG2D. *J Immunol* 2004;**173**(4):2470–8.
148. Colucci F, Schweighoffer E, Tomasello E, Turner M, Ortaldo JR, Vivier E, et al. Natural cytotoxicity uncoupled from the Syk and ZAP-70 intracellular kinases. *Nat Immunol* 2002;**3**(3):288–94.
149. Groh V, Rhinehart R, Randolph-Habecker J, Topp MS, Riddell SR, Spies T. Costimulation of CD8 αβ T cells by NKG2D via engagement by MIC induced on virus-infected cells. *Nat Immunol* 2001;**2**(3):255–60.
150. Jamieson AM, Diefenbach A, McMahon CW, Xiong N, Carlyle JR, Raulet DH. The role of the NKG2D immunoreceptor in immune cell activation and natural killing. *Immunity* 2002;**17**(1):19–29.
151. Diefenbach A, Jensen ER, Jamieson AM, Raulet DH. Rae1 and H60 ligands of the NKG2D receptor stimulate tumour immunity. *Nature* 2001;**413**(6852):165–71.
152. Giorda R, Rudert WA, Vavassori C, Chambers WH, Hiserodt JC, Trucco M. NKR-P1, a signal transduction molecule on natural killer cells. *Science* 1990;**249**(4974):1298–300.
153. Koo GC, Dumont FJ, Tutt M, Hackett Jr J, Kumar V. The NK-1.1(–) mouse: a model to study differentiation of murine NK cells. *J Immunol* 1986;**137**:3742–7.
154. Bahram S, Bresnahan M, Geraghty DE, Spies T. A second lineage of mammalian major histocompatibility complex class I genes. *Proc Natl Acad Sci USA* 1994;**91**(14):6259–63.
155. Steinle A, Groh V, Spies T. Diversification, expression, and γδ T cell recognition of evolutionarily distant members of the MIC family of major histocompatibility complex class I-related molecules. *Proc Natl Acad Sci USA* 1998;**95**(21):12510–5.
156. Bauer S, Groh V, Wu J, Steinle A, Phillips JH, Lanier LL, et al. Activation of NK cells and T cells by NKG2D, a receptor for stress-inducible MICA. *Science* 1999;**285**(5428):727–9.
157. Groh V, Bahram S, Bauer S, Herman A, Beauchamp M, Spies T. Cell stress-regulated human major histocompatibility complex class I gene expressed in gastrointestinal epithelium. *Proc Natl Acad Sci USA* 1996;**93**(22):12445–50.
158. Groh V, Steinle A, Bauer S, Spies T. Recognition of stress-induced MHC molecules by intestinal epithelial γδ T cells. *Science* 1998;**279**(5357):1737–40.
159. Wu J, Groh V, Spies T. T cell antigen receptor engagement and specificity in the recognition of stress-inducible MHC class I-related chains by human epithelial gamma delta T cells. *J Immunol* 2002;**169**(3):1236–40.
160. Amadou C, Kumánovics A, Jones EP, Lambracht-Washington D, Yoshino M, Lindahl KF. The mouse major histocompatibility complex: some assembly required. *Immunol Rev* 1999;**167**(5):211–21.
161. Diefenbach A, Raulet DH. Strategies for target cell recognition by natural killer cells. *Immunol Rev* 2001;**181**:170–84.
162. Cerwenka A, Bakker ABH, McClanahan T, Wagner J, Wu J, Phillips JH, et al. Retinoic acid early inducible genes define a ligand family for the activating NKG2D receptor in mice. *Immunity* 2000;**12**(6):721–7.
163. Diefenbach A, Jamieson AM, Liu SD, Shastri N, Raulet DH. Ligands for the murine NKG2D receptor: expression by tumor cells and activation of NK cells and macrophages. *Nat Immunol* 2000;**1**(2):119–26.
164. Diefenbach A, Hsia JK, Hsiung MYB, Raulet DH. A new ligand for the NKG2D receptor activates NK cells and macrophages and induces tumor immunity. *Eur J Immunol* 2003;**33**:381–91.

165. Carayannopoulos LN, Naidenko OV, Fremont DH, Yokoyama WM. Cutting edge: murine UL16-binding protein-like transcript 1: a newly described transcript encoding a high-affinity ligand for murine NKG2D. *J Immunol* 2002;**169**(8):4079–83.
166. Takada A, Yoshida S, Kajikawa M, Miyatake Y, Tomaru U, Sakai M, et al. Two novel NKG2D ligands of the mouse H60 family with differential expression patterns and binding affinities to NKG2D. *J Immunol* 2008;**180**(3):1678–85.
167. Cosman D, Müllberg J, Sutherland CL, Chin W, Armitage R, Fanslow W, et al. ULBPs, novel MHC class I-related molecules, bind to CMV glycoprotein UL16 and stimulate NK cytotoxicity through the NKG2D receptor. *Immunity* 2001;**14**:123–33.
168. Radosavljevic M, Cuillerier B, Wilson MJ, Clement O, Wicker S, Gilfillan S, et al. A cluster of ten novel MHC class I related genes on human chromosome 6q24.2–q25.3. *Genomics* 2002;**79**(1):114–23.
169. Steinle A, Li P, Morris DL, Groh V, Lanier LL, Strong RK, et al. Interactions of human NKG2D with its ligands MICA, MICB, and homologs of the mouse RAE-1 protein family. *Immunogenetics* 2001;**53**(4):279–87.
170. Sutherland CL, Chalupny NJ, Schooley K, VandenBos T, Kubin M, Cosman D. UL16-binding proteins, novel MHC class I-related proteins, bind to NKG2D and activate multiple signaling pathways in primary NK cells. *J Immunol* 2002;**168**(2):671–9.
171. Li P, McDermott G, Strong RK. Crystal structures of RAE-1β and its complex with the activating immunoreceptor NKG2D. *Immunity* 2002;**16**(1):77–86.
172. Radaev S, Rostro B, Brooks AG, Colonna M, Sun PD. Conformational plasticity revealed by the cocrystal structure of NKG2D and its class I MHC-like ligand ULBP3. *Immunity* 2001;**15**(6):1039–49.
173. Carayannopoulos LN, Naidenko OV, Kinder J, Ho EL, Fremont DH, Yokoyama WM. Ligands for murine NKG2D display heterogeneous binding behavior. *Eur J Immunol* 2002;**32**(3):597–605.
174. O'Callaghan CA, Cerwenka A, Willcox BE, Lanier LL, Bjorkman PJ. Molecular competition for NKG2D: H60 and RAE1 compete unequally for NKG2D with dominance of H60. *Immunity* 2001;**15**(2):201–11.
175. Krmpotic A, Busch DH, Bubic I, Gebhardt F, Hengel H, Hasan M, et al. MCMV glycoprotein gp40 confers virus resistance to CD8+ T cells and NK cells *in vivo*. *Nat Immunol* 2002;**3**(6):529–35.
176. Lodoen M, Ogasawara K, Hamerman JA, Arase H, Houchins JP, Mocarski ES, et al. NKG2D-mediated natural killer cell protection against cytomegalovirus is impaired by viral gp40 modulation of retinoic acid early inducible 1 gene molecules. *J Exp Med* 2003;**197**(10):1245–53.
177. Krmpotic A, Hasan M, Loewendorf A, Saulig T, Halenius A, Lenac T, et al. NK cell activation through the NKG2D ligand MULT-1 is selectively prevented by the glycoprotein encoded by mouse cytomegalovirus gene m145. *J Exp Med* 2005;**201**(2):211–20.
178. Cerwenka A, Baron JL, Lanier LL. Ectopic expression of retinoic acid early inducible-1 gene (RAE-1) permits natural killer cell-mediated rejection of a MHC class I-bearing tumor *in vivo*. *Proc Natl Acad Sci USA* 2001;**98**(20):11521–6.
179. Raulet DH. Roles of the NKG2D immunoreceptor and its ligands. *Nat Rev Immunol* 2003;**3**(10):781–90.
180. Diefenbach A, Raulet DH. The innate immune response to tumors and its role in the induction of T cell immunity. *Immunol Rev* 2002;**188**:9–21.
181. Medzhitov R, Janeway Jr CA. Decoding the patterns of self and nonself by the innate immune system. *Science* 2002;**296**(5566):298–300.
182. Diefenbach A, Raulet DH. Innate immune recognition by stimulatory immunoreceptors. *Curr Opin Immunol* 2003;**15**(1):37–44.
183. Guerra N, Tan YX, Joncker NT, Choy A, Gallardo F, Xiong N, et al. NKG2D-deficient mice are defective in tumor surveillance in models of spontaneous malignancy. *Immunity* 2008;**28**(4):571–80.
184. Venkataraman GM, Suciu D, Groh V, Boss JM, Spies T. Promoter region architecture and transcriptional regulation of the genes for the MHC class I-related chain A and B ligands of NKG2D. *J Immunol* 2007;**178**(2):961–9.
185. Gasser S, Orsulic S, Brown EJ, Raulet DH. The DNA damage pathway regulates innate immune system ligands of the NKG2D receptor. *Nature* 2005;**436**(7054):1186–90.
186. Raulet DH, Guerra N. Oncogenic stress sensed by the immune system: role of natural killer cell receptors. *Nat Rev Immunol* 2009;**9**(8):568–80.
187. Raulet DH, Gasser S, Gowen BG, Deng W, Jung H. Regulation of ligands for the NKG2D activating receptor. *Annu Rev Immunol* 2013;**31**:413–41.
188. Krizhanovsky V, Yon M, Dickins RA, Hearn S, Simon J, Miething C, et al. Senescence of activated stellate cells limits liver fibrosis. *Cell* 2008;**134**(4):657–67.
189. Groh V, Wu J, Yee C, Spies T. Tumour-derived soluble MIC ligands impair expression of NKG2D and T-cell activation. *Nature* 2002;**419**(6908):734–8.
190. Kaiser BK, Yim D, Chow IT, Gonzalez S, Dai Z, Mann HH, et al. Disulphide-isomerase-enabled shedding of tumour-associated NKG2D ligands. *Nature* 2007;**447**(7143):482–6.
191. Waldhauer I, Goehlsdorf D, Gieseke F, Weinschenk T, Wittenbrink M, Ludwig A, et al. Tumor-associated MICA is shed by ADAM proteases. *Cancer Res* 2008;**68**(15):6368–76.

192. Boutet P, Aguera-Gonzalez S, Atkinson S, Pennington CJ, Edwards DR, Murphy G, et al. Cutting edge: the metalloproteinase ADAM17/TNF-alpha-converting enzyme regulates proteolytic shedding of the MHC class I-related chain B protein. *J Immunol* 2009;**182**(1):49–53.
193. Fernandez-Messina L, Ashiru O, Boutet P, Aguera-Gonzalez S, Skepper JN, Reyburn HT, et al. Differential mechanisms of shedding of the glycosylphosphatidylinositol (GPI)-anchored NKG2D ligands. *J Biol Chem* 2010;**285**(12):8543–51.
194. Armeanu S, Bitzer M, Lauer UM, Venturelli S, Pathil A, Krusch M, et al. Natural killer cell-mediated lysis of hepatoma cells via specific induction of NKG2D ligands by the histone deacetylase inhibitor sodium valproate. *Cancer Res* 2005;**65**(14):6321–9.
195. Skov S, Pedersen MT, Andresen L, Straten PT, Woetmann A, Odum N. Cancer cells become susceptible to natural killer cell killing after exposure to histone deacetylase inhibitors due to glycogen synthase kinase-3-dependent expression of MHC class I-related chain A and B. *Cancer Res* 2005;**65**(23):11136–45.
196. Lopez-Soto A, Folgueras AR, Seto E, Gonzalez S. HDAC3 represses the expression of NKG2D ligands ULBPs in epithelial tumour cells: potential implications for the immunosurveillance of cancer. *Oncogene* 2009;**28**(25):2370–82.
197. Gonzalez S, Lopez-Soto A, Suarez-Alvarez B, Lopez-Vazquez A, Lopez-Larrea C. NKG2D ligands: key targets of the immune response. *Trends Immunol* 2008;**29**(8):397–403.
198. Lucas M, Schachterle W, Oberle K, Aichele P, Diefenbach A. Dendritic cells prime natural killer cells by *trans*-presenting interleukin 15. *Immunity* 2007;**26**(4):503–17.
199. Fehniger TA, Cai SF, Cao X, Bredemeyer AJ, Presti RM, French AR, et al. Acquisition of murine NK cell cytotoxicity requires the translation of a pre-existing pool of granzyme B and perforin mRNAs. *Immunity* 2007;**26**(6):798–811.
200. Fernandez NC, Lozier A, Flament C, Ricciardi-Castagnoli P, Bellet D, Suter M, et al. Dendritic cells directly trigger NK cell functions: cross-talk relevant in innate anti-tumor immune responses *in vivo*. *Nat Med* 1999;**5**(4):405–11.
201. Andrews DM, Scalzo AA, Yokoyama WM, Smyth MJ, Degli-Esposti MA. Functional interactions between dendritic cells and NK cells during viral infection. *Nat Immunol* 2003;**4**(2):175–81.
202. Arase H, Mocarski ES, Campbell AE, Hill AB, Lanier LL. Direct recognition of cytomegalovirus by activating and inhibitory NK cell receptors. *Science* 2002;**296**(5571):1323–6.
203. Smith HR, Heusel JW, Mehta IK, Kim S, Dorner BG, Naidenko OV, et al. Recognition of a virus-encoded ligand by a natural killer cell activation receptor. *Proc Natl Acad Sci USA* 2002;**99**(13):8826–31.
204. Ferlazzo G, Pack M, Thomas D, Paludan C, Schmid D, Strowig T, et al. Distinct roles of IL-12 and IL-15 in human natural killer cell activation by dendritic cells from secondary lymphoid organs. *Proc Natl Acad Sci USA* 2004;**101**(47):16606–11.
205. Martin-Fontecha A, Thomsen LL, Brett S, Gerard C, Lipp M, Lanzavecchia A, et al. Induced recruitment of NK cells to lymph nodes provides IFN-gamma for T(H)1 priming. *Nat Immunol* 2004;**5**(12):1260–5.
206. Jung S, Unutmaz D, Wong P, Sano G, De los Santos K, Sparwasser T, et al. *In vivo* depletion of CD11c+ dendritic cells abrogates priming of CD8+ T cells by exogenous cell-associated antigens. *Immunity* 2002;**17**:211–20.
207. Hochweller K, Striegler J, Hammerling GJ, Garbi N. A novel CD11c.DTR transgenic mouse for depletion of dendritic cells reveals their requirement for homeostatic proliferation of natural killer cells. *Eur J Immunol* 2008;**38**(10):2776–83.
208. Schleicher U, Liese J, Knippertz I, Kurzmann C, Hesse A, Heit A, et al. NK cell activation in visceral leishmaniasis requires TLR9, myeloid DCs, and IL-12, but is independent of plasmacytoid DCs. *J Exp Med* 2007;**204**(4):893–906.
209. Biassoni R, Falco M, Cambiaggi A, Costa P, Verdiani S, Pende D, et al. Amino acid substitutions can influence the natural killer (NK)-mediated recognition of HLA-C molecules. Role of serine-77 and lysine-80 in the target cell protection from lysis mediated by "group 2" or "group 1" NK clones. *J Exp Med* 1995;**182**(2):605–9.
210. Bihl F, Pecheur J, Breart B, Poupon G, Cazareth J, Julia V, et al. Primed antigen-specific CD4+ T cells are required for NK cell activation *in vivo* upon *Leishmania major* infection. *J Immunol* 2010;**185**(4):2174–81.
211. McCartney S, Vermi W, Gilfillan S, Cella M, Murphy TL, Schreiber RD, et al. Distinct and complementary functions of MDA5 and TLR3 in poly(I:C)-mediated activation of mouse NK cells. *J Exp Med* 2009;**206**(13):2967–76.
212. Baranek T, Manh TP, Alexandre Y, Maqbool MA, Cabeza JZ, Tomasello E, et al. Differential responses of immune cells to type I interferon contribute to host resistance to viral infection. *Cell Host Microbe* 2012;**12**(4):571–84.
213. Mattei F, Schiavoni G, Belardelli F, Tough DF. IL-15 is expressed by dendritic cells in response to type I IFN, double-stranded RNA, or lipopolysaccharide and promotes dendritic cell activation. *J Immunol* 2001;**167**(3):1179–87.

214. Koka R, Burkett P, Chien M, Chai S, Boone DL, Ma A. Cutting edge: murine dendritic cells require IL-15R alpha to prime NK cells. *J Immunol* 2004;**173**(6):3594–8.
215. Mortier E, Woo T, Advincula R, Gozalo S, Ma A. IL-15Rα chaperones IL-15 to stable dendritic cell membrane complexes that activate NK cells via *trans* presentation. *J Exp Med* 2008;**205**(5):1213–25.
216. Jaeger BN, Donadieu J, Cognet C, Bernat C, Ordonez-Rueda D, Barlogis V, et al. Neutrophil depletion impairs natural killer cell maturation, function, and homeostasis. *J Exp Med* 2012;**209**(3):565–80.
217. Schulthess J, Meresse B, Ramiro-Puig E, Montcuquet N, Darche S, Begue B, et al. Interleukin-15-dependent NKp46+ innate lymphoid cells control intestinal inflammation by recruiting inflammatory monocytes. *Immunity* 2012;**37**(1):108–21.
218. Coombes JL, Han SJ, van Rooijen N, Raulet DH, Robey EA. Infection-induced regulation of natural killer cells by macrophages and collagen at the lymph node subcapsular sinus. *Cell Reports* 2012;**2**(1):124–35.
219. Scalzo AA, Fitzgerald NA, Simmons A, La Vista AB, Shellam GR. Cmv-1, a genetic locus that controls murine cytomegalovirus replication in the spleen. *J Exp Med* 1990;**171**(5):1469–83.
220. Tay CH, Welsh RM. Distinct organ-dependent mechanisms for the control of murine cytomegalovirus infection by natural killer cells. *J Virol* 1997;**71**(1):267–75.
221. Scalzo AA, Lyons PA, Fitzgerald NA, Forbes CA, Yokoyama WM, Shellam GR. Genetic mapping of Cmv1 in the region of mouse chromosome 6 encoding the NK gene complex-associated loci Ly49 and musNKR-P1. *Genomics* 1995;**27**(3):435–41.
222. Forbes CA, Brown MG, Cho R, Shellam GR, Yokoyama WM, Scalzo AA. The Cmv1 host resistance locus is closely linked to the Ly49 multigene family within the natural killer cell gene complex on chromosome 6. *Genomics* 1997;**41**:406–13.
223. Depatie C, Lee SH, Stafford A, Avner P, Belouchi A, Gros P, et al. Sequence-ready BAC contig, physical, and transcriptional map of a 2-Mb region overlapping the mouse chromosome 6 host-resistance locus Cmv1. *Genomics* 2000;**66**(2):161–74.
224. Brown MG, Dokun AO, Heusel JW, Smith HR, Beckman DL, Blattenberger EA, et al. Vital involvement of a natural killer cell activation receptor in resistance to viral infection. *Science* 2001;**292**(5518):934–7.
225. Lee SH, Girard S, Macina D, Busa M, Zafer A, Belouchi A, et al. Susceptibility to mouse cytomegalovirus is associated with deletion of an activating natural killer cell receptor of the C-type lectin superfamily. *Nat Genet* 2001;**28**(1):42–5.
226. Tomasello E, Desmoulins PO, Chemin K, Guia S, Cremer H, Ortaldo J, et al. Combined natural killer cell and dendritic cell functional deficiency in KARAP/DAP12 loss-of-function mutant mice. *Immunity* 2000;**13**:355–64.
227. Bakker ABH, Hoek RM, Cerwenka A, Blom B, Lucian L, McNeil T, et al. DAP12-deficient mice fail to develop autoimmunity due to impaired antigen priming. *Immunity* 2000;**13**:345–53.
228. Sun JC, Beilke JN, Lanier LL. Adaptive immune features of natural killer cells. *Nature* 2009;**457**(7229):557–61.
229. Sun JC, Madera S, Bezman NA, Beilke JN, Kaplan MH, Lanier LL. Proinflammatory cytokine signaling required for the generation of natural killer cell memory. *J Exp Med* 2012;**209**(5):947–54.
230. Cooper MA, Elliott JM, Keyel PA, Yang L, Carrero JA, Yokoyama WM. Cytokine-induced memory-like natural killer cells. *Proc Natl Acad Sci USA* 2009;**106**(6):1915–9.
231. Ni J, Miller M, Stojanovic A, Garbi N, Cerwenka A. Sustained effector function of IL-12/15/18-preactivated NK cells against established tumors. *J Exp Med* 2012;**209**(13):2351–65.
232. Bjorkstrom NK, Lindgren T, Stoltz M, Fauriat C, Braun M, Evander M, et al. Rapid expansion and long-term persistence of elevated NK cell numbers in humans infected with hantavirus. *J Exp Med* 2011;**208**(1):13–21.
233. O'Leary JG, Goodarzi M, Drayton DL, von Andrian UH. T cell- and B cell-independent adaptive immunity mediated by natural killer cells. *Nat Immunol* 2006;**7**(5):507–16.
234. Paust S, Gill HS, Wang BZ, Flynn MP, Moseman EA, Senman B, et al. Critical role for the chemokine receptor CXCR6 in NK cell-mediated antigen-specific memory of haptens and viruses. *Nat Immunol* 2010;**11**(12):1127–35.

CHAPTER

5

Phagocytes and Immunoglobulins

Luisa Martinez-Pomares

Faculty of Medicine and Health Sciences, University of Nottingham, Queen's Medical Centre, Nottingham, United Kingdom

ANTIBODIES IN THE CONTEXT OF INNATE AND ACQUIRED IMMUNE RECOGNITION

Soluble and cellular components of the innate immune system in collaboration sense changes in the physiological status of tissues caused by infection or trauma and orchestrate inflammatory responses that facilitate containment of the infectious agent and restoration of tissue integrity.[1–3] Antibodies are normally considered part of the acquired immune response, as most are produced in an antigen-specific fashion by plasma cells, but natural immunoglobulin M (IgM), produced by innate B-cell populations,[4] is now recognized as a *bona fide* component of the innate immune system. Natural IgM is poly-reactive and cross-reacts with endogenouos antigens, such as apoptotic cells, and pathogens.[4,5] Early detection of conserved microbial components by natural IgM promotes early complement activation through the classical pathway and mediates protection against multiple infectious agents such as influenza virus *Pseudomonas aeruginosa* and *Toxoplasma gondii*. Once acquired immunity is engaged, antigen-specific antibodies increase the effectiveness of the inflammatory response by promoting targeted killing and phagocytosis of the infectious agent or infected/damaged cells through antibody-dependent cell-mediated cytotoxicity (ADCC), antibody-dependent cellular phagocytosis (ADCP), or antibody-dependent, complement-dependent cytotoxicity (ADCDC).

GENERAL CHARACTERISTICS OF MONONUCLEAR PHAGOCYTES: MACROPHAGES, MONOCYTES, AND DENDRITIC CELLS

Mononuclear phagocytes are comprised of three major cellular subsets: macrophages, dendritic cells, and monocytes. Macrophages are widely distributed throughout tissues where they perform important clearance functions necessary for maintenance of tissue homeostasis such as uptake of apoptotic cells and effete red blood cells and clearance of serum components.[6] These cells originate from precursors in the bone marrow and adopt tissue-specific characteristics that depend on the cues provided by the environment.[7] Dendritic cells

(DCs) share numerous phenotypic characteristics with macrophages but are uniquely specialized for the presentation of antigen to naive T cells and the initiation and regulation of adaptive immunity. There are several subsets of DCs, including conventional DCs (cDCs), originally found in lymphoid organs and detected at low levels in blood; Langerhans cells that reside in the epidermis; plasmacytoid DCs specialized in type I IFN production; and inflammatory DC or Tip-DCs. Macrophages and DCs are derived from a common hematopoietic precursor (macrophage/DC precursor, or MDP) that gives rise to cDCs, plasmacytoid DCs, and monocytes. Monocytes will differentiate into macrophages, Langerhans cells, and inflammatory DCs.[7,8] Blood monocytes represent the circulating precursors of most tissue macrophages and inflammatory DCs but also act as important effector cells in their own right; they can be considered as the "blood-resident macrophages," with subtypes specialized in patrolling blood vessels (see below). Monocytes account for 10% of human and 4% of mouse blood leukocytes, and their differentiation from MDCP is driven by M-CSF (also termed CSF-1).[8] Expression of the FcγR CD16 was originally used to identify subsets of human monocytes.[9] $CD14^+CD16^{++}$ monocytes were initially considered distinct from the $CD14^+CD16^-$ subset and as the human counterpart of mouse $Gr1^-$ monocytes.[9] Recent evidence suggests that CD16 may be a marker of activation and that $CD14^+$ monocytes (both, $CD16^-$ and $CD16^+$) correspond to mouse $Gr1^+$ monocytes and specialize in phagocytosis and production of radical oxygen species (ROS) and proinflammatory cytokines.[10–12] $CD14^{dim}$ human monocytes, which also express CD16, correspond to $Gr1^-$ mouse monocytes, patrol blood vessels, and appear to survey tissue for signs of viral infection or tissue damage.[10] Monocytes of atopic individuals have been shown to express functional high-affinity IgE receptors (FcεRI).[13] Receptors for IgA are also expressed by myeloid cells, particularly neutrophils and eosinophils, as well as subpopulations of monocytes/macrophages and dendritic cells.[14] Tissue specialization in macrophages is clearly illustrated in the mouse by the differential expression of cellular markers, some with macrophage-restricted expression.[6,15] Numbers of macrophages increase during inflammation, in most cases through the recruitment of monocytes and their differentiation into elicited macrophages (see below), but under Th2-driven inflammation this can occur through cellular proliferation (see Table 5.1).[16]

GENERAL CHARACTERISTICS OF GRANULOCYTES

Granulocytes are generally absent from healthy tissues but are readily recruited upon inflammation. Additional pools of granulocytes will be mobilized from the bone marrow during inflammatory conditions as a means to provide sustainable recruitment of these short-lived cells. Based on their affinities for histological stains and their nuclear morphology, granulocytes are divided into neutrophils, eosinophils, and basophis. Eosinophil granules are strongly labeled with eosin, whereas basophils contain granules that can be stained with basophilic aniline dyes. Neutrophils present a segmented nucleus and their granular contents are neutrophilic.

In general, neutrophils are the first cells recruited in response to an immunological insult such as trauma or bacterial infection, while eosinophils are recruited under selected circumstances such as parasitic infections and allergic responses. In addition to their recruitment being promoted by Th2-driven responses, eosinophils are themselves sources of IL4.[17–20] This property, together with the ability to express indoleamine 2,3-dioxygease (IDO)[21] and eosinophil-derived neurotoxin,[22] places eosinophils as key promoters of Th2 immunity.

Under steady-state conditions, eosinophils reside in the gastrointestinal track, uterus,

TABLE 5.1 General Characteristics of Macrophages and Neutrophils

Neutrophils	Macrophages
Both arise from a common precursors in the bone marrow Both regulate innate and adaptive immune responses Both collaborate in inflammatory sites without the contribution of the adaptive immune system Both undergo enhanced activation in response to cytokines (e.g., GM-CSF) and engagement of pattern recognition receptors Both have high phagocytic activity, both opsonic and non-opsonic	
Short lived	**Long lived**
Absence in healthy tissues Recruited during inflammation	Present in tissues as resident macrophages Primary inducers of an inflammatory response Mediate recruitment of neutrophils
Key growth factor: G-CSF	Key growth factor: M-CSF
Preformed antimicrobial peptides and proteases already stored in granules	Antimicrobial products need to be synthesized upon activation In general less microbicidal and cytotoxic
Low numbers in blood, fast mobilization from the bone marrow upon inflammation	Elicited macrophages (and inflammatory DCs) generated in tissues from monocytes during inflammation
Rapid production of oxygen radicals Reactive oxygen species and hypochlorous acid still regarded as the critical killing mechanism	Production of reactive nitrogen species
Can generate extracellular traps (NETs) Their action has to be tightly controlled to avoid excessive tissue damage	Key role in restoring tissue homeostasis after inflammation; uptake of apoptotic neutrophils contributes to this role

thymus, mammary glands, and bone marrow, where they might contribute to important homeostatic processes such as preparation of the mature uterus for pregnancy, postnatal mammary gland development, maintenance of the epithelial cell barrier, maintenance of plasma cells in bone marrow, and MHC class I (MHC-I)-restricted thymocyte deletion. Eosinophils express MHC class II (MHC-II) co-stimulatory molecules, are capable of migrating to T-cell areas of draining lymph nodes, and can present antigen to T cells *in vitro*. Additionally, eosinophils are important sources of cytokines such as IL-3 and GM-CSF and, through the production of TGF-β, osteopontin, vascular endothelial cell growth factor, and metalloproteases, and could contribute to tissue remodelling.[23]

The effector functions of eosinophils are mediated through the release of the granule contents including cytotoxic proteins such as major basic protein, eosinophil cationic protein and eosinophil peroxidase. Lipid mediators include leukotriene (LT) C4 that is processed into LTD4 and LTE4. These mediators promote contraction of smooth muscle cells, mucus secretion, modulation of vascular permeability, and recruitment of neutrophils and eosinophils.[23]

Eosinophils can undergo innate immune stimulation; they express several Toll-like receptors (TLRs, see below) and protease-activated receptors that are activated by proteolytic enzymes produced by microbes and allergens. Eosinophil degranulation can be induced by sepharose beads coated with IgG, IgA, and secreted IgA (sIgA). sIgA was found to be a very potent stimulus, which may be caused by the existence of a binding site for the secretory component. Human eosinophils express CD89 (FcαR)[24] and CD32 (FcγRII),[25] raising the possibility that IgA and IgG could promote eosinophil degranulation at mucosal sites. There is controversy regarding the role that IgE might play on eosinophil degranulation in spite of the fact that eosinophils can potentially express the three IgE receptors (high- and low-affinity FcεR) and the lectin receptor CD23.[26] β_2 integrins (mostly Mac-1, CD11b/CD18$\alpha_M\beta_2$) appear to be important in controlling the consequences of eosinophil activation, being cytokine production versus degranulation.[27] This observation correlates with findings relating the size of the surface to which Ig (IgG or IgA) is attached and their capacity to induce degranulation. In hypereosinophilic patients, eosinophils express FcRεRI. In these cells, FcRεRI is involved in eosinophil degranulation and could contribute to cytotoxic responses against *Schistosoma mansoni*.[28]

Basophils are less abundant than neutrophils and eosinophils. In spite of their similarity to tissue mast cells, basophils are not considered their precursors and are rarely found in tissues. Their numbers increase during Th2-driven inflammatory responses. Basophils produce a wide range of immune modulators, including histamine and platelet-activating factor (PAF), leukotriene C4, and the Th2-associated cytokines IL-4 and IL-13, and they express the $\alpha\beta\gamma_2$ form of the high-affinity receptor for IgE (FcεRI).[29,30]

Neutrophils are the most abundant immune cell type. Under physiological conditions most neutrophils are in the bone marrow, with only 2% being present in blood. During inflammation the number of circulating neutrophils is increased through the action of granulocyte-colony stimulating factor (G-CSF).[31] Neutrophils play a key role in host defense as exemplified by the life-threatening effects of deficiencies in neutrophil recruitment and function.[32] Neutrophils are highly active phagocytic cells and have the capacity to produce cytokines and chemokines.[33] The most characteristic role of neutrophils is their ability to undergo the extracellular respiratory burst consisting of a non-mitochondrial reduction of oxygen to forms less reduced but more reactive than water (reactive oxygen intermediates, or ROIs) that can interact with macromolecules, leading to their oxidation and lack of function. These include superoxide, singlet oxygen, ozone, hydrogen peroxide (H_2O_2), hypohalous acids, chloramines, and hydroxyl radicals. In phagocytes (neutrohils and macrophages) superoxide is generated by the phagocyte NAPDH oxidase (phox), which consists of the membrane-bound gp91^{phox}–p22^{phox} heterodimer (the catalytic cytochrome *b*559) and the regulatory cytosolic subunits p67^{phox}, p47^{phox}, p40^{phox}, and small GTPase Rac1/2.[34,35]

Neutrophils store microbicidal products in three sets of granules that are discharged in the following order: secondary and tertiary first and primary or azurophilic later. Secondary and tertiary granules contain lactoferrin, lipocalin, and the chemotatic and microbicidal peptide LL37 as well as metalloproteases 8, 9, and 25, which facilitate tissue degradation. Azurophilic granules contain myeloperoxidase; defensins; bactericidal permeability increasing (BPI) protein that binds to lipopolysaccharide (LPS); serprocidins, including the serine proteinases cathepsin G; proteinase 3; and neutrophil elastase and azurocidin or CAP54. Myeloperoxidase converts H_2O_2 into hypochlorous acid (HOCl), hypobromous acid (HOBr), and hypoiodous acid (HOI).[35]

During inflammation, neutrophils can undergo NETosis, which is a form of cell death that leads to the formation of neutrophil extracellular traps (NETs). NETs consist of nuclear components associated with proteins derived from the different neutrophil granules. NET formation favors the trapping of microorganisms and their exposure to granule contents (see Table 5.1).[33]

OPSONIC AND NON-OPSONIC RECOGNITION IN PHAGOCYTES

The distinction between non-opsonic and opsonic recognition by macrophages and granulocytes provides a useful framework to discuss the role of complement and immunoglobulin in the facilitation of antigen recognition by phagocytes. Phagocytes can bind antigens directly (non-opsonic recognition) or indirectly via a bridging molecule (opsonic recognition). The bridging molecule could be a complement fragment, usually iC3b recognized through complement receptors, or an antibody, recognized by FcRs. Main characteristics of non-opsonic and opsonic recognition are presented below.

NON-OPSONIC RECOGNITION: PATTERN RECOGNITION RECEPTORS

Macrophages can ascertain the health status of tissues through the expression of a wide range of non-opsonic receptors called *pattern-recognition receptors* (PRRs),[36–38] that recognize molecules associated with the presence of microbes (microbe-associated molecular patterns, or MAMPs) or cellular damage (damage associated molecular patterns, or DAMPs).[1,2,36–40] In the case of MAMPs, PRRs generally recognize components highly conserved and essential for microbial fitness such as lipopolysaccharide, a key component of the outer cell membrane of Gram-negative bacteria,[41] and flagellin, the main component of bacterial flagellum, as well as characteristics unique to bacterial DNA and proteins such as the absence of methyl groups in CpG motifs or formyl peptides, respectively.[42] DAMPs are generally considered to be components of healthy tissues that because of trauma or stress are relocated or modified and become available for detection by PRRs. Examples of DAMPs include the highly proinflammatory nuclear component high-mobility group box 1 protein (HMGB1), oligonucleotides, polynucleotides, nucleosides, and urate.[1,2,43,44] PRRs are present at different subcellular locations (plasma membrane, endosomes, and cytoplasm), and this enables detection of a broad range of pathogens or pathogen-associated tissue damage caused by virulence factors.[38] See Table 5.2 for further details.

PRRs can do double duty as uptake and signaling receptors, with their individual contribution to ligand uptake or cellular activation being determined by the motifs present at their intracellular domain. While some PRRs (canonical PRRs) have a dominant signaling role, as shown for Toll-like receptors (TLRs) or nucleotide binding and oligomerization domain (NOD)-like receptors (NLRs), others, such as scavenger receptors[45] and lectin receptors,[46–50] are major mediators of ligand uptake and can function as facilitators of ligand recognition by the canonical PRRs or as modifiers of PRR-induced signaling. In some instances, PRRs can mediate phagocytic uptake of particulate ligands, as demonstrated in the case of scavenger receptor class A[51] and the lectin Dectin-1.[48,52] Both receptors promote phagocytic uptake when expressed in non-professional phagocytic cells.

PHAGOCYTE ACTIVATION IN RESPONSE TO NON-OPSONIC RECOGNITION

Engagement of PRRs triggers a wide range of signaling events, but activation of the family of transcription factors NF-κB (nuclear factor kappa B) is considered central to the activation of innate immune cells.[53] The NF-κB proteins form numerous homo- and heterodimers that can regulate target gene transcription differentially; they consist of five members: NF-κB1

TABLE 5.2 Major Pattern Recognition Systems in Phagocytes

Location	Recognition Systems	General Characteristics
Plasma membrane	Toll-like receptors (1, 2, 4, 5, 6)	TLR1/2 heterodimers bind tri-acyl lipoprotein and signal through MyD88. TLR2/6 heterodimers bind di-acyl lipoprotein and signal through MyD88. TLR4 together with MD2 form the LPS–receptor complex. TLR4 signals through MyD88 and TRIF. TLR5 binds flagellin and signals through MyD88.
	Lectin receptors	Mannose receptor has three binding sites for sulfated glycans, collagen, and mannosylated glycans, respectively. DC-SIGN requires Raf1 for signaling; modulates TLR signaling. Dectin-1 binds β-glucan, signals through Syk-CARD9. Dectin-2 binds mannosylated compounds, signals through Syk-CARD9.
	Scavenger receptors	Bind selected polyanionic molecules and modified lipids Collaborate with TLRs for bacterial recognition
	CD14	GPI-linked Increases sensitivity to endotoxin
Endosomes	Toll-like receptors (3, 7, 8, 9)	Recognition of nucleic acids TLR3 binds dsRNA and signals through TRIF. TLR7 and 8 ssRNA signal through MyD88. TLR9 recognizes unmethylated CpG and signals through MyD88.
Cytosol	NOD1 and NOD2	Belong to the NLR family Recognize peptidoglycan and activate NF-κB through RICK.
	Inflammasomes	Receptors belong to the NLR family and upon ligand recognition promote formation of protein complex that activates caspase I. Sense cell damage, uric acid crystals, bacterial toxins, flagellum. Activated caspase I mediates cytokine production and inflammatory cell death (pyroptosis).
	RLRs[a] RIG1, MDA-5	Helicase activity Signal through IPS-1 located at the mitochondrial surface RIG-I: Short dsRNA, 5′-triphosphate dsRNA MDA-5: Long dsRNA

[a]*RLR, retinoic acid-inducible gene (RIG)-I-like receptors.*

(p105/p50), NF-κB2 (p100/p52), RelA (p65), RelB, and c-Rel. NF-κB controls the synthesis of proinflammatory cytokines and promotes cell survival. Under steady-state conditions, NF-κB dimers are retained in the cytoplasm by IκBs, which are specific inhibitors that bind to the Rel-homology domain and interfere with its nuclear localization function. In the canonical pathway of NF-κB activation caused by proinflammatory cytokines and PRR engagement, the IκB kinase (IKK) complex is activated. IKK is comprised of the catalytic subunits IKKα and IKKβ and the regulatory subunit IKKγ. The activated IKK complex, in an IKKγ-dependent manner, catalyzes the phosphorylation of IκBs leading to its polyubiquitination and subsequent degradation by the 26S proteasome.[53,54] In this way the NF-κB dimers are released and translocate to the nucleus, bind DNA, and activate gene transcription. Negative feedback mechanisms ensure that potential damaging effects of NF-κB activation are under control. One of these mechanisms is mediated by NF-κB as genes encoding the inhibitory

IκBs are themselves NF-κB targets. NF-κB activation leads to production of proinflammatory cytokines such as TNF-α and IL-6 and chemokines such as CXCL8. In the case of IL-1β and IL-18, NF-κB activation induces synthesis of the precursors pro-IL-1β and pro-IL-18. Both cytokines require further processing by active caspase I into mature IL-1β and IL-18. Caspase I activation takes place through the formation of a multi-protein complex triggered through engagement of members of a group of cytosolic PRRs belonging to the NLR family that include NALP1, NALP3, and IPAF. These molecules sense bacterial components or cellular damage that causes mitochondrial ROS production.[55,56] Caspase I activation can also lead to an inflammatory form of cell death termed *pyroptosis*.[57,58]

Some PRRs have a unique ability to activate the transcription factors IRF-3 and -7. IRF-3 and -7 lead to production of type I interferons which is critical for protection against viral infections.[59,60] Type I IFN induces the synthesis of cellular antiviral mechanisms in an autocrine and paracrine fashion through engagement of the IFNR. It is fitting that the PRRs that selectively promote IFN synthesis are those associated with the recognition of nucleic acids such as TLR 3, 7, 8. and 9 (see Table 5.2), as well as the helicases retinoic acid-inducible gene I (RIG-1) and melanoma differentiation-associated gene 5 (MDA-5),[61] as the presence of unique nucleic acids such as unmethylated CpG, dsRNA, and RNA bearing 5′-triphosphate are signature signs of viral infection.

The breadth of responses induced by PRR engagement is further increased by their ability to activate MAP kinases, in particular ERK, JNK, and p38,[62] as well as Syk (see below).

OPSONIC RECOGNITION: FcRs AND COMPLEMENT RECEPTORS

Phagocytes interact with the Fc region of Ig through FcR. Together with basophils and mast cells, monocytes, macrophages, DCs, and neutrophils express both activating and inhibitory FcRs.[63] Human neutrophils express a unique receptor (FcγRIIIB) that is attached to the cells through a GPI link. In mice, resident monocytes and macrophages express all activating and inhibitory FcγRs (FcγRI–FcγRIV), inflammatory monocytes express FcγRI and FcγRIII, neutrophils mainly express the activating receptors FcγRIII and FcγRIV, and DCs express FcγRI, FcγRIIB, and FcγRIII. In this regard, caution is advised as the breadth of activation states displayed by phagocytes is likely to translate into changes in the expression profiles of FcRs. For instance, monocytes from systemic lupus erythematosus patients have increased FcγRI and reduced FcγRII.[64]

In mice, all activating receptors are composed of an α-chain that mediates ligand binding and lacks signaling motifs associated with the common γ-chain that bears the immunoreceptor tyrosine-based activation motif (ITAM, Tyr-X-X-(Leu/Ile)-X6-12-Tyr-X-X). In humans, the activating receptors FcγRIIA and FcγRIIC are composed of a single ligand-binding chain that contains the ITAM. Inhibitory receptors consist of a single chain that contains an immunoreceptor tyrosine-based inhibitory motif (ITIM, (Ile/Val/ Leu/Ser)-X-Tyr-X-X-(Leu/Val)).[63]

The kinase Syk mediates signaling triggered by the recognition of immunocomplexes by activating FcγRs.[63,65] Receptor cross-linking induces phosphorylation of the ITAMs by members of the SRC tyrosine kinase family. Phosphorylation in both Tyr residues within the ITAM leads to the recruitment of Syk, which binds to phosphorylated ITAMs through its Src homology 2 (SH2) domains. SH2 binding facilitates adoption of an active conformation and autophosphorylation. Phosphorylated SyK, through its numerous partners, induces a wide range of cellular responses, such as production of ROIs, cytoskeletal changes (see below section on FcR-mediated phagocytosis and endocytosis), and production of proinflammatory cytokines.[65]

The recent findings of lectin PRRs signaling through Syk either through engagement of the common γ-chain as in the case of Dectin-2 and Mincle or of the adaptor DAP-12 in the case of CLEC5a. Direct signaling occurs in the case of Dectin-1 because of the presence of hemi-TAMs (a single Tyr residue is phosphorylated, Tyr-X-X-Leu) in the cytosolic domain. These findings place Syk as a key regulator of innate immune activation in phagocytes beyond the recognition of immunocomplexes.[49,65] Syk-associated lectins have been implicated in recognition of fungi, mycobacteria, and allergens, and Mincle can sense necrotic cells through its recognition of SAP130, a DAMP. In the case of hemiITAMs, it is assumed that engagement of two phosphorylated motifs in tandem engages the two SH2 domains of Syk. Among the Syk-dependent signaling events triggered in response to Dectin-1, Dectin-2, and Mincle engagement, NF-κB-mediated activation depends on caspase recruitment domain-containing protein 9 (CARD9), which is consistent with the association between CARD9 deficiency and susceptibility to fungal infection.[66] Syk has also been implicated in the activation of the NLRP3 inflammasome following yeast infection.[67]

Inhibitory FcγRIIB plays a key role in establishing the threshold of activation of phagocytes.[63,68] In these cells, FcγRIIB inhibits events triggered by activating FcγRs, such as phagocytosis and release of proinflammatory cytokines.[69] In B cells, simultaneous stimulation of the BCR and FcγRIIB leads to ITIM phosphorylation by LYN, which causes recruitment of SRC-homology-2-domain-containing inositol-5-phosphatase (SHIP) and hydrolysis of phosphatidylinositol-3,4,5-triphosphate into phosphatidylinositol-4,5-biphosphate, which inhibit recruitment of signal transducers such as BTK and PLCγ.[69] It is likely that a similar scenario occurs in myeloid cells upon co-engagement of activating receptors (FcRs and PRRs) and FcγRIIB.

Phagocytes express complement C3 receptors (CRs). CR1, a member of the SCR (short consensus repeat) family, mediates phagocytosis by neutrophils but not by tissue macrophages. CR1 recognizes C3b and C4b and is a potent inhibitor of complement activation. CR3 and CR4 are integrins (CD11b/CD18, $\alpha_M\beta_2$ and CD11c/CD18, $\alpha_x\beta_2$) and are involved in binding to extracellular matrix in addition to mediating recognition of iC3b. Integrin activity is regulated through "inside-out signaling," which transforms the integrins from a low-affinity to a high-affinity binding state. CRIg belongs to the immunoglobulin superfamily, binds C3b, and is expressed by selected tissue macrophages.[70]

PHAGOCYTE COOPERATION DURING INFLAMMATION

The complementary properties displayed by neutrophils and macrophages regarding life span, presence of antimicrobial products, specific requirements for extravasation, ability to degranulate and form extracellular NETs, and production of metalloproteases, proinflammatory and antiinflammatory cytokines, and lipid mediators make them excellent partners for a coordinated response during inflammation (see Table 5.1 and Figure 5.1).[71,72] This response, when appropriately gauged, can lead to elimination of the triggering stimulus, followed by a resolution phase and restoration of organ function. While the emphasis in innate immunity and phagocyte biology has been on the events triggering inflammation, the prevalence of inflammatory diseases, in many cases driven or associated with the presence of pathological Ig, makes understanding the mechanism controlling inflammation of clinical importance.[3,73,74] In the context of Ig-driven inflammation, understanding how cellular activation could be dampened through engagement of inhibitory Fc receptors[3] or bystander activation of lectin receptors or TLRs (see below) would have significant therapeutic relevance.

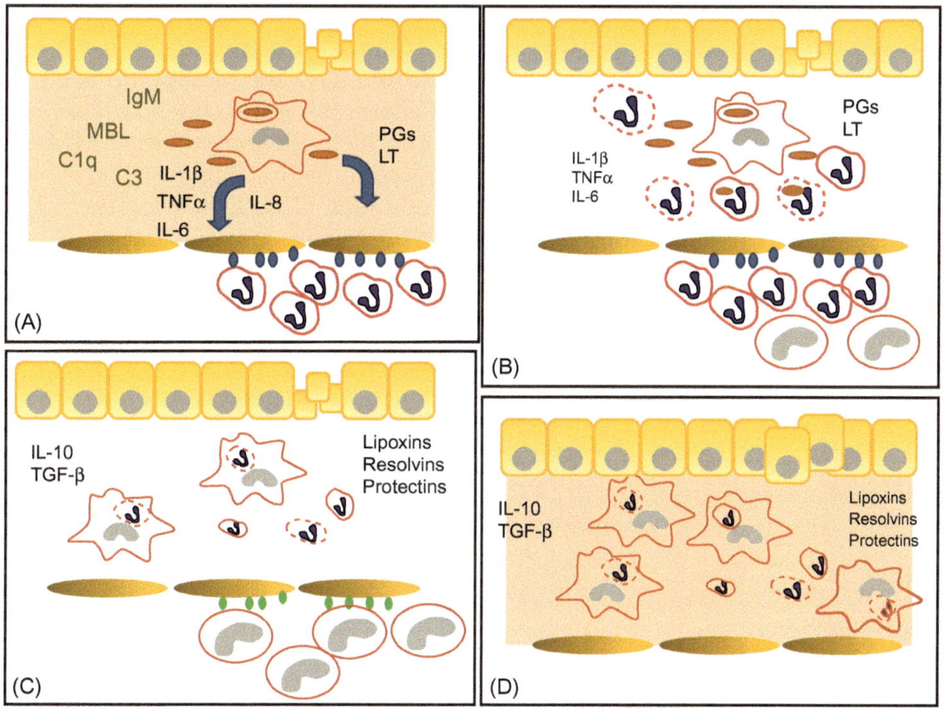

FIGURE 5.1 **Cooperation between macrophages and neutrophils during inflammation.** (A) Cellular damage and presence of infectious agents stimulate resident tissue macrophages through pattern recognition receptors and induce production of proinflammatory mediators such as the cytokines IL-1β, TNF-α, and IL-6; the chemokine IL-8; and lipid mediators prostaglandins and leukotrienes. Soluble components of the immune system, such as mannose-binding lectin (MBL), natural IgM, and complement components C1q and C3, are also involved in innate–opsonic recognition of damage and pathogens. Inflammatory mediators activate and induce expression of adhesion molecules in the endothelial cells that promote recruitment of neutrophils that are attracted to the inflammatory site following a chemokine gradient. (B) Macrophages and neutrophils collaborate in the clearance of the infection. Both cell types are highly phagocytic but neutrophils are unique in their capacity to release the content of their granules, causing effectively the liquefaction of tissues, and form NETs. Under highly proinflammatory conditions the half-life of neutrophils is extended. (C) Microbial clearance and reduced stimulation induce a shift in lipid being produced, and pro-resolving lipids are synthesized by neutrophils and macrophages. There is also a change in the pattern of adhesion molecules in the endothelial cells, and preferential recruitment of monocytes takes place. Neutrophil apoptosis increases, and the uptake of apoptotic neutrophils by macrophages shifts the phenotype of these cells towards an antiinflammatory state characterized by the production of IL-10 and TGF-β. (D) Once the inflammatory insult is cleared macrophages promote wound healing through the production, among others, of pro-angiogenic growth factors.

Initiation of inflammation is orchestrated by resident macrophages. Through engagement of PRRs, macrophages respond to changes in the physiological status of the tissues.[6,71] Macrophage activation would be more acute if activation involves the engagement of FcRs. Macrophage activation leads to production of cytokines and chemokines and of proinflammatory lipid mediators (prostaglandins and leukotrienes) by the action of cytosolic phospholipase A_2 and the cycloxigenase and lipoxigenase pathways.[6,71] Proinflammatory prostanglandins control blood flow and vascular dilation and permeability at the site of inflammation.[75] Neutrophil recruitment is promoted by CXCL5 and CXCL8 and is enhanced by MMP8 and MMP9, which cleave chemokines and enhance their chemotactic activity.

There is a shift from a neutrophil-dominated inflammatory response to a monocyte-dominated inflammation that is promoted by activated neutrophils. IL-6Rα is shed from the surface of activated neutrophils, while IL-6 is produced by macrophages and endothelial cells. sIL-6R–IL-6 complexes bind gp130 on endothelial cells and induce expression of V-CAM (a ligand for the integrin VLA-4 (α_4-β_1) expressed by monocytes) and CCL2, a chemotactic factor for monocytes. Shedding of IL-6Rα by neutrophils is also induced by apoptosis. Protease-mediated cleavage of chemokines increases their affinity for CCR1 and promotes monocyte recruitment.[71]

Killing of pathogens is achieved through phagocytosis by neutrophils and macrophages, and there is increased evidence in support of a collaborative effort between both cell types in microbial clearance.[72] During phagocytosis, activated neutrophils can deliver the content of their granules to phagosomes or can release it to the extracellular milieu.[35,71] Finally, the formation of NETs by neutrophils also promotes microbial killing.[33]

During resolution, neutrophil infiltration stops, neutrophil apoptosis increases, and lipid mediator class-switch takes place.[75,76] At this stage, prostaglandins and leukotrienes are replaced by lipoxins, resolvins, and protectins. Platelets and epithelial cells provide metabolic precursors for lipoxin synthesis by neutrophils. Macrophages synthesize lipoxins upon uptake of apoptotic cells. Lipoxin A4 facilitates resolution of inflammation by reducing neutrophil activity and uptake of apoptotic neutrophils, favoring monocyte migration and inhibiting CXCL8 synthesis. Clearance of CXCL3 and CXCL5 is promoted by resolvin E1 and protectin D1. These lipids increase the expression of CXCR5 in apoptotic neutrophils, which acts as a trap for its ligands CXCL3 and CXCL5. Additionally, the ability of CXC chemokines to promote neutrophil recruitment is reduced through cleavage by selected MMPs. Uptake of apoptotic neutrophils by macrophages inhibits production of IL-23, a cytokine involved in promoting granulopoiesis, and promotes synthesis of IL-10 and TGF-β, which are potent antiinflammatory cytokines.[71]

PHAGOCYTOSIS

The capacity of phagocytes to effectively internalize material through phagocytosis results from the combined effect of expressing phagocytic receptors and having a highly developed endosomal compartment capable of supporting the membrane redistribution required for the uptake process. Indeed, although the expression of phagocytic receptors in non-professional phagocytes enables phagocytic uptake, the levels of phagocytosis are lower than those achieved by professional cells.[51]

The best characterized model of phagocytosis is the FcRγR-mediated phagocytic process. In this model, use of IgG-opsonized material, such as erythrocytes and beads, has been useful in delineating the contribution of different FcγRs and the effect of IgG density and particle size on the internalization process. The early identification of morphological differences between the internalization of IgG versus C3b-opsonized particles[77] and the increasing understanding of the role of non-opsonic recognition in immunity indicate that the particle internalization process and ensuing phagosome maturation might be greatly influenced by the receptors engaged at the plasma membrane, the cargo, and cellular activation. For instance, the maturation of apoptotic cell phagosomes is faster than in the case of FcR-mediated uptake.[78] Also, the cell type might have an effect, as phagosomal acidification (apoptotic cells) in DCs is

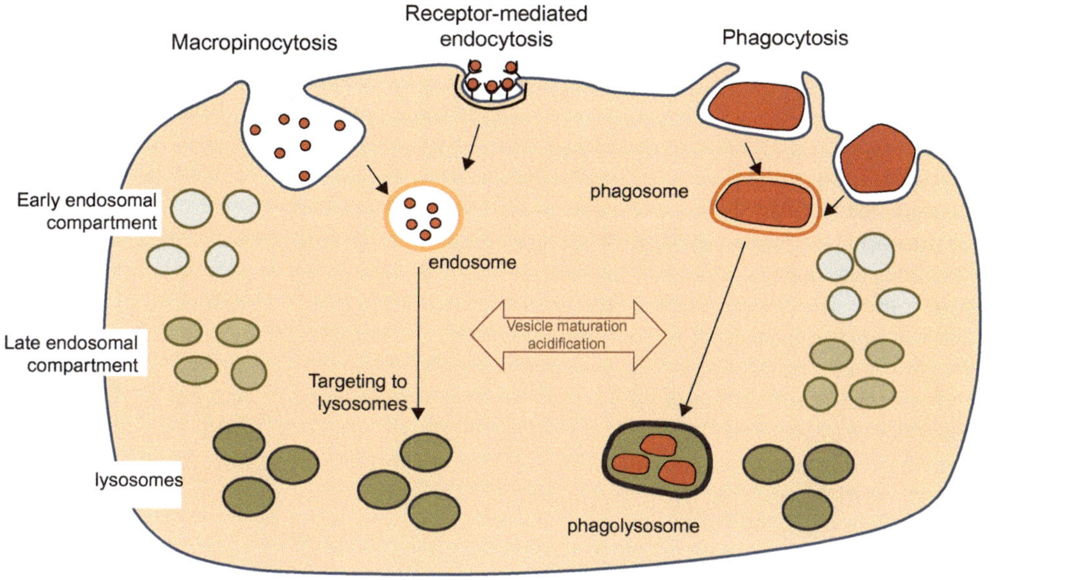

FIGURE 5.2 **The phagocytic process.** Macrophages have highly developed endocytic compartments and are very active endocytic and phagocytic cells. Uptake of soluble components by macropinocytosis or receptor-mediated endocytosis leads to the formation of endosomes that follow a maturation process characterized by a reduction of luminal pH and the acquisition of lytic enzymes. Maturation is achieved through sequential fusion events with vesicles from the early and late endosomal compartment and, finally, lysosomes. Particle uptake leads to the formation of phagosomes. There is clear evidence indicating that the phagocytic process is highly influenced by the receptors engaged during uptake, with early studies showing distinct differences between FcγR-mediated phagocytosis (formation of pseudopodia, left) and complement receptor-mediated phagocytosis (sinking process, right). Phagosomes follow a maturation process similar to endosomes that culminates in their fusion with lysosomes and the formation of phagolysosomes. Phagolysosomes are highly acidic and contain a complex cocktail of proteases and antimicrobial products.

not as efficient as in macrophages and neutrophils. This is considered a strategy to maximise cross-presentation (see below).[79] There have also been reports of TLRs influencing the phagosome maturation process in a phagosome autonomous fashion and of preferential MHC-II-mediated presentation of the cargo of phagosomes containing TLR ligands.[80] Disruption of the phagosome maturation process is used by numerous microorganisms as an evasion strategy.[81,82] Engagement of the mannose receptor, a lectin receptor, during the phagocytic uptake of *Mycobacterium tuberculosis* delays phagosome maturation.[83,84]

The phagocytosis process resembles that of endocytosis in that newly formed vesicles mature through fusion with different components of the endosomal compartment (see Figure 5.2).[81,85] Rho GTP-binding proteins are critical for the reorganization of actin during phagocytosis. When activated and bound to GTP, these proteins facilitate recruitment of Arp2/3 and actin polymerisation. Rac1 and cell division control protein 42 (CdC42) are essential for the formation of the characteristic actin cups during FcγR-mediated phagoocytosis.[86] Uptake of antibody-coated particles occurs through the formation of pseudopodia following a zip-like mechanism with close contact between the particles, and the plasma membrane particles end up coated by the pseudopods that fuse at the leading edge, resulting in the formation of a phagosome. FcγR-mediated phagocytosis induces phagocyte activation and leads to the production of ROIs through the action of Syk.

Complement opsonised particles are also efficiently internalized by phagocytes. Recognition of iC3b-coated material does not activate phagocytes and an additional signal is required, although monocytes do not seem to have the same requirement. It is noteworthy to mention that CR3 is an integrin and as such can be activated through an "inside-out" mechanism; the small G-protein Rap1 is sufficient to activate CR3 and is necessary for CR3 activation in response to inflammatory mediators.[86] Uptake of iC3b-coated particle occurs through sinking of the particle into the cells, does not require tyrosine phosphorylation, and involves the activation of the Rho-family protein, RhoA.[86] Both FcγR and CR3-mediated uptake require RhoG.[87]

It is highly plausible that Ig-opsonized material will also bear C3 fragments, and interest has increased in understanding how co-engagement of FcγR and CR could affect particle internalization. The presence of C3 has been shown to reduce the amount of IgG required for particle ingestion by monocytes,[88] and FcγR stimulation influences CR3 function. Co-stimulation of CR3 and FcγRI using monomeric IgG inhibits CR3-mediated endocytosis, while the opposite is true when CR3 and FcγRIIA are co-stimulated.[88]

As in the case of endocytosis, phagosomes undergo a maturation process through fusion with vesicles from early endosomes, late endosomes, and lysosomes. In neutrophils, granule content can be delivered to the phagosomes. These docking-fusion events are controlled by SNARES. Vesicle SNARES can selectively interact with cognate SNARES on the target membrane.[85] The small GTPase Rab5 (an early endosomal marker) is involved in the fusion of phagosomes with early endosomes. This is accompanied by acidification of the lumen and changes in its composition. Early phagosomes are mildly acidic (pH 6.1–6.5). In addition to fusion, fision events take place so that membranes are recycled back to the plasma membrane. Budding vesicles are also targeted to the endosomes and the *trans*-Golgi network. Membrane that needs to be degraded is diverted into the lumen, leading to the formation of multivesicular bodies. Late phagosomes have a more acidic lumen (pH 5.5–6.0) because of the presence of V-ATPases that pump protons into the lumen. There is also enrichment of proteases and lysosomal-associated membrane proteins (LAMPs). The small GTPase Rab7 (a late endosomal marker) is involved in the fusion of late phagosomes with late endosomes and lysosomes. The maturation process ends with the formation of the phagolysosome through the fusion of late phagosomes with lysosomes. Phagolysosomes are highly acidic (pH 4.5) because of the recruitment of additional V-ATPases and are characterized by a high content of cathepsins and lack of mannose-6-phosphate receptors. Proteases are delivered to the phagosome sequentially, and cathepsin H can be found in early endosomes while cathepsin S is mostly found in late phagosomes. These proteases, together with defensins, cathelicidins, lysozymes, and lipases, cause direct damage to microorganisms.[81] Acidic pH affects bacterial metabolism and favors the activity of acid hydrolytic enzymes, and it is intrinsic to the maturation process. Combined action of NOX (see neutrophils) and high H^+ levels provided by the V-ATPases enable the formation of more complex oxygen species that kill intraphagosomal organisms.[81]

Macrophages have the capacity to produce reactive nitrogen species (RNS) through the action of the inducible nitrogen synthase (NOS2). This only occurs upon activation, as NOS2 must be synthesised *de novo*. NOS2 mediates the processing of L-arginine into NO and citrulline in the presence of oxygen. NO is synthesized in the cytosol but diffuses into the phagosome where in the presence of ROIs converts to a series of RNS. ROIs and RNS have synergistic toxic effects by targeting thiol groups, metal centers, Tyr residues, nucleid acids, and lipids.[81]

An additional mechanism that limits bacterial growth involves the sequestration of key nutrients by lactoferrin (Fe^{2+}) or NRAMP1, which extrudes Fe^{2+}, Zn^{2+}, and Mn^{2+} from the lumen.[81]

ANTIGEN PRESENTATION BY DCs, ROLE OF FcγRs

As mentioned earlier, DCs are phagocytes uniquely suited for the activation of naïve T cells.[89–91] The current paradigm states that three signals are required for T-cell activation: (1) peptide–MHC complexes, (2) co-stimulation, and (3) cytokines. MHC–peptide complexes interact with the T-cell receptor complex and determine the specificity of the T-cell response. Co-stimulation refers to the expression at the DC cell surface of co-stimulatory molecules (B7-1/CD80, B7-2/CD86) that interact with CD28 at the surface of T cells and promote T-cell activation. The absence of co-stimulation leads to T-cell anergy. Other members of this family of molecules, instead of promoting T-cell activation, deliver inhibitory signals such as PD-L1 (B7-H1/CD274) and PD-L2 (B7-DC/CD273) that interact with PD-1 on activated T cells and inhibit T-cell proliferation and cytokine production.[92] This mechanism, together with the ability of CD80 and CD86 to engage the inhibitory receptor CTLA-4[93] on T cells, ensures that T-cell activation does not lead to overly exuberant pathological responses.

DCs undergo a maturation process by which immature DC specialized in antigen uptake and with poor T-cell activation capacity become mature DCs with high levels of MHC-II–peptide complexes and co-stimulatory molecules at the cell surface. DC maturation is promoted by engagement of PRRs and FcRs and is associated with cytokine production. The conditions leading to DC activation have a marked influence on the ensuing T-cell response.[94] IL-12 promotes Th1 differentiation, and the absence of IL-12 and exogenous production of IL-4 by mast cells, eosinophils, or basophils promote Th2 differentiation. T cells can also adopt a Th17 phenotype that requires IL-1β and IL-6 in humans[95] and TGF-β and IL-6 in mice. Regulatory T cells can also be generated after the encounter of DCs and naive T cells.[91] These cells display immunosuppresive activities and are key players in the maintenance of tolerance.

Endocytosed proteins are processed in the endosomal compartment, leading to the generation of peptides that are subsequently loaded on MHC-II molecules. DCs, as all cells except red blood cells, express MHC-I molecules that mediate the presentation of proteins synthesized within the cell, both host- and pathogen-derived, to CD8 T cells. These proteins are processed in the cytosol, and the resulting peptides are transported into the endoplasmic reticulum through specialized transporters (TAP-1/TAP-2) where they are loaded onto newly synthesised MHCI molecules.[89] A third route of Ag processing is cross-presentation, by which internalized material is presented through the MHC-I presentation pathway.[89,96] Cross-presentation can occur following a TAP-1/TAP-2-dependent or a TAP-1/TAP-2-independent pathway.[89] Although highly ineffective *in vitro*, this pathway enables the generation of cytotoxic T-cell responses against viruses or other intracellular pathogens that do not infect DCs *in vivo*. The endocytic pathway used for internalization as well as the activation state of the DCs strongly influence the effectiveness of the cross-presentation process.

Antigen uptake by DCs is favored by endocytic receptors. While the initial uptake of antigens in the absence of an established immune response is largely mediated by non-opsonic receptors such as lectin and scavenger receptors, once antigen-specific IgG is generated then uptake of immunocomplexes by activating FcγRs will increase antigen presentation and work as a feedback loop for the promotion of robust immune recognition. Antigen uptake through FcγRs leads to increased presentation through the exogenous (MHC-II) and cross-presentation pathways by effectively targeting antigen to lysosomal compartments and improves activation of CD4 and CD8 T cells, respectively.[97–100] Additionally, engagement of activating FcγRs induces Syk-dependent DC maturation and can lead to the breakdown of T-cell tolerance and induction of autoimmune disease.[101] Inhibitory FcγR plays an important role in the modulation of DC-mediated T-cell activation; it has been shown to inhibit TLR-4-induced DC activation[102] and antigen presentation through activation of FcγR.[68] One of the mechanisms involved in this inhibitory effect could involve the opposite roles of activating and inhibitory receptors in the regulation of type I-IFN signaling.[103] FcγR-mediated activation leads to the activation of type I-IFN responsive genes which is required for DC maturation. Accordingly, FcγRIIB is upregulated in rheumatoid arthritis patients with quiescent disease.[102] The unique ability of activating FcγRs to promote T-cell activation is being exploited for the generation of novel vaccine preparations that through the targeting of these receptors aim at the induction of antigen-specific T-cell responses against tumors of infectious agents. These reagents include gold nanoparticles and liposomes bearing the Fc portion of human IgG_1[104] and DNA encoding chimeric antibodies in which the CRD region has been replaced with CTL and T cell-helper epitopes.[105]

COLLABORATION BETWEEN FcR AND NON-OPSONIC RECEPTORS

Current literature emphasizes the importance of the cross-talk between PRRs and FcRs. As mentioned above, inhibitory FcγR has been shown to inhibit TLR-4 activation in DCs.[102] Historically, macrophages have been considered to be major effector cells during Th1-driven immune responses because of their enhanced ability to kill intracellular pathogens through the production of reactive nitrogen species, ability to present antigen to activated T cells, and ability to produce a wide range of proinflammatory cytokines. This pattern of macrophage activation (M1-like or classical activation) contrasts with the phenotype of macrophages observed during helminth infection (M2-like or alternative activation) or treated with IL-4 *in vitro* which are characterized by the production of a subset of effector molecules such as arginase I, which reduces the availability of arginine and has a major effect on T-cell activation.[106,107] These macrophages are associated with wound healing responses required during parasitic infections as a means to minimize tissue damage.[108] Within the spectrum of M2 activation,[109] some authors single out a subgroup of regulatory macrophages characterized by high production of IL-10 but that, in contrast to *bona fide* M2 macrophages, express co-stimulatory molecules and lack arginase expression.[110] These cells are similar to macrophages treated with apoptotic cells or glucocorticoids and are termed *regulatory macrophages*.[109] Regulatory macrophages can be also generated by ligation of FcγRs in the presence of endotoxin; immunocomplexes inhibit IL-12 production and induce IL-10 synthesis by mouse macrophages in response to LPS.

Because of the IgG glycosylation changes that take place during immune responses, lectins expressed by macrophages and DCs could contribute to IgG-mediated responses. For instance, the antiinflammatory activity of intravenous Ig is mediated by a small pool of IgG molecules bearing α2,6-linked sialic acid in the Fc portion, and SIGNR1 has been identified as the lectin responsible for this effect.[111,112] This was a surprising result because SIGNR-1 was not considered a sialic-acid binding lectin, and it is thought that a unique binding for SIGNR1 is generated in sialylated Fc.[112] Additionally, the mannose receptor has been involved in immunocomplex-induced glomerulonephritis using a mouse model. Mice deficient in mannose receptor are protected against nephrotoxic serum-induced glomerulonephritis.[113] This result correlates with two independent effects caused by mannose receptor deficiency. First is the reduced Fc-mediated activation observed in mannose receptor-deficient macrophages and kidney mesangial cells. Second is the increased apoptosis observed in mannose receptor-deficient mesangial cells and a more antiinflammatory phenotype of mannose receptor-deficient macrophages after uptake of apoptotic mesangial cells.[113] These results correlate with the ability of mannose receptors to bind Fab fragments of whole sheep nephrotoxic globulin. This is not the first example of MR involvement in Ig-induced pathology, as it has been previously shown to interact with the pathological G_0 IgG form associated with rheumatoiod arthritis.[114]

These results highlight the importance of understanding post-translational modifications of immunocomplexes, as the presence of selected glycoforms could have major effects on their biological activities through their ability to interact with lectin receptors on phagocytes.

CONCLUDING REMARKS

Phagocytes exert their important immunological functions in the absence of acquired immunity through their ability to sense, through PRRs, and through changes in the physiological status of tissues induced by infectious agents and/or cellular stress. PRR engagement induces an inflammatory response that will endeavor to clear the initial insult and repair tissue. This effective, although unspecific, response is greatly boosted by the tools offered by the acquired immunity that include the presence of antigen-specific antibodies and activated T cells. Activating FcRs expressed by phagocytes promotes antigen uptake and cellular activation, leading to increased phagocytosis, cellular recruitment, and T-cell activation. This positive feedback circle of activation is kept under control by inhibitory FcγRs, which function as buffers of the immune system and negatively regulate cellular activation in response to PRRs and activating FcRs. In this manner, inhibitory FcγRs minimize the potential for pathological immune responses that could compromise organ function. Further understanding of the interplay between phagocyte receptors will enable the design of novel therapeutic agents aimed at blunting immune complex-induced pathologies and vaccination strategies that could exploit activating FcγRs for the elicitation of robust humoral and T cell-mediated immune responses.

References

1. Chen GY, Nunez G. Sterile inflammation: sensing and reacting to damage. *Nat Rev Immunol* 2010;**10**(12):826–37.
2. Green DR, Ferguson T, Zitvogel L, Kroemer G. Immunogenic and tolerogenic cell death. *Nat Rev Immunol* 2009;**9**(5):353–63.
3. Nathan C, Ding A. Nonresolving inflammation. *Cell* 2010;**140**(6):871–82.
4. Baumgarth N. The double life of a B-1 cell: self-reactivity selects for protective effector functions. *Nat Rev Immunol* 2011;**11**(1):34–46.
5. Ehrenstein MR, Notley CA. The importance of natural IgM: scavenger, protector and regulator. *Nat Rev Immunol* 2010;**10**(11):778–86.
6. Taylor PR, Martinez-Pomares L, Stacey M, Lin HH, Brown GD, Gordon S. Macrophage receptors and immune recognition. *Annu Rev Immunol* 2005;**23**:901–44.
7. Auffray C, Sieweke MH, Geissmann F. Blood monocytes: development, heterogeneity, and relationship with dendritic cells. *Annu Rev Immunol* 2009;**27**:669–92.
8. Geissmann F, Manz MG, Jung S, Sieweke MH, Merad M, Ley K. Development of monocytes, macrophages, and dendritic cells. *Science* 2010;**327**(5966):656–61.
9. Geissmann F, Jung S, Littman DR. Blood monocytes consist of two principal subsets with distinct migratory properties. *Immunity* 2003;**19**(1):71–82.

10. Cros J, Cagnard N, Woollard K, Patey N, Zhang SY, Senechal B, et al. Human CD14dim monocytes patrol and sense nucleic acids and viruses via TLR7 and TLR8 receptors. *Immunity* 2010;**33**(3):375–86.
11. Grage-Griebenow E, Flad HD, Ernst M. Heterogeneity of human peripheral blood monocyte subsets. *J Leukoc Biol* 2001;**69**(1):11–20.
12. Saha P, Geissmann F. Toward a functional characterization of blood monocytes. *Immunol Cell Biol* 2011;**89**(1):2–4.
13. Maurer D, Fiebiger E, Reininger B, Wolff-Winiski B, Jouvin MH, Kilgus O, et al. Expression of functional high affinity immunoglobulin E receptors (Fc epsilon RI) on monocytes of atopic individuals. *J Exp Med* 1994;**179**(2):745–50.
14. Monteiro RC, Van De Winkel JG. IgA Fc receptors. *Annu Rev Immunol* 2003;**21**:177–204.
15. Martinez-Pomares L, Gordon S. CD169(+) macrophages at the crossroads of antigen presentation. *Trends Immunol* 2012;**33**(2):66–70.
16. Jenkins SJ, Ruckerl D, Cook PC, Jones LH, Finkelman FD, van Rooijen N, et al. Local macrophage proliferation, rather than recruitment from the blood, is a signature of TH2 inflammation. *Science* 2011;**332**(6035):1284–8.
17. Reese TA, Liang HE, Tager AM, Luster AD, Van Rooijen N, Voehringer D, et al. Chitin induces accumulation in tissue of innate immune cells associated with allergy. *Nature* 2007;**447**(7140):92–6.
18. Van Dyken SJ, Garcia D, Porter P, Huang X, Quinlan PJ, Blanc PD, et al. Fungal chitin from asthma-associated home environments induces eosinophilic lung infiltration. *J Immunol* 2011;**187**(5):2261–7.
19. Voehringer D, van Rooijen N, Locksley RM. Eosinophils develop in distinct stages and are recruited to peripheral sites by alternatively activated macrophages. *J Leukoc Biol* 2007;**81**(6):1434–44.
20. Wu D, Molofsky AB, Liang HE, Ricardo-Gonzalez RR, Jouihan HA, Bando JK, et al. Eosinophils sustain adipose alternatively activated macrophages associated with glucose homeostasis. *Science* 2011;**332**(6026):243–7.
21. Odemuyiwa SO, Ghahary A, Li Y, Puttagunta L, Lee JE, Musat-Marcu S, et al. Cutting edge: human eosinophils regulate T cell subset selection through indoleamine 2,3-dioxygenase. *J Immunol* 2004;**173**(10):5909–13.
22. Yang D, Chen Q, Su SB, Zhang P, Kurosaka K, Caspi RR, et al. Eosinophil-derived neurotoxin acts as an alarmin to activate the TLR2–MyD88 signal pathway in dendritic cells and enhances Th2 immune responses. *J Exp Med* 2008;**205**(1):79–90.
23. Kita H. Eosinophils: multifaceted biological properties and roles in health and disease. *Immunol Rev* 2011;**242**(1):161–77.
24. Monteiro RC, Hostoffer RW, Cooper MD, Bonner JR, Gartland GL, Kubagawa H. Definition of immunoglobulin A receptors on eosinophils and their enhanced expression in allergic individuals. *J Clin Invest* 1993;**92**(4):1681–5.
25. van de Winkel JG, Capel PJ. Human IgG Fc receptor heterogeneity: molecular aspects and clinical implications. *Immunol Today* 1993;**14**(5):215–21.
26. Truong MJ, Gruart V, Liu FT, Prin L, Capron A, Capron M. IgE-binding molecules (Mac-2/epsilon BP) expressed by human eosinophils. Implication in IgE-dependent eosinophil cytotoxicity. *Eur J Immunol* 1993;**23**(12):3230–5.
27. Kato M, Abraham RT, Okada S, Kita H. Ligation of the beta2 integrin triggers activation and degranulation of human eosinophils. *Am J Respir Cell Mol Biol* 1998;**18**(5):675–86.
28. Gounni AS, Lamkhioued B, Ochiai K, Tanaka Y, Delaporte E, Capron A, et al. High-affinity IgE receptor on eosinophils is involved in defence against parasites. *Nature* 1994;**367**(6459):183–6.
29. Min B. Basophils: what they "can do" versus what they "actually do." *Nat Immunol* 2008;**9**(12):1333–9.
30. Schroeder JT. Basophils: emerging roles in the pathogenesis of allergic disease. *Immunol Rev* 2011;**242**(1):144–60.
31. Sadik CD, Kim ND, Luster AD. Neutrophils cascading their way to inflammation. *Trends Immunol* 2011;**32**(10):452–60.
32. Lekstrom-Himes JA, Gallin JI. Immunodeficiency diseases caused by defects in phagocytes. *N Engl J Med* 2000;**343**(23):1703–14.
33. Mantovani A, Cassatella MA, Costantini C, Jaillon S. Neutrophils in the activation and regulation of innate and adaptive immunity. *Nat Rev Immunol* 2011;**11**(8):519–31.
34. Lambeth JD. NOX enzymes and the biology of reactive oxygen. *Nat Rev Immunol* 2004;**4**(3):181–9.
35. Nathan C. Neutrophils and immunity: challenges and opportunities. *Nat Rev Immunol* 2006;**6**(3):173–82.
36. Janeway Jr CA, Medzhitov R. Innate immune recognition. *Annu Rev Immunol* 2002;**20**:197–216.
37. Medzhitov R, Janeway Jr. CA. Decoding the patterns of self and nonself by the innate immune system. *Science* 2002;**296**(5566):298–300.
38. Takeuchi O, Akira S. Pattern recognition receptors and inflammation. *Cell* 2010;**140**(6):805–20.
39. Loo YM, Gale Jr. M. Immune signaling by RIG-I-like receptors. *Immunity* 2011;**34**(5):680–92.
40. Franchi L, Warner N, Viani K, Nunez G. Function of Nod-like receptors in microbial recognition and host defense. *Immunol Rev* 2009;**227**(1):106–28.
41. Bryant CE, Spring DR, Gangloff M, Gay NJ. The molecular basis of the host response to lipopolysaccharide. *Nat Rev Microbiol* 2010;**8**(1):8–14.
42. Zhang Q, Raoof M, Chen Y, Sumi Y, Sursal T, Junger W, et al. Circulating mitochondrial DAMPs

cause inflammatory responses to injury. *Nature* 2010;**464**(7285):104–7.
43. Bianchi ME, Manfredi AA. High-mobility group box 1 (HMGB1) protein at the crossroads between innate and adaptive immunity. *Immunol Rev* 2007;**220**:35–46.
44. Hanley PJ, Musset B, Renigunta V, Limberg SH, Dalpke AH, Sus R, et al. Extracellular ATP induces oscillations of intracellular Ca^{2+} and membrane potential and promotes transcription of IL-6 in macrophages. *Proc Natl Acad Sci USA* 2004;**101**(25):9479–84.
45. Mukhopadhyay S, Gordon S. The role of scavenger receptors in pathogen recognition and innate immunity. *Immunobiology* 2004;**209**(1–2):39–49.
46. Gazi U, Martinez-Pomares L. Influence of the mannose receptor in host immune responses. *Immunobiology* 2009;**214**(7):554–61.
47. Geijtenbeek TB, Gringhuis SI. Signalling through C-type lectin receptors: shaping immune responses. *Nat Rev Immunol* 2009;**9**(7):465–79.
48. Kerrigan AM, Brown GD. C-type lectins and phagocytosis. *Immunobiology* 2009;**214**(7):562–75.
49. Kerrigan AM, Brown GD. Syk-coupled C-type lectins in immunity. *Trends Immunol* 2011;**32**(4):151–6.
50. Osorio F, Reis e Sousa C. Myeloid C-type lectin receptors in pathogen recognition and host defense. *Immunity* 2011;**34**(5):651–64.
51. Peiser L, Gough PJ, Kodama T, Gordon S. Macrophage class A scavenger receptor-mediated phagocytosis of *Escherichia coli*: role of cell heterogeneity, microbial strain, and culture conditions *in vitro*. *Infect Immun* 2000;**68**(4):1953–63.
52. Herre J, Marshall AS, Caron E, Edwards AD, Williams DL, Schweighoffer E, et al. Dectin-1 uses novel mechanisms for yeast phagocytosis in macrophages. *Blood* 2004;**104**(13):4038–45.
53. Bonizzi G, Karin M. The two NF-kappaB activation pathways and their role in innate and adaptive immunity. *Trends Immunol* 2004;**25**(6):280–8.
54. Wertz IE, Dixit VM. Signaling to NF-kappaB: regulation by ubiquitination. *Cold Spring Harb Perspect Biol* 2010;**2**(3):a003350.
55. Martinon F, Mayor A, Tschopp J. The inflammasomes: guardians of the body. *Annu Rev Immunol* 2009;**27**:229–65.
56. Schroder K, Tschopp J. The inflammasomes. *Cell* 2010;**140**(6):821–32.
57. Bergsbaken T, Fink SL, Cookson BT. Pyroptosis: host cell death and inflammation. *Nat Rev Microbiol* 2009;**7**(2):99–109.
58. Bergsbaken T, Fink SL, den Hartigh AB, Loomis WP, Cookson BT. Coordinated host responses during pyroptosis: caspase-1-dependent lysosome exocytosis and inflammatory cytokine maturation. *J Immunol* 2011;**187**(5):2748–54.
59. Bowie AG, Unterholzner L. Viral evasion and subversion of pattern-recognition receptor signalling. *Nat Rev Immunol* 2008;**8**(12):911–22.
60. Wilkins C, Gale Jr. M. Recognition of viruses by cytoplasmic sensors. *Curr Opin Immunol* 2010;**22**(1):41–7.
61. Takeuchi O, Akira S. MDA5/RIG-I and virus recognition. *Curr Opin Immunol* 2008;**20**(1):17–22.
62. Zhang YL, Dong C. MAP kinases in immune responses. *Cell Mol Immunol* 2005;**2**(1):20–7.
63. Nimmerjahn F, Ravetch JV. Fcgamma receptors as regulators of immune responses. *Nat Rev Immunol* 2008;**8**(1):34–47.
64. Steinbach F, Henke F, Krause B, Thiele B, Burmester GR, Hiepe F. Monocytes from systemic lupus erythematous patients are severely altered in phenotype and lineage flexibility. *Ann Rheum Dis* 2000;**59**(4):283–8.
65. Mocsai A, Ruland J, Tybulewicz VL. The SYK tyrosine kinase: a crucial player in diverse biological functions. *Nat Rev Immunol* 2010;**10**(6):387–402.
66. Glocker EO, Hennigs A, Nabavi M, Schaffer AA, Woellner C, Salzer U, et al. A homozygous CARD9 mutation in a family with susceptibility to fungal infections. *N Engl J Med* 2009;**361**(18):1727–35.
67. Gross O, Poeck H, Bscheider M, Dostert C, Hannesschlager N, Endres S, et al. Syk kinase signalling couples to the Nlrp3 inflammasome for anti-fungal host defence. *Nature* 2009;**459**(7245):433–6.
68. Boruchov AM, Heller G, Veri MC, Bonvini E, Ravetch JV, Young JW. Activating and inhibitory IgG Fc receptors on human DCs mediate opposing functions. *J Clin Invest* 2005;**115**(10):2914–23.
69. Smith KG, Clatworthy MR. FcgammaRIIB in autoimmunity and infection: evolutionary and therapeutic implications. *Nat Rev Immunol* 2010;**10**(5):328–43.
70. van Lookeren Campagne M, Wiesmann C, Brown EJ. Macrophage complement receptors and pathogen clearance. *Cell Microbiol* 2007;**9**(9):2095–102.
71. Soehnlein O, Lindbom L. Phagocyte partnership during the onset and resolution of inflammation. *Nat Rev Immunol* 2010;**10**(6):427–39.
72. Silva MT. When two is better than one: macrophages and neutrophils work in concert in innate immunity as complementary and cooperative partners of a myeloid phagocyte system. *J Leukoc Biol* 2010;**87**(1):93–106.
73. Han J, Ulevitch RJ. Limiting inflammatory responses during activation of innate immunity. *Nat Immunol* 2005;**6**(12):1198–205.
74. Lawrence T, Gilroy DW. Chronic inflammation: a failure of resolution?. *Int J Exp Pathol* 2007;**88**(2):85–94.
75. Serhan CN, Savill J. Resolution of inflammation: the beginning programs the end. *Nat Immunol* 2005;**6**(12):1191–7.
76. Serhan CN, Yacoubian S, Yang R. Anti-inflammatory and proresolving lipid mediators. *Annu Rev Pathol* 2008;**3**:279–312.

77. Caron E, Hall A. Identification of two distinct mechanisms of phagocytosis controlled by different Rho GTPases. *Science* 1998;**282**(5394):1717–21.
78. Erwig LP, McPhilips KA, Wynes MW, Ivetic A, Ridley AJ, Henson PM. Differential regulation of phagosome maturation in macrophages and dendritic cells mediated by Rho GTPases and ezrin–radixin–moesin (ERM) proteins. *Proc Natl Acad Sci USA* 2006;**103**(34):12825–30.
79. Zhou Z, Yu X. Phagosome maturation during the removal of apoptotic cells: receptors lead the way. *Trends Cell Biol* 2008;**18**(10):474–85.
80. Blander JM, Medzhitov R. On regulation of phagosome maturation and antigen presentation. *Nat Immunol* 2006;**7**(10):1029–35.
81. Flannagan RS, Cosio G, Grinstein S. Antimicrobial mechanisms of phagocytes and bacterial evasion strategies. *Nat Rev Microbiol* 2009;**7**(5):355–66.
82. Kumar Y, Valdivia RH. Leading a sheltered life: intracellular pathogens and maintenance of vacuolar compartments. *Cell Host Microbe* 2009;**5**(6):593–601.
83. Kang PB, Azad AK, Torrelles JB, Kaufman TM, Beharka A, Tibesar E, et al. The human macrophage mannose receptor directs *Mycobacterium tuberculosis* lipoarabinomannan-mediated phagosome biogenesis. *J Exp Med* 2005;**202**(7):987–99.
84. Sweet L, Singh PP, Azad AK, Rajaram MV, Schlesinger LS, Schorey JS. Mannose receptor-dependent delay in phagosome maturation by *Mycobacterium avium* glycopeptidolipids. *Infect Immun* 2010;**78**(1):518–26.
85. Vieira OV, Botelho RJ, Grinstein S. Phagosome maturation: aging gracefully. *Biochem J* 2002;**366**(Pt 3):689–704.
86. Groves E, Dart AE, Covarelli V, Caron E. Molecular mechanisms of phagocytic uptake in mammalian cells. *Cell Mol Life Sci* 2008;**65**(13):1957–76.
87. Tzircotis G, Braga VM, Caron E. RhoG is required for both FcgammaR- and CR3-mediated phagocytosis. *J Cell Sci* 2011;**124**(Pt 17):2897–902.
88. Huang ZY, Hunter S, Chien P, Kim MK, Han-Kim TH, Indik ZK, et al. Interaction of two phagocytic host defense systems: Fcgamma receptors and complement receptor 3. *J Biol Chem* 2011;**286**(1):160–8.
89. Delamarre L, Mellman I. Harnessing dendritic cells for immunotherapy. *Semin Immunol* 2011;**23**(1):2–11.
90. Steinman RM. Dendritic cells: understanding immunogenicity. *Eur J Immunol* 2007;**37**(Suppl. 1):S53–60.
91. Maldonado RA, von Andrian UH. How tolerogenic dendritic cells induce regulatory T cells. *Adv Immunol* 2010;**108**:111–65.
92. Keir ME, Butte MJ, Freeman GJ, Sharpe AH. PD-1 and its ligands in tolerance and immunity. *Annu Rev Immunol* 2008;**26**:677–704.
93. Wing K, Yamaguchi T, Sakaguchi S. Cell-autonomous and -non-autonomous roles of CTLA-4 in immune regulation. *Trends Immunol* 2011;**32**(9):428–33.
94. Zhu J, Yamane H, Paul WE. Differentiation of effector CD4 T cell populations (*). *Annu Rev Immunol* 2010;**28**:445–89.
95. Acosta-Rodriguez EV, Napolitani G, Lanzavecchia A, Sallusto F. Interleukins 1beta and 6 but not transforming growth factor-beta are essential for the differentiation of interleukin 17-producing human T helper cells. *Nat Immunol* 2007;**8**(9):942–9.
96. Amigorena S, Savina A. Intracellular mechanisms of antigen cross presentation in dendritic cells. *Curr Opin Immunol* 2010;**22**(1):109–17.
97. Fanger NA, Wardwell K, Shen L, Tedder TF, Guyre PM. Type I (CD64) and type II (CD32) Fc gamma receptor-mediated phagocytosis by human blood dendritic cells. *J Immunol* 1996;**157**(2):541–8.
98. Dhodapkar KM, Krasovsky J, Williamson B, Dhodapkar MV. Antitumor monoclonal antibodies enhance cross-presentation of cellular antigens and the generation of myeloma-specific killer T cells by dendritic cells. *J Exp Med* 2002;**195**(1):125–33.
99. Regnault A, Lankar D, Lacabanne V, Rodriguez A, Thery C, Rescigno M, et al. Fcgamma receptor-mediated induction of dendritic cell maturation and major histocompatibility complex class I-restricted antigen presentation after immune complex internalization. *J Exp Med* 1999;**189**(2):371–80.
100. Kalergis AM, Ravetch JV. Inducing tumor immunity through the selective engagement of activating Fcgamma receptors on dendritic cells. *J Exp Med* 2002;**195**(12):1653–9.
101. Harbers SO, Crocker A, Catalano G, D'Agati V, Jung S, Desai DD, et al. Antibody-enhanced cross-presentation of self antigen breaks T cell tolerance. *J Clin Invest* 2007;**117**(5):1361–9.
102. Wenink MH, Santegoets KC, Roelofs MF, Huijbens R, Koenen HJ, van Beek R, et al. The inhibitory Fc gamma IIb receptor dampens TLR4-mediated immune responses and is selectively up-regulated on dendritic cells from rheumatoid arthritis patients with quiescent disease. *J Immunol* 2009;**183**(7):4509–20.
103. Dhodapkar KM, Banerjee D, Connolly J, Kukreja A, Matayeva E, Veri MC, et al. Selective blockade of the inhibitory Fcgamma receptor (FcgammaRIIB) in human dendritic cells and monocytes induces a type I interferon response program. *J Exp Med* 2007;**204**(6):1359–69.
104. Cruz LJ, Rueda F, Cordobilla B, Simon L, Hosta L, Albericio F, et al. Targeting nanosystems to human DCs via Fc receptor as an effective strategy to deliver antigen for immunotherapy. *Mol Pharm* 2011;**8**(1):104–16.
105. Durrant LG, Pudney VA, Spendlove I. Using monoclonal antibodies to stimulate antitumor cellular immunity. *Expert Rev Vaccines* 2011;**10**(7):1093–106.

106. Murray PJ, Wynn TA. Protective and pathogenic functions of macrophage subsets. *Nat Rev Immunol* 2011;**11**(11):723–37.
107. Gordon S, Martinez FO. Alternative activation of macrophages: mechanism and functions. *Immunity* 2010;**32**(5):593–604.
108. Allen JE, Wynn TA. Evolution of Th2 immunity: a rapid repair response to tissue destructive pathogens. *PLoS Pathog* 2011;**7**(5):e1002003.
109. Mosser DM, Edwards JP. Exploring the full spectrum of macrophage activation. *Nat Rev Immunol* 2008;**8**(12):958–69.
110. Edwards JP, Zhang X, Frauwirth KA, Mosser DM. Biochemical and functional characterization of three activated macrophage populations. *J Leukoc Biol* 2006;**80**(6):1298–307.
111. Anthony RM, Nimmerjahn F, Ashline DJ, Reinhold VN, Paulson JC, Ravetch JV. Recapitulation of IVIG anti-inflammatory activity with a recombinant IgG Fc. *Science* 2008;**320**(5874):373–6.
112. Anthony RM, Wermeling F, Karlsson MC, Ravetch JV. Identification of a receptor required for the anti-inflammatory activity of IVIG. *Proc Natl Acad Sci USA* 2008;**105**(50):19571–8.
113. Chavele KM, Martinez-Pomares L, Domin J, Pemberton S, Haslam SM, Dell A, et al. Mannose receptor interacts with Fc receptors and is critical for the development of crescentic glomerulonephritis in mice. *J Clin Invest* 2010;**120**(5):1469–78.
114. Dong X, Storkus WJ, Salter RD. Binding and uptake of agalactosyl IgG by mannose receptor on macrophages and dendritic cells. *J Immunol* 1999;**163**(10):5427–34.

CHAPTER

6

B Cells

Development, Differentiation, and Regulation by Fcγ Receptor IIB in the Humoral Immune Response

*Elizabeth R. Walsh and Silvia Bolland**

Laboratory of Immunogenetics, National Institute of Allergy and Infectious Diseases, National Institutes of Health, Rockville, Maryland

B CELL DEVELOPMENT AND SELECTION IN THE BONE MARROW

B cells develop in the bone marrow from a common progenitor shared with T, NK, and some DC subsets. Throughout development, B cells migrate to different niches in the bone marrow and are dependent on contact with stromal cells that secrete survival and differentiation factors such as Flt3, CXCL12, and IL-7.[1] Progenitor B cells progress through the early stages of maturation, rearranging heavy- and light-chain genes at the pro- to pre-B cell stage until they express rearranged IgM receptors on the cell surface as immature B cells, at which point they exit the bone marrow to continue maturation in the peripheral immune system.

The first major checkpoint that occurs during the B-cell development process in the bone marrow is rearrangement of the μ heavy chain gene at the pro-B-cell stage.[2,3] If this is successful, it combines with surrogate light chains to form the pre-B cell receptor, which causes transition into the pre-B cell stage, where heavy chain rearrangement ceases and provides allelic exclusion.[4,5] The expression of the pre-B cell receptor also causes pre-B cell proliferation, creating a pool of B-cell clones that can attempt light chain rearrangement.[6] If light chain rearrangement is successful, a complete IgM receptor is formed; however, at this stage of receptor rearrangement it is possible for autoreactive specificities to arise that could potentially cause a break in self-tolerance and lead to the development of autoimmunity. Precautionary measures to safeguard against self-reactive B cells achieving full maturity have evolved alongside adaptive immunity to ensure that this does not occur with regularity, although there is a fine line between excluding enough self-reactive specificities to prevent autoimmunity and compromising the level of diversity necessary for pathogen responses by eliminating too many receptors.

* Corresponding Author

B cells are subject to several different regulatory checkpoints during light chain rearrangement to maintain tolerance in the bone marrow as well as to prevent autoreactivity and to ensure that B cells are expressing a functional antigen receptor. A B cell that rearranges an IgM receptor that interacts strongly with self antigen has one of two fates. It will either undergo clonal deletion, particularly if the self antigen is multivalent, or it will continue to rearrange its Ig light chain genes to produce a non self-reactive receptor in a process called receptor editing.[7–9] Autoreactive B cells with lower avidity self-antigen interactions, usually with small soluble self proteins, are able to escape clonal deletion in the bone marrow but then are likely to become inactivated and enter a state of anergy.[10] However, in some instances, self-reactive B cells do not encounter their specific antigens and remain in a state of immunological ignorance, due either to the specific antigen not being strongly stimulatory or limited accessibility of antigen in the bone marrow.[10] Regardless, not all self-reactive B cells are deleted in the bone marrow, and those that escape to the periphery are subject to additional regulatory mechanisms that shorten the lifespan of anergized B cells and are effective means of maintaining peripheral tolerance.

B CELL SELECTION, ACTIVATION, AND TOLERANCE IN THE PERIPHERAL IMMUNE SYSTEM

Upon exiting the bone marrow, B cells are still immature, expressing high levels of surface IgM but little IgD, whereas mature B cells express high levels of IgD.[11,12] Most of these B cells are destined for apoptosis after failing to be positively selected by T cells. B cells enter the periarteriolar sheath from high endothelial venules (HEVs), wherein they undergo further selection in a competitive process involving the B-cell receptor (BCR) and B-cell activating factor (BAFF).[13–15] In this area, B cells require interaction with T cells and T-cell-derived cytokine signals in order to survive. Anergic B cells have desensitized antigen receptors, limiting T-cell interactions, and respond poorly to cytokines, leading to a shortened lifespan and an increased propensity to undergo cell death.[16,17] Tolerized self-reactive B cells often do not escape the periarteriolar sheath due to these factors and can also be induced into programmed cell death (PCD) by T cells if they engage with them in a suboptimal interaction that does not properly activate the T cell.[18,19] Productive interactions in this zone enable B cells to enter into the B-cell follicle and become recirculating B cells.

Once a B cell starts recirculating, it has a half-life of about three days unless antigen is encountered.[20] The B cell traverses follicles once about every 24 hours and can encounter antigen in a variety of ways. They exit the bloodstream via HEVs and localize to the B-cell follicle, driven under the impetus of the chemokine CXCL13 produced by a specialized subset of B-cell follicle resident dendritic cells, follicular dendritic cells (FDCs), as well as other stromal cells.[21,22] CXCR5 receptor expressed on follicular B cells allows them to respond to CXCL13 chemokines and is one means that helps the B cell traverse the follicle.[22] In addition to responding to FDC-derived chemokines, B cells travel along the dendritic processes of these cells as a mode of transit throughout the follicle.[23] FDCs are centrally localized in primary follicles and serve as a repository for immune-complexed antigen, using complement receptors CD21 and CD35, as well as FcγRIIB, to capture antigen and retain it on the cell surface.[24–26] These immune complexes can remain on display on the cell surface long term for months and perhaps even years.[27] In an elegant *in vivo* imaging study using the hen egg lysozyme model antigen, it was shown that fluorescently labeled naïve B cells bearing a HEL-specific receptor adoptively transferred into mice that had been immunized with HEL antigen nine days prior to B-cell transfer were able to acquire antigen directly from the FDC cell surface.[28] Large particulate antigens cannot be shuttled through conduits and require accessory cells such as non-recirculating marginal zone B cells to transport them from the blood to FDCs for presentation.[29,30] Specialized macrophages in the marginal sinus are responsible for sampling blood-derived antigen and presenting it on the cell surface for delivery to B cells.[31–33] Noncognate B cells can acquire antigen via their complement receptors and then shuttle it to the follicle for presentation on FDCs.[20,30,31] However, if a cognate B cell comes in contact with marginal sinus macrophages it can be directly activated, which induces upregulation of CCR7 on the B-cell surface and migration to the T:B zone border to present antigen to T cells.[31–33] CCL21, the chemokine ligand for CCR7, is expressed by stromal cells and dendritic cells in the T-cell zone and attracts B cells expressing CCR7 to the T:B zone boundary.[22,31] Activated B cells also upregulate EBI2 receptor, which assists in arranging B cells along the T:B zone border.[34] Conversely, naïve T cells localized in the T-cell zone express high levels of CCR7 until they are activated by dendritic cells, which prompts them to downregulate CCR7, upregulate CXCR5, and, in response to CXCL13 produced in the B-cell follicle, migrate to the T:B zone boundary to interact with B cells.[35,36] These T cells are a specialized subset of helper cell called *T follicular helper cells* that are designed to support B-cell differentiation and proliferation in the follicle.

After acquiring antigen via its BCR, the B cell must internalize and process it through the endocytic processing pathway and present the resulting peptides in the context of MHC class II to T cells. Antigen-stimulated B cells that do not encounter a T cell of the same specificity die within 24 hours. Cognate CD4+ T helper cell binding to the peptide–MHC along with costimulatory molecule binding such as CD40L deliver activating signals to the B cell that enable it to proliferate and further differentiate.[37,38] Some of these B cells proliferate rapidly and migrate to an outer-follicular zone where they differentiate into plasmablasts in an early extrafollicular response. These cells become plasma cells that produce antibodies in a quick response to invading pathogens; however, it is believed that these antibodies are generally lower affinity than those produced by plasma cells that exit the germinal center (GC).[39] Most of these cells produce antibodies and then die by apoptosis after three days, although some exit to the bone marrow to compete for niches there as long-lived plasma cells.

Alternately, activated B cells at the T:B zone border will downregulate CCR7, upregulate CXCR5, migrate into the follicle, and enter a GC.[40] At the same time, productive interactions with B cells can induce T_{FH} cells to migrate into the germinal center and provide further support for dividing and differentiating B cells.[35] Tolerance mechanisms are in place at this juncture as well, to prevent an autoimmune response from taking place and will be discussed later.

GENERATION OF PLASMA CELLS AND MEMORY B CELLS IN THE GERMINAL CENTER

B cells that have productive interactions with T cells move to the B-cell follicle, where they become centrocytes that undergo clonal expansion, somatic hypermutation, and affinity maturation in GCs within secondary B-cell follicles. GCs are transient formations that generally disappear within 15 to 21 days of the first recognition of antigen, though the duration is highly dependent on the model system studied.[41] These are the principle sites where activated B cells differentiate into long-term memory cells and effector plasma cells. These processes provide yet another instance where self-reactive lymphocytes can be generated and must be tightly regulated in order to maintain tolerance.

How and when the fate of a B cell entering the germinal center is determined are questions that have puzzled scientists for decades. It has never been clear whether a B cell is preordained to become an antibody-producing plasma cell versus a memory B cell or if the fate of each cell is random. Recent studies suggest that timing is key to the generation of each of these prospective differentiation pathways. It appears that memory B cells are generated early on in GC formation, whereas plasma cells are preferentially produced later in the GC response.[42] Examination of memory BCR sequences revealed that these receptors have significantly fewer mutations than those of plasma cells and that memory BCR sequences matched those of early-stage GC B cells. Along with this, long-lived plasma cells found in the bone marrow bore BCRs similar to those found in late-stage GC B cells, suggesting that plasma cells are produced later in GC reactions.[42] Regardless of how these two cell types are produced, both persist after an antigenic response is resolved in order to be able to react to future antigenic challenges, and it is clear that the germinal center plays a primary role in their generation.

Activated B cells entering the secondary follicle rapidly expand, displacing resting follicular B cells, which get pushed to the periphery of the follicle and form a mantle zone around the dividing B cells, which express SIPR2, which inhibits B-cell migration out of the GC.[43] The GC is divided into a light zone and a dark zone based on immunohistochemical observations of spleen sections that noted light and dark areas in the germinal center. The light zone is proximal to the marginal sinus in the spleen, while the dark zone is most distal to the marginal sinus. The events that take place in the dark versus light zone have created controversy as to whether migration occurs between the two zones or whether each zone can support B-cell selection and proliferation independently of one another; however, recent data indicate that the classical view of interzonal migration is more likely to be correct. The light zone and dark zones contain distinct populations of nondividing centrocytes and mitotically active centroblasts, respectively. It was once thought that these two populations could be distinguished by size, with centroblasts being larger than centrocytes, but it is now known that cells in both zones are of similar size and shape.[44] After proliferation and somatic hypermutation in the dark zone, centroblasts travel to the light zone to capture antigen from follicular dendritic cells and undergo selection by T_{FH} cells. *In vivo* imaging studies have shown that there is a bias for travel from the dark zone to the light zone, as about 50% of B cells in the dark zone migrate to the light zone within four hours in a nonrandom manner,[44–46] but only about 15% of centrocytes in the light zone migrate to the dark zone. This does theoretically agree with the idea that after somatic hypermutation in the dark zone B cells migrate to the light zone to undergo selection by T cells. Most B cells would have unsuccessful interactions with T cells and apoptose, thus reducing the number of B cells available to return to the dark zone to undergo more rounds of proliferation and somatic hypermutation. Migration between the two zones is mediated by chemokine gradients. B cells centralized in the dark zone express chemokine receptor CXCR4 and chemotax toward SDF-1 produced by stromal cells.[47] In order to migrate to the light zone, B cells downregulate CXCR4, upregulate expression of CXCR5, and are attracted to CXCL13 produced by FDCs in the light zone.[47]

Somatic hypermutation and class switch recombination occur primarily in the dark zone of the GCs. Somatic hypermutation is a means of diversification of the antibody repertoire that is accomplished by introducing single base-pair substitutions, and rarely insertions or deletions into the variable regions of antibody gene segments.[48] This process is driven by activation-induced cytidine deaminase (AID), which selectively binds and deaminates only actively transcribed single-stranded DNA and introduces a lesion that must be repaired.[48] The mode of repair determines the variety of mutation that is introduced and the resulting antibody specificity. At each cell division, there is about a 50% chance that a centroblast will acquire a mutation in its receptor, and if the mutation increases the centroblast's ability to bind antigen then this clone proliferates and further mutations can occur.[49] In this manner, one BCR can accumulate many mutations, so long as the ability to bind antigen is maintained. Most mutations are deleterious to antigen binding, and these B cells are eliminated via apoptosis. Autoreactive specificities can also arise during this process, although not much is understood about how tolerance is maintained during a GC reaction. Two recent reports have found a population of regulatory T cells in the GC that express both Foxp3 and CXCR5 and have been termed T_{FR} cells.[50,51] Both studies concluded that these cells were important in regulating B cells and T cells in the GC, but whether this was from inhibition of T_{FH} cells or direct interaction with GC B cells was not clear. Future studies will tell us whether T_{FR} cells are also necessary for preventing autoreactive plasma cells and memory B cells from escaping the GC.

In order to continue to survive, B cells require continued interactions with the small population of T_{FH} that make up about 5% of the cells in the GC.[52] However, it is also assumed that there is limited antigen available for B cells to process and present to T cells, such that those B cells able to bind antigen with higher affinity have a selective advantage over those with low antigen affinity, either in their ability to acquire and retain antigen or in the amount that they are able to capture and present on the cell surface.[52] The better ability of B cells bearing high-affinity receptors to capture and present antigen to T cells ensures that these B cells will survive, while those bearing low-affinity receptors will not, and in this way affinity maturation of Ig receptors takes place.

The importance of T_{FH} cells to the generation, selection, and maintenance of GC B cells cannot be stressed enough. Both B cells and T cells in the germinal center express the transcription factor Bcl-6, which promotes cell cycle progression and proliferation and represses cellular responses to DNA damage so somatic hypermutation can occur.[53–55] In the absence of Bcl-6, GC formation in T-dependent responses is extremely poor. GC formation is also dependent on costimulatory T_{FH} cell signals through ICOS to promote expression of Bcl-6 and through CD40L to provide proliferation and survival signals.[56–58] It has been found that these costimulatory molecules are vital to proper function of T_{FH} cells that support GC B cells. Signaling through SAP downstream of SLAM receptors is also integral to formation of proper GCs. In the absence of SAP, production of T_{FH} cells is compromised, germinal center formation is disrupted, and the antibody responses generated are very poor.[59,60] SLAM family member CD84 is particularly important to B cell–T cell interactions in the germinal centers as CD84–CD84 binding stabilizes B cell–T cell conjugates.[60] In the absence of CD84 binding, B cell–T cell conjugates can only be maintained for a short time, germinal centers are much smaller, and plasma cells exiting the GC are of much lower affinity than normal. In the absence of IL-21, which is produced primarily by T_{FH} cells, germinal centers are smaller, B cells have defects in class-switching to IgG_1, and the duration of the GC is shortened.[49] This last feature is likely responsible for the reduced affinity maturation that takes place in IL-21-deficient environments. Because the longevity of the GC is shortened, this could limit the number of rounds of proliferation and somatic hypermutation that B cells can undergo before exiting the GC.

After 5 to 10 rounds of division and undergoing somatic hypermutation, class switching, and affinity maturation, memory B cells and plasma cells exit the GC to their respective fates. Memory B cells take up residence in secondary lymphoid tissue, where they can exist for several months. Short-lived plasma cells produce antibody and die in a few days. Long-lived plasma cells migrate to the bone marrow, where they compete for residence in specialized niches that provide survival factors to these cells. Plasma cells can persist for decades in the bone marrow and maintain antibodies to specific antigens at about 10% of the level reached at the peak of the germinal center response.[61]

FcγRIIB REGULATES B-CELL ACTIVATION AND APOPTOSIS

There are many different forms of regulation in maintaining humoral tolerance throughout the development of B cells and differentiation of antibody-producing plasma cells. Some of those regulatory mechanisms to avoid autoreactivity have already been discussed, such as clonal deletion and receptor editing in the bone marrow and B-cell selection by T cells in the peripheral immune system. Most of these regulatory mechanisms involve recognizing and eliminating B cells that have autoreactive BCRs. As stated previously, however, not all autoreactive B cells are removed from the repertoire, so additional methods of maintaining tolerance are put in place to prevent the development of autoimmune responses. B cells express both positive and negative co-receptors on the cell surface. These molecules exist to help balance the threshold of activation through the BCR. Receptors such as CD40 and TLRs expressed on B cells can contribute to reducing the threshold for activation through the BCR,[62] while inhibitory receptors such as CD22, CD72, and FcγRIIB increase the threshold for activation.[63] These negative regulatory receptors are important in preventing overstimulation of B cells and also in preventing low-affinity, self-reactive BCRs from being activated. FcγRIIB is particularly important in maintaining humoral tolerance in the periphery and is the primary focus of discussion here.

FcγRIIB expression is found on most immune cells, with the exception of T and NK cells. It contains an extracellular IgG-binding domain that is highly homologous to activating Fcγ receptors; however, the cytoplasmic tail contains an immunoreceptor tyrosine-based inhibitory motif (ITIM), which restricts signals leading to cell activation.[64] FcγRIIB is the only known inhibitory Fc receptor that binds IgG, though there are other FcR-like inhibitory molecules (FcRX and FcRH1-5) for which no ligands have yet been found.[65] Two membrane-bound isoforms of FcγRIIB that are encoded from the same gene are displayed on different cell types and have dichotomous functions. Immune cells other than B cells express FcγRIIB-2, which induces endocytosis or phagocytosis upon receptor cross-linking with IgG immune complexes.[66] However, FcγRIIB-1 expression is unique to B cells and only weakly induces internalization of IgG immune complexes. This isoform is generated by alternative mRNA splicing that results in a 47-amino-acid cytoplasmic insertion upstream of the ITIM motif that inhibits endocytosis by preventing receptor accumulation in clathrin pits.[67] FcγRIIB-1 is the sole Fc receptor expressed on B cells and plays a significant role as a regulator of B-cell activation and as a distal checkpoint in regulation of humoral tolerance.

FcγRIIB is expressed on all mature B cells and also on pre-B cells, though data from FcγRIIB-deficient mice suggest that it does not affect early maturation of B cells in the bone marrow, playing no known role in receptor editing, clonal deletion, or anergy.[68] It is also dispensable for some early peripheral checkpoints, as the absence or presence of FcγRIIB does not affect the generation of self-reactive IgM+ plasma cells, although this could be due to production of IgM+ short-lived plasmablasts occurring before the requisite IgG for FcγRIIB ligation is produced.[69–71] However, some research suggests that FcγRIIB could be important in preventing autoreactive B cells from gaining access to B-cell follicles in the spleen after exiting from the bone marrow. 3H9 transgenic mice have self-reactive B cells that escape into the periphery but then are denied access to the B-cell follicle and accumulate at the interface between the T-cell zone and B-cell follicle.[72] When these mice are crossed onto an FcγRIIB-deficient background, these B cells are able to gain access to the follicle, suggesting that the absence of FcγRIIB removes this peripheral checkpoint, perhaps by lowering the threshold for B-cell activation in self-reactive B cells, allowing them to migrate into the follicle.[72]

FcγRIIB utilizes multiple mechanisms to inhibit B-cell signaling, two that are dependent on ITIMs to dampen cellular activation and proliferation and two that are independent of this motif and instead act by disrupting immune synapse formation and inducing apoptosis in B cells respectively (Figure 6.1). Co-ligation of FcγRIIB with the BCR is able to disrupt early B-cell activation events upstream of inhibitory signaling through ITIMs, preventing BCR oligomerization, disrupting BCR transformation from a closed to an open signaling conformation, and altering the BCR-lipid raft environment.[73–76] Co-aggregation of FcγRIIB with the B-cell receptor activates an inhibitory signaling cascade that increases the threshold for activation through the BCR, ensuring that only high-affinity, non-self interactions lead to B-cell activation. Phosphorylation of tyrosine by Lyn in the cytoplasmic tail of FcγRIIB induces recruitment of SH2-domain-containing phosphatase SHIP-1, which blocks membrane recruitment of molecules that participate in BCR signaling and calcium mobilization (Btk and PLCγ, respectively).[77,78] An ITIM-dependent pathway is also used to arrest B-cell proliferation, although in this case the signaling mechanism is dependent on molecules such as Dok and MAP kinases.[77] B-cell synergistic activation via the BCR and endosomal TLR pathways is also subject to modulation by FcγRIIB.[79] B-cell responses to weakly immunostimulatory immune complexes containing CpG-poor dsDNA fragments were heightened in the absence of FcγRIIB, although the expression or lack thereof of FcγRIIB on B cells made no difference in B-cell responses to immune complexes containing CpG-rich dsDNA.[79]

FcγRIIB is also a strong inducer of apoptosis in B cells. Clustering of the FcγRIIB receptor on the B-cell surface leads to proapoptotic signals that activate caspases and induce cytochrome *c* release, although these signals can be partially blocked by co-ligation of FcγRIIB to the BCR and recruitment of SHIP.[80,81] FcγRIIB-induced apoptosis occurs independently of ITIM and SHIP-1 phosphatase and is reliant on c-Abl-mediated mechanisms for phosphorylation of membrane-proximal tyrosine phosphorylation of the cytoplasmic tail and downstream activation of MAP kinases.[81] Aggregation of FcγRIIB independent of the BCR allows for deletion of B cells that lose antigen specificity while undergoing somatic hypermutation during germinal center expansion, as well as those B cells that acquire self-reactive specificities. This is a particularly important checkpoint considering that the pathogenic potential of IgG autoantibodies is much higher than that of self-reactive IgM antibodies.

FcγRIIB INHIBITS AUTOANTIBODY PRODUCTION

Events such as somatic hypermutation in the germinal center allow for *de novo* generation of self-reactive B cells that are not subject to central tolerance mechanisms that take place in the bone marrow. Under normal circumstances, high-affinity, self-reactive lymphocytes that are generated during somatic hypermutation are deleted or tolerized, although the mechanisms

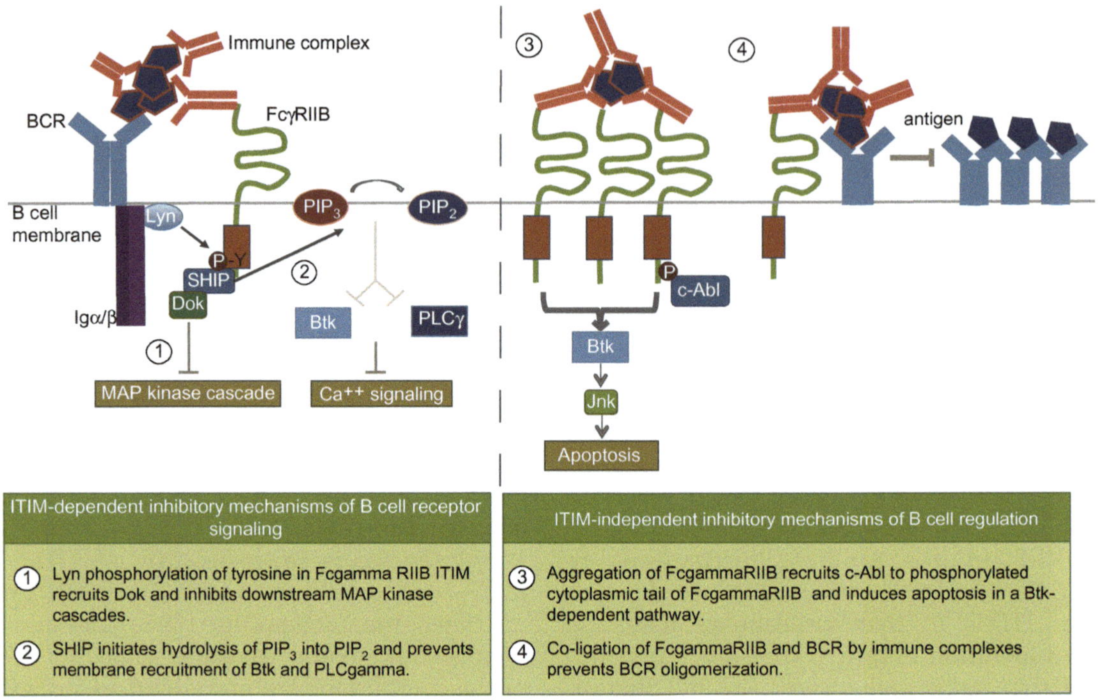

FIGURE 6.1 **FcγRIIB inhibitory mechanisms of B-cell signaling.** (1) Crosslinking of the B-cell receptor (BCR) with FcγRIIB by immune complexes leads to phosphorylation of ITIM in the cytoplasmic tail of FcγRIIB by Lyn. This induces recruitment of SRC-homology 2-domain-containing inositol-5 phosphatase (SHIP-1), which in turn could recruit docking protein (Dok) into close proximity with Lyn. Lyn activation of Dok leads to downstream arrest of MAP kinase activation and B-cell proliferation. (2) SHIP-1 association with phosphorylated ITIM in FcγRIIB blocks membrane recruitment of molecules that participate in BCR signaling and calcium mobilization, Bruton's tyrosine kinase (Btk) and phospholipase C gamma (PLCγ), respectively. (3) Aggregation of FcγRIIB on the surface of plasma cells activates an ITIM-independent pathway that relies upon c-Abl recruitment to a phosphorylated residue in the cytoplasmic tail of FcγRIIB. This pathway is also dependent upon Btk and c-Jun N terminal kinase (Jnk) activation for apoptosis induction. (4) Co-ligation of FcγRIIB and BCR by immune complexes sequesters BCRs and prevents them from oligomerizing in the membrane.

by which these occur in the GCs are not clear. However, B cells are still subject to selection checkpoints by T cells, requiring both cell contact with these cells as well as T cell-derived cytokine help to survive. In order for a B cell to present antigen to T cells and avoid apoptosis, negative signaling through FcγRIIB must be overcome. GC B cells normally express high levels of this receptor on their cell surfaces.[82–85] In the absence of FcγRIIB, GC B cells are enriched for somatically mutated self-reactive specificities, including anti-dsDNA and kidney reactivity, indicating that FcγRIIB plays a significant regulatory role in the GC.[8,86–89] Cytokine production of IL-4 by T cells has been shown to reduce the levels of FcγRIIB on the B-cell surface, lowering the threshold for activation and perhaps enhancing antigen presentation to T cells.[90] Conversely, high levels of FcγRIIB expression downregulate costimulatory molecules on the B-cell surface, such as CD86, and reduce antigen presenting capability.[69,91]

Setting a sufficiently high threshold of activation for B cells ensures both that low-affinity autoreactive B cells will be eliminated via deletion and that B cells bearing BCRs with the highest affinity for antigen have the potential to differentiate into antibody-producing cells. This idea is corroborated by evidence from mouse models deficient in FcγRIIB, in which the germinal center B-cell and plasma-cell compartments are expanded, but the quality of antibody-producing cells is compromised. These mice develop hypergammaglobulinaemia and spontaneously produce low-affinity polyreactive antibodies to a wide range of specificities, many of which are self-reactive; this leads to a lupus-like disease that eventually causes death due to glomerulonephritis.[89,92,93] Initial studies investigating immunization of FcγRIIB-deficient mice determined that T-dependent responses against sheep red blood cells (SRBCs) and trinitrophenol keyhole limpet (TNP-KLH), as well as T-independent responses against trinitrophenol lipopolysaccharide (THP-LPS) or trinitrophenol-Ficoll (TNP-Ficoll), elicited higher antibody titers of IgM, IgG_1, $IgG_{2a/b}$, IgG_3, and IgA than similarly immunized WT mice.[70] However, in this instance, autoimmune antibody specificities were not examined. It is important to note that strain differences in FcγRIIB-deficient mice do exist that affect the development of autoimmunity. Unlike C57BL/6 mice, Balb/c mice lacking FcγRIIB do not develop spontaneous disease, indicating the importance of strain-specific epistatic effects in the development of autoimmunity.[87] Receptor editing is also more efficient in Balb/c mice and may contribute to an increased resistance to developing autoimmunity. Balb/c.56R mice, which are transgenic for the expression of an anti-DNA heavy chain, effectively edit BCR light chains to circumvent the generation of DNA-binding BCR specificities and maintain tolerance.[94] However, this same transgene in the C57Bl/6 background exhibits anti-DNA antibodies in the serum, indicating that receptor editing is less efficient in this strain.[94] Furthermore, when C57Bl/6.56R mice are crossed with FcγRIIB-deficient mice, the production of anti-DNA antibodies is exacerbated, and these mice develop lupus-like disease.[94] In an extension of these studies, it was found that generation of pathogenic anti-DNA $IgG_{2a/b}$ antibodies in the C57Bl/6.56R FcγRIIB-deficient mice is dependent on signaling through MyD88 and TLR9.[88] In the absence of either of these signaling molecules, both of these subclasses of antibodies were reduced, while less pathogenic IgG_1 antibody production was more or less intact.[88]

In line with this result, autoimmune-prone strains such as NZB, NOD, and BXSB express lower levels of FcγRIIB on the activated and GC B-cell surface, which has been linked to polymorphisms in the promoter of this gene.[82–84,95] These polymorphisms lead to decreased transcription of FcγRIIB and subsequently reduced surface expression, resulting in a lower threshold for B-cell activation. Polymorphisms in the promoter region of human systemic lupus erythematosus (SLE) patients have also been identified, and lower expression of FcγRIIB on activated B-cell subsets has been confirmed.[96,97] Humanized mice harboring human B cells bearing naturally occurring and functionally impaired variants of FcγRIIB develop autoantibodies and have higher serum IgM and IgG titers, indicating that FcγRIIB plays an important role in humoral tolerance in humans as well.[86]

Although FcγRIIB is expressed on many immune cells, it is believed that autoimmunity arises in FcγRIIB-deficient mice from B cell-dependent breaks in tolerance, as this molecule has the potential to regulate B cells on several levels (Figure 6.2). Irradiated B cell-deficient mice reconstituted with bone marrow from FcγRIIB-deficient mice develop autoantibodies and autoimmunity, despite the fact that all immune cells other than B cells are able to express FcγRIIB.[87] Also, increasing B-cell

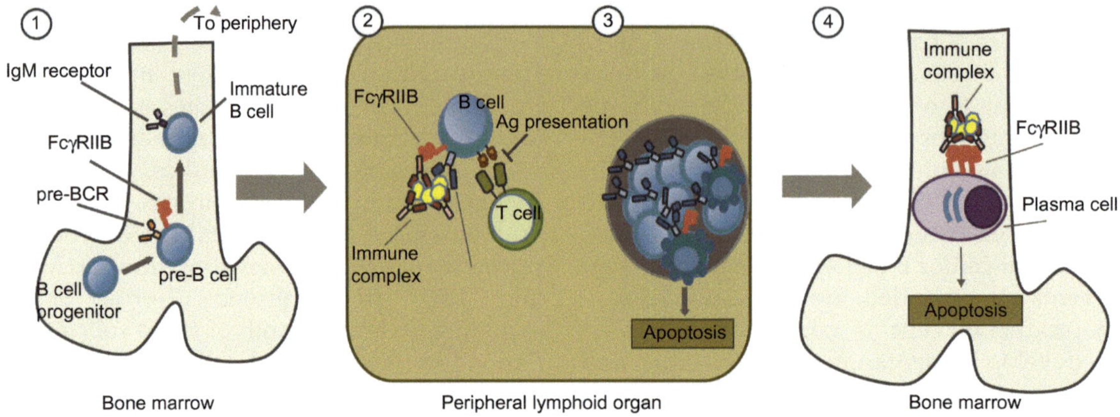

Developmental Stage	Location	FcγRIIB Proposed Function
(1) pre-B cell	Bone marrow	-Negative regulation of pre-BCR signals
(2) Mature B cell	Peripheral lymph node	-Prevent antigen presentation to T cell by stopping antigen internalization -Negative regulation of B cell activation -Possible role in follicular exclusion
(3) GC B cell	Germinal center	-Deletion of autoreactive specificities created by somatic hypermutation
(4) Long-lived plasma cell	Bone marrow	-Induce apoptosis upon immune complex engagement

FIGURE 6.2 **FcγRIIB functions in maintaining tolerance throughout B-cell development and differentiation.** (1) B cells undergo development in the bone marrow from a common lymphoid progenitor, developing into pre-B cells that express a pre-B cell receptor and then immature B cells expressing rearranged IgM receptors that exit the bone marrow to go to peripheral lymphoid organs. FcγRIIB is expressed at the pre-B cell stage, potentially negatively regulating the strength of pre-BCR signals to prevent apoptosis. (2) Once immature B cells enter a lymphoid organ, they must interact with and present antigen to T cells in order to receive cytokines vital to survival. Expression of high levels of FcγRIIB on B cells can reduce efficiency of antigen internalization and presentation to T cells or raise the BCR signal threshold to prevent activation of B cells that bind antigen with low affinity. These processes can lead to apoptosis of B cells or induction of anergy and exclude access to the B-cell follicle. (3) B cells in the germinal center (GC) undergo somatic hypermutation that can give rise to autoreactive specificities. High expression levels of FcγRIIB on GC B cells may be important in induction of apoptosis in *de novo*-generated autoreactive B cells. (4) After exiting the germinal center some B cells differentiate into plasma cells that home to the bone marrow for long-term survival. Plasma cells express little BCR but express high levels of FcγRIIB. Aggregation of FcγRIIB on the cell surface and interaction with immune complexes lead to plasma cell apoptosis.

expression of FcγRIIB to wild-type levels by retroviral transduction of bone marrow from autoimmune-prone mouse strains is able to prevent autoantibody production.[98] Finally, these data suggesting that expression of FcγRIIB in B cells is necessary to suppress autoimmunity were confirmed through cell-specific overexpression of FcγRIIB in a model of Mrl/*lpr* spontaneous autoimmunity.[69] B-cell overexpression of FcγRIIB likely increased the threshold for activation in these cells and prevented autoimmunity. These mice also produced higher affinity antibodies in T-dependent responses, reinforcing the importance of this molecule in generating an effective antibody repertoire. In contrast, overexpression of FcγRIIB in macrophages in Mrl/*lpr* mice was unable to suppress autoimmune disease, indicating that FcγRIIB on B cells but not macrophages is a key to preventing autoantibody production.

FcγRIIB AS A REGULATOR OF LONG-TERM SURVIVAL OF PLASMA CELLS IN THE BONE MARROW

Plasma cells play a vital role in the maintenance of humoral immunity by producing serum IgG antibodies, the bulk of which are made by a subset of long-lived plasma cells that reside in the bone marrow. Following primary T-dependent activation, B cells undergo class switch and somatic hypermutation in the germinal center. Some of these cells differentiate into a population of memory B cells that have high-affinity receptors and can be reactivated quickly upon secondary antigenic challenge. Interestingly, in humans, recirculating memory B-cell populations are enriched for poly- and self-reactive specificities, which is thought to be some sort of survival mechanism.[99] Other cells that exit from the GC become plasma cells, most of which rapidly secrete antibody and die after a few days; however, a small proportion of plasma cells with high-affinity receptors randomly produced in the germinal center migrate to the bone marrow, where they receive specialized survival signals to help them fully differentiate and become part of the long-lived plasma cell repertoire.[61] Unlike memory B cells, which are thought to maintain self-reactive specificities as a survival mechanism, poly- and self-reactive plasma cells are excluded from the bone marrow environment.[100] How these plasma cells are regulated and maintained in their specialized niches in the bone marrow after antigen resolution is still an area that is full of more questions than answers, but it is clear that FcγRIIB is integral to the regulation of this important population.

Long-lived plasma cells require survival signals from stromal cells and eosinophils, such as chemokine CXCL12 and cytokines IL-6, B cell-activating factor, APRIL, and tumor necrosis factor, in order to survive long term in the bone marrow.[61] Plasma cells make up roughly a tenth of a percent of all bone marrow populations, suggesting that there are a limited number of niches that can support plasma cell survival. How humoral tolerance is maintained over time and how space in the bone marrow is made for new plasma cells after each immune challenge remains an unsolved puzzle. Recent evidence has suggested that FcγRIIB is involved in homeostasis of these cells.[71] Plasma cells express little or no BCR on the cell surface but continuously transcribe FcγRIIB and express high levels of this receptor.[71] Cross-linking FcγRIIB on plasma cells with IgG immune complexes *in vitro* induces apoptosis in a BCL-2-interacting mediator of cell death (BIM)-dependent manner.[71] In a suggested model involving FcγRIIB in plasma cell turnover in the bone marrow, immune complexes generated during an immune response would cross-link FcγRIIB on some plasma cells, inducing apoptosis and creating space in bone marrow niches for new long-lived plasma cells. In support of this, secondary immunization studies in mice have shown that using a different antigen from the one mice were originally primed with reduces the antibody titers and number of circulating plasmablasts that are specific for the primary immunization antigen in an FcγRIIB-dependent manner.[71] FcγRIIB-deficient mice have increased numbers of plasma cells that are resistant to apoptosis, most likely contributing to the higher autoantibody titers found in the serum and induction of autoimmunity.[70,71,94]

Rescuing the expression of FcγRIIB by transducing deficient bone marrow cells with a retrovirus encoding FcγRIIB reduces the titers of autoreactive IgG in the serum.[98] Only 40% of the B cells were transduced in this model, indicating that even moderate increases in FcγRIIB expression can have therapeutic benefits. Corroborating these results, many autoimmune-prone strains with high levels of autoantibodies in the serum have B cells with unusually low expression of FcγRIIB on the cell surface.[82–84,95] Rectifying this phenotype by crossing some of these strains to a transgenic mouse overexpressing FcγRIIB on the surface of B cells results in lower serum IgG autoantibody titers and prolonged survival of these mice.[69] These studies point to FcγRIIB as a promising target for developing therapies for diseases involving dysregulation of plasma cells and IgG antibodies. Clinical studies manipulating FcγRIIB as a therapeutic agent are currently underway for treatment of a myriad of autoimmune diseases, lymphomas, and myelomas.

References

1. Nagasawa T. Microenvironmental niches in the bone marrow required for B-cell development. *Nat Rev Immunol* 2006;**6**:107–16.
2. Allman D, Li J, Hardy RR. Commitment to the B lymphoid lineage occurs before DH-JH recombination. *J Exp Med* 1999;**189**:735–40.
3. Hardy RR, Carmack CE, Shinton SA, et al. Resolution and characterization of pro-B and pre-pro-B cell stages in normal mouse bone marrow. *J Exp Med* 1991;**173**:1213–25.
4. Loffert D, Ehlich A, Muller W, et al. Surrogate light chain expression is required to establish immunoglobulin heavy chain allelic exclusion during early B cell development. *Immunity* 1996;**4**:133–44.
5. Geier JK, Schlissel MS. Pre-BCR signals and the control of Ig gene rearrangements. *Semin Immunol* 2006;**18**:31–9.
6. Sleckman BP, Gorman JR, Alt FW. Accessibility control of antigen-receptor variable-region gene assembly: role of cis-acting elements. *Annu Rev Immunol* 1996;**14**:459–81.
7. Casellas R, Shih TA, Kleinewietfeld M, et al. Contribution of receptor editing to the antibody repertoire. *Science* 2001;**291**:1541–4.
8. Chen C, Nagy Z, Radic MZ, et al. The site and stage of anti-DNA B-cell deletion. *Nature* 1995;**373**:252–5.
9. Cornall RJ, Goodnow CC, Cyster JG. The regulation of self-reactive B cells. *Curr Opin Immunol* 1995;**7**:804–11.
10. Pillai S, Mattoo H, Cariappa A. B cells and autoimmunity. *Curr Opin Immunol*. 2011;**23**:721–31.
11. Carsetti R, Kohler G, Lamers MC. Transitional B cells are the target of negative selection in the B cell compartment. *J Exp Med* 1995;**181**:2129–40.
12. Jacobsen K, Osmond DG. Microenvironmental organization and stromal cell associations of B lymphocyte precursor cells in mouse bone marrow. *Eur J Immunol* 1990;**20**:2395–404.
13. Marchesi VT, Gowans JL. The migration of lymphocytes through the endothelium of venules in lymph nodes: an electron microscope study. *Proc R Soc Lond B Biol Sci* 1964;**159**:283–90.
14. Girard JP, Springer TA. High endothelial venules (HEVs): specialized endothelium for lymphocyte migration. *Immunol Today* 1995;**16**:449–57.
15. Stadanlick JE, Cancro MP. BAFF and the plasticity of peripheral B cell tolerance. *Curr Opin Immunol* 2008;**20**:158–61.
16. Goodnow CC, Crosbie J, Adelstein S, et al. Altered immunoglobulin expression and functional silencing of self-reactive B lymphocytes in transgenic mice. *Nature* 1988;**334**:676–82.
17. Cooke MP, Heath AW, Shokat KM, et al. Immunoglobulin signal transduction guides the specificity of B cell–T cell interactions and is blocked in tolerant self-reactive B cells. *J Exp Med* 1994;**179**:425–38.
18. Rathmell JC, Cooke MP, Ho WY, et al. CD95 (Fas)-dependent elimination of self-reactive B cells upon interaction with CD4+ T cells. *Nature* 1995;**376**:181–4.
19. Foote LC, Marshak-Rothstein A, Rothstein TL. Tolerant B lymphocytes acquire resistance to Fas-mediated apoptosis after treatment with interleukin 4 but not after treatment with specific antigen unless a surface immunoglobulin threshold is exceeded. *J Exp Med* 1998;**187**:847–53.
20. Gonzalez SF, Degn SE, Pitcher LA, et al. Trafficking of B cell antigen in lymph nodes. *Annu Rev Immunol* 2011;**29**:215–33.
21. Gunn MD, Ngo VN, Ansel KM, et al. A B-cell-homing chemokine made in lymphoid follicles activates Burkitt's lymphoma receptor-1. *Nature* 1998;**391**:799–803.
22. Reif K, Ekland EH, Ohl L, et al. Balanced responsiveness to chemoattractants from adjacent zones determines B-cell position. *Nature* 2002;**416**:94–9.
23. Bajenoff M, Egen JG, Koo LY, et al. Stromal cell networks regulate lymphocyte entry, migration, and territoriality in lymph nodes. *Immunity* 2006;**25**:989–1001.
24. Molina H, Holers VM, Li B, et al. Markedly impaired humoral immune response in mice deficient in

complement receptors 1 and 2. *Proc Natl Acad Sci USA* 1996;**93**:3357–61.
25. Ahearn JM, Fischer MB, Croix D, et al. Disruption of the Cr2 locus results in a reduction in B-1a cells and in an impaired B cell response to T-dependent antigen. *Immunity* 1996;**4**:251–62.
26. El Shikh ME, El Sayed R, Szakal AK, et al. Follicular dendritic cell (FDC)-FcgammaRIIB engagement via immune complexes induces the activated FDC phenotype associated with secondary follicle development. *Eur J Immunol* 2006;**36**:2715–24.
27. Tew JG, Mandel TE. Prolonged antigen half-life in the lymphoid follicles of specifically immunized mice. *Immunology* 1979;**37**:69–76.
28. Suzuki K, Grigorova I, Phan TG, et al. Visualizing B cell capture of cognate antigen from follicular dendritic cells. *J Exp Med* 2009;**206**:1485–93.
29. Roozendaal R, Mempel TR, Pitcher LA, et al. Conduits mediate transport of low-molecular-weight antigen to lymph node follicles. *Immunity* 2009;**30**:264–76.
30. Cinamon G, Zachariah MA, Lam OM, et al. Follicular shuttling of marginal zone B cells facilitates antigen transport. *Nat Immunol* 2008;**9**:54–62.
31. Phan TG, Grigorova I, Okada T, et al. Subcapsular encounter and complement-dependent transport of immune complexes by lymph node B cells. *Nat Immunol* 2007;**8**:992–1000.
32. Junt T, Moseman EA, Iannacone M, et al. Subcapsular sinus macrophages in lymph nodes clear lymph-borne viruses and present them to antiviral B cells. *Nature* 2007;**450**:110–4.
33. Carrasco YR, Batista FD. B cells acquire particulate antigen in a macrophage-rich area at the boundary between the follicle and the subcapsular sinus of the lymph node. *Immunity* 2007;**27**:160–71.
34. Pereira JP, Kelly LM, Xu Y, et al. EBI2 mediates B cell segregation between the outer and centre follicle. *Nature* 2009;**460**:1122–6.
35. Haynes NM, Allen CD, Lesley R, et al. Role of CXCR5 and CCR7 in follicular Th cell positioning and appearance of a programmed cell death gene-1 high germinal center-associated subpopulation. *J Immunol* 2007;**179**:5099–108.
36. Vinuesa CG, Cyster JG. How T cells earn the follicular rite of passage. *Immunity* 2011;**35**:671–80.
37. Jaiswal AI, Croft M. CD40 ligand induction on T cell subsets by peptide-presenting B cells: implications for development of the primary T and B cell response. *J Immunol* 1997;**159**:2282–91.
38. Grewal IS, Flavell RA. The role of CD40 ligand in costimulation and T-cell activation. *Immunol Rev* 1996;**153**:85–106.
39. Shih TA, Meffre E, Roederer M, et al. Role of BCR affinity in T cell dependent antibody responses *in vivo*. *Nat Immunol* 2002;**3**:570–5.
40. Gatto D, Wood K, Brink R. EBI2 operates independently of but in cooperation with CXCR5 and CCR7 to direct B cell migration and organization in follicles and the germinal center. *J Immunol* 2011;**187**:4621–8.
41. Allen CD, Okada T, Cyster JG. Germinal-center organization and cellular dynamics. *Immunity* 2007;**27**:190–202.
42. Takahashi Y, Ohta H, Takemori T. Fas is required for clonal selection in germinal centers and the subsequent establishment of the memory B cell repertoire. *Immunity* 2001;**14**:181–92.
43. Green JA, Suzuki K, Cho B, et al. The sphingosine 1-phosphate receptor S1P maintains the homeostasis of germinal center B cells and promotes niche confinement. *Nat Immunol* 2011;**12**:672–80.
44. Victora GD, Schwickert TA, Fooksman DR, et al. Germinal center dynamics revealed by multiphoton microscopy with a photoactivatable fluorescent reporter. *Cell* 2010;**143**:592–605.
45. Figge MT, Garin A, Gunzer M, et al. Deriving a germinal center lymphocyte migration model from two-photon data. *J Exp Med* 2008;**205**:3019–29.
46. Beltman JB, Allen CD, Cyster JG, et al. B cells within germinal centers migrate preferentially from dark to light zone. *Proc Natl Acad Sci USA* 2011;**108**:8755–60.
47. Allen CD, Ansel KM, Low C, et al. Germinal center dark and light zone organization is mediated by CXCR4 and CXCR5. *Nat Immunol* 2004;**5**:943–52.
48. Maul RW, Gearhart PJ. AID and somatic hypermutation. *Adv Immunol* 2010;**105**:159–91.
49. Vinuesa CG, Linterman MA, Goodnow CC, et al. T cells and follicular dendritic cells in germinal center B-cell formation and selection. *Immunol Rev* 2010;**237**:72–89.
50. Wollenberg I, Agua-Doce A, Hernandez A, et al. Regulation of the germinal center reaction by Foxp3+ follicular regulatory T cells. *J Immunol* 2011;**187**:4553–60.
51. Linterman MA, Pierson W, Lee SK, et al. Foxp3+ follicular regulatory T cells control the germinal center response. *Nat Med* 2011;**17**:975–82.
52. Tarlinton DM. Evolution in miniature: selection, survival and distribution of antigen reactive cells in the germinal centre. *Immunol Cell Biol* 2008;**86**:133–8.
53. Shaffer AL, Yu X, He Y, et al. BCL-6 represses genes that function in lymphocyte differentiation, inflammation, and cell cycle control. *Immunity* 2000;**13**:199–212.
54. Johnston RJ, Poholek AC, DiToro D, et al. Bcl6 and Blimp-1 are reciprocal and antagonistic regulators of T follicular helper cell differentiation. *Science* 2009;**325**:1006–10.
55. Nurieva RI, Chung Y, Martinez GJ, et al. Bcl6 mediates the development of T follicular helper cells. *Science* 2009;**325**:1001–5.

56. Choi YS, Kageyama R, Eto D, et al. ICOS receptor instructs T follicular helper cell versus effector cell differentiation via induction of the transcriptional repressor Bcl6. *Immunity* 2011;**34**:932–46.
57. Crotty S. Follicular helper CD4 T cells (TFH). *Annu Rev Immunol* 2011;**29**:621–63.
58. Good-Jacobson KL, Shlomchik MJ. Plasticity and heterogeneity in the generation of memory B cells and long-lived plasma cells: the influence of germinal center interactions and dynamics. *J Immunol* 2010;**185**:3117–25.
59. Qi H, Cannons JL, Klauschen F, et al. SAP-controlled T-B cell interactions underlie germinal centre formation. *Nature* 2008;**455**:764–9.
60. Cannons JL, Qi H, Lu KT, et al. Optimal germinal center responses require a multistage T cell:B cell adhesion process involving integrins, SLAM-associated protein, and CD84. *Immunity* 2010;**32**:253–65.
61. Radbruch A, Muehlinghaus G, Luger EO, et al. Competence and competition: the challenge of becoming a long-lived plasma cell. *Nat Rev Immunol* 2006;**6**:741–50.
62. Cerutti A, Puga I, Cols M. Innate control of B cell responses. *Trends Immunol* 2011;**32**:202–11.
63. Nitschke L. The role of CD22 and other inhibitory co-receptors in B-cell activation. *Curr Opin Immunol* 2005;**17**:290–7.
64. Ravetch JV, Kinet JP. Fc receptors. *Annu Rev Immunol* 1991;**9**:457–92.
65. Davis RS, Ehrhardt GR, Leu CM, et al. An extended family of Fc receptor relatives. *Eur J Immunol* 2005;**35**:674–80.
66. Miettinen HM, Rose JK, Mellman I. Fc receptor isoforms exhibit distinct abilities for coated pit localization as a result of cytoplasmic domain heterogeneity. *Cell* 1989;**58**:317–27.
67. Miettinen HM, Matter K, Hunziker W, et al. Fc receptor endocytosis is controlled by a cytoplasmic domain determinant that actively prevents coated pit localization. *J Cell Biol* 1992;**116**:875–88.
68. Brauweiler AM, Cambier JC. Autonomous SHIP-dependent FcgammaR signaling in pre-B cells leads to inhibition of cell migration and induction of cell death. *Immunol Lett* 2004;**92**:75–81.
69. Brownlie RJ, Lawlor KE, Niederer HA, et al. Distinct cell-specific control of autoimmunity and infection by FcgammaRIIb. *J Exp Med* 2008;**205**:883–95.
70. Takai T, Ono M, Hikida M, et al. Augmented humoral and anaphylactic responses in Fc gamma RII-deficient mice. *Nature* 1996;**379**:346–9.
71. Xiang Z, Cutler AJ, Brownlie RJ, et al. FcgammaRIIb controls bone marrow plasma cell persistence and apoptosis. *Nat Immunol* 2007;**8**:419–29.
72. Paul E, Nelde A, Verschoor A, et al. Follicular exclusion of autoreactive B cells requires FcgammaRIIb. *Int Immunol* 2007;**19**:365–73.
73. Liu W, Won Sohn H, Tolar P, et al. Antigen-induced oligomerization of the B cell receptor is an early target of Fc gamma RIIB inhibition. *J Immunol* 2010;**184**:1977–89.
74. Sohn HW, Pierce SK, Tzeng SJ. Live cell imaging reveals that the inhibitory FcgammaRIIB destabilizes B cell receptor membrane-lipid interactions and blocks immune synapse formation. *J Immunol* 2008;**180**:793–9.
75. Kono H, Kyogoku C, Suzuki T, et al. FcgammaRIIB Ile232Thr transmembrane polymorphism associated with human systemic lupus erythematosus decreases affinity to lipid rafts and attenuates inhibitory effects on B cell receptor signaling. *Hum Mol Genet* 2005;**14**:2881–92.
76. Floto RA, Clatworthy MR, Heilbronn KR, et al. Loss of function of a lupus-associated FcgammaRIIb polymorphism through exclusion from lipid rafts. *Nat Med* 2005;**11**:1056–8.
77. Bolland S, Ravetch JV. Inhibitory pathways triggered by ITIM-containing receptors. *Adv Immunol* 1999;**72**:149–77.
78. Ono M, Okada H, Bolland S, et al. Deletion of SHIP or SHP-1 reveals two distinct pathways for inhibitory signaling. *Cell* 1997;**90**:293–301.
79. Avalos AM, Uccellini MB, Lenert P, et al. FcγRIIB regulation of BCR/TLR-dependent autoreactive B-cell responses. *Eur J Immunol* 2010;**40**:2692–8.
80. Pearse RN, Kawabe T, Bolland S, et al. SHIP recruitment attenuates Fc gamma RIIB-induced B cell apoptosis. *Immunity* 1999;**10**:753–60.
81. Tzeng SJ, Bolland S, Inabe K, et al. The B cell inhibitory Fc receptor triggers apoptosis by a novel c-Abl family kinase-dependent pathway. *J Biol Chem* 2005;**280**:35247–54.
82. Jiang Y, Hirose S, Abe M, et al. Polymorphisms in IgG Fc receptor IIB regulatory regions associated with autoimmune susceptibility. *Immunogenetics* 2000;**51**:429–35.
83. Jiang Y, Hirose S, Sanokawa-Akakura R, et al. Genetically determined aberrant down-regulation of FcgammaRIIB1 in germinal center B cells associated with hyper-IgG and IgG autoantibodies in murine systemic lupus erythematosus. *Int Immunol* 1999;**11**:1685–91.
84. Pritchard NR, Cutler AJ, Uribe S, et al. Autoimmune-prone mice share a promoter haplotype associated with reduced expression and function of the Fc receptor FcγRII. *Curr Biol* 2000;**10**:227–30.
85. Xiu Y, Nakamura K, Abe M, et al. Transcriptional regulation of Fcgr2b gene by polymorphic promoter region and its contribution to humoral immune responses. *J Immunol* 2002;**169**:4340–6.
86. Baerenwaldt A, Lux A, Danzer H, et al. Fcgamma receptor IIB (FcgammaRIIB) maintains humoral tolerance in the human immune system in vivo. *Proc Natl Acad Sci USA* 2011;**108**:18772–7.
87. Bolland S, Ravetch JV. Spontaneous autoimmune disease in Fc(gamma)RIIB-deficient mice results from strain-specific epistasis. *Immunity* 2000;**13**:277–85.

88. Ehlers M, Fukuyama H, McGaha TL, et al. TLR9/MyD88 signaling is required for class switching to pathogenic IgG2a and 2b autoantibodies in SLE. *J Exp Med* 2006;**203**:553–61.
89. Tiller T, Kofer J, Kreschel C, et al. Development of self-reactive germinal center B cells and plasma cells in autoimmune Fc gammaRIIB-deficient mice. *J Exp Med* 2010;**207**:2767–78.
90. Rudge EU, Cutler AJ, Pritchard NR, et al. Interleukin 4 reduces expression of inhibitory receptors on B cells and abolishes CD22 and Fc gamma RII-mediated B cell suppression. *J Exp Med* 2002;**195**:1079–85.
91. Smith KG, Clatworthy MR. FcγRIIB in autoimmunity and infection: evolutionary and therapeutic implications. *Nat Rev Immunol* 2010;**10**:328–43.
92. Mackay M, Stanevsky A, Wang T, et al. Selective dysregulation of the FcgammaIIB receptor on memory B cells in SLE. *J Exp Med* 2006;**203**:2157–64.
93. Tackenberg B, Jelcic I, Baerenwaldt A, et al. Impaired inhibitory Fcgamma receptor IIB expression on B cells in chronic inflammatory demyelinating polyneuropathy. *Proc Natl Acad Sci USA* 2009;**106**:4788–92.
94. Fukuyama H, Nimmerjahn F, Ravetch JV. The inhibitory Fcgamma receptor modulates autoimmunity by limiting the accumulation of immunoglobulin G+ anti-DNA plasma cells. *Nat Immunol* 2005;**6**:99–106.
95. Luan JJ, Monteiro RC, Sautes C, et al. Defective Fc gamma RII gene expression in macrophages of NOD mice: genetic linkage with up-regulation of IgG1 and IgG2b in serum. *J Immunol* 1996;**157**:4707–16.
96. Kyogoku C, Dijstelbloem HM, Tsuchiya N, et al. Fcgamma receptor gene polymorphisms in Japanese patients with systemic lupus erythematosus: contribution of FCGR2B to genetic susceptibility. *Arthritis Rheum* 2002;**46**:1242–54.
97. Willcocks LC, Carr EJ, Niederer HA, et al. A defunctioning polymorphism in FCGR2B is associated with protection against malaria but susceptibility to systemic lupus erythematosus. *Proc Natl Acad Sci USA* 2010;**107**:7881–5.
98. McGaha TL, Sorrentino B, Ravetch JV. Restoration of tolerance in lupus by targeted inhibitory receptor expression. *Science* 2005;**307**:590–3.
99. Tiller T, Tsuiji M, Yurasov S, et al. Autoreactivity in human IgG+ memory B cells. *Immunity* 2007;**26**:205–13.
100. Scheid JF, Mouquet H, Kofer J, et al. Differential regulation of self-reactivity discriminates between IgG+ human circulating memory B cells and bone marrow plasma cells. *Proc Natl Acad Sci USA* 2011;**108**:18044–8.

CHAPTER

7

Structural Recognition of Immunoglobulins by Fcγ Receptors

Peter Sun

Laboratory of Immunogenetics, National Institute of Allergy and Infectious Diseases, National Institutes of Health, Rockville, Maryland

INTRODUCTION

Immunoglobulin Fc receptors (FcRs) are expressed on all hematopoietic cells and play crucial roles in antibody-mediated immune responses.[1–3] Binding of immune complexes to FcR activates effector cells, leading to phagocytosis, endocytosis of IgG-opsonized particles, releases of inflammatory mediators, and antibody-dependent cellular cytotoxicity (ADCC).[4–8] Fc receptors have been described for all classes of immunoglobulins: FcγR and neonatal FcR (FcRn) for IgG, FcεR for IgE, FcαR for IgA, FcδR for IgD, and FcμR for IgM.[3,9–16] Of these receptors, leucocyte FcγR and FcεR are characterized most extensively. Structurally, all known Fc receptors belong to the immunoglobulin superfamily, except for FcRn and FcεRII, which are structurally related to class I major histocompatibility antigens and C-type lectins, respectively. Among them, FcγRI and FcεRI are high-affinity Fc receptors with dissociation constants ranging from 10^{-8} to 10^{-10}M.[12,17] All other IgG receptors, such as FcγRII and FcγRIII, are low-affinity receptors with dissociation constants in the range of 10^{-5} to 10^{-7}M. The high-affinity receptors FcεRI and FcγRI are activated by monomeric immunoglobulins. Under physiological conditions, the low-affinity receptors FcγRII and FcγRIII require multivalent immune complexes for their activation. In addition to the affinity variations among the receptors, each Fcγ receptor displays distinct IgG subtype specificities; for example, FcγRIII binds IgG_1 and IgG_3 better than IgG_2 and IgG_4.[18] Structural knowledge regarding antibody recognition by Fc receptors is critically important to antibody-mediated immune therapeutics. This review focuses on the structures of Fcγ receptors and their recognition of IgGs, as well as more recent findings of pentraxin recognition by Fc receptors.

STRUCTURES OF Fcγ RECEPTORS

In humans, three classes of receptors, FcγRI, FcγRII, and FcγRIII, have been described.[3] All Fcγ receptors are type I transmembrane glycoproteins with a ligand-binding α-subunit consisting of two (FcγRIIA,B,C and FcγRIIIA,B) or three (FcγRIA,B,C) C2-type immunoglobulin-like domains. All Fcγ receptors show a high degree of sequence identity in their extracellular portion (50 to 96%) but differ significantly in their cytoplasmic domains.[12] Some Fcγ receptors contain the immunoreceptor tyrosine-based activation motif (ITAM) (FcγRIIA,C) or the corresponding inhibitory motif (ITIM) (FcγRIIB) in their cytoplasmic tails. Others (FcγRI and FcγRIIIA) require the association of the ITAM-containing Fc receptor common γ-chain or T-cell receptor ζ-chain for signaling.[19] Activating and inhibitory Fcγ receptors are co-expressed on macrophages, monocytes, neutrophils, and eosonophils.[13] Different from other Fcγ receptors, FcγRIIIB is expressed exclusively on neutrophils. It contains no signaling component and is anchored to the plasma membrane via a glycosylphosphatidylinositol anchor. Presumably, FcγRIIIB acts synergistically with other receptors like FcγRIIA and uses their signaling apparatus for signal transduction and cell activation.[20–22] A soluble form of FcγRIIIB was reported to activate CR3 complement receptor-dependent inflammatory pathways.

IgG binding affinities vary considerably among Fcγ receptors (Table 7.1).[11,18,23,24] In solution, human FcγRI binds to IgG_1, IgG_3, and IgG_4 with similar affinities between 10 and 100 nM.

TABLE 7.1 Solution IgG and Pentraxins Binding Affinities for Human FcγRs (10^{-6} M)

	FcγRI	FcγRII	FcγRIII
IgG1	10^{-8}–10^{-7} (M)	10^{-7}–10^{-6} (M)	10^{-6}–10^{-5} (M)
IgG2	$>10^{-6}$ (M)	$>10^{-5}$ (M)	$>10^{-5}$ (M)
IgG3	10^{-8}–10^{-7} (M)	10^{-6} (M)	10^{-6}–10^{-5} (M)
IgG4	10^{-8}–10^{-7} (M)	10^{-6} (M)	10^{-6} (M)
CRP	10^{-6} (M)	10^{-6} (M)	10^{-6} (M)
SAP	10^{-7} (M)	10^{-6} (M)	10^{-6} (M)
PTX3	N.D.	N.D.	10^{-6} (M)

FcγRIIA displays intermediate IgG binding affinities between 10^{-7} and 10^{-6} M. FcγRIIB and FcγRIII are low-affinity IgG receptors with affinities generally around 10^{-6} M; however, these affinities also vary depending on FcγR allotype. In addition, FcγRs also discriminate an individual subclass of IgGs. In general, IgG_1 and IgG_3 display similar affinities toward each FcγR isoforms, whereas IgG_2 has the lowest affinity for FcγRs. These differential receptor binding affinities suggest that (1) FcγRI on circulating leukocytes is likely pre-occupied by IgGs; (2) antibodies of IgG_1 and IgG_3 subclasses trigger better effector cell responses; and (3) activation of Fcγ receptors, especially FcγRII and FcγRIII, requires immune complex formation.

The crystal structures of the extracellular portion of four ligand-free Fcγ receptors (FcγRIA, FcγRIIA, FcγRIIB, and FcγRIII), as well as the structure of ligand-free FcεRI, have been solved to date.[24–29] FcγRI is the only Fcγ receptor with three extracellular Ig-like domains, and its structure shows that the N-terminal two domains, D1 and D2, act as structural equivalents of the two domain receptors.[24] Overall, all FcγRs display very similar D1 and D2 domain structures that can be superimposed with root-mean-square (r.m.s.) deviations of 0.9 to 1.1 Å. Both D1 and D2 domains belong to variations of a C2-type Ig-like structure with two β-sheets packing against each other and stabilized by a disulfide bond between the sheets (Figure 7.1A). One β-sheet consists of strands A-A′-B-E and the other of strands C′-C′-F-G. The disulfide bond, common to the Ig-fold, cross-links strands B and F. There is only one short α-helix in each domain in the EF loop. This short α-helix is not part of the Ig-fold but has been observed in many Ig-like structures. A subtle difference between the D1 and D2 domains is the splitting of the G-strand into G and G′ strands in D2 but not D1 domains (Figure 7.1B). A feature common to all known Ig-like Fc receptors is the peculiar hinge angle

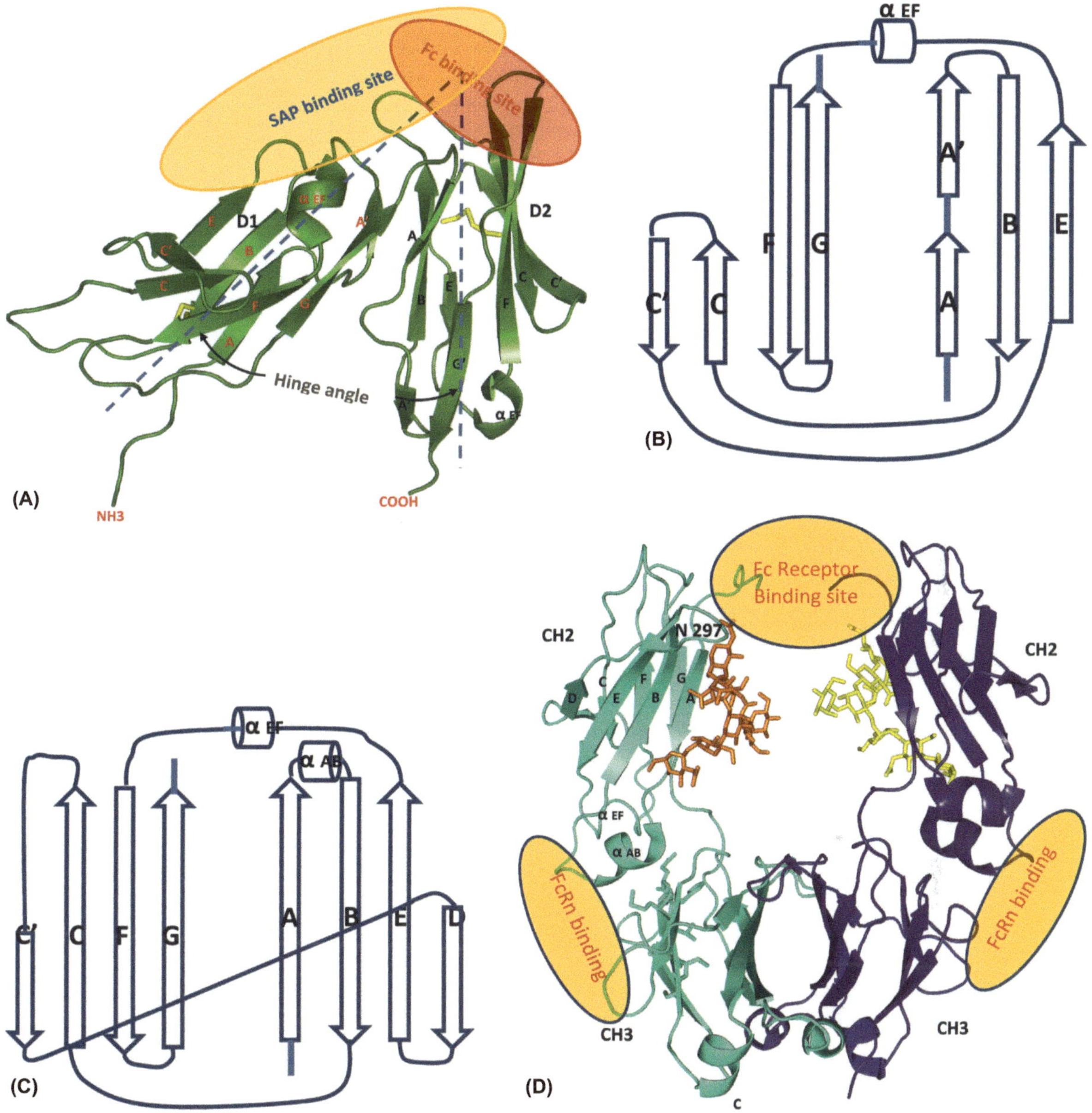

FIGURE 7.1 **Structures of Fcγ receptor and IgG–Fc.** (A) Illustration of FcγRIIIB structure with α-strands labeled. The receptor binding sites for IgG–Fc and pentraxins are indicated. (B, C) Secondary structure diagram of Fcγ receptor (B) and Fc (C). (D) Structure of IgG–Fc with the two chains are colored cyan and blue. The glycans attached to Asn 297 of each chain are shown in orange and yellow stick models. Fc receptors bind at the lower hinge region close to the N-terminal of the C_H2 domains of Fc. FcRn binds at the junction between C_H2 and C_H3 domains.

between D1 and D2 domains. This hinge angle is approximately 50° to 55° for FcγRII and FcγRIII.[27,30] Compared to other Ig-like structures, such as the hematopoietic receptors, natural killer cell killer immunoglobulin-like receptors (KIRs) and adhesion receptors, Fc receptors not only have smaller hinge angles but the juxtaposition of their N-terminal (D1) domain with respect to the C-terminal (D2) domain is also opposite to other receptors.[30] This opposite D1 and D2 domain orientation in Fc receptor structures is likely due to a shorter interdomain linker found in Fc receptors as compared to those in KIR and growth hormone receptors. The D1–D2 hinge angle is stabilized by both hydrophobic and charged interactions. Interestingly, the D1–D2 hinge angles observed in the structures of high-affinity FcγRI and FcεRI are significantly smaller than those in low-affinity receptor structures. Both FcγRI and FcεRI display the D1–D2 hinge angle of about 35°.[24] It is unclear, however, if smaller hinge angles contribute to their high affinity for antibody.

STRUCTURE OF THE IgG Fc DOMAIN

The IgG heavy chain consists of four regions: V_H1, C_H1, C_H2, and C_H3. V_H1 and C_H1 pair with IgG light chains to form Fab domains. C_H2 and C_H3 self dimerize to form a disulfide-bonded Fc domain. The structures of several Fc fragments have been determined.[31–37] Both C_H2 and C_H3 domains of Fc are C1-type immunoglobulin domains with their β-strands A-B-E-D packed against C′-C-F-G to form a β-sandwich (Figure 7.1C). There are two short α-helices in each domain, one in the loop connecting strands A and B and one in the loop connecting strands E and F. Like other Ig-folds, both C_H2 and C_H3 domains are stabilized by a disulfide bond between their B and F strands. The overall shape of Fc resembles a horseshoe, with the two C_H3 domains packed tightly against each other at the bottom of the horseshoe and the two C_H2 domains forming the opening of the horseshoe at the hinge region (Figure 7.1D). The intact Fc portion of an antibody shows an intrinsic twofold symmetry relating the two chains. A unique feature among Fc structures is their ordered carbohydrate moieties associated with the conserved glycosylation residue Asn 297 on both chains of Fc. Unlike most glycosylated proteins, Asn 297 is strictly conserved among all subtypes of IgGs and is present also in IgA, IgE, and IgM. In general, N-linked glycans are exposed on the protein surface and structurally disordered. Glycan associated with Asn 297, however, is partially ordered in all known Fc structures. Carbohydrate residues from the two chains of Fc pack against each other in the center of the CH_2 dimer, forming a surrogate hydrophobic core in the C_H2 domain (Figure 7.1D). Removing glycan by peptide *N*-glycanase digestion reduces IgG binding to most FcγR and results in a more closed conformation of Fc.[38,39] Indeed, the specific glycan structure is known to influence receptor binding affinity. Different regions of Fc are known to bind to different receptors. While Fcγ receptors bind to the lower hinge region immediately preceding the C_H2 domain, neonatal FcRn as well as bacterial protein A and protein G bind to the C_H2–C_H3 joint region (Figure 7.1D).[31,40]

STRUCTURE OF FcγRIII–Fc COMPLEX

In general, Fcγ receptors respond to immune complexes rather than monomeric antibody–antigen complex. The need to form multivalent antibody–antigen complexes reflects the low binding affinity between IgGs and Fc receptors. Earlier mutational work on IgG-Fc identified the lower hinge region, particularly residues between C_H1 and C_H2 domains of IgG-Fc, as being critical for Fcγ receptor

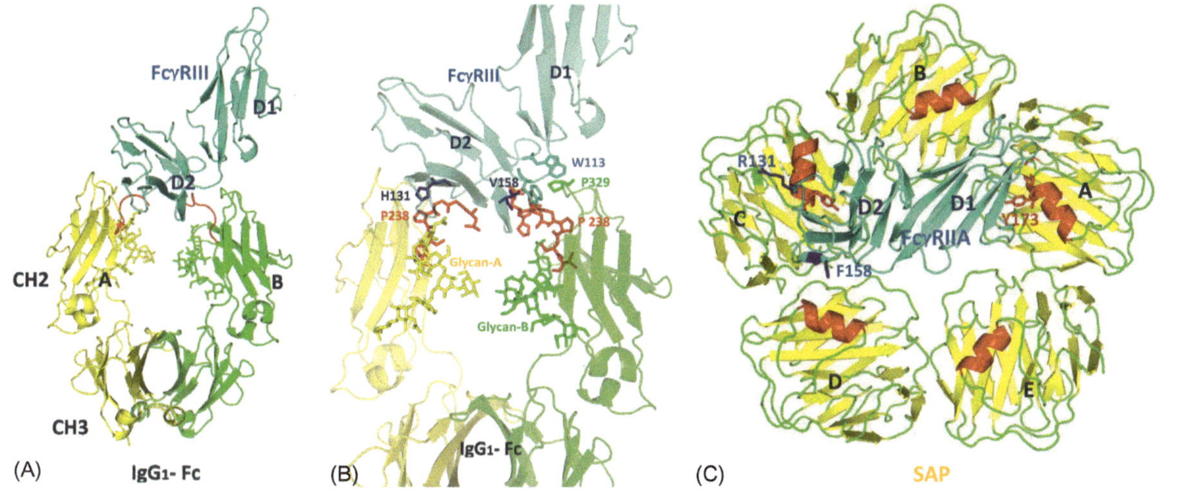

FIGURE 7.2 **Structures of the FcγRIII in complex with Fc portion of IgG$_1$ (A, B) and FcγRIIA in complex with SAP (C).** (A) FcγRIII is shown in cyan and Fc in yellow and green for chains A and B, respectively. The lower hinge regions of Fc are colored in red. The C$_H$2 and C$_H$3 domains of Fc are marked. Carbohydrate moieties attached to the conserved glycosylation site Asn297 on each Fc chains are shown in yellow and green stick models. (B) Zoom-in view of the panel (A) with interface residues labeled. The polymorphic residue V158 of FcγRIII and the corresponding H131 of FcγRIIA are shown and labeled in blue. (C) Crystal structure of FcγRIIA (cyan) in complex with SAP (yellow). The short interface α-helix on SAP is shown in red. Fc receptor contacts the A and C subunits of SAP. The polymorphic residue R131 of FcγRIIA and the corresponding F158 of FcγRIII are shown and labeled in blue.

binding.[17,41] Similar work has identified the membrane proximal domain of FcγRIIIB as the principle antibody binding domain.[41] It was not clear, however, prior to the publication of crystal structures, if each IgG bound to one or two Fcγ receptor molecules. Because Fc is a disulfide-bonded dimer, both 1:1 (Fc:FcγR) and 1:2 models of binding were proposed.[25,27] The crystal structures of IgG bound to its Fcγ receptors were determined in multiple crystal forms using the Fc portion of a human IgG$_1$ bound to a recombinant extracellular domain of human FcγRIII (Figure 7.2A).[35,36] The structures showed clearly the receptor to Fc binding stoichiometry to be 1:1, consistent with earlier binding studies using non-equilibrium and equilibrium gel filtration experiments.[27] The conformation of the FcγRIII–Fc complex, including the carbohydrate moieties attached to the glycosylation site on Fc, is essentially identical between the crystal forms. In all cases, FcγRIII binds to the horseshoe opening of the antibody constant domain at its lower hinge region and makes contact with both chains of the Fc (Figure 7.2). This asymmetric interaction, in which unrelated surfaces of the receptor bind to identical residues from both chains of Fc, breaks down the dyad symmetry of Fc. It also excludes the possibility of having a second receptor interact with the same Fc molecule, resulting in a 1:1 stoichiometry for receptor–Fc recognition. The binding mode of FcγR is distinct from that of FcRn, which binds to Fc at the junction between C$_H$2 and C$_H$3 regions.[40] Thus, the 1:1 binding stoichiometry of FcγR to IgG-Fc is also in contrast to the 2:1 stoichiometry of FcRn (Figure 7.1D). A similar binding mode was also observed between IgE and FcεRI in the structure of an IgE–Fc in complex with its high-affinity ligand binding α-chain

FcεRI.[42] In addition to clarifying receptor binding stoichiometry, the crystal structures also settled another important issue regarding Fc receptor activation—that is, whether receptor activation involved antibody-binding-induced receptor conformational change, a popular theory for cytoplasmic signaling machinery to sense ligand binding to extracellular receptor domains across the cell membrane. This mode of signaling was proved not to be the case, as no significant conformational changes in the Fc receptors from their ligand-free structures were observed upon complex formations. Thus, structural evidence supports receptor clustering as the main mechanism for intracellular activation.

FcγRIII–Fc BINDING INTERFACE

Many questions have been raised since the cloning of Fcγ receptors as to the use of the effectors for antibody functions. For example, how do Fc receptors distinguish subclasses of IgGs? What interactions determine the IgG affinity for Fcγ receptors? Do the conserved glycosylation on the C_H2 domain of Fc contribute to the receptor recognition? Is the known association in FcγRIIA polymorphism and risk of autoimmune diseases and infections directly related to receptor–Fc recognition? The answers to these questions are key to understanding the antibody function at cellular and molecular levels and thus would make it possible to design an entire novel class of therapeutic compounds targeted at Fcγ receptors for autoimmune diseases. Many but not all of these questions were resolved by structural studies. The formation of the FcγRIII–Fc complex buries approximately 1800 Å^2 of the solvent-accessible area.[24,35] All receptor contacts to Fc are made exclusively through the D2 domain of FcγRIII. The receptor N-terminal D1 domain is positioned in close proximity but makes no contact with Fc (Figure 7.2A). The interface of the complex consists of the hinge loop between the D1 and D2 domain of the receptor; the BC, C′E, and FG loops; and the C′ β-strand of the D2 domain. If the two chains of IgG–Fc are designated as A and B, with the A-chain situated close to the membrane-proximal region of the receptor and the B-chain in close proximity to the membrane-distal D1 domain of the receptor. The BC loop is positioned across the horseshoe opening of Fc, making contact with residues from both hinge A and hinge B. The C′ strand is situated atop the chain A of the Fc, positioning the C′E loop into contact with the residues of hinge A. The receptor FG loop protrudes into the opening between the two chains of Fc. All three receptor loops (BC, C′E, and FG) were implicated in Fc binding through the studies of chimeric FcγRII /FcεRI receptors and through site-directed mutagenesis.[17,43,44] On the Fc side of the complex, interactions with the receptor are dominated by residues Leu 234–Ser 239 (Leu–Leu–Gly–Gly–Pro–Ser) from the lower hinge region, consistent with the results from earlier mutational studies.[18] Together, hinges A and B contribute approximately 60% of the overall receptor–Fc interface area. Fc receptor binding clearly ordered the lower hinge loops as both hinge A and hinge B are disordered in all unbound Fc structures, including the structure of an intact mouse IgG2a.[31–34] In contrast, the same hinge A and hinge B in the FcγRIII-complexed Fc structures are clearly visible in the electron density maps, suggesting that the binding of FcγRIII stabilizes the lower hinge conformation of Fc.

Overall, the key features of the receptor–Fc interface are well preserved among all Fc receptors, with possible hinge conformational adjustment for each receptor–Fc pair. The interface between FcγRIII and the A-chain of Fc is dominated by hydrogen bonding interactions, whereas hydrophobic interactions occur primarily between the FcγRIII and the B-chain of Fc. A network of nine hydrogen bonds, including both main-chain and side-chain bonds, is formed between the receptor and Fc. Seven of them are distributed across the receptor and Fc-A interface and two are at the receptor and Fc-B interface. An H134A mutant of FcγRII that has been shown experimentally to reduce the Fc binding drastically would result in the loss of two interface hydrogen bonds, illustrating the importance of the interface hydrogen bonding network to the stability of the complex. A proline sandwich is formed between Trp 90 and Trp 113 of the receptor, both conserved in all human Fcγ and Fcε receptors sequences, and an invariant proline residue, Pro 329 (B-chain). This hydrophobic core extends further to include Val 158, the aliphatic side-chain of Lys 161 from the receptor, and Leu 235 from hinge B. Mutations of both Trp 113 and Lys 161 in FcγRIII lead to a loss in receptor function.[41,45] The side-chain of Leu 235 from the Fc B-chain packs tightly against Gly 159 of the receptor, leaving little space to accommodate any residues larger than Gly at this position. A Gly-to-Ala mutation on the chimeric FcγRII resulted in complete disruption of Fc binding, highlighting the steric constraints imposed on Gly 159.[17] Of particular interest is Trp 113 of the receptor, for which a Phe substitution resulted in the loss of Fc binding. In addition, in order to be a part of the hydrophobic core of the binding interface, this tryptophan is also positioned as a wedge inserted into the D1 domain to provide pivotal interactions that stabilize the acute receptor D1/D2 domain hinge angle. A W113F mutation would relieve the pivotal wedge and lead to a disruption in binding by altering the orientation between the D1 and D2 domains.

FcγR SPECIFICITIES FOR IgG SUBCLASSES

Fcγ receptors display IgG subclass specificities. For example, human FcγRIII binds IgG_1 and IgG_3 tighter than IgG_2 and IgG_4.[12,18] Mutational studies of IgG_2 binding to human high-affinity receptor FcγRI concluded that the entire lower hinge sequence was required to restore the IgG_1 binding affinity in IgG_2, whereas point mutations in IgG_1 hinge residues resulted in a loss of the receptor binding.[46] Most of the Fc residues of the contact region are conserved among the IgG sequences, suggesting a conserved binding site for all four subclasses of human IgGs. These binding residues, with the exception of a Glu 269 to Asp replacement, are also conserved in murine IgG2a, consistent with its ability to act as a ligand for human Fcγ receptors. The lower hinge region of IgG_1 (in particular, residues L234–L235–G236–G237–P238) was earlier identified as crucial for binding to FcγR. Human IgG_2 has a Val–Ala at positions 234 and 235, instead of Leu–Leu, as observed in IgG_1 and IgG_3, and a single residue deletion at position 237 of the corresponding IgG_1. Human IgG_4 has a Phe at position 234. In addition, IgG_2 and IgG_4 sequences contain a three-residue deletion relative to IgG_1 at the N-terminal end of the lower hinge adjacent to the receptor contact area, thus possibly restricting the lower hinge conformation.

A study of the ability of peptides with the sequences of lower hinges of IgG_1, IgG_2, and IgG_4 (denoted as $pIgG_1$, $pIgG_2$, and $pIgG_4$) to bind to FcγRIII was carried out in an attempt to explain the receptor binding specificities.[38] In this case, individual amino acid contribution to receptor affinity was separated from the effect of their environment—namely, the length of the lower hinge in an intact antibody. The receptor–peptide binding constants ranged from 100 μM to 400 μM, with $pIgG_2$ and $pIgG_4$ displaying nearly the same affinity to FcγRIII as $pIgG_1$. Replacing Leu with Phe in $pIgG_4$ or changing Glu–Leu–Leu–Gly to Pro–Val–Ala in $pIgG_2$ in addition to a single residue deletion made little difference in their affinity to the receptor. This result suggests that factors other than the contact amino acids of Fc play an important role in determining the weaker binding affinity of IgG_2 and IgG_4 to FcγRIII (as compared to IgG_1).

It has been proposed that the overall length of the lower hinge may be important to the receptor IgG subclass specificity,[18] since the hinges of IgG_1 and IgG_3 are about three residues longer than those of IgG_2 and IgG_4. It is possible that the shorter lower hinges of IgG_2 and IgG_4 are constrained in a conformation less optimum for the receptor binding.

Fc RECEPTOR ISOFORM AFFINITIES TO IgG

The IgG binding affinities vary significantly among the three subtypes of Fcγ receptors. In both human and mouse, FcγRI is the high-affinity IgG receptor, with ~10^{-8} M dissociation constants (Table 7.1). FcγRII and RIII display intermediate to low affinities to IgG. There is no significant difference in IgG binding affinities between the activating FcγRIIA and inhibitory FcγRIIB forms. It was not immediately clear from the crystal structure of the FcγRIII–Fc complex what distinguishes the high-affinity FcγRI from the low-affinity FcγRIII. A unique feature of the high-affinity FcγRI is its three extracellular Ig-like domains rather than the two in all low-affinity Fcγ receptors.[47] The presence of a third Ig-like domain (D3) has been proposed to be responsible for the high affinity of the receptor.[48] However, the high-affinity FcεRI contains only two extracellular Ig-like domains similar to those in the low-affinity Fcγ receptors, suggesting that high-affinity binding can be achieved by the N-terminal two Ig-like receptor domains. Indeed, the crystal structure of the extracellular domains of human FcγRI showed that the disposition of the third Ig-like domain of the receptor is too distant from the putative antibody binding region to contact Fc.[24] The FcγRIII–Fc and FcεRI–Fc complexes show a similar mode of receptor–ligand recognition.[35,42] The two complexes can be superimposed with r.m.s. deviations of 1.5 Å between all the Cα atoms, and the overall pattern of the receptor–Fc interactions is preserved between the FcγRIII–Fc and FcεRI–Fc complexes.

The interface between FcεRI and IgE–Fc, however, contains more extensive hydrophobic interactions, as well as additional hydrogen bonds and salt bridges as compared to the interface between FcγRIII and IgG–Fc. For example, two salt bridges are observed between FcεRI and Fc but only one of them is preserved between FcγRIII and Fc. The known structures also show that the D2 domain FG-loop on both FcγRI and FcγRIII form many critical interface contacts with Fc. Interestingly, the D2 domain FG-loop of FcγRI (^{171}M-GKHRY^{176}) is one residue shorter than that of FcγRII/FcγRIII. This deletion is present in all species from human to mouse. Indeed, a simple swap of FcγRI FG-loop (^{171}M-GKHRY^{176}) into FcγRIII resulted in a 15-fold increase in IgG_1 binding. This FG-loop swapped FcγRIII bound to IgG_1 with 100-nM affinity. Further, if the corresponding Valine residue, observed in the FG-loop of FcγRIII but missing in FcγRI, is inserted into the swapped FcγRI loop (^{171}MVGKHRY^{177}), IgG_1 binding affinity is reduced to that of FcγRIII.[24] This mutational work supports the importance of the D2 domain FG-loop, in particular its shorter length, in contributing to the high-affinity IgG binding by FcγRI.

INFLUENCE OF FcR POLYMORPHISM ON IgG RECOGNITION

Fcγ receptor genes exhibit functional polymorphisms that are often associated with risk of infection or autoimmune disease.[49] The best-studied polymorphic locations are residue 131 (R/H form) of FcγRIIA and 158 (V/F form) of FcγRIIIA. Both mutations result in point mutations in the receptors' extracellular membrane proximal domains. Biochemically, the R131 form of FcγRIIA displays lower binding affinity to all IgG subtypes than the H131 form of the receptor. The affinity differences can be significant; for example, human IgG_2 can only be recognized by the H131 but not R131 form of FcγRIIA.[49,50] Because the IgG_2 response appears to be important against infections by encapsulated bacteria, such as *Streptococcus pneumoniae*, the binding disparity resulting from this genetic polymorphism may result in a functional deficiency in clearance of the infections in R131/R131 homozygous individuals.[51] Alternatively, while the H131 isoform of FcγRIIA has advantages in phagocytosis and the clearance of pathogens, it may pose risks in certain autoimmune diseases due to its tighter binding to antibodies. Indeed, FcγRIIA H131 has been associated with the severity of Guillain–Barré syndrome (GBS).[52] To date, there is no high-resolution structure of IgG in complex with FcγRIIA; however, the IgG_1–Fc-complexed FcγRIII structure, which has a histidine at the equivalent position, provides some structural insight into the effect of this genetic polymorphism at residue 131 of FcγRIIA. The histidine is located at the IgG–Fc interface and makes a hydrogen bond between its side-chain and Ser 267 on the CH_2 domain of the Fc. An arginine residue at this position is most likely too large to retain the hydrogen bond, and thus becomes less stable than the H131 isoform.[35] V158 of FcγRIII is also located at the IgG binding interface and directly interacts with Leu 235 of the lower hinge between the CH_1 and CH_2 domains of IgG. The tight packing of V158 against the lower hinge of Fc suggests that a bulky F158 substitution may disrupt the packing between IgG–Fc and FcγRIIIA, thus destabilizing the complex. The V158 isoform of FcγRIIIA binds IgG better and is associated with increased ADCC activity on NK cells relative to the F158 isoform.[53] Conversely, the V158 allele has been linked to increased risk in autoimmune disorders, such as rheumatoid arthritis (RA).[54,55]

ROLE OF Fc GLYCOSYLATION IN THE RECOGNITION OF ANTIBODIES BY Fcγ RECEPTORS

The contribution of glycosylation of Fc to the function of immunoglobulins has been debated over the years.[56–59] Early studies have demonstrated that, compared to the native murine IgG_{2a}, deglycosylated IgG_{2a} caused a mild reduction in the activation of complement component C1 and a drastic reduction in the activation of Fcγ receptors.[58,60] Later it was found that deglycosylated IgG_3 retained 80% capability of trigging human phagocyte respiratory burst despite a severe impairment in ADCC.[59] However, unlike the impairment to the Fcγ receptor function, the removal of carbohydrates of IgE did not cause significant loss in FcεRI recognition.[57,61] Structurally, the oligosaccharides attached to the conserved Asn 297 of IgG are a biantennary type with a core heptasaccharide, consisting of three *N*-acetylglucosamine (GlcNac) and three manose (Man), and variable fucose additions to the core. The preferential recognition of Fcγ receptors to non-fucosylated Fc was shown to be due to potential structural hindrance of branched fucose to Fc receptor contacting residues.[35,36,62] Unlike most glycans, these carbohydrates occupy a space between two chains of Fc, and they appear to be well ordered in all crystal structures of Fc, with electron densities visible for most of the core sugar moieties.[31,34,35] In both FcγRIII–Fc and FcεRI–Fc complex structures, the carbohydrates make no direct interactions with the receptors.[35,36,42] Nevertheless, enzymatically deglycosylated IgG_1 exhibits 10- to 15-fold decreases in solution binding affinity to FcγRIII.[38] Because the carbohydrates make no direct contact with the receptor, one possible role for the carbohydrates is to function as a surrogate hydrophobic core between the two chains of Fc, thereby stabilizing the IgG lower hinge in an active receptor binding conformation. Indeed, both biochemical and structural evidence showed that the removal of the Fc-glycan resulted in a conformational transition in Fc from an open to a closed form.[38,39] Despite their well-ordered structure in Fc, recent NMR evidence suggests that the termini of both Asn 297-associated glycans display considerable dynamic flexibilities,[63] consistent with their accessibility to deglycosylation enzymes. In addition, N-linked glycans on FcγRIIa also modulated antibody binding affinity.[64,65]

RECOGNITION OF Fc RECEPTORS BY PENTRAXINS

Until recently, antibodies were the only known ligands for Fc receptors. In recent years, however, pentraxins have emerged as a new family of Fc receptor ligands.[66] Pentraxins are secreted pattern recognition proteins involved in pathogen recognition during infection.[67,68] Members of the family contain a highly conserved pentraxin domain that is roughly 200 amino acids in length. Most research into this family has been focused on the function of two short-chain pentraxins: C-reactive protein (CRP) and serum amyloid P component (SAP). Both are present as plasma proteins in humans. CRP is also an acute-phase protein whose concentration is dramatically elevated during infections and thus becomes a clinical marker for infections.[69–71] CRP recognizes phosphorylcholine moieties associated with microbial polysaccharides or necrotic cells and certain nuclear antigens, such as small nuclear ribonucleoprotein and chromatin subunits, in a calcium-dependent manner.[67,72–77] SAP is known to bind phosphorylethanolamine (PE), lipopolysaccharide (LPS), and other bacteria and yeast surface components, as well as nuclear antigens, in a calcium-dependent manner.[68,73,78,79] Both CRP and SAP can opsonize microbial pathogens or apoptotic cells effectively and promote pathogen clearance through complement activations.[80–83] Both CRP and SAP form pentamers of identical subunits with individual pentraxin domain exhibiting a β-sandwich fold from two opposing β-sheets each consisting of 7 β-strands.[84–86] The two opposite faces of the donut-shaped pentamers of CRP and SAP are termed ligand and effector binding faces, respectively, for pattern recognition and effector C1q binding. Similar to antibodies, pentraxins display broad binding specificities for all isoforms of Fcγ receptors (Table 7.1). In solution, CRP displays similar binding affinities of 2 to 4 μM to all FcγRs. SAP has a slight preference for FcγRI, with a binding affinity of 0.5 μM, three to five times higher than its binding to other FcγRs. The measured solution binding affinities between pentraxins and FcγRs are similar to those between IgG and their low-affinity Fcγ receptors. This suggests that circulating pentraxins in healthy individuals are too low in concentration to activate Fc receptors, and the receptor activation most likely requires higher concentrations of pentraxins as measured in acute inflammation and target opsonization.

The recent crystal structure of human SAP in complex with the extracellular domain of FcγRIIA provided structural support for pentraxin binding to Fcγ receptors.[87] FcγRIIA is bound at the effector face of SAP, diagonally across the pentameric subunits. The complex formation does not induce significant conformational changes in SAP or the receptor. The Fcγ receptor contact areas are approximately equally divided between the two diagonal SAP subunits, which use similar residues, including Tyr 173 and Gln 174, to contact FcγRIIA. Additional contacts involve the C-terminal residues 200 to 204 of SAP and the D2 domain of the Fc receptor. Mutations of the putative interface residues on CRP significantly impaired its binding to Fcγ receptors, suggesting that CRP binds FcγR in a similar structural mode. The crystal structure of the SAP and FcγRIIA complex also shows that the pentraxin binding site partially overlaps that of IgG on the Fcγ receptor; namely, antibodies and pentraxins are bound in closely related orientations with respect to Fcγ receptors, suggesting the potential for synergistic Fc receptor activation in situations where a pathogenic surface is coated with both antibodies and pentraxins. On the other hand, the overlapping binding site between IgG–Fc and SAP also predicts a direct competition between their binding to Fc receptors. Indeed, free IgGs and soluble pentraxins competed for FcγR binding both in solution and in phagocytosis assays. Despite the structural differences between antibodies and pentraxins, their recognition by Fcγ receptors shares common features. Both antibodies and pentraxins are homooligomers, dimers, and pentamers. Yet, each antibody or SAP interacts with only one Fcγ receptor molecule. The receptor binds to symmetrically located sites from two subunits of antibody–Fc and SAP, such that each receptor binding precludes additional receptors from binding to the same ligand. The receptor binding stoichiometry obligates immune complex formation or pentraxin opsonization for Fc receptor activation. Functionally, pentraxin binding to Fcγ receptors leads to monocyte and macrophage activation and cytokine production.[87] Further, CRP treatment in autoimmune ITP (immune thrombocytopenia) mice was shown to protect the animal against antibody-induced thrombocytopenia similar to that of IVIg treatment.[88]

More recently, pentraxins have been shown to bind and activate the human type I IgA receptor, FcγRI (CD89).[89] Like FcγRs, FcγRI (CD89) also signals through the common FcR γ-chain but, unlike Fcγ receptors, it resides in a region of chromosome close to the leukocyte receptor complex (LRC), which encodes killer cell Ig-like receptors (KIR) and an activating NK cell receptor, NKp46. FcγRI also shares ~30% sequence identity with KIR and NKp46. In solution, both CRP and SAP bind with μM affinities to soluble FcγRI but not to its closely related KIR and NKp46.[89] In humans, FcγRI is expressed primarily on circulating neutrophils and monocytes, and CRP cross-linking on neutrophils induced cell surface relocation of intracellular FcγRI, phagocytosis, and TNF-α production. Similar to Fcγ receptors, the observed μM affinity between pentraxins and FcγRI means that target opsonization and acute inflammation are required for pentraxins to activate FcγRI.

CONCLUSIONS

Through the effort of many laboratories, great progress has been made toward understanding the structural mechanism of antibody function, especially engagement with Fc receptors leading to the activation of effector functions. This structural knowledge informed not only our understanding of antibody functions and their role in diseases but also directly facilitated efforts to engineer better antibodies with the desired properties for therapeutic benefit. With the recent successes of antibody immunotherapy, structure-based antibody engineering is becoming an important part of drug development.

References

1. Nimmerjahn F, Ravetch JV. FcgammaRs in health and disease. *Curr Top Microbiol Immunol* 2011;**350**:105–25.
2. Powell MS, Hogarth PM. Fc receptors. *Adv Exp Med Biol* 2008;**640**:22–34.
3. Daeron M. Fc receptor biology. *Annu Rev Immunol* 1997;**15**:203–34.
4. Young JD, Ko SS, Cohn ZA. The increase in intracellular free calcium associated with IgG gamma 2b/gamma 1 Fc receptor–ligand interactions: role in phagocytosis. *Proc Natl Acad Sci USA* 1984;**81**(17):5430–4.
5. Anderson CL, Shen L, Eicher DM, Wewers MD, Gill JK. Phagocytosis mediated by three distinct Fc gamma receptor classes on human leukocytes. *J Exp Med* 1990;**171**(4):1333–45.
6. Titus JA, Perez P, Kaubisch A, Garrido MA, Segal DM. Human K/natural killer cells targeted with hetero-cross-linked antibodies specifically lyse tumor cells *in vitro* and prevent tumor growth *in vivo*. *J Immunol* 1987;**139**(9):3153–8.

7. Chan PL, Sinclair NR. Regulation of the immune response V. An analysis of the function of the Fc portion of antibody in suppression of an immune response with respect to interaction with components of the lymphoid system. *Immunology* 1971;**21**(6):967–81.
8. Phillips NE, Parker DC. Fc-dependent inhibition of mouse B cell activation by whole anti-mu antibodies. *J Immunol* 1983;**130**(2):602–6.
9. Unkeless JC, Scigliano E, Freedman VH. Structure and function of human and murine receptors for IgG. *Annu Rev Immunol* 1988;**6**:251–81.
10. Fridman WH. Fc receptors and immunoglobulin binding factors. *Faseb J* 1991;**5**(12):2684–90.
11. Hulett MD, Hogarth PM. Molecular basis of Fc receptor function. *Adv Immunol* 1994;**57**:1–127.
12. Ravetch JV, Kinet JP. Fc receptors. *Annu Rev Immunol* 1991;**9**:457–92.
13. Ravetch JV, Bolland S. IgG Fc receptors. *Annu Rev Immunol* 2001;**19**:275–90.
14. Mostov KE, Blobel G. A transmembrane precursor of secretory component. The receptor for transcellular transport of polymeric immunoglobulins. *J Biol Chem* 1982;**257**(19):11816–21.
15. Shibuya A, Sakamoto N, Shimizu Y, Shibuya K, Osawa M, Hiroyama T, et al. Fc alpha/mu receptor mediates endocytosis of IgM-coated microbes. *Nat Immunol* 2000;**1**(5):441–6.
16. Kubagawa H, Oka S, Kubagawa Y, Torii I, Takayama E, Kang DW, et al. Identity of the elusive IgM Fc receptor (FcmuR) in humans. *J Exp Med* 2009;**206**(12):2779–93.
17. Hulett MD, Witort E, Brinkworth RI, McKenzie IF, Hogarth PM. Identification of the IgG binding site of the human low affinity receptor for IgG Fc gamma RII. Enhancement and ablation of binding by site-directed mutagenesis. *J Biol Chem* 1994;**269**(21):15287–93.
18. Tamm A, Schmidt RE. IgG binding sites on human Fc gamma receptors. *Int Rev Immunol* 1997;**16**(1–2):57–85.
19. van der Poel CE, Spaapen RM, van de Winkel JG, Leusen JH. Functional characteristics of the high affinity IgG receptor, FcγRI. *J Immunol* 2011;**186**(5):2699–704.
20. Unkeless JC, Shen Z, Lin CW, DeBeus E. Function of human Fc gamma RIIA and Fc gamma RIIIB. *Semin Immunol* 1995;**7**(1):37–44.
21. Kimberly RP, Ahlstrom JW, Click ME, Edberg JC. The glycosyl phosphatidylinositol-linked Fc gamma RIIIPMN mediates transmembrane signaling events distinct from Fc gamma RII. *J Exp Med* 1990;**171**(4):1239–55.
22. Galon J, Gauchat JF, Mazieres N, Spagnoli R, Storkus W, Lotze M, et al. Soluble Fcgamma receptor type III (FcgammaRIII, CD16) triggers cell activation through interaction with complement receptors. *J Immunol* 1996;**157**(3):1184–92.
23. Bruhns P, Iannascoli B, England P, Mancardi DA, Fernandez N, Jorieux S, et al. Specificity and affinity of human Fcgamma receptors and their polymorphic variants for human IgG subclasses. *Blood* 2009;**113**(16):3716–25.
24. Lu J, Ellsworth JL, Hamacher N, Oak SW, Sun PD. Crystal structure of FcγRI and its implication in high affinity γ-immunoglobulin G binding. *J Biol Chem* 2011;**286**(47):40608–13.
25. Sondermann P, Huber R, Jacob U. Crystal structure of the soluble form of the human fcgamma-receptor IIb: a new member of the immunoglobulin superfamily at 1.7 A resolution. *Embo J* 1999;**18**(5):1095–103.
26. Maxwell KF, Powell MS, Hulett MD, Barton PA, McKenzie IF, Garrett TP, et al. Crystal structure of the human leukocyte Fc receptor, Fc gammaRIIa. *Nat Struct Biol* 1999;**6**(5):437–42.
27. Zhang Y, Boesen CC, Radaev S, Brooks AG, Fridman WH, Sautes-Fridman C, et al. Crystal structure of the extracellular domain of a human Fc gamma RIII. *Immunity* 2000;**13**(3):387–95.
28. Sondermann P, Kaiser J, Jacob U. Molecular basis for immune complex recognition: a comparison of Fc-receptor structures. *J Mol Biol* 2001;**309**(3):737–49.
29. Garman SC, Kinet JP, Jardetzky TS. Crystal structure of the human high-affinity IgE receptor. *Cell* 1998;**95**(7):951–61.
30. Snyder GA, Brooks AG, Sun PD. Crystal structure of the HLA-Cw3 allotype-specific killer cell inhibitory receptor KIR2DL2. *Proc Natl Acad Sci USA* 1999;**96**(7):3864–9.
31. Deisenhofer J. Crystallographic refinement and atomic models of a human Fc fragment and its complex with fragment B of protein A from *Staphylococcus aureus* at 2.9- and 2.8-A resolution. *Biochemistry* 1981;**20**(9):2361–70.
32. Harris LJ, Larson SB, Hasel KW, Day J, Greenwood A, McPherson A. The three-dimensional structure of an intact monoclonal antibody for canine lymphoma. *Nature* 1992;**360**(6402):369–72.
33. Sauer-Eriksson AE, Kleywegt GJ, Uhlen M, Jones TA. Crystal structure of the C2 fragment of streptococcal protein G in complex with the Fc domain of human IgG. *Structure* 1995;**3**(3):265–78.
34. DeLano WL, Ultsch MH, de Vos AM, Wells JA. Convergent solutions to binding at a protein-protein interface. *Science* 2000;**287**(5456):1279–83.
35. Radaev S, Motyka S, Fridman WH, Sautes-Fridman C, Sun PD. The structure of a human type III Fcgamma receptor in complex with Fc. *J Biol Chem* 2001;**276**(19):16469–77.
36. Sondermann P, Huber R, Oosthuizen V, Jacob U. The 3.2-A crystal structure of the human IgG_1 Fc fragment–Fc gammaRIII complex. *Nature* 2000;**406**(6793):267–73.
37. Ramsland PA, Farrugia W, Bradford TM, Sardjono CT, Esparon S, Trist HM, et al. Structural basis for Fc

gammaRIIa recognition of human IgG and formation of inflammatory signaling complexes. *J Immunol* 2011;**187**(6):3208–17.
38. Radaev S, Sun PD. Recognition of IgG by Fcgamma receptor. The role of Fc glycosylation and the binding of peptide inhibitors. *J Biol Chem* 2001;**276**(19):16478–83.
39. Feige MJ, Nath S, Catharino SR, Weinfurtner D, Steinbacher S, Buchner J. Structure of the murine unglycosylated IgG_1 Fc fragment. *J Mol Biol* 2009;**391**(3):599–608.
40. Burmeister WP, Gastinel LN, Simister NE, Blum ML, Bjorkman PJ. Crystal structure at 2.2 A resolution of the MHC-related neonatal Fc receptor. *Nature* 1994;**372**(6504):336–43.
41. Tamm A, Kister A, Nolte KU, Gessner JE, Schmidt RE. The IgG binding site of human FcgammaRIIIB receptor involves CC′ and FG loops of the membrane-proximal domain. *J Biol Chem* 1996;**271**(7):3659–66.
42. Garman SC, Wurzburg BA, Tarchevskaya SS, Kinet JP, Jardetzky TS. Structure of the Fc fragment of human IgE bound to its high-affinity receptor Fc epsilonRI alpha. *Nature* 2000;**406**(6793):259–66.
43. Hulett MD, Witort E, Brinkworth RI, McKenzie IF, Hogarth PM. Multiple regions of human Fc gamma RII (CD32) contribute to the binding of IgG. *J Biol Chem* 1995;**270**(36):21188–94.
44. Cook JP, Henry AJ, McDonnell JM, Owens RJ, Sutton BJ, Gould HJ. Identification of contact residues in the IgE binding site of human FcepsilonRIalpha. *Biochemistry* 1997;**36**(50):15579–88.
45. Hibbs ML, Tolvanen M, Carpen O. Membrane-proximal Ig-like domain of Fc gamma RIII (CD16) contains residues critical for ligand binding. *J Immunol* 1994;**152**(9):4466–74.
46. Chappel MS, Isenman DE, Everett M, Xu YY, Dorrington KJ, Klein MH. Identification of the Fc gamma receptor class I binding site in human IgG through the use of recombinant IgG_1/IgG_2 hybrid and point-mutated antibodies. *Proc Natl Acad Sci USA* 1991;**88**(20):9036–40.
47. Allen JM, Seed B. Isolation and expression of functional high-affinity Fc receptor complementary DNAs. *Science* 1989;**243**(4889):378–81.
48. Hulett MD, Hogarth PM. The second and third extracellular domains of FcgammaRI (CD64) confer the unique high affinity binding of IgG_{2a}. *Mol Immunol* 1998;**35**(14–15):989–96.
49. van Sorge NM, van der Pol WL, van de Winkel JG. FcgammaR polymorphisms: implications for function, disease susceptibility and immunotherapy. *Tissue Antigens* 2003;**61**(3):189–202.
50. Parren PW, Warmerdam PA, Boeije LC, Arts J, Westerdaal NA, Vlug A, et al. On the interaction of IgG subclasses with the low affinity Fc gamma RIIa (CD32) on human monocytes, neutrophils, and platelets. Analysis of a functional polymorphism to human IgG_2. *J Clin Invest* 1992;**90**(4):1537–46.
51. Sanders LA, van de Winkel JG, Rijkers GT, Voorhorst-Ogink MM, de Haas M, Capel PJ, et al. Fc gamma receptor IIa (CD32) heterogeneity in patients with recurrent bacterial respiratory tract infections. *J Infect Dis* 1994;**170**(4):854–61.
52. van der Pol WL, van den Berg LH, Scheepers RH, van der Bom JG, van Doorn PA, van Koningsveld R, et al. IgG receptor IIa alleles determine susceptibility and severity of Guillain–Barre syndrome. *Neurology* 2000;**54**(8):1661–5.
53. Koene HR, Kleijer M, Algra J, Roos D, von dem Borne AE, de Haas M. Fc gammaRIIIa-158V/F polymorphism influences the binding of IgG by natural killer cell Fc gammaRIIIa, independently of the Fc gammaRIIIa-48L/R/H phenotype. *Blood* 1997;**90**(3):1109–14.
54. Nieto A, Caliz R, Pascual M, Mataran L, Garcia S, Martin J. Involvement of Fc gamma receptor IIIA genotypes in susceptibility to rheumatoid arthritis. *Arthritis Rheum* 2000;**43**(4):735–9.
55. Morgan AW, Griffiths B, Ponchel F, Montague BM, Ali M, Gardner PP, et al. Fcgamma receptor type IIIA is associated with rheumatoid arthritis in two distinct ethnic groups. *Arthritis Rheum* 2000;**43**(10):2328–34.
56. Jefferis R, Lund J, Pound JD. IgG–Fc-mediated effector functions: molecular definition of interaction sites for effector ligands and the role of glycosylation. *Immunol Rev* 1998;**163**:59–76.
57. Kulczycki Jr A, Vallina VL. Specific binding of non-glycosylated IgE to Fc epsilon receptor. *Mol Immunol* 1981;**18**(8):723–31.
58. Lund J, Tanaka T, Takahashi N, Sarmay G, Arata Y, Jefferis R. A protein structural change in aglycosylated IgG_3 correlates with loss of huFc gamma R1 and huFc gamma R111 binding and/or activation. *Mol Immunol* 1990;**27**(11):1145–53.
59. Pound JD, Lund J, Jefferis R. Aglycosylated chimaeric human IgG_3 can trigger the human phagocyte respiratory burst. *Mol Immunol* 1993;**30**(3):233–41.
60. Leatherbarrow RJ, Rademacher TW, Dwek RA, Woof JM, Clark A, Burton DR, et al. Effector functions of a monoclonal aglycosylated mouse IgG_{2a}: binding and activation of complement component C1 and interaction with human monocyte Fc receptor. *Mol Immunol* 1985;**224**:407–15.
61. Basu M, Hakimi J, Dharm E, Kondas JA, Tsien WH, Pilson RS, et al. Purification and characterization of human recombinant IgE–Fc fragments that bind to the human high affinity IgE receptor. *J Biol Chem* 1993;**268**(18):13118–27.
62. Mizushima T, Yagi H, Takemoto E, Shibata-Koyama M, Isoda Y, Iida S, et al. Structural basis for improved

efficacy of therapeutic antibodies on defucosylation of their Fc glycans. *Genes Cells* 2011;**16**(11):1071–80.

63. Barb AW, Prestegard JH. NMR analysis demonstrates immunoglobulin G N-glycans are accessible and dynamic. *Nat Chem Biol* 2011;**7**(3):147–53.
64. Ferrara C, Stuart F, Sondermann P, Brunker P, Umana P. The carbohydrate at FcgammaRIIIa Asn-162. An element required for high affinity binding to non-fucosylated IgG glycoforms. *J Biol Chem* 2006;**281**(8):5032–6.
65. Shibata-Koyama M, Iida S, Okazaki A, Mori K, Kitajima-Miyama K, Saitou S, et al. The N-linked oligosaccharide at Fc gamma RIIIa Asn-45: an inhibitory element for high Fc gamma RIIIa binding affinity to IgG glycoforms lacking core fucosylation. *Glycobiology* 2009;**19**(2):126–34.
66. Du Clos TW, Mold C. Pentraxins (CRP, SAP) in the process of complement activation and clearance of apoptotic bodies through Fcγ receptors. *Curr Opin Organ Transplant* 2010; Dec 9.
67. Volanakis JE, Kaplan MH. Specificity of C-reactive protein for choline phosphate residues of pneumococcal C-polysaccharide. *Proc Soc Exp Biol Med* 1971;**136**(2):612–4.
68. Pepys MB, Butler PJ. Serum amyloid P component is the major calcium-dependent specific DNA binding protein of the serum. *Biochem Biophys Res Commun* 1987;**148**(1):308–13.
69. Ganapathi MK, Rzewnicki D, Samols D, Jiang SL, Kushner I. Effect of combinations of cytokines and hormones on synthesis of serum amyloid A and C-reactive protein in Hep 3B cells. *J Immunol* 1991;**147**(4):1261–5.
70. Du Clos TW, Mold C. C-reactive protein: an activator of innate immunity and a modulator of adaptive immunity. *Immunol Res* 2004;**30**(3):261–77.
71. Ganapathi MK, May LT, Schultz D, Brabenec A, Weinstein J, Sehgal PB, et al. Role of interleukin-6 in regulating synthesis of C-reactive protein and serum amyloid A in human hepatoma cell lines. *Biochem Biophys Res Commun* 1988;**157**(1):271–7.
72. Mold C, Baca R, Du Clos TW. Serum amyloid P component and C-reactive protein opsonize apoptotic cells for phagocytosis through Fcgamma receptors. *J Autoimmun* 2002;**19**(3):147–54.
73. Du Clos TW. The interaction of C-reactive protein and serum amyloid P component with nuclear antigens. *Mol Biol Rep* 1996;**23**(3–4):253–60.
74. Du Clos TW. C-reactive protein reacts with the U1 small nuclear ribonucleoprotein. *J Immunol* 1989;**143**(8):2553–9.
75. Du Clos TW, Zlock LT, Rubin RL. Analysis of the binding of C-reactive protein to histones and chromatin. *J Immunol* 1988;**141**(12):4266–70.
76. Pepys MB, Booth SE, Tennent GA, Butler PJ, Williams DG. Binding of pentraxins to different nuclear structures: C-reactive protein binds to small nuclear ribonucleoprotein particles, serum amyloid P component binds to chromatin and nucleoli. *Clin Exp Immunol* 1994;**97**(1):152–7.
77. Du Clos TW, Marnell L, Zlock LR, Burlingame RW. Analysis of the binding of C-reactive protein to chromatin subunits. *J Immunol* 1991;**146**(4):1220–5.
78. Schwalbe RA, Dahlback B, Coe JE, Nelsestuen GL. Pentraxin family of proteins interact specifically with phosphorylcholine and/or phosphorylethanolamine. *Biochemistry* 1992;**31**(20):4907–15.
79. Dong A, Caughey WS, Du Clos TW. Effects of calcium, magnesium, and phosphorylcholine on secondary structures of human C-reactive protein and serum amyloid P component observed by infrared spectroscopy. *J Biol Chem* 1994;**269**(9):6424–30.
80. Kaplan MH, Volanakis JE. Interaction of C-reactive protein complexes with the complement system. I. Consumption of human complement associated with the reaction of C-reactive protein with pneumococcal C-polysaccharide and with the choline phosphatides, lecithin and sphingomyelin. *J Immunol* 1974;**112**(6):2135–47.
81. Hutchinson WL, Noble GE, Hawkins PN, Pepys MB. The pentraxins, C-reactive protein and serum amyloid P component, are cleared and catabolized by hepatocytes *in vivo*. *J Clin Invest* 1994;**94**(4):1390–6.
82. Du Clos TW. Function of C-reactive protein. *Ann Med* 2000;**32**(4):274–8.
83. Mold C, Gewurz H, Du Clos TW. Regulation of complement activation by C-reactive protein. *Immunopharmacology* 1999;**42**(1–3):23–30.
84. Thompson D, Pepys MB, Wood SP. The physiological structure of human C-reactive protein and its complex with phosphocholine. *Structure* 1999;**7**(2):169–77.
85. Shrive AK, Cheetham GM, Holden D, Myles DA, Turnell WG, Volanakis JE, et al. Three dimensional structure of human C-reactive protein. *Nat Struct Biol* 1996;**3**(4):346–54.
86. Emsley J, White HE, O'Hara BP, Oliva G, Srinivasan N, Tickle IJ, et al. Structure of pentameric human serum amyloid P component. *Nature* 1994;**367**(6461):338–45.
87. Lu J, Marnell LL, Marjon KD, Mold C, Du Clos TW, Sun PD. Structural recognition and functional activation of FcgammaR by innate pentraxins. *Nature* 2008;**456**(7224):989–92.
88. Marjon KD, Marnell LL, Mold C, Du Clos TW. Macrophages activated by C-reactive protein through FcγRI transfer suppression of immune thrombocytopenia. *J Immunol* 2009;**182**(3):1397–403.
89. Lu J, Marjon KD, Marnell LL, Wang R, Mold C, Du Clos TW, et al. Recognition and functional activation of the human IgA receptor (FcalphaRI) by C-reactive protein. *Proc Natl Acad Sci USA* 2011;**108**(12):4974–9.

CHAPTER

8

FcγRs Across Species

Brian Moldt[a] *and Ann J. Hessell*[b]

[a]Department of Immunology and Microbial Science, The Scripps Research Institute, La Jolla, California, [b]Oregon National Primate Research Center and Vaccine & Gene Therapy Institute, Oregon Health & Science University, Beaverton, Oregon

INTRODUCTION

Fc receptors for immunoglobulins are expressed on most innate and adaptive immune cells and are an integrated part of a response against invading pathogens and of immune homeostasis.[1] Immunoglobulin G (IgG) is the most abundant antibody isotype in serum and a highly potent effector molecule. The cellular receptors for IgG, responsible for mediating the connection between the humoral response and cellular effector functions, belong to the Fcγ receptor (FcγR) family. To date, four classes of Fcγ receptors have been identified; FcγRI (CD64), FcγRII (CD32), FcγRIII (CD16), and FcγRIV, all structurally part of the immunoglobulin superfamily. The receptor genes are conserved between species and are clustered on chromosome 1 in humans, chimpanzees, macaques, and mice (FcγRI is located on chromosome 3); on chromosome 13 in rats; and on chromosome 38 in dogs.[2] Functionally, the Fcγ receptors can be divided into activating and inhibitory receptors depending on whether the cellular signal transmits through an immunoreceptor tyrosine-based activation motif (ITAM) or inhibitory motif (ITIM).[3–6] The formation of immune complexes by cross-linking and aggregation of the receptors is crucial for the signaling and function of all receptors except for the high-affinity receptor FcγRI. Key effects mediated by Fcγ receptors include antibody-dependent cellular cytotoxicity (ADCC), antibody-dependent cellular phagocytosis (ADCP), antibody-dependent complement dependent cytotoxicity (ADCDC), cytokine and chemokine release, and inhibition of B-cell activation.

Animal models have been used extensively to study the interaction between Fcγ receptors and IgG. Specifically, the mouse has been an invaluable tool and has been the origin of most of our knowledge about Fcγ receptors. Nevertheless, despite an overall similarity between human and mouse Fcγ receptors, species diversification has resulted in the evolution of a much more complex system in humans.[2,7] Extrapolation of data generated in mice, in terms of predicting the biological effect of Fcγ receptors and antibodies in humans, may therefore be a challenging endeavor. Compared to the mouse, less is known about the Fcγ receptors in nonhuman primates, including Old

World monkeys such as the rhesus and cynomolgus macaque that are particularly valuable models for human therapeutics and AIDS research. It is now apparent that the close similarity between humans and macaques compared to humans and mice make the model very attractive not only in the study of Fcγ receptors but also in biomedical research in general. This chapter describes Fcγ receptors in humans, mice, and rhesus macaques, with specific focus on the similarities and differences for the animal models in comparison to the human receptors.

HUMAN FcγRs

The human (h) Fcγ receptor family consists of three classes (I, II, III) with a total of six members. hFcγRI, hFcγRIIA, hFcγRIIC, and hFcγRIIIA are activating receptors, whereas hFcγRIIB is an inhibitory receptor. The remaining receptor, hFcγRIIIB, is of unknown function (Figure 8.1 and Table 8.1).

hFcγRI (hFcγRIA) is a 374-amino-acid residue protein and is composed of three extracellular Ig-like domains, a transmembrane (TM) domain, and a cytoplasmic (CY) tail. To transmit a cell-activating signal, hFcγRI depends on interaction with the ITAM-bearing FcRγ (Fcer1g).[9] hFcγRIA is expressed by monocytes, macrophages, and dendritic cells (DCs), in addition to inducible expression on neutrophils and mast cells; in contrast to hFcγRII and hFcγRIII, hFcγRIA binds its ligands, IgG_1, IgG_3, and IgG_4, with high affinity.[8,10,11] Two other FcγRI genes (hFcγRIB and hFcγRIC) have been described; however, they presumably do not encode functional proteins.[12]

The three members of the hFcγRII class are comprised of two extracellular Ig-like domains, a TM domain, and a CY domain containing a signal-transducing motif. They share a high level of homology in the extracellular domain with more than 90% similarity. hFcγRIIA is a 316-amino-acids residue protein, hFcγRIIB consists of 310 amino acids, and hFcγRIIC consists of 323 amino acids. For hFcγRIIA and hFcγRIIC, the signal-transducing motif is an ITAM, whereas for hFcγRIIB it is an ITIM. hFcγRIIA is expressed by monocytes/macrophages, neutrophils, DCs, basophils, eosinophils, mast cells, and platelets.[7] hFcγRIIA occurs in two allelic forms, with a single amino acid substitution in the extracellular domain (H131 and R131), which influence binding to IgG_2. The inhibitory receptor hFcγRIIB is the only Fcγ receptor on circulating B cells where it is highly expressed. hFcγRIIB is also highly expressed on basophils, moderately expressed on DCs and tissue macrophages, and expressed at much lower levels on a small subset of monocytes and neutrophils.[13–15] hFcγRIIB downregulates cell activation and proliferation when co-aggregated with an activating FcγR.[16,17] hFcγRIIC is expressed on NK cells, monocytes/macrophages, and neutrophils but appears in only 20 to 30% of the population because of an allelic polymorphism stop codon in the third exon.[18–20] Members of the hFcγRII class bind IgG_1, IgG_3, and IgG_4 with low affinity; hFcγRIIA also binds IgG_2 with low affinity (H131 allele binds with fivefold higher affinity than R131 allele); and hFcγRIIB and hFcγRIIC bind IgG_2 with very low affinity.[8]

The hFcγRIIIA protein is composed of 254 amino acid residues forming two extracellular Ig-like domains, a TM domain, and a CY tail. Similar to hFcγRI, hFcγRIIIA depends on interaction with the ITAM-bearing FcRγ to transmit a cellular activation signal.[9] hFcγRIIIA appears in two allelic forms with a single amino acid substitution in the extracellular domain (F158 and V158) and is expressed on NK cells and monocytes/macrophages.[7] hFcγRIIIB consists of two extracellular Ig-like domains attached to the plasma membrane by an alpha-GPI anchor. In contrast to hFcγRIIIA (and all other hFcγRs), hFcγRIIIB does not contain a cytoplasmic domain and is therefore slightly smaller than hFcγRIIIA at 233 amino acids. The receptor is

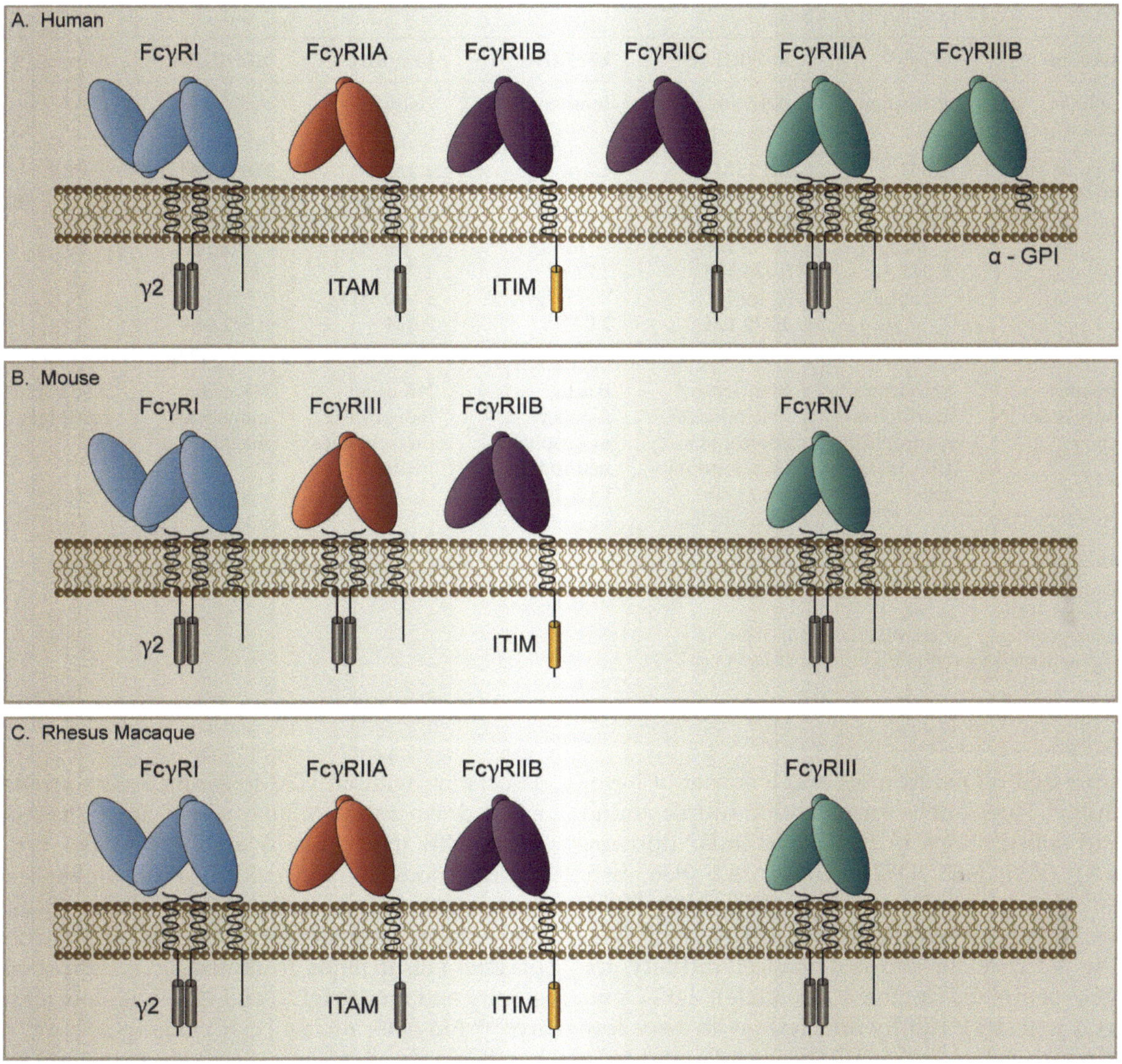

FIGURE 8.1 **Schematic representation of human, mouse and rhesus macaque Fcγ receptors.** (A) The human Fcγ receptor family consists of three classes with six members: the activating hFcγRI, hFcγRIIA, hFcγRIIC, hFcγRIIIA, the inhibitory hFcγRIIB and hFcγRIIIB with unknown function. (B) The mouse Fcγ receptor family consists of four classes with four members: the activating moFcγRI, moFcγRIII, moFcγRIV, and the inhibitory moFcγRIIB. (C) The rhesus macaque Fcγ receptor family consists of three classes with four members: the activating macFcγRI, macFcγRIIA, macFcγRIII and the inhibitory macFcγRIIB. Orthologous receptors between the three species are aligned in the same column. γ2 represents the ITAM bearing FcRγ; gray bars represent an ITAM, and the yellow bars represent an ITIM. See text and tables for details.

TABLE 8.1 Human Fcγ Receptors

Receptor	hFcγRI	hFcγRIIA[b]	hFcγRIIB	hFcγRIIC	hFcγRIIIA[c]	hFcγRIIIB
Cellular activation type	Activating	Activating	Inhibitory	Activating	Activating	Unknown
Ligands and affinity[a]	$650 M^{-1}$ for IgG_1 $610 M^{-1}$ for IgG_3 $340 M^{-1}$ for IgG_4	$52/35 M^{-1}$ for IgG_1 $4.5/1.0 M^{-1}$ for IgG_2 $8.9/9.1 M^{-1}$ for IgG_3 $1.7/2.1 M^{-1}$ for IgG_4	$1.2 M^{-1}$ for IgG_1 $0.2 M^{-1}$ for IgG_2 $1.7 M^{-1}$ for IgG_3 $2.0 M^{-1}$ for IgG_4	$1.2 M^{-1}$ for IgG_1 $0.2 M^{-1}$ for IgG_2 $1.7 M^{-1}$ for IgG_3 $2.0 M^{-1}$ for IgG_4	$20/11.7 M^{-1}$ for IgG_1 $0.7/0.3 M^{-1}$ for IgG_2 $98/77 M^{-1}$ for IgG_3 $2.5/2.0 M^{-1}$ for IgG_4	$2.0 M^{-1}$ for IgG_1 $10 M^{-1}$ for IgG_3
Cellular expression	Monocytes/ macrophages, neutrophils DCs, mast cells	Monocytes/ macrophages, neutrophils, DCs, basophils, mast cells, eosinophils, platelets	B cells, monocytes/ macrophages, neutrophils, DCs, basophils	NK cells, monocytes/ macrophages, neutrophils	NK cells, monocytes/ macrophages	Neutrophils, basophils

Source: Bruhns et al.[8]
[a]*Affinity constants,* K_A *(×* 10^5*).*
[b]*Affinity numbers are for hFcγRIIA H131/R131 alleles.*
[c]*Affinity numbers are for hFcγRIIIA V158/P158 alleles.*

expressed on neutrophils and a subset of basophils.[21] Three allelic forms with multiple amino acid substitutions in the extracellular domain, NA1 (R36, N65, D82, V106), NA2 (S36, S65, N82, I106), and SH (S36, S65, D78, N82, I106), are known for hFcγRIIIB. hFcγRIIIA binds IgG_1 (the V158 allele shows enhanced affinity for IgG_1 compared to the F158 allele), IgG_3, and IgG_4 with low affinity and IgG_2 with very low affinity, whereas hFcγRIIIB binds IgG_1 and IgG_3 with low affinity.[8]

MOUSE FcγRs

In mice, four classes of Fcγ receptors have been described: the activating FcγRI, FcγRIII, and FcγRIV and the inhibitory FcγRIIB (Figure 8.1 and Table 8.2). The activating mouse (mo) FcγRs (moFcγRI, moFcγRIII, moFcγRIV) require association with an ITAM-bearing FcRγ to transmit a downstream cellular signal, in contrast to moFcγRIIB that contains an ITIM in the cytoplasmic domain.[9] moFcγRI is a 404-amino-acid protein consisting of three extracellular Ig-like domains, a transmembrane domain, and a cytoplasmic tail. It binds to mouse IgG_{2a} with high affinity and mouse IgG_{2b} and IgG_3 with low affinity.[24,25] No other mouse FcγR binds IgG_3. mFcγRI has been found to be exclusively expressed on monocyte-derived dendritic cells.[26,27]

The inhibitory moFcγRIIB is a 329-amino-acid-residue protein composed of two extracellular Ig-like domains, a TM domain, and a CY domain. Several polymorphic variants have been described for moFcγRIIB; however, none has been shown to have any effect on binding to its ligands.[7] moFcγRIIB binds mouse IgG_1, IgG_{2a}, and IgG_{2b}, as well as mouse IgE, all with low affinity.[28,29] The inhibitory receptor is expressed

TABLE 8.2 Mouse Fcγ Receptors

Receptor	moFcγRI	moFcγRIIB	moFcγRIII	moFcγRIV
Cellular activation type	Activating	Inhibitory	Activating	Activating
Ligands and affinity[a]	38 n*M* for IgG_{2a} Also binds IgG_{2b} and IgG_3 with low affinity	301 n*M* for IgG_1 2.39 μ*M* for IgG_{2a} 448 n*M* for IgG_{2b} 50 μ*M* for IgE	3.2 μ*M* for IgG_1 1.46 μ*M* for IgG_{2a} 1.55 μ*M* for IgG_{2b} 51 μ*M* for IgE	34.5 n*M* for IgG_{2a} 59 n*M* for IgG_{2b} 4.2 μ*M* for IgE
Cellular expression	Monocyte-derived DCs	B cells, monocytes/ macrophages, neutrophils, DCs, basophils, mast cells, eosinophils	NK cells, monocytes/ macrophages, neutrophils, DCs, basophils, mast cells, eosinophils	Monocytes/ macrophages, neutrophils
Sequence homology to human extracellular domain	75% homology to human FcγRI (EC and TM domain)	63% homology to human FcγRIIB	—	65% homology to human FcγRIIIA

Sources: Amigorena et al.,[3] Mancardi et al.,[22] Nimmerjahn et al.[23]
[a]*Affinity constants* K_D.

on B cells, monocytes/macrophages, neutrophils, DCs, basophils, mast cells, and eosinophils.[11]

moFcγRIII contains 267 amino acids which compose two extracellular Ig-like domains, a TM domain, and CY tail. moFcγRIII is a low-affinity receptor for mouse IgG_1, IgG_{2a}, IgG_{2b}, and IgE and is the only activating mouse FcγR that binds mouse IgG_1.[28,29] As seen for moFcγRIIB, several polymorphic variants have been reported for moFcγRIII but none has been shown to impact the binding affinities for any of its ligands.[7] moFcγRIII is expressed on all myeloid cells (monocytes/macrophages, neutrophils, basophils, eosinophils, dendritic cells, and mast cells) as well as NK and NKT cells.[11,30]

moFcγRIV is the most recent mouse Fcγ receptor to be described.[23] It is a 240-amino-acid-residue protein structurally similar to moFcγRIII with two extracellular Ig-like domains, a TM domain, and CY tail. However, moFcγRIV differs from moFcγRIII in affinity for its ligands, binding mouse IgG_{2a} and IgG_{2b} with high affinity and IgE with low affinity.[23,25] It is expressed on monocytes/macrophages and neutrophils.[25,31]

HUMAN *VERSUS* MOUSE FcγRs

Despite three classes of Fcγ receptors in human and four classes in mouse, amino acid sequence analysis has shown the presence of orthologous proteins in the two species. A direct comparison, however, is not without caveats as the function and expression pattern of the identified orthologous Fcγ receptors can be significantly different (Table 8.3). It should also be noted that the differences between human and mouse IgG subclasses add additional complications for evaluating the orthologous receptors.

The orthologous receptor for human FcγRI is moFcγRI, with which it shares 75% amino acid sequence similarity in the extracellular domains and the TM domain.[32,33] However, the human form is a high-affinity receptor for three IgG subclasses and is expressed on multiple cell types, whereas the mouse form is a high-affinity receptor for only one IgG subclass, and cellular expression is restricted to monocyte-derived dendritic cells.[8,10,11,26,27]

TABLE 8.3 Comparison of Orthologous Human and Mouse Fc Receptors

Human Receptor	Orthologous Receptor	Main Similarities	Main Differences
hFcγRI	moFcγRI	High-affinity receptor No ITAM in cytoplasmic domain	hFcγRI binds IgG_1, IgG_3, and IgG_4 moFcγRI binds IgG_{2a} (binds IgG_{2b} and IgG_3 with low affinity) hFcγRI is expressed on multiple cell types moFcγRI is only expressed on monocyte-derived dendritic cells
hFcγRIIA	moFcγRIII	Low-affinity receptor Expressed on monocytes, macrophages, neutrophils, DCs, basophils, mast cells, eosinophils	hFcγRIIA contains an ITAM in cytoplasmic domain hFcγRIIA is expressed on platelets moFcγRIII is expressed on NK cells hFcγRIIA has two allelic forms that influence binding affinities moFcγRIII binds IgE
hFcγRIIB	moFcγRIIB	Low-affinity receptor Expressed on B cells, basophils, DCs Expressed on monocytes, macrophages, neutrophils (see text for details) Contains an ITIM in cytoplasmic domain	moFcγRIIB is expressed on mast cells and eosinophils hFcγRIIB has lower ligand affinity than human activation receptors moFcγRIIB has similar ligand affinity as mouse activating receptors moFcγRIIB binds IgE
hFcγRIIC	Not present in mouse	—	—
hFcγRIIIA	moFcγRIV	Expressed on monocytes and macrophages Binds defucosylated IgG with higher affinity No ITAM in cytoplasmic domain	hFcγRIIIA is expressed on NK cells moFcγRIV is expressed on neutrophils hFcγRIIIA has two allelic forms that influence binding affinities moFcγRIV is a high-affinity receptor moFcγRIV binds IgE
hFcγRIIIB	Not present in mouse	—	—

For human FcγRIIA, the orthologous mouse receptor is moFcγRIII. However, human FcγRIIA differs from mouse FcγRIII in that the human receptor contains its own ITAM whereas the mouse FcγRIII relies on interaction with FcγR. The human FcγRIIA is also not expressed on NK cells in contrast to mouse FcγRIII, and mouse FcγRIII is not expressed on platelets in contrast to human FcγRIIA.[7,11,30] Moreover, human FcγRIIA exists in two allelic forms with different affinity for specific IgG subclasses that do not appear for mouse FcγRIII.[8]

The orthologous mouse receptor for human FcγRIIIA is moFcγRIV with which it shares 65% amino acid homology in the extracellular domain.[34] In terms of cellular expression a significant difference between the receptors is that human FcγRIIIA is expressed on NK cells while the mouse receptor is not, and, in contrast, mouse FcγRIV is expressed on neutrophils whereas human FcγRIIIA is not.[7,25,31] They are both expressed on monocytes/macrophages and bind defucosylated IgG with higher affinity. In addition, moFcγRIV binds its ligands with high affinity in contrast to human FcγRIIIA which is a low affinity receptor.[8,23]

The human inhibitory receptor hFcγRIIB shares 63% amino acid homology in the extracellular domain with the orthologous moFcγRIIB.[35] Interestingly, human FcγRIIB has lower affinity for IgG_1, IgG_2, and IgG_3 compared to the activating human Fcγ receptors.[8,23] This is not observed in mice, where mouse FcγRIIB has similar affinity for IgG_1 and IgG_{2b} compared to the activating mouse Fcγ receptors. The human receptor also appears to be more restricted in terms of cellular expression than the mouse receptor, as high expression is only seen on circulating B cells and basophils.[11,21]

No orthologous mouse proteins exist for human FcγRIIC and FcγIIIB, indicating a higher level of complexity of the human Fcγ receptor system.[11] An additional noticeable difference between the human and mouse Fcγ receptors is that none of the human receptors binds IgE, whereas mouse FcγRIIB, FcγRIII, and FcγRIV do.[8,25,29] In summary, significant discrepancies exist between human and mouse Fcγ receptors, and defining the orthologous proteins on sequence homology is not without complications. Hence, human and mouse Fcγ receptor systems are not identical, and caution should be taken when making direct comparisons or extrapolations based on experiments in one species compared to the other.

On a final note, mouse Fcγ receptors bind human IgG subclasses with various affinities, whereas human Fcγ receptors either do not bind or only bind with low affinity to mouse IgG subclasses.[22,36,37] From a biomedical research perspective this is noteworthy, as many human antibodies with potential therapeutic application are evaluated using mouse models. Hence, potential effects (target and off-target) of the mouse FcγR–human IgG interaction are challenging to predict and obtained results are difficult to translate into a human clinical setting. To partially bypass this issue, transgenic mice have been developed to express single human FcγRs.[37] Recently, further progress in the field of mouse engineering has resulted in the development of a fully humanized Fcγ receptor mouse expressing hFcγRI, hFcγRIIA, hFcγRIIB, hFcγRIIIA, hFcγRIIIB and none of the endogenous mouse Fcγ receptors.[37,38] Another approach has been to use immunodeficient mice and repopulate the hematopoietic cell lineages with human PBMCs or human hematopoietic stem cells after irradiation (reviewed in Shultz et al.[39]).

MACAQUE FcγRs

The macaque (mac) Fcγ receptor family consists of three classes (I, II, III) with a total of four members: macFcγRI, macFcγRIIA, macFcγRIIB, and macFcγRIII. macFcγRI, macFcγRIIA, and macFcγRIII are activating receptors; macFcγRIIB is an inhibitory receptor (Figure 8.1 and Table 8.4). macFcγRI is a 342-amino-acid-residue polypeptide composed of three extracellular Ig-like domains, a transmembrane domain, and a cytoplasmic tail. To date, only partial sequences of the cytoplasmic region are available to verify the type or number of cell-activating signals. However, it is assumed that macFcγRI, as seen in hFcγRI, depends on interaction with the ITAM-bearing FcRγ due to the ligand-binding profiles. macFcγRI binds its ligands, IgG_1, IgG_2, IgG_3, and IgG_4, with high affinity.[40] Three allelic polymorphic residues (V6G, Q18R, and V60A) have been identified in macFcγRI, all occurring in the first and most membrane-distal extracellular domain.[41] The cellular expression pattern of macFcγRI has not been investigated thoroughly; however, based on the high similarity it is assumed to mimic the human pattern (monocytes/macrophages, dendritic cells, neutrophils, and mast cells).

macFcγRIIA is comprised of two extracellular Ig-like domains, a TM domain, and a CY domain containing a signal-transducing ITAM. The 288-amino-acid-residue protein (Uniprot: AAL92096, 1-210) contains a 12-amino-acid

TABLE 8.4 Macaque Fcγ Receptors

Receptor	macFcγRI	macFcγRIIA	macFcγRIIB	macFcγRIII
Cellular activation type	Activating	Activating	Inhibitory	Activating
Ligands and affinity	Cellular binding to cyno FcγRI:	Cyno FcγRIIA K_D =	Cyno FcγRIIB K_D =	Cyno FcγRIII K_D =
	0.14 *nM* for IgG_1	1.07 μ*M* for IgG_1	1.17 μM for IgG_1	0.48 μ*M* for IgG_1
	0.40 *nM* for IgG_2	2.13 μ*M* for IgG_2	1.92 μM for IgG_2	2.38 μ*M* for IgG_2
	0.31 *nM* for IgG_3	1.94 μ*M* for IgG_3	3.59 μM for IgG_3	0.62 μ*M* for IgG_3
	0.30 *nM* for IgG_4	2.72 μ*M* for IgG_4	4.94 μM for IgG_4	2.84 μ*M* for IgG_4
Cellular expression[a]	Unknown but presumable same as human FcγRI (monocytes/macrophages, dendritic cells, neutrophils and mast cells)	NK cells, monocytes/macrophages. Expressed at high levels on cynomolgus granulocytes (neutrophils, eosinophils)		NK cells, monocytes/macrophages
Sequence homology to human	94–95% homology to human FcγRI	88–90% homology to human FcγRIIA	88–90% homology to human FcγRIIA	Rhesus is 91.7% and cynomolgus is 91.3% homologous with human FcγRIIIA

Source: Warncke et al.[40]
[a]*Specific cellular expression profiles for macFcγRIIA and macFcγRIIB are not available.*

N-terminal leader region followed by the extracellular portion consisting of 176 amino acids. macFcγRIIB, the inhibitory receptor, is a 294-amino-acid protein (Uniprot: AAL92097, 1-226) of similar structure but contains an ITIM. macFcγRII is known to be expressed by NK cells, monocytes/macrophages, neutrophils, and eosinophils. It binds macaque IgG_1, IgG_2, IgG_3, and IgG_4 with low affinity. Nine allelic polymorphic residues (M55R, V791, T93P, A119T, K1251, S126A, N128K, N113D, and Q142R) have been identified in macFcγRII. Seven of these nine polymorphic sites appear in a cluster within a short segment of the second extracellular domain.[41] Potential differences on ligand affinities are currently unknown for the macFcγRII alleles.

macFcγRIII is composed of two extracellular Ig-like domains, a TM domain, and a CY tail. Similar to hFcγRIIIA, macFcγRIII depends on interaction with the ITAM containing FcRγ to transmit a cellular activation signal. macFcγRIII binds IgG_1, IgG_2, and IgG_4 with low affinity and is expressed on NK cells and monocytes. Several macFcγRIII polymorphisms have been identified, some of which were determined to affect treatment with a monoclonal antibody.[41–43] However, the affects on ligand affinities, if any, are unknown.

HUMAN *VERSUS* MACAQUE FcγRs

Based on rhesus and cynomolgus macaque sequences, the predicted structures of the three classes of macaque receptors, macFcγRI, macFcγRII, and macFcγRIII, have been found to be highly similar to the orthologous human FcγRs (Table 8.5). Both species exhibit the same mRNA primary structure and are overall about 90% similar in sequence. However,

TABLE 8.5 Comparison of Orthologous Human and Macaque Fc Receptors

Human Receptor	Orthologous Receptor	Main Similarities	Main Differences
hFcγRI	macFcγRI	High-affinity receptor Binds IgG_1, IgG_3, and IgG_4 No ITAM in cytoplasmic domain	macFcγRI binds IgG_2 macFcγRI has higher affinity for IgG_4
hFcγRIIA	macFcγRIIA	Low-affinity receptor Contains an ITAM in cytoplasmic domain	hFcγRIIA has two allelic forms that influence binding affinities macFcγRII expression is higher on granulocytes
hFcγRIIB	macFcγRIIB	Low-affinity receptor Contains an ITIM in cytoplasmic domain	macFcγRIIB has higher affinity for ligands than hFcγRIIB macFcγRIIB binds IgG_2 macFcγRII expression is higher on granulocytes
hFcγRIIC	Not present in macaque	—	—
hFcγRIIIA	macFcγRIII	Low-affinity receptor Binds defucosylated IgG with higher affinity No ITAM in cytoplasmic domain	hFcγRIIA has two allelic forms that influence binding affinities macFcγRIII has higher affinity for IgG_2 and IgG_4
hFcγRIIIB	Not present in macaque	—	—

notwithstanding the high degree of homology, there is notably a high degree of genetic heterogeneity, as well. For example, while cysteines are conserved between the species, the macaque FcγRs show a high level of polymorphism and number variations in potential *N*-linked glycosylation sites (PNGs). All activating ITAM-bearing FcγRs of human and cynomolgus origin show very comparable binding profiles, but the inhibitory macFcγRIIB displays strikingly different Fcγ binding characteristics compared to hFcγRIIB.

The macFcγRI sequence is extensively similar to hFcγRI mRNA structure and typical of the type I membrane Ig-like domain proteins with six conserved cysteines (C26, C68, C107, C151, C195, C243) forming the disulfide bonds of the three extracellular domains.[44] The macFcγRI shares 94 to 95% homology with hFcγRI within the entire 267-amino-acid extracellular region. However, the homology between the two species is strongest, with fewer amino acid differences in the third extracellular domain compared to the first two extracellular regions.[41] Unlike hFcγRI that contains seven potential *N*-linked glycosylation sites, macFcγRI contains only four (N44, N95, N6, N80). Two glycosylation sites are replaced with other amino acids in macFcγRI, and a substitution at position 101 breaks the motif at position 99. Together, these sequence differences suggest that the functional differences between the receptors could result from this interspecies variation.[41]

The specific residues crucial for ligand binding by hFcγRI are unknown. Nonetheless, at least three invariant amino acids within the binding interface (W3, W26, K77) are fully conserved between hFcγRI and macFcγRI.[41,45] Binding studies with human and cynomolgus macFcγRI indicate no binding to human IgG_2, but both receptors show nanomolar affinity to cynomolgus IgG_2.[40] Also, due to a slower off-rate, the affinity of cynomolgus macaque IgG_4 is tenfold higher for macFcγRI than is seen in the human molecules.[40] Yet, human and cynomolgus IgG_1 and IgG_3 have almost identical binding to human and cynomolgus macFcγRI.

macFcγRII is 88% to 90% homologous to hFcγRII within the entire extracellular region and varies by only five amino acid residues within the TM region.[41] Three PNGs are conserved between hFcγRII and macFcγRII.[44] Two are located in the extracellular regions and the third one is located in the cytoplasmic tail with no known functional significance.[41] The macFcγRII also contains two PNGs in the second extracellular domain that are a result of amino acid differences from hFcγRII. The first, N77, is polymorphic in macaques and is not always present. The second, N88, is always present in macaques but polymorphic in humans, only sometimes having an *N*-glycosylation site.[41,46]

Only a single amino acid residue in macFcγRII that is critical for IgG binding[47] differs compared to hFcγRII. In macFcγRII, the residue at position 81 in the second extracellular domain is M, but in hFcγRII it is L. The conserved residues that are presumed to directly contact the IgG Fc ligand are K29, P30, S79, D82, and Y113. Residues that may affect conformation of the loops are L36, P87, and I108.[41]

Noticeable differences between hFcγRII and macFcγRII are found in cellular expression and in IgG affinity. Although no distinction is made between FcγRIIA and FcγRIIB, granulocytes of cynomolgus macaque were found to express threefold higher levels of macFcγRII compared to hFcγRII expression.[40] In contrast macFcγRII expression on cynomolgus monocytes was found to be equal to that of hFcγRII on human monocytes. A distinction between FcγRIIA and FcγRIIB is made with the cynomolgus inhibitory FcγRIIB regarding its ligand binding. macFcγRIIB binds IgG_2 with substantially higher affinity than hFcγRIIB. This difference is likely due to a difference in sequence in the Fc binding region of the macFcγRIIB. Unlike hFcγRII, which is polymorphic at amino acid residue H131 defining the specificity of the human receptor for IgG_2, there is no allelic variation in macFcγRII. Instead, all macFcγRII sequences contain H80 that corresponds to the H131 residue in hFcγRIIA. When the amino acid at position 131 is a histidine in the activating hFcγRIIA, it has a higher affinity to IgG_2. Comparably, macFcγRIIB has a high-affinity-conferring histidine at this position and thus shows a tenfold higher affinity to cynomolgus IgG_2. For hFcγRIIB, the amino acid at position 131 is an arginine, thus leading to low-affinity binding of IgG_2.[40,41] It has been hypothesized that the differences in cellular FcγR expression between humans and macaques may have evolved due to variation in requirements for phagocytosis and neutralization of bacteria and parasites. Thus, the enhanced activity of IgG_2 and IgG_4 that evolved in cynomolgus macaques is counterbalanced by increased inhibitory activity of the cynomolgus FcγRIIB toward IgG_2 that is known to prefer binding to repetitive sugar antigens on bacteria.[40,48,49] This increased inhibitory activity of macFcγRIIB extends to IgG_4, an isotype that primarily binds parasites and allergens.[50,51] Thus, it is possible that the macaque species developed a different strategy compared to humans to balance activating and inhibitory IgG/FcγR interactions by simply co-evolving activating IgG isotypes and the inhibitory rhFcγRIIB.[40] If this alternative regulatory strategy is overlooked, testing various human immunoglobulin isotypes in macaques could lead to unpredicted complications and misinterpretations of outcomes.

Rhesus and cynomolgus macaque macFcγRIII are 91.7% and 91.3% identical, respectively, to hFcγRIIIA. An orthologous receptor to human FcγRIIIB has not been identified in macaques.[43] Instead of the allotypic variation seen in hFcγRIIIA with V158 conferring a high-affinity phenotype and F158 conferring a lower affinity phenotype, macFcγRIII contains an isoleucine at position 158, more similar to the high-affinity phenotype of the V158 in hFcγRIIIA. Also, the D147 present in hFcγRIIIB is not present in macFcγRIII, but instead is a glycine matching that of hFcγRIIIA.[43] Interestingly, cynomolgus macFcγRIII binds IgG_2 and IgG_4 with five to ten times higher affinity than its human counterparts. This is likely because of the amino acid sequences within the C_H2 domain of the cynomolgus IgG_2 and IgG_4 that contain residues matching those of the human IgG_1 and IgG_3.[40] Also, one of the residues (F203) that is critical to the expression of hFcγRIIIB as a GP-linked protein is in macFcγRIII a serine.[52] All other residues at positions that define a difference between hFcγRIIIA and hFcγRIIIB are conserved in nonhuman primates, including, most residues that involve hFcγRIII contact with IgG_1. Only three substitutions are found in macFcγRIII: A135, H153, and V176 become Leu, Glu, and Ile, respectively.[40]

Four of the five *N*-glycosylation sites that occur in hFcγRIII are conserved in nonhuman primates and one additional motif is present in macFcγRIII.[43] As in humans, the macaque FcγRIII is expressed on NK cells and monocytes,[53–55] with similar cellular expression patterns and levels of hFcγRIIIA.

CONCLUSIONS

As documented above, there are appreciable differences among human, mouse, and macaque Fcγ receptors, including cellular expression, cell activation signaling, ligand binding, glycosylation, and balancing the regulation of activating and inhibitory functions. Improvements to mouse models, specifically the newly developed transgenic mouse expressing all of the human Fcγ receptors may solve some of the limitations using the murine models. Ongoing research will further evaluate and characterize nonhuman primate Fcγ receptors. Due to their close evolutionary relationship with humans, rhesus and cynomolgus macaques are logical choices to model preclinical therapeutic effects in a variety of human diseases and for assessing vaccines, especially in AIDS research. Irrespective of which mammalian model is used, cautious assessment of experimental outcomes regarding mechanism and efficacy is prudent when translating to humans for treatment of infectious diseases, cancer, and AIDS pathogenesis.

ACKNOWLEDGMENTS

The authors would like to thank Christina Corbaci for assistance with graphics. Financial support was provided by the Lundbeck Foundation (BM).

References

1. Nimmerjahn F, Ravetch JV. Fcgamma receptors as regulators of immune responses. *Nat Rev. Immunol* 2008;**8**:34–47.
2. Nimmerjahn F, Ravetch JV. Fcgamma receptors: old friends and new family members. *Immunity* 2006;**24**:19–28.
3. Amigorena S, Bonnerot C, Drake JR, Choquet D, Hunziker W, Guillet J-G, et al. Cytoplasmic domain heterogeneity and functions of IgG Fc receptors in B lymphocytes. *Science* 1992;**256**:1808–12.
4. Daeron M, Latour S, Malbec O, Espinosa E, Pina P, Pasmans S, et al. The same tyrosine-based inhibition motif, in the intracytoplasmic domain of Fc gamma RIIB, regulates negatively BCR-, TCR-, and FcR-dependent cell activation. *Immunity* 1995;**3**:635–46.
5. Muta T, Kurosaki T, Misulovin Z, Sanchez M, Nussenzweig MC, Ravetch JVA. 13-amino-acid motif in the cytoplasmic domain of Fc gamma RIIB modulates B-cell receptor signalling. *Nature* 1994;**368**:70–3.
6. Vely F, Vivier E. Conservation of structural features reveals the existence of a large family of inhibitory cell surface receptors and noninhibitory/activatory counterparts. *J Immunol* 1997;**159**:2075–7.
7. Bruhns P. Properties of mouse and human IgG receptors and their contribution to disease models. *Blood* 2012;**119**:5640–9.
8. Bruhns P, Iannascoli B, England P, Mancardi DA, Fernandez N, Jorieux S, et al. Specificity and affinity of human Fcgamma receptors and their polymorphic variants for human IgG subclasses. *Blood* 2009;**113**:3716–25.

9. Ra C, Jouvin MH, Blank U, Kinet JP. A macrophage Fc gamma receptor and the mast cell receptor for IgE share an identical subunit. *Nature* 1989;**341**:752–4.
10. Okayama Y, Kirshenbaum AS, Metcalfe DD. Expression of a functional high-affinity IgG receptor, Fc gamma RI, on human mast cells: up-regulation by IFN-gamma. *J Immunol* 2000;**164**:4332–9.
11. Ravetch JV, Kinet JP. Fc receptors. *Annu Rev Immunol.* 1991;**9**:457–92.
12. Maresco DL, Chang E, Theil KS, Francke U, Anderson CL. The three genes of the human FCGR1 gene family encoding Fc gamma RI flank the centromere of chromosome 1 at 1p12 and 1q21. *Cytogenet Cell Genet* 1996;**73**:157–63.
13. Cassard L, Jonsson F, Arnaud S, Daeron M. Fcgamma receptors inhibit mouse and human basophil activation. *J Immunol* 2012;**189**:2995–3006.
14. Magnusson SE, Engstrom M, Jacob U, Ulfgren AK, Kleinau S. High synovial expression of the inhibitory FcgammaRIIb in rheumatoid arthritis. *Arthritis Res Ther* 2007;**9**:R51.
15. Veri MC, Gorlatov S, Li H, Burke S, Johnson S, et al. Monoclonal antibodies capable of discriminating the human inhibitory Fcgamma-receptor IIB (CD32B) from the activating Fcgamma-receptor IIA (CD32A): biochemical, biological and functional characterization. *Immunology* 2007;**121**:392–404.
16. Hunter S, Indik ZK, Kim MK, Cauley MD, Park JG, Schreiber AD. Inhibition of Fcgamma receptor-mediated phagocytosis by a nonphagocytic Fcgamma receptor. *Blood* 1998;**91**:1762–8.
17. Liu Y, Masuda E, Blank MC, Kirou KA, Gao X, Park MS, et al. Cytokine-mediated regulation of activating and inhibitory Fc gamma receptors in human monocytes. *J Leukocyte Biol* 2005;**77**:767–76.
18. Breunis WB, van Mirre E, Bruin M, Geissler J, de Boer M, et al. Copy number variation of the activating FCGR2C gene predisposes to idiopathic thrombocytopenic purpura. *Blood* 2008;**111**:1029–38.
19. Metes D, Ernst LK, Chambers WH, Sulica A, Herberman RB, Morel PA. Expression of functional CD32 molecules on human NK cells is determined by an allelic polymorphism of the FcgammaRIIC gene. *Blood* 1998;**91**:2369–80.
20. van der Heijden J, Breunis WB, Geissler J, de Boer M, van den Berg TK, Kuijpers TW. Phenotypic variation in IgG receptors by nonclassical FCGR2C alleles. *J Immunol* 2012;**188**:1318–24.
21. Meknache N, Jonsson F, Laurent J, Guinnepain MT, Daeron M. Human basophils express the glycosylphosphatidylinositol-anchored low-affinity IgG receptor FcgammaRIIIB (CD16B). *J Immunol* 2009;**182**:2542–50.
22. Mancardi DA, Albanesi M, Jonsson F, Iannascoli B, Van Rooijen N, et al. The high-affinity human IgG receptor FcgammaRI (CD64) promotes IgG-mediated inflammation, anaphylaxis, and antitumor immunotherapy. *Blood* 2013;**121**:1563–73.
23. Nimmerjahn F, Bruhns P, Horiuchi K, Ravetch JV. FcgammaRIV: a novel FcR with distinct IgG subclass specificity. *Immunity* 2005;**23**:41–51.
24. Gavin AL, Barnes N, Dijstelbloem HM, Hogarth PM. Identification of the mouse IgG3 receptor: implications for antibody effector function at the interface between innate and adaptive immunity. *J Immunol* 1998;**160**:20–3.
25. Mancardi DA, Iannascoli B, Hoos S, England P, Daeron M, Bruhns P. FcgammaRIV is a mouse IgE receptor that resembles macrophage FcepsilonRI in humans and promotes IgE-induced lung inflammation. *J Clin Invest* 2008;**118**:3738–50.
26. Langlet C, Tamoutounour S, Henri S, Luche H, Ardouin L, et al. CD64 expression distinguishes monocyte-derived and conventional dendritic cells and reveals their distinct role during intramuscular immunization. *J Immunol* 2012;**188**:1751–60.
27. Tan PS, Gavin AL, Barnes N, Sears DW, Vremec D, Shortman K, et al. Unique monoclonal antibodies define expression of Fc gamma RI on macrophages and mast cell lines and demonstrate heterogeneity among subcutaneous and other dendritic cells. *J Immunol* 2003;**170**:2549–56.
28. Daeron M. Fc receptor biology. *Annu Rev Immunol.* 1997;**15**:203–34.
29. Takizawa F, Adamczewski M, Kinet JP. Identification of the low affinity receptor for immunoglobulin E on mouse mast cells and macrophages as Fc gamma RII and Fc gamma RIII. *J Exp Med* 1992;**176**:469–75.
30. Kim HY, Kim S, Chung DH. FcgammaRIII engagement provides activating signals to NKT cells in antibody-induced joint inflammation. *J Clin Invest* 2006;**116**:2484–92.
31. Biburger M, Aschermann S, Schwab I, Lux A, Albert H, Danzer H, et al. Monocyte subsets responsible for immunoglobulin G-dependent effector functions *in vivo*. *Immunity* 2011;**35**:932–44.
32. Sears DW, Osman N, Tate B, McKenzie IF, Hogarth PM. Molecular cloning and expression of the mouse high affinity Fc receptor for IgG. *J Immunol* 1990;**144**:371–8.
33. Zidovetzki R, Rost B, Armstrong DL, Pecht I. Transmembrane domains in the functions of Fc receptors. *Biophys Chem* 2003;**100**:555–75.
34. Mechetina LV, Najakshin AM, Alabyev BY, Chikaev NA, Taranin AV. Identification of CD16-2, a novel mouse receptor homologous to CD16/Fc gamma RIII. *Immunogenetics* 2002;**54**:463–8.
35. Brooks DG, Qiu WQ, Luster AD, Ravetch JV. Structure and expression of human IgG FcRII(CD32). Functional heterogeneity is encoded by the alternatively

spliced products of multiple genes. *J Exp Med* 1989;**170**:1369–85.
36. Jonsson F, Mancardi DA, Kita Y, Karasuyama H, Iannascoli B, et al. Mouse and human neutrophils induce anaphylaxis. *J Clin Invest* 2011;**121**:1484–96.
37. Lux A, Nimmerjahn F. Of mice and men: the need for humanized mouse models to study human IgG activity *in vivo*. *J Clin Immunol* 2013;**33**(Suppl 1):S4–S8.
38. Smith P, DiLillo DJ, Bournazos S, Li F, Ravetch JV. Mouse model recapitulating human Fcgamma receptor structural and functional diversity. *Proc Natl Acad Sci USA* 2012;**109**:6181–6.
39. Shultz LD, Brehm MA, Garcia-Martinez JV, Greiner DL. Humanized mice for immune system investigation: progress, promise and challenges. *Nat Rev Immunol* 2012;**12**:786–98.
40. Warncke M, Calzascia T, Coulot M, Balke N, Touil R, Kolbinger F, et al. Different adaptations of IgG effector function in human and nonhuman primates and implications for therapeutic antibody treatment. *J Immunol* 2012;**188**:4405–11.
41. Nguyen DC, Scinicariello F, Attanasio R. Characterization and allelic polymorphisms of rhesus macaque (*Macaca mulatta*) IgG Fc receptor genes. *Immunogenetics* 2011;**63**:351–62.
42. Miller CJ, Genesca M, Abel K, Montefiori D, Forthal D, et al. Antiviral antibodies are necessary for control of simian immunodeficiency virus replication. *J Virol* 2007;**81**:5024–35.
43. Rogers KA, Scinicariello F, Attanasio R. IgG Fc receptor III homologues in nonhuman primate species: genetic characterization and ligand interactions. *J Immunol* 2006;**177**:3848–56.
44. Lefranc MP, Pommie C, Kaas Q, Duprat E, Bosc N, et al. IMGT unique numbering for immunoglobulin and T cell receptor constant domains and Ig superfamily C-like domains. *Dev Comp Immunol* 2005;**29**:185–203.
45. Radaev S, Sun P. Recognition of immunoglobulins by Fcgamma receptors. *Mol Immunol* 2002;**38**:1073–83.
46. Ehrenmann F, Kaas Q, Lefranc MP. IMGT/3Dstructure-DB and IMGT/DomainGapAlign: a database and a tool for immunoglobulins or antibodies, T cell receptors, MHC, IgSF and MhcSF. *Nucleic Acids Res* 2010;**38**:D301–7.
47. Maxwell KF, Powell MS, Hulett MD, Barton PA, McKenzie IF, Garrett TP, et al. Crystal structure of the human leukocyte Fc receptor, Fc gammaRIIa. *Nat Struct Biol* 1999;**6**:437–42.
48. Barrett DJ, Ayoub EM. IgG2 subclass restriction of antibody to pneumococcal polysaccharides. *Clin Exp Immunol* 1986;**63**:127–34.
49. Yount WJ, Dorner MM, Kunkel HG, Kabat EA. Studies on human antibodies. VI. Selective variations in subgroup composition and genetic markers. *J Exp Med* 1968;**127**:633–46.
50. Carballido JM, Carballido-Perrig N, Oberli-Schrammli A, Heusser CH, Blaser K. Regulation of IgE and IgG4 responses by allergen specific T-cell clones to bee venom phospholipase A2 *in vitro*. *J Allergy Clin Immunol* 1994;**93**:758–67.
51. Maizels RM. Exploring the immunology of parasitism—from surface antigens to the hygiene hypothesis. *Parasitology* 2009;**136**:1549–64.
52. Kurosaki T, Ravetch JV. A single amino acid in the glycosyl phosphatidylinositol attachment domain determines the membrane topology of Fc gamma RIII. *Nature* 1989;**342**:805–7.
53. Carter DL, Shieh TM, Blosser RL, Chadwick KR, Margolick JB, Hildreth JE, et al. CD56 identifies monocytes and not natural killer cells in rhesus macaques. *Cytometry* 1999;**37**:41–50.
54. Reimann KA, Waite BC, Lee-Parritz DE, Lin W, Uchanska-Ziegler B, O'Connell MJ, et al. Use of human leukocyte-specific monoclonal antibodies for clinically immunophenotyping lymphocytes of rhesus monkeys. *Cytometry* 1994;**17**:102–8.
55. Sopper S, Stahl-Hennig C, Demuth M, Johnston IC, Dorries R, ter Meulen V. Lymphocyte subsets and expression of differentiation markers in blood and lymphoid organs of rhesus monkeys. *Cytometry* 1997;**29**:351–62.

CHAPTER

9

Human IgG Subclasses

Theo Rispens[a] *and Gestur Vidarsson*[b]

[a]Department of Immunopathology, and [b]Department of Experimental Immunohematology, Sanquin Research, and Landsteiner Laboratory, Academic Medical Center, University of Amsterdam, The Netherlands

INTRODUCTION: IMMUNOGLOBULINS AND HUMORAL IMMUNITY

Immunoglobulins are a group of closely related glycoproteins composed of 82 to 96% protein and 4 to 18% carbohydrate. In humans, there are five classes of immunoglobulins, which differ in heavy-chain structure. Immunoglobulin G (IgG) is the major class of immunoglobulins in blood and can be further subdivided in subclasses. The four subclasses of IgG were discovered in the 1960s following extensive studies using specific rabbit antisera against human IgG myeloma proteins.[1] They are designated IgG_1, IgG_2, IgG_3, and IgG_4, in order of decreasing abundance. Several decades of research has revealed subtle but profound differences among the subclasses. Each subclass has a unique profile with respect to antigen binding, immune complex formation, complement activation, triggering of effector cells, and placental transport (Table 9.1). In addition, IgG antibody responses to different types of antigens or pathogens often lead to marked skewing toward one of the subclasses. On the other hand, selective subclass deficiencies are usually not detrimental to the individual but do sometimes lead to enhanced susceptibility toward specific classes of pathogens. All in all, the acquired variability within the Ig locus seems to have selected for beneficial changes during evolution for optimizing or fine-tuning the antibody-mediated immune response.

GENETICS

Immunoglobulins are encoded by three non-linked clusters of autosomal genes, one cluster coding for heavy (H) chains, a second one for κ-light chains and a third one for λ-light chains. In humans, the H gene family is on chromosome 14 (Figure 9.1A), the κ gene family is on chromosome 2, and the λ gene family is on chromosome 22. A unique variable region is created within developing B cells early in their development by the random recombination of three distinct types of gene segments for the heavy chain—designated VH (variable), D (diversity), and JH (joining)—and two for the light chain (VL and JL). Each B cell only

TABLE 9.1 Properties of Human IgG Subclasses

	IgG1	IgG2	IgG3	IgG4
General				
Molecular mass (kD)	146	146	170	146
Amino acids in hinge region	15	12	62[a]	12
Inter-heavy chain disulfide bonds	2	4[b]	11[a]	2
Susceptibility to proteolytic enzymes	++	+/−	+++	+
Mean adult serum level (g/l)	6.98	3.8	0.51	0.56
Proportion of total IgG (%)	60	32	4	4
Half-life (days)	21	21	7/~21[a]	21
Placental transfer	++++	++	++	+++
Antibody response to:				
Proteins	++	+/−	++	++[e]
Polysaccharides	+	+++	+/−	+/−
Allergens	+	(−)	(−)	++
Complement activation				
C1q binding	++	+	+++	−
Fc receptors				
FcγRI	+++[c]	−	++++	++
	65[d]	−	61	34
FcγRIIa$_{H131}$	+++	++	++++	++
	5.2	0.45	0.89	0.17
FcγRIIa$_{R131}$	+++	+	++++	++
	3.5	0.10	0.91	0.21
FcγRIIb/c	+	−	++	+
	0.12	0.02	0.17	0.20
FcγRIIIa$_{F158}$	++	−	++++	−
	1.2	0.03	7.7	0.20
FcγRIIIa$_{V158}$	+++	+	++++	++
	2.0	0.07	9.8	0.25
FcγRIIIb	+++	−	++++	−
	0.2	−	1.1	−
FcRn (at pH<6.5)	+++	+++	++/+++[a]	+++

(Continued)

TABLE 9.1 (Continued)

	IgG1	IgG2	IgG3	IgG4
Prot A/G				
Protein A binding	+++	+++	–[a]	++
Protein G binding	+++	+++	+++	+++

Notes:
[a] Depends on allotype
[b] For A2 isomer.
[c] Multivalent binding to transfected cells
[d] Association constants for monovalent binding as measured with Biacore (10^{-6} M^{-1}) [61]
[e] After repeated encounters with protein antigens, often allergens

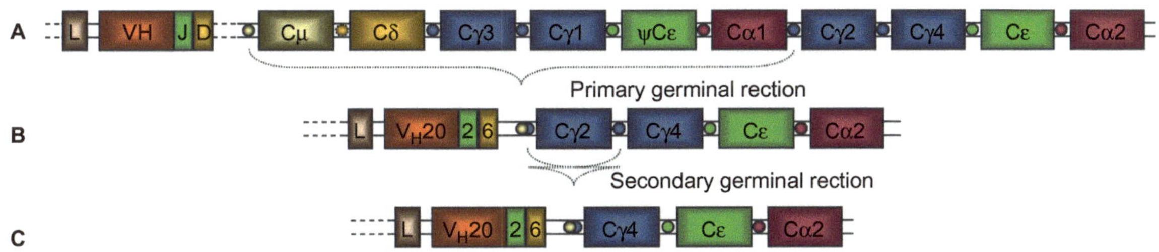

FIGURE 9.1 **Heavy-chain locus on chromosome 14.** (A) Pre- (VDJ)-arranged heavy chain locus of a naïve B cell. A functional RNA is transcribed from the promoter upstream of the V region, leading to a long transcript that can be spliced into mRNA encoding for either IgM or IgD. In naïve B cells, this mRNA encodes for Ig with transmembrane regions, giving rise to the B-cell receptor that forms the "sensing" part of the B cell. Upon recognition of its cognate antigen, the B cell becomes activated, proliferates, and initiates alternative splicing mechanisms, splicing out the transmembrane part of IgM, leading to secretion of IgM. (B) Upon further stimulus, the B cell may undergo class switching by excision of chromosomal DNA between that of the switch region (small circles upstream of H chain locuses) of IgM and downstream heavy-chain loci. This leads to loss of heavy-chain loci between IgM and the target heavy-chain locus. (C) Upon even further stimulus, subsequent class switching may occur. For protein antigens, a common result is class switching to IgG_4, the most 3′ of the IgG locuses.

expresses one allele of the recombined VDJ gene (the product of which is the VH segment) and one allele of either the κ or the λ locus (the product of which is the VL segment), ensuring the clonal specificity of the naïve B cell when it exits the bone marrow. These processes (i.e., VDJ recombination and clonal specificity through allelic exclusion) are extensively reviewed elsewhere.[2]

Early on, the B cell expresses its fully formed immunoglobulin using the V-gene proximal constant region—that is, IgM and IgD (through alternative splicing) as membrane-bound receptors (Figure 9.1). Once cross-linked by exogenous antigen, given the appropriate environment (e.g., stimulation through Toll-like receptors), the B cell may start secreting IgM by alternative splicing, resulting in the absence of the transmembrane region of IgM. If T cell help and other immune stimuli are applied (as for most protein antigens), class switching can occur, resulting in loss of the IgM and other intervening heavy-chain constant regions between IgM and the target constant (C) locus (Figure 9.1B). The choice of this locus is not random, as it is preceded by sterile transcription of

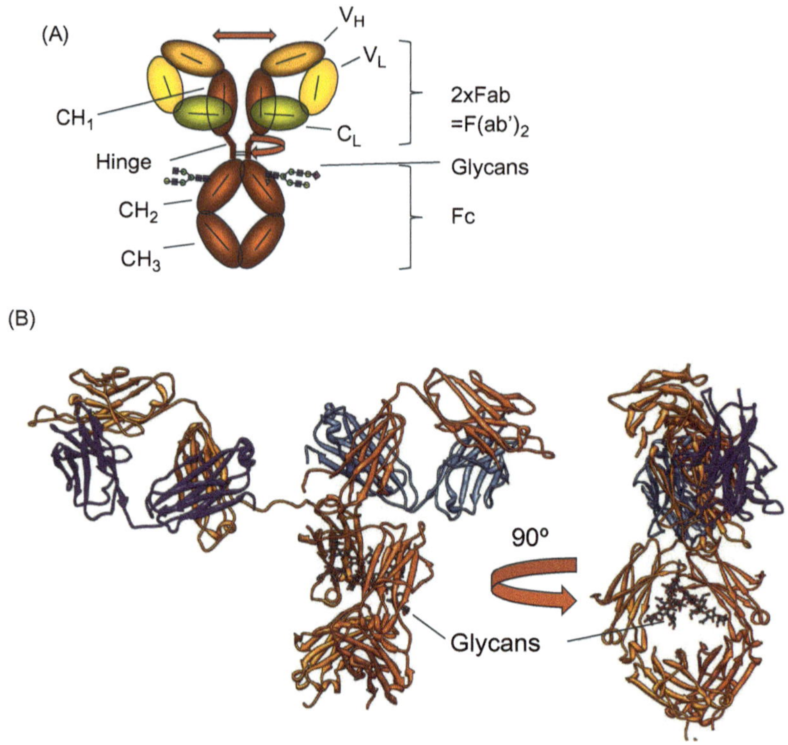

FIGURE 9.2 **Structure of IgG.** (A) Illustration of the structure of an IgG molecule with the different domains indicated. Inter- and intra-chain disulfide bonds are indicated with black lines within Ig-like domains or between the two heavy chains in the hinge region. (B) Crystal structure of an IgG molecule (1HZH) viewed from two different angles, demonstrating the flexibility of the two Fab fragments with respect to each other and the Fc tail. The location of the glycan attached to each of the heavy chains (N297) is also indicated.

the targeted locus.[3] The opening of those loci is guided by the cytokine environment and the cellular niche in which the B cell resides during its encounter with the corresponding antigen in the germinal reaction. This genetic excision reaction (class switching) has also been extensively reviewed elsewhere.[4]

STRUCTURE[5–7]

The basic immunoglobulin molecule has a four-chain structure, comprised of two identical γ heavy (H) chains and two identical κ or λ light (L) chains, linked together by inter-chain disulfide bonds. Each heavy chain consists of an N-terminal variable domain (VH) and three constant domains (CH1, CH2, CH3), with an additional hinge region between CH1 and CH2 (Figure 9.2). Light chains consist of an N-terminal variable domain (VL) and a constant domain (CL) and are associated with the VH and CH1 domains to form a Fab (fragment antigen-binding) arm. Functionally, the V regions are involved in antigen binding. Two heavy-chain/light-chain heterodimers (HL) are combined into a single antibody molecule (H_2L_2) via disulfide bonds in the hinge region and non-covalent interactions between the CH3 domains. The part of the antibody formed by the lower hinge region and the CH2/CH3 domains is called fragment crystalline (*Fc*); it is formed after mild proteolysis using papain, which cleaves intact IgG molecules into two Fab fragments and an Fc fragment. The latter fragment crystallizes easily, hence its designation. The Fc part is responsible for effector functions of antibodies, as it contains a largly overlapping binding site for C1q (complement) and IgG–Fc receptors (FcγR) on effector cells of the innate immune system. It is also contains the binding site for the neonatal Fc receptor (FcRn) that is responsible for the prolonged half-life of IgG antibodies and placental passage. The highly conserved glycosylation site N297 is located at the interface between the two CH2/CH3, forming the Fc of an IgG molecule (Figure 9.2) that is responsible for subtle but important changes of quaternary structure of the Fc, allowing for a more exposed docking site for FcγR. As discussed in other chapters in this book, these glycans also directly participate in FcγR binding, but they can also modulate these interactions through highly specific modifications of the N297 glycan—changes that seem to be regulated during specific immune responses in humans.[8] Although this glycosylation site is considered to be the single glycosylation site in IgG, the V region of approximately 30% of all antibodies has also been found to be glycosylated, sometimes arising through VDJ recombination or somatic hypermutation, and this glycosylation has been reported to affect antibody binding characteristics.[9,10]

The global structures of the four human IgG subclasses are very similar but with important differences that affect the functionality of each subclass (Figure 9.3A). The four subclasses show over 90% homology in amino acid sequence, with differences that are not randomly distributed. Much variation is found in the hinge region and N-terminal CH2 domain, whereas fewer amino acid differences are found in the other domains. Of these, least is known about the functional consequences (if any) of structural variations found within the CH1 domain. On the other hand, structural differences in the CH2/CH3 domains, forming the Fc tail, are relatively well studied. The binding profiles of the subclasses to FcγR and C1q are quite different and have been investigated in detail. Differences in the primary sequences of the IgG subclasses (Fc and hinge) lead to variations in tertiary structural elements, thereby critically influencing the properties of each subclass, as discussed in greater detail below.

Structural Variation in the Hinge Region

The hinge region forms a flexible linker between the Fab arms and the Fc part. Length and flexibility of the hinge region vary extensively among the IgG subclasses.[7] This length variation has consequences for the possible conformations of the Fab arms relative to the Fc domain as well as to each other. The hinge region of IgG_1 encompasses 15 amino acids and is very flexible. IgG_2 has a shorter hinge than IgG_1, with 12 amino acid residues. The lower hinge region of IgG_2 (actually encoded by the CH2 region) also has a one amino acid deletion (G236) and contains a rigid polyproline double helix, stabilized by four extra inter-heavy-chain disulfide bridges (Figure 9.1). These properties restrict the flexibility of the IgG_2 molecule. IgG_3 has a much longer hinge region than any other IgG subclasses or Ig human isotype; it is about four times as long as the IgG_1 hinge, containing 62 amino acids (including 21 prolines and 11 cysteines) and forming a polyproline double helix with limited flexibility.[11,12] In IgG_3, the Fab fragments are relatively far away from the Fc fragment, giving the molecule a greater flexibility. This long hinge of IgG_3 is a result of duplications of the hinge exon, encoded by one exon in IgG_1, IgG_2, and IgG_4 but up to four exons in IgG_3. One of those exons is common to all IgG_3 allotypes, but IgG_3 also has one

(A)

CH1

	131	133	137	138	189	192	193	196	199	203	214
IgG1	S	K	G	G	P	S	L	Q	I	N	K
IgG2	C	R	E	S	P	N	F	Q	T	D	T
IgG3	C	R	G	G	P	S	L	Q	T	N	R
IgG4	C	R	E	S	P	S	L	K	T	D	R

hinge

	*	217	219	220	221	222	223	224	225	228
IgG1		P	S	C	D	K	T	H	T	P
IgG2		R	C	C	.	.	V	.	E	P
IgG3	*	P	S	C	D	T	P	P	P	R
IgG4		S	.	.	.	Y	G	P	P	S
										fae

CH2

	233	234	235	236	268	274	276	282	291	292	296	300	309	327	330	331	339
IgG1	E	L	L	G	H	K	N	V	P	R	Y	Y	L	A	A	P	A
IgG2	P	V	A	.	H	Q	N	V	P	R	F	F	V	G	A	P	T
IgG3	E	L	L	G	H	Q	K	V	P	R	Y	F	L	A	A	P	T
IgG4	E	F	L	G	Q	Q	N	V	P	R	F	Y	L	G	S	S	A
	γ	γ	c/γ	γ					r				r	γ	γ	c	

CH3

	355	356	358	379	384	397	409	419	422	431	435	436	445
IgG1	R	D	L	V	N	V	K	Q	V	A	H	Y	P
IgG2	R	E	M	V	N	M	K	Q	V	A	H	Y	P
IgG3	R	E	M	V	S	M	K	Q	I	A	R	F	P
IgG4	Q	E	M	V	N	V	R	E	V	A	H	Y	L
							fae				r	r	

(B)

IgG1	CH1 214	CH3→ 356	358	431
z,a	K	D	L	A
z,a,x	K	D	L	G
f	R	E	M	A
f,a	R	D	L	A
	↓ z (K)/ f (R)	↓ a	↓ a	↓ x

IgG2	CH1 189	CH2 282
n	T	M
..	P	V

IgG4	CH2 309	CH3 409
4a I	L	R
4a II	L	K
4b	V	R
	↓ 4a (L)/ 4b (V)	

IgG3	CH2→ 291	292	CH3→ 379	384	397	409	419	422	435	436
b*	P	R	V	S	M	K	Q	I	R	F
c3*	P	R	V	S	M	K	E	I	R	F
c3c5*	P	R	V	S	V	R	E	V	R	F
s*	P	R	M	S	V	K	Q	I	H	Y
st*	P	W	M	S	V	K	Q	I	H	Y
g*	L	R	V	N	M	K	Q	I	R	Y
	↓ g1	↓ t	↓ s				↓ c3	↓ c5	↓ g5	↓ b1

b* = b0,b1,b3,b4,b5,u,v
c3* = b0,b1,c3,b5,u,v
c3c5* = b0,b1,c3,u,c5
s* = b0,b3,b5,s,v
st* = b0,b3,b5,s,t,v
g* = g1,g5,u,v

FIGURE 9.3 **Variations in IgG between subclasses and individuals.** (A) Overview of the amino acid differences between the four IgG subclasses per domain. Residues also known to differ between individuals (allotypic residues) are indicated in green (IgG_1), magenta (IgG_2), blue (IgG_3), and red (IgG_4). Displayed allotypes are G1m(za), G2m(..), G3m(b*), and nGm4(a). The amino acid positions involved in differential binding of the subclasses to C1q, FcγR, and FcRn, are indicated below each sequence alignment with c, γ, and r, respectively. Residue positions marked with "fae" are involved in the Fab arm exchange of IgG_4. Hinge exons 1 to 3 for IgG_3 are not displayed. See text for more details. (B) Allotypes of the different IgG subclasses as classified by the alphabetical classification (genetic marker, Gm) system. For IgG_3, the allotypes indicated in the table represent a summary of the most frequently occurring alleles; the individual allotypes corresponding to these alleles are indicated below the table. The amino acids encoding for a particular allotype, providing the anti-allotype epitope, are indicated below each allotype with the corresponding alphabetical numbering.

to three copies of a homologous second type of IgG_3 hinge exon. The elongated hinge in IgG_3 is also responsible for its higher molecular weight compared to the other subclasses. The hinge region of IgG_4 is 12 amino acids long and thus shorter than that of IgG_1. Its flexibility is intermediate between that of IgG_1 and IgG_2.[13] The difference in hinge flexibility influences the relative orientation and movement of the Fab arms and Fc tail of the IgG antibody.

Binding sites for C1q and/or FcγR may be partially or completely shielded by Fab arms. Furthermore, the relative flexibility that both Fab arms may have with respect to each other differs between subclasses as follows: $IgG_3 > IgG_1 > IgG_4 > IgG_2$.[13,14] This flexibility affects antigen-binding capacity, immune complex formation, and C1q and FcγR binding.

Inter-Chain Disulfide Bonds

The four IgG subclasses also differ with respect to the number of inter-heavy-chain disulfide bonds in the hinge region (Table 9.1). In addition, both IgG_2 and IgG_4 may be found as several isomers in which the hinge disulfide bonds are connected in different ways (see below). Another structural difference between the human IgG subclasses is the linkage of the heavy and light chain by a disulfide bond. This bond links the carboxy-terminal cysteine of the light chain to the cysteine at position 220 (in IgG_1) or at position 131 (in IgG_2, IgG_3, and IgG_4) in the CH1 domain. These two positions are spatially juxtaposed, and the essential structure and function of the molecule appears to be conserved between the two types of linkage between heavy and light chain.

Hinge Isomers in IgG_2 and IgG_4

In IgG_2, structural hinge isomers have been observed as a result of alternative formation of disulfide bonds between the cysteines in the hinge region of the heavy chains and those involved in the formation of disulfide bonds between light and heavy chains.[15,16] These isomers were found for IgG_2 antibodies with κ light chains but were absent for λ light chains. The major forms are the classical A form with four disulfide bridges between the two IgG_2 heavy chains and the B form in which hinge cysteine instead forms a disulfide bond with the light chain, although multiple other configurations exist.[16] These isoforms apparently form independently of each other, giving rise to A/A, B/B, and A/B isoforms. Fc receptor binding does not seem to be different for the different isomers.[17] IgG_2 has also been reported to form covalent dimers,[18] which might be regarded as an additional isomer.

Two isomers of IgG_4 differing in the disulfide bonding of hinge cysteines coexist. The core hinge of IgG is formed by a CXXC motif also found in redox-reactive proteins such as thioredoxins.[19] Compared to IgG_1, with a relatively rigid CPPC motif,[20] intra-chain disulfide bonds are more easily formed between cysteines 226 and 229 in IgG_4, which possesses a CPSC core hinge. The result is an observable amount of non-covalently linked half-molecules (HL, as opposed to H_2L_2), in addition to covalently linked inter-chain isomers.[21,22] An S228P mutant of IgG_4 does not form half-molecules, in agreement with the finding that this species does not occur in IgG_1. The process is reversible but depends on redox conditions. Formation of the intra-chain isomer (half-molecules) is an important step in Fab arm exchange (see below).

IgG_4 Fab Arm Exchange

In vivo, half-molecules of IgG_4 recombine randomly with half-molecules of other IgG_4, combining specificities from one IgG_4 with the specificities of another IgG_4 and effectively resulting in monovalent antibodies.[23,24] This process is controlled by redox conditions.[22] The unique S228 in the core hinge of IgG_4 allows formation of the intra-chain isomer, and R409 (rather than the equivalent lysine in IgG_1) results in weaker CH3–CH3 interactions.[25] Both determinants appear to be required to observe Fab arm exchange *in vivo*.[22]

Proteolysis

The structural differences between the IgG subclasses are also reflected in their susceptibility to proteolytic enzymes including papain,[26,27] plasmin,[28] trypsin,[29] and pepsin.[30] IgG_3 is more susceptible to cleavage by these enzymes, whereas IgG_2 is relatively resistant, and IgG_1 and IgG_4 generally exhibit an intermediary sensitivity. Because these proteolytic enzymes all cleave IgG molecules near or within the hinge region, it is likely that protease sensitivity is related to hinge accessibility and conformational flexibility.[31] Because such proteolytic enzymes are utilized by numerous bacteria, the relatively resistant IgG_2 antibodies, often elicited to bacterial polysaccharides, may represent a host response to counteract the effects of these Fc-restricting enzymes.

Allotypes

In addition to isotypic variation, allelic variation is found among the subclasses (Figure 9.3). Allotypes are defined as the polymorphic epitopes of immunoglobulins[32] that were originally discovered on the basis of serological findings.[33] Immunogenic determinants were found on IgG from some individuals but not others. Subsequently, allotypic variations were genetically analyzed and a number of structural determinants identified.[34–37] A large number of polymorphisms were found for IgG, a finding made useful in, for example, paternity testing and forensic medicine before HLA typing became available.[33] Exposure of an individual to a non-self allotype can induce an anti-allotype response and may occur in transfused individuals.[33] However, not all variations in IgG amino acid sequence lead to determinants that are immunogenic because some determinants are found in other isotypes and are therefore called *isoallotypic* variants. The allotypes that were originally typed serologically, resulting originally in the alphabetical designation system (Gm, or genetic marker, including subclass designations such as G1m for IgG[33]), do not fully cover the structural variation among different allelic forms of IgG subclasses, particularly IgG_3, which shows extensive polymorphisms, often of isoallotypic origin (Figure 9.3B).[34] An example is the non-a or nG1m(a) determinant that can also be found on IgG_2, IgG_3, and IgG_4.[32]

The main allelic forms for IgG_1 (Figure 9.3B) are $G1m^{za}$, $G1m^{f}$, and $G1m^{fa}$.[32] The $G1m^{f}$ allele is only found in Caucasians, whereas the $G1m^{fa}$ allele is common in Asian populations. Two allelic forms of IgG_2 are known, whereas many allelic forms of IgG_3 are known; the most important ones are shown in Figure 9.3B. Because some allotypes have proven to be immunogenic, they may be relevant to consider when developing therapeutic antibodies. Treatment using therapeutic monoclonal antibodies can in principle also lead to an anti-allotype response; however, to date, little evidence has been found for significant anti-allotype responses (e.g., adalimumab[38] or infliximab[39]). There are no known allotypic variations that result in a functionally different antibody, except for IgG_3, for which a few isoallotypic variants result in an extended half-life (discussed below). Interestingly, plasma IgG concentrations of an individual appear to correlate with Gm allotype.[40–42]

BINDING TO EFFECTOR MOLECULES

Antibodies link the adaptive immune system with the effector mechanisms of the innate immune system. They literally form a bridge by combining in one molecule antigen-binding sites and binding sites for a range of innate receptors and adaptor molecules. The effector mechanisms that will be triggered vary between the different immunoglobulin classes and subclasses. Broadly speaking, IgG_1 and IgG_3 are potent triggers of effector mechanisms, whereas IgG_2 and IgG_4 are not and may induce responses only in certain cases; however, these antibodies remain capable of neutralizing virus particles and toxins. Below, binding to C1q and Fc receptors is discussed, with a focus on the structural aspects that differ among the subclasses (Table 9.1).

C1q

IgG, as well as IgM, can activate complement once bound to target surfaces. This occurs through binding and subsequent activation of C1q, leading to deposition of C3b to further opsonize the target, as well as to the formation of the membrane attack complex (C5–C9), causing disruption of the targeted bilipid membranes.[43] IgG_1 and IgG_3 are efficient in triggering this classical route of complement,[44] but IgG_2 and IgG_4 are not. This is due in large part to the reduced binding of C1q to the latter subclasses,[44–46] although it has also been observed that, in addition to C1q binding, downstream events of the complement cascade (C4b deposition) are differentially affected by IgG subclass.[44] Residues in the CH2 region important for C1q binding include L235, D270, K322, P329, and P331.[46–49] In IgG_2, A235 (Leu in other subclasses) appears to account for reduced C1q binding,[48] whereas in IgG_4 P331 is (at least in part) responsible for the reduced or absent binding of C1q (Figure 9.3A).[46,49] Structural determinants in the middle, or core, hinge region (residues 226 to 230) can influence the binding of C1q;[50] rigidity in this region contributes favorably to C1q binding, whereas removal of cysteine bonds negatively affects binding. It has also been suggested that the relatively long hinge of IgG_3 makes the C1q binding site more accessible, resulting in more efficient complement activation.[51,52] However, IgG_3 engineered with a short IgG_4 hinge binds C1q efficiently, although complement activation was somewhat reduced.[53] Interestingly, engineered $IgG_{1/3}$ hybrids with an IgG_1 CH1 and hinge region were found to be more potent in complement activation compared to wild-type IgG_3, with the largest contribution arising from the CH1 domain swap.[54] The binding of C1q to IgG_4 may conversely be influenced by shielding of the potential binding site by Fab arms.[22,52,55,56] IgG_4 also results in less complement activation by forming small immune complexes and in this way can even reduce complement activation by IgG_1 antibodies.[57] Although the short hinge of IgG_2 may lead to similar shielding of the potential C1q binding site, a notion that fits with its general poor activation of the classical complement cascade, IgG_2 can activate this cascade at high densities of surface antigens, as is the case for polysaccharides, to which IgG_2 antibodies tend to form.[58–60]

Fcγ-Receptors

FcγR bind to a region partially overlapping the C1q binding site and are responsible for many of the effector functions of IgG as discussed elsewhere in this book. The binding of IgG to these receptors has been studied in detail. Each of the IgG subclasses has a unique binding profile to each FcγR (Table 9.1).[61] A major distinction can be made between IgG_1/IgG_3, which interact efficiently with most FcγR, and IgG_2/IgG_4, which show reduced affinity to a number of FcγR. Furthermore, monomeric IgG_3 binds more efficient than monomeric IgG_1 to FcγRIIa, FcγRIIIa, and FcγRIIIb; also, the binding efficiency of complexed IgG_3 to all Fc receptors exceeds that of IgG_1.[61] Structural determinants responsible for the differences between IgG_1 and IgG_3 are not well defined, although one might expect the length of the hinge to be of crucial importance. Below, structural differences that determine the subclass-specific variations are discussed. For all FcγR interactions, the stretch of amino acids comprising the N-terminus of the CH2 domains and strands adjacent in the three-dimensional immunoglobulin fold are important for binding. In general, this encompasses amino acids 234 to 239, 265 to 269, 297 to 299 and 327 to 330.[62,63] Subclass-specific variations in these regions are responsible for the weaker binding of IgG_2 in particular, but also of IgG_4 to all FcγR.

FcγRI

This receptor binds all human IgG subclasses except IgG_2 and, unlike the other FcγR, contains a unique third membrane-proximal immunoglobulin domain that probably is also responsible for its higher affinity to IgG. Mutations of IgG_1 in the lower hinge to the IgG_2 equivalents, particularly E233P, L235A, and G236Delta, will abrogate binding.[64–68] Binding to FcγRI is reduced for IgG_4,[61] and both P331S and L234F are implicated to account for the reduced binding in comparison to IgG_3,[67] but P331 may not be important for binding of IgG_1.[66,68] An IgG_3 with a partially deleted hinge was found to have reduced binding to FcγRI and FcγRIIa.[69]

FcγRIIa

FcγRIIa is the only FcγR with significant binding to IgG_2.[61,70–72] Binding is more efficient for the 131H (low-responder, LR) variant than the 131R (high-responder, HR) variant (nomenclature based on differential binding to mouse IgG_1 which binds the HR much better).[70] Binding affinity varies among subclasses as follows: $IgG_3>IgG_1>IgG_4=IgG_2$. Recently, a crystal structure of the complex of IgG_1 Fc with FcγRIIa was published,[62] and contact residues relating to differences in subclass binding include L234, L235, and G236 in the lower hinge and the structurally adjacent A327. Significantly, the 131R site in FcγRIIa is also in close proximity to the lower hinge in this co-crystal structure. Thus, the lowered binding affinity of IgG_2 to FcγRIIa and the differential binding to the HR/LR form of FcγRIIa may also be attributed to differences in the hinge of IgG_2.

FcγRIIb/IIc

The extracellular domain of the inhibiting FcγRIIb is identical to the activating FcγRIIc that is expressed in some individuals.[73] Binding to the inhibitory receptor FcγRIIb or FcγRIIc is weak for all subclasses, generally preferring $IgG_3=IgG_1=IgG_4>IgG_2$. Interestingly, dissociation constants for binding of monomeric IgG_1 and IgG_3 are similar, but immune complexes of IgG_3 seem to bind more efficiently compared to IgG_1.[61] Binding to most activating Fc receptors is lower for IgG_4 compared to IgG_1, but this is not the case for the inhibitory receptor FcγRIIb. This altered balance between binding to activatory receptors in comparison to inhibitory receptors may be an important feature of IgG_4 that contributes to its low proinflammatory capacity.

FcγRIIIa

Two allotypic variants of FcγRIIIa exist: F158 and V158. The V158 variant has greater affinity for all subclasses, and for IgG_3 binding efficiency approaches that of FcγRI,[61] with general affinities following $IgG_3>IgG_1 >> IgG_4>IgG_2$. Besides changing amino acids 233 to 236 from IgG_1 to the IgG_2 equivalents, A327G (Ala present in IgG_1 and IgG_3; Gly in IgG_2 and IgG_4) also results in decreased binding.[66] The binding affinity of FcγRIIIa seems to be particularly sensitive to core fucosylation of the N-linked glycan at N297 of the Fc tail of IgG, as its binding affinity can be enhanced up to 50 times—with corresponding increase in effector function—if the Fc tail is not fucosylated.[74,75] Recent work by Ferrara et al.[76] has pinpointed this interaction to be due to carbohydrate–carbohydrate interactions between the glycan on N297 of the heavy chain and glycosylation of FcγRIIIa at position 162, a position unique to both FcγRIIIa and FcγRIIIb.

FcγRIIIb

There are also functional allotypic variations of the neutrophil FcγRIIIb, referred to as human neutrophil antigen 1 (NA1/HNA1a) and neutrophil antigen 2 (NA2/HNA1b).[77] The FcγRIIIb-NA1 form is capable of better ingestion of IgG_1- or IgG_3-opsonized particles than FcγRIIIb-NA2.[78] FcγRIIIb generally bind IgG_1 and IgG_3 but not IgG_2 and IgG_4, with IgG_3 binding being better than IgG_1.[61] A crystal structure of the complex of IgG_1 Fc with FcγRIIIb reveals amino acids 234 to 238 to be important contact residues, and the subclass-specific variation in this area again can explain the lack of binding of IgG_2 and IgG_4 to this receptor.[63,79]

FcRn

In the 1960s, the existence of a functionally distinct FcγR was first proposed by Brambell,[80,81] who suggested that the unusually long half-life of immunoglobulin G (three weeks; see Table 9.1) and efficient transport from mother to young were mediated by a single receptor. This was later confirmed by various groups.[82–85] Structurally, the neonatal IgG receptor, or FcRn, is strikingly similar to MHC-class I molecules.[86,87] Like MHC class-I and CD1, FcRn is coexpressed with the non-glycosylated 12-kD β_2-microglobulin encoded on chromosome 15. The α-chain of human FcRn, a 45-kD polypeptide chain, is encoded on chromosome 19 in the vicinity of various other immune receptors (e.g., KIR, LAIR-1, CD89, CEACAM). Unlike FcRn from mice and rat, human FcRn has only one potential glycosylation site (N102). It is located on the face opposite the IgG-binding site and is also shared with that of all known FcRn sequences (mouse, rat, human, macaque, pig, sheep, bovine, dromedary, and possum). FcRn does not bind its ligand at physiological pH (7.4). Only in the acidic environment of endocytic vacuoles ($pH \leq 6.5$), where solvent-exposed histidine residues in IgG are protonated, does binding to FcRn take place.[85,88,89] Histidine residues within the Fc tail of IgG (CH2–CH3 interface) are critical for high-affinity binding to residues within β_2M and FcRn α-chain.[66,86,87] H435 sits at the heart of this interface, and the lowered affinity of R435-containing allotypes of IgG_3 to FcRn likely explains their shortened half-life (see Table 9.1), as H435-containing IgG_3 allotypes have a normal half-life of three weeks.[90]

On mucosal cells, FcRn has been found to transport IgG and be involved in antigen sampling,[91–93] and its expression on phagocytic cells[91,94] has recently been found to enhance the phagocytosis capacity of IgG-opsonized particles.[95,96] On antigen-presenting cells, this ingestion of IgG complexes can lead to enhanced presentation.[97–99] Similar to phagocytosis responses, the enhanced presentation likely requires external sensing and cellular activation through FcγR and pattern-recognition receptors and handing the IgG–antigen cargo over to FcRn at low pH.[96,97,100] Thus, immunoglobulin activities including extended half-life, transport to young, and antigen sampling seem to be orchestrated through a single receptor, the MHC-class I-like FcRn. In contrast, other effector functions of IgG, such as phagocytosis and antigen-presentation seem to be mediated by both FcRn and classical FcγRs.

Protein A and Protein G

Protein A and protein G are bacterial proteins that bind human IgG, but also IgG from various other species. The proteins are widely used as affinity matrices for purification of IgG. For both proteins, the major binding site in IgG is located in the Fc part of the antibody at the CH2–CH3 interface and overlaps with the FcRn binding site.[101–103] Protein G binds all human subclasses (Kd ~2×10^{-10} M),[104,105] whereas protein A generally only binds IgG_1, IgG_2, and IgG_4 (Kd ~2×10^{-9} M), but not IgG_3. Because Arg435 in IgG_3 is responsible for the lack of binding to protein A, IgG_3 allotypes with a histidine rather than arginine at position 435 do bind protein A.[106] In addition to the high-affinity Fc binding site, protein G binds to a low-affinity site in the CH1 domain of IgG[107,108] that apparently is not present in IgG_2.[109] Protein A also binds variable domains from the VH3 family.[110]

IgG ANTIBODY RESPONSES

The nature of the antigen and the route by which it enters the body govern and steer the (secondary) immune reaction into preferential patterns of class switching. In addition to direct B-cell triggering by the antigen itself, a number of secondary signals will also influence differentiation of the B cell, including ligands for

Toll-like receptors and cytokines produced by other lymphocytes and antigen-presenting cells. For example, protein antigens usually trigger B cells receiving T-cell help through MHC-class II expressed by the B cell. For those antigens, class switching tends to be IgG_1 or IgG_3, but can also be IgG_4 or IgE. On the other hand, in the absence of T-cell help, polysaccharide antigens may induce class switching to IgG_2 in particular. B cells that have undergone class switching in a primary or secondary immune reaction can also go through subsequent class switching,[111] but those events are limited by the availability of remaining heavy-chain genes. The relatively terminal position of the Cγ4 cassette may be one of the reasons why IgG_4 responses tend to occur after repeated antigen exposure (Figure 9.1C).

Selective deficiency of one or more subclasses may occur in individuals. A complete isotype or subclass deficiency caused by deletions in chromosome 14 loci is rare.[112] More often, one or more of the IgG subclass levels (predominantly IgG_2 and/or IgG_4) are below the normal range in healthy individuals,[113] which sometimes leads to an impaired response to infections with encapsulated bacteria, as will be discussed below.

IgG_1

Antibody responses to soluble protein antigens such as tetanus toxoid and membrane proteins primarily induce IgG_1 but are accompanied by lower levels of the other subclasses.[114] IgG_1 deficiencies are seen in a variety of primary and secondary antibody deficiencies and, because of its high titer, result in a decreased level of total IgG levels (hypogammaglobulinemia). IgG_1 deficiencies alone, but also in combination with deficiencies of other subclasses, are associated with recurrent infections.[115] IgG_1 responses are often, but not always, formed together with IgG_3 and sometimes IgG_4. The latter case usually results from chronic or repeated antigen stimulation (see below).

IgG_2

Antibody responses to bacterial capsular polysaccharide antigens can be almost completely restricted to IgG_2,[114,116–118] and IgG_2 deficiency may result in the virtual absence of IgG anti-carbohydrate antibodies.[119] An increased susceptibility to certain bacterial infections is associated with IgG_2 deficiency, suggesting a role of IgG_2 in the defense to these pathogens.[120] Low concentrations of IgG_2 often occur in association with a deficiency in IgG_4 and IgA_1 and IgA_2. An extensive analysis of anti-carbohydrate reactivities in intravenous immunoglobulin revealed that, although IgG_2 indeed represents the bulk of the reactivity to many glycans, this is not always the case,[121] as IgG_1 antibodies can also prevail—for instance, to *Haemophilus influenza* b polysaccharide during natural infections.[114]

IgG_3

IgG_3 antibodies are particularly effective in the induction of effector functions. Being a potent proinflammatory antibody, its shorter half-life may function to limit the potential of excessive inflammatory responses. However, the finding that some individuals bearing the sG3m allotypic marker also have IgG_3 with a prolonged half-life may challenge that assumption.[90] Curiously, IgG_3 levels in these individuals do not seem to be increased, which may be explained by γ_3-promotor polymorphisms known to affect the frequency of class switching to IgG_3 in G3m(g) allotypes, explaining the low concentration in most G3m(g) homozygous individuals.[42,122] Viral infections in general lead to IgG antibodies of the IgG_1 and IgG_3 subclasses, with IgG_3 antibodies appearing first in the course of the infection.[114] IgG_3-dominated responses appear to be rare. A curious example is so-called anti-hinge antibodies,[123] which bind to the hinge region of Fab2 fragments but not intact IgG antibodies. Also, antibodies to P and P^k blood group antigens are largely restricted to IgG_3.[124] Decreased IgG_3 levels are frequently associated with other IgG subclass deficiencies.[40]

IgG_4

Allergens are often good inducers of IgG_1 and IgG_4, in addition to IgE. IgG_4 antibodies are often formed following repeated or long-term exposure to antigen in a non-infectious setting and may become the dominant subclass. Examples are long-term beekeepers and allergic individuals who underwent immune therapy.[125–128] In immunotherapy, relief of symptoms appears to correlate with IgG_4 induction. Switching to IgG_4 may be modulated by IL-10, linking this subclass downregulation of immune responses or tolerance induction.[128,129] IgG_4 may also represent the dominant antibody subclass in immune responses to therapeutic proteins such as factor VIII and IX[130–132] and adalimumab.[133] Furthermore, helminth or filarial parasite infections may result in the formation of IgG_4 antibodies,[134,135] and high IgG_4 titers can be associated with an asymptomatic infection.[136]

Isolated IgG_4 deficiencies are rare and the consequences uncertain. On the other hand, a group of disorders today referred to as IgG_4-related diseases (IgG_4RD) is characterized by elevated serum IgG_4 concentration and tissue infiltration by IgG_4-positive plasma cells and may affect a number of organs.[137,138] The spectrum of IgG_4RD is wide and includes patients with autoimmune pancreatitis (AIP), Mikulicz's disease, hypophysitis, Riedel thyroiditis, interstitial pneumonitis, interstitial nephritis, prostatitis, lymphadenopathy, retroperitoneal fibrosis, inflammatory aortic aneurysm, and inflammatory pseudotumor. In AIP patients, serum IgG_4 elevations (>1.4 g/L) are seen in 70 to 80% of the cases and in 10% of pancreatic cancer patients. However, as 5% of the normal population also have elevated IgG_4 levels, this makes it an unsuitable single marker for diagnosis. When combined with other features of AIP, it can be of great diagnostic value, although its utility in the monitoring of therapy or as a marker or predictor of relapse is limited.

THERAPEUTIC CONSIDERATIONS

In order to develop therapeutic antibodies with improved effector function profiles, binding profiles to FcγR, FcRn, and C1q have been optimized by engineering the constant domains of the heavy chains. Antibodies with improved CDC activity[54] have been developed by combining structural elements from different subclasses to achieve enhanced effector functions (e.g., IgG_1 with elements from IgG_3). Likewise, attempts have been made to alleviate binding to the effector arm of these molecules (FcγR and C1q) by transferring amino acids found in IgG_2 and IgG_4 onto an IgG_1 backbone.[68,139–143] Similarly, antibodies engineered with increased affinity for FcRn, aimed to increase the half-life of IgG for increased bioavailability of therapeutic antibodies, may eventually lead to IgG molecules with increased half-life, but these may come at a cost because they have mutations that are not naturally occurring and may have immunogenicity issues.[144,145] Some of these modifications also increased binding at pH 7.5, actually resulting in blockade of FcRn; thus, they may have therapeutic benefits on their own by blocking recycling of endogenous autoantibodies.[146] In contrast, reduced affinity to FcRn may also be beneficial in imaging applications due to the increased rate of clearance of non-binding excess antibody and label.[147] In conclusion, tailored effector functions of IgG may be achieved while avoiding immunogenicity by making use of isotypic and isoallotypic variations existing within all individuals. This seems to have been achieved for IgG_1, with IgG_2/IgG_4 containing alterations for diminished activities,[68,143] but also for isoallotypic variants of IgG_3 with long half-lives and improved effector functions compared to IgG_1.[90] Importantly, glyco-engineering of IgG may also be used to fine-tune IgG effetor functions (discussed elsewhere in this book). Blocking antibodies based on an IgG_4 backbone may participate in Fab arm exchange *in vivo*, resulting in monovalent IgG_4. This may not be problematic and may even be beneficial, provided that the affinity is sufficient, as seems to be the case for the blocking anti-α_4-integrin IgG_4 antibody (natalizumab), which is used with success for the treatment of remitting-relapsing multiple sclerosis.[148] To avoid Fab arm exchange, an S228P mutation and/or the isoallotypic R409K can be introduced (Figure 9.3B),[149] which appears to be sufficient for abrogating Fab arm exchange *in vivo*.[22,25,150,151]

Acknowledgment

The authors would like to thank Ed Nieuwenhuys for his critical reading of the manuscript.

References

1. Schur PH. IgG subclasses. A historical perspective. *Monogr Allergy* 1988;**23**:1–11.
2. Schatz DG, Swanson PC. V(D)J recombination: mechanisms of initiation. *Annu Rev Genet* 2011;**45**:167–202.
3. Bachl J, Turck CW, Wabl M. Translatable immunoglobulin germ-line transcript. *Eur J Immunol* 1996;**26**(4):870–4.
4. Kracker S, Durandy A. Insights into the B cell specific process of immunoglobulin class switch recombination. *Immunol Lett* 2011;**138**(2):97–103.
5. Nezlin R. *The Immunoglobulins*. New York: Academic Press; 1998.
6. Schroeder Jr HW, Cavacini L. Structure and function of immunoglobulins. *J Allergy Clin Immunol* 2010;**125** (2 Suppl. 2):S41–52.
7. Hamilton RG. Human IgG subclass measurements in the clinical laboratory. *Clin Chem* 1987;**33**(10):1707–25.
8. Wuhrer M, Porcelijn L, Kapur R, Koeleman CA, Deelder A, de Haas M, et al. Regulated glycosylation patterns of IgG during alloimmune responses against human platelet antigens. *J Proteome Res* 2009;**8**(2):450–6.
9. Guhr T, Bloem J, Derksen NI, Wuhrer M, Koenderman AH, Aalberse RC, et al. Enrichment of sialylated IgG by lectin fractionation does not enhance the efficacy of immunoglobulin G in a murine model of immune thrombocytopenia. *PLoS One* 2011;**6**(6):e21246.
10. Stadlmann J, Weber A, Pabst M, Anderle H, Kunert R, Ehrlich HJ, et al. A close look at human IgG sialylation and subclass distribution after lectin fractionation. *Proteomics* 2009;**9**(17):4143–53.
11. Michaelsen TE, Naess LM, Aase A. Human IgG3 is decreased and IgG1, IgG2 and IgG4 are unchanged in molecular size by mild reduction and reoxidation without any major change in effector functions. *Mol Immunol* 1993;**30**(1):35–45.
12. Saluk PH, Clem LW. The unique molecular weight of the heavy chain from human IgG3. *J Immunol* 1971;**107**(1):298–301.
13. Roux KH, Strelets L, Michaelsen TE. Flexibility of human IgG subclasses. *J Immunol* 1997;**159**(7):3372–82.
14. Carrasco B, Garcia de la Torre J, Davis KG, Jones S, Athwal D, Walters C, et al. Crystallohydrodynamics for solving the hydration problem for multi-domain proteins: open physiological conformations for human IgG. *Biophys Chem* 2001;**93**(2–3):181–96.
15. Wypych J, Li M, Guo A, Zhang Z, Martinez T, Allen MJ, et al. Human IgG2 antibodies display disulfide-mediated structural isoforms. *J Biol Chem* 2008;**283**(23):16194–205.
16. Zhang B, Harder AG, Connelly HM, Maheu LL, Cockrill SL. Determination of Fab-hinge disulfide connectivity in structural isoforms of a recombinant human immunoglobulin G2 antibody. *Anal Chem* 2010;**82**(3):1090–9.
17. Lightle S, Aykent S, Lacher N, Mitaksov V, Wells K, Zobel J, et al. Mutations within a human IgG2 antibody form distinct and homogeneous disulfide isomers but do not affect Fc gamma receptor or C1q binding. *Protein Sci* 2010;**19**(4):753–62.
18. Yoo EM, Wims LA, Chan LA, Morrison SL. Human IgG2 can form covalent dimers. *J Immunol* 2003;**170**(6):3134–8.
19. Chivers PT, Prehoda KE, Raines RT. The CXXC motif: a rheostat in the active site 2. *Biochemistry* 1997;**36**(14):4061–6.
20. Bloom JW, Madanat MS, Marriott D, Wong T, Chan SY. Intrachain disulfide bond in the core hinge region of human IgG4. *Protein Sci* 1997;**6**(2):407–15.
21. Angal S, King DJ, Bodmer MW, Turner A, Lawson AD, Roberts G, et al. A single amino acid substitution abolishes the heterogeneity of chimeric mouse/human (IgG4) antibody. *Mol Immunol* 1993;**30**(1):105–8.
22. Rispens T, Ooijevaar-de HP, Bende O, Aalberse RC. Mechanism of immunoglobulin G4 Fab-arm exchange. *J Am Chem Soc* 2011;**133**(26):10302–11.
23. Van der Zee JS, Van Swieten P, Aalberse RC. Serologic aspects of IgG4 antibodies. II. IgG4 antibodies form small, nonprecipitating immune complexes due to functional monovalency. *J Immunol* 1986;**137**(11):3566–71.

24. van der Neut KM, Schuurman J, Losen M, Bleeker WK, Martinez-Martinez P, Vermeulen E, et al. Anti-inflammatory activity of human IgG4 antibodies by dynamic Fab arm exchange. *Science* 2007;**317**(5844):1554–7.
25. Labrijn AF, Rispens T, Meesters J, Rose RJ, den Bleker TH, Loverix S, et al. Species-specific determinants in the IgG CH3 domain enable Fab-arm exchange by affecting the noncovalent CH3–CH3 interaction strength. *J Immunol* 2011;**187**(6):3238–46.
26. Gergely J, Fudenberg HH, Van LE. The papain susceptibility of IgG myeloma proteins of different heavy chain subclasses. *Immunochemistry* 1970;**7**(1):1–6.
27. Gergely J, Stanworth DR, Jefferis R, Normansell DE, Henney CS, Pardo GI. Structural studies of immunoglobulins. I. The role of cysteine in papain hydrolysis. *Immunochemistry* 1967;**4**:101–11.
28. Skvaril F, Theilkas L, Probst M, Morell A, Barundun S. IgG subclass composition and immunochemical characteristics of plasmin-treated human gamma-globulin. *Vox Sang* 1976;**30**:334–8.
29. Gergely J, Medgyesi GA, Wang AC, Fudenberg HH. IgG myeloma subclass-typing by tryptic digestion of whole sera. *Immunochemistry* 1972;**9**(5):589–92.
30. Medgyesi GA, Gergely J. Structural studies of immunoglobulins. 3. Susceptibility of human gamma G globulins to peptic hydrolysis and papain sensitivity of F(ab′)2 fragments. *Immunochemistry* 1969;**6**(3):473–9.
31. Ryan MH, Petrone D, Nemeth JF, Barnathan E, Bjorck L, Jordan RE. Proteolysis of purified IgGs by human and bacterial enzymes *in vitro* and the detection of specific proteolytic fragments of endogenous IgG in rheumatoid synovial fluid 3. *Mol Immunol* 2008;**45**(7):1837–46.
32. de Lange GG. Polymorphisms of human immunoglobulins: Gm, Am, Em and Km allotypes. *Exp Clin Immunogenet* 1989;**6**(1):7–17.
33. Jefferis R, Lefranc MP. Human immunoglobulin allotypes: possible implications for immunogenicity. *MAbs* 2009;**1**(4):332–8.
34. Dard P, Lefranc MP, Osipova L, Sanchez-Mazas A. DNA sequence variability of IGHG3 alleles associated to the main G3m haplotypes in human populations. *Eur J Hum Genet* 2001;**9**(10):765–72.
35. Brusco A, Saviozzi S, Cinque F, DeMarchi M, Boccazzi C, De LG, et al. Molecular characterization of immunoglobulin G4 gene isoallotypes. *Eur J Immunogenet* 1998;**25**(5):349–55.
36. Brusco A, de Lange GG, Boccazzi C, Carbonara AO. Molecular characterization of Gm(n+) and G2m(n–) allotypes. *Immunogenetics* 1995;**42**(5):414–7.
37. de Lange G. *Monoclonal antibodies against human immunoglobulin allotypes*. PhD thesis, University of London, 1988.
38. Bartelds GM, de GE, Nurmohamed MT, Hart MH, van Eede PH, Wijbrandts CA, et al. Surprising negative association between IgG1 allotype disparity and anti-adalimumab formation: a cohort study 1. *Arthritis Res Ther* 2010;**12**(6):R221.
39. Magdelaine-Beuzelin C, Vermeire S, Goodall M, Baert F, Noman M, Assche GV, et al. IgG1 heavy chain-coding gene polymorphism (G1m allotypes) and development of antibodies-to-infliximab 8. *Pharmacogenet Genomics* 2009;**19**(5):383–7.
40. Meyts I, Bossuyt X, Proesmans M, Boeck KD. Isolated IgG3 deficiency in children: to treat or not to treat? Case presentation and review of the literature. *Pediatr Allergy Immunol* 2012;**2006**(17):544–50.
41. Morell A, Skvaril F, Steinberg AG, Van LE, Terry WD. Correlations between the concentrations of the four sub-classes of IgG and Gm allotypes in normal human sera. *J Immunol* 1972;**108**(1):195–206.
42. Seppala IJ, Sarvas H, Makela O. Low concentrations of Gm allotypic subsets G3 mg and G1 mf in homozygotes and heterozygotes. *J Immunol* 1993;**151**(5):2529–37.
43. Sarma JV, Ward PA. The complement system. *Cell Tissue Res* 2011;**343**(1):227–35.
44. Bindon CI, Hale G, Bruggemann M, Waldmann H. Human monoclonal IgG isotypes differ in complement activating function at the level of C4 as well as C1q. *J Exp Med* 1988;**168**(1):127–42.
45. Schumaker VN, Calcott MA, Spiegelberg HL, Muller-Eberhard HJ. Ultracentifuge studies of the binding of IgG of different subclasses to the Clq subunit of the first component of complement. *Biochemistry* 1976;**15**(23):5175–81.
46. Tao MH, Smith RI, Morrison SL. Structural features of human immunoglobulin G that determine isotype-specific differences in complement activation. *J Exp Med* 1993;**178**(2):661–7.
47. Idusogie EE, Presta LG, Gazzano-Santoro H, Totpal K, Wong PY, Ultsch M, et al. Mapping of the C1q binding site on rituxan, a chimeric antibody with a human IgG1 Fc. *J Immunol* 2000;**164**(8):4178–84.
48. Morgan A, Jones ND, Nesbitt AM, Chaplin L, Bodmer MW, Emtage JS. The N-terminal end of the CH2 domain of chimeric human IgG1 anti-HLA-DR is necessary for C1q, Fc gamma RI and Fc gamma RIII binding. *Immunology* 1995;**86**(2):319–24.
49. Brekke OH, Michaelsen TE, Aase A, Sandin RH, Sandlie I. Human IgG isotype-specific amino acid residues affecting complement-mediated cell lysis and phagocytosis. *Eur J Immunol* 1994;**24**(10):2542–7.
50. Dall'Acqua WF, Cook KE, Damschroder MM, Woods RM, Wu H. Modulation of the effector functions of a human IgG1 through engineering of its hinge region. *J Immunol* 2006;**177**(2):1129–38.
51. Dangl JL, Wensel TG, Morrison SL, Stryer L, Herzenberg LA, Oi VT. Segmental flexibility and

complement fixation of genetically engineered chimeric human, rabbit and mouse antibodies. *EMBO J* 1988;**7**(7):1989–94.
52. Lu Y, Harding SE, Michaelsen TE, Longman E, Davis KG, Ortega A, et al. Solution conformation of wild-type and mutant IgG3 and IgG4 immunoglobulins using crystallohydrodynamics: possible implications for complement activation. *Biophys J* 2007;**93**(11):3733–44.
53. Tan LK, Shopes RJ, Oi VT, Morrison SL. Influence of the hinge region on complement activation, C1q binding, and segmental flexibility in chimeric human immunoglobulins. *Proc Natl Acad Sci USA* 1990;**87**(1):162–6.
54. Natsume A, In M, Takamura H, Nakagawa T, Shimizu Y, Kitajima Engineered antibodies of IgG1/IgG3 mixed isotype with enhanced cytotoxic activities. *Cancer Res* 2008;**68**(10):3863–72.
55. Aalberse RC, Schuurman J. IgG4 breaking the rules. *Immunology* 2002;**105**(1):9–19.
56. Abe Y, Gor J, Bracewell DG, Perkins SJ, Dalby PA. Masking of the Fc region in human IgG4 by constrained x-ray scattering modelling: implications for antibody function and therapy 1. *Biochem J* 2010;**432**(1):101–11.
57. Van der Zee JS, Van Swieten P, Aalberse RC. Inhibition of complement activation by IgG4 antibodies. *Clin Exp Immunol* 1986;**64**(2):415–22.
58. Saeland E, Vidarsson G, Leusen JH, Van Garderen E, Nahm MH, Vile-Weekhout H, et al. Central role of complement in passive protection by human IgG1 and IgG2 anti-pneumococcal antibodies in mice. *J Immunol* 2003;**170**(12):6158–64.
59. Vidarsson G, Sigurdardottir ST, Gudnason T, Kjartansson S, Kristinsson KG, Ingolfsdottir G, et al. Isotypes and opsonophagocytosis of pneumococcus type 6B antibodies elicited in infants and adults by an experimental pneumococcus type 6B-tetanus toxoid vaccine. *Infect Immun* 1998;**66**(6):2866–70.
60. Vidarsson G, Jonsdottir I, Jonsson S, Valdimarsson H. Opsonization and antibodies to capsular and cell wall polysaccharides of *Streptococcus pneumoniae*. *J Infect Dis* 1994;**170**:592–9.
61. Bruhns P, Iannascoli B, England P, Mancardi DA, Fernandez N, Jorieux S, et al. Specificity and affinity of human Fcgamma receptors and their polymorphic variants for human IgG subclasses. *Blood* 2009;**113**(16):3716–25.
62. Ramsland PA, Farrugia W, Bradford TM, Sardjono CT, Esparon S, Trist HM, et al. Structural basis for Fc gammaRIIa recognition of human IgG and formation of inflammatory signaling complexes. *J Immunol* 2011;**187**(6):3208–17.
63. Sondermann P, Huber R, Oosthuizen V, Jacob U. The 3.2-A crystal structure of the human IgG1 Fc fragment–Fc gammaRIII complex. *Nature* 2000;**406**(6793):267–73.
64. Canfield SM, Morrison SL. The binding affinity of human IgG for its high affinity Fc receptor is determined by multiple amino acids in the CH2 domain and is modulated by the hinge region. *J Exp Med* 1991;**173**(6):1483–91.
65. Chappel MS, Isenman DE, Everett M, Xu YY, Dorrington KJ, Klein MH. Identification of the Fc gamma receptor class I binding site in human IgG through the use of recombinant IgG1/IgG2 hybrid and point-mutated antibodies. *Proc Natl Acad Sci USA* 1991;**88**(20):9036–40.
66. Shields RL, Namenuk AK, Hong K, Meng YG, Rae J, Briggs J, et al. High resolution mapping of the binding site on human IgG1 for Fc gamma RI, Fc gamma RII, Fc gamma RIII, and FcRn and design of IgG1 variants with improved binding to the Fc gamma R. *J Biol Chem* 2001;**276**(9):6591–604.
67. Lund J, Winter G, Jones PT, Pound JD, Tanaka T, Walker MR, et al. Human Fc gamma RI and Fc gamma RII interact with distinct but overlapping sites on human IgG. *J Immunol* 1991;**147**(8):2657–62.
68. Armour KL, Clark MR, Hadley AG, Williamson LM. Recombinant human IgG molecules lacking Fcgamma receptor I binding and monocyte triggering activities. *Eur J Immunol* 1999;**29**(8):2613–24.
69. Redpath S, Michaelsen TE, Sandlie I, Clark MR. The influence of the hinge region length in binding of human IgG to human Fcgamma receptors. *Hum Immunol* 1998;**59**(11):720–7.
70. Parren PW, Warmerdam PA, Boeije LC, Arts J, Westerdaal NA, Vlug A, et al. On the interaction of IgG subclasses with the low affinity Fc gamma RIIa (CD32) on human monocytes, neutrophils, and platelets. Analysis of a functional polymorphism to human IgG2. *J Clin Invest* 1992;**90**(4):1537–46.
71. Armour KL, van de Winkel JG, Williamson LM, Clark MR. Differential binding to human FcgammaRIIa and FcgammaRIIb receptors by human IgG wildtype and mutant antibodies. *Mol Immunol* 2003;**40**(9):585–93.
72. Wines BD, Powell MS, Parren PW, Barnes N, Hogarth PM. The IgG Fc contains distinct Fc receptor (FcR) binding sites: the leukocyte receptors Fc gamma RI and Fc gamma RIIa bind to a region in the Fc distinct from that recognized by neonatal FcR and protein A. *J Immunol* 2000;**164**(10):5313–8.
73. Breunis WB, van ME, Bruin M, Geissler J, de BM, Peters M, et al. Copy number variation of the activating FCGR2C gene predisposes to idiopathic thrombocytopenic purpura. *Blood* 2008;**111**(3):1029–38.
74. Li H, Sethuraman N, Stadheim TA, Zha D, Prinz B, Ballew N, et al. Optimization of humanized IgGs in glycoengineered *Pichia pastoris*. *Nat Biotechnol* 2006;**24**(2):210–5.
75. Siberil S, de Romeuf C, Bihoreau N, Fernandez N, Meterreau JL, Regenman A, et al. Selection of a

human anti-RhD monoclonal antibody for therapeutic use: impact of IgG glycosylation on activating and inhibitory Fc gamma R functions. *Clin Immunol* 2006;**118**(2–3):170–9.

76. Ferrara C, Grau S, Jager C, Sondermann P, Brunker P, Waldhauer I, et al. Unique carbohydrate-carbohydrate interactions are required for high affinity binding between FcgammaRIII and antibodies lacking core fucose. *Proc Natl Acad Sci USA* 2011;**108**(31):12669–74.
77. Huizinga TW, Kleijer M, Tetteroo PA, Roos D, von dem Borne AE. Biallelic neutrophil Na-antigen system is associated with a polymorphism on the phospho-inositol-linked Fc gamma receptor III (CD16). *Blood* 1990;**75**(1):213–7.
78. Huizinga TW, Kerst M, Nuyens JH, Vlug A, von dem Borne AE, Roos D, et al. Binding characteristics of dimeric IgG subclass complexes to human neutrophils. *J Immunol* 1989;**142**(7):2359–64.
79. Radaev S, Motyka S, Fridman WH, Sautes-Fridman C, Sun PD. The structure of a human type III Fcgamma receptor in complex with Fc. *J Biol Chem* 2001;**276**(19):16469–77.
80. Brambell FW, Hemmings WA, Morris IG. A theoretical model of gamma-globulin catabolism. *Nature* 1964;**203**:1352–4.
81. Brambell FW. The transmission of immunity from mother to young and the catabolism of immunoglobulins. *Lancet* 1966;**2**(7473):1087–93.
82. Ghetie V, Hubbard JG, Kim JK, Tsen MF, Lee Y, Ward ES. Abnormally short serum half-lives of IgG in beta 2-microglobulin-deficient mice. *Eur J Immunol* 1996;**26**(3):690–6.
83. Israel EJ, Wilsker DF, Hayes KC, Schoenfeld D, Simister NE. Increased clearance of IgG in mice that lack beta 2-microglobulin: possible protective role of FcRn. *Immunology* 1996;**89**(4):573–8.
84. Junghans RP, Anderson CL. The protection receptor for IgG catabolism is the beta2-microglobulin-containing neonatal intestinal transport receptor. *Proc Natl Acad Sci USA* 1996;**93**(11):5512–6.
85. Roopenian DC, Christianson GJ, Sproule TJ, Brown AC, Akilesh S, Jung N, et al. The MHC class i-like IgG receptor controls perinatal IgG transport, IgG homeostasis, and fate of IgG-Fc-coupled drugs. *J Immunol* 2003;**170**(7):3528–33.
86. Burmeister WP, Gastinel LN, Simister NE, Blum ML, Bjorkman PJ. Crystal structure at 2.2 A resolution of the MHC-related neonatal Fc receptor. *Nature* 1994;**372**(6504):336–43.
87. West Jr AP, Bjorkman PJ. Crystal structure and immunoglobulin G binding properties of the human major histocompatibility complex-related Fc receptor. *Biochemistry* 2000;**39**(32):9698–708.
88. Chaudhury C, Mehnaz S, Robinson JM, Hayton WL, Pearl DK, Roopenian DC, et al. The major histocompatibility complex-related Fc receptor for IgG (FcRn) binds albumin and prolongs its lifespan. *J Exp Med* 2003;**197**(3):315–22.
89. Gastinel LN, Simister NE, Bjorkman PJ. Expression and crystallization of a soluble and functional form of an Fc receptor related to class I histocompatibility molecules. *Proc Natl Acad Sci USA* 1992;**89**(2):638–42.
90. Stapleton NM, Andersen JT, Stemerding AM, Bjarnarson SP, Verheul RC, Gerritsen J, et al. Competition for FcRn-mediated transport gives rise to short half-life of human IgG3 and offers therapeutic potential. *Nat Commun* 2011;**5**:599.
91. Spiekermann GM, Finn PW, Ward ES, Dumont J, Dickinson BL, Blumberg RS, et al. Receptor-mediated immunoglobulin G transport across mucosal barriers in adult life: functional expression of FcRn in the mammalian lung. *J Exp Med* 2002;**196**(3):303–10.
92. Yoshida M, Claypool SM, Wagner JS, Mizoguchi E, Mizoguchi A, Roopenian DC, et al. Human neonatal Fc receptor mediates transport of IgG into luminal secretions for delivery of antigens to mucosal dendritic cells. *Immunity* 2004;**20**(6):769–83.
93. Yoshida M, Kobayashi K, Kuo TT, Bry L, Glickman JN, Claypool SM, et al. Neonatal Fc receptor for IgG regulates mucosal immune responses to luminal bacteria. *J Clin Invest* 2006;**116**(8):2142–51.
94. Zhu X, Meng G, Dickinson BL, Li X, Mizoguchi E, Miao L, et al. MHC class I-related neonatal Fc receptor for IgG is functionally expressed in monocytes, intestinal macrophages, and dendritic cells. *J Immunol* 2001;**166**(5):3266–76.
95. Cervenak J, Bender B, Schneider Z, Magna M, Carstea BV, Liliom K, et al. Neonatal FcR overexpression boosts humoral immune response in transgenic mice. *J Immunol* 2011;**186**(2):959–68.
96. Vidarsson G, Stemerding AM, Stapleton NM, Spliethoff SE, Janssen H, Rebers FE, et al. FcRn: an IgG receptor on phagocytes with a novel role in phagocytosis. *Blood* 2006;**108**(10):3573–9.
97. Baker K, Qiao SW, Kuo TT, Aveson VG, Platzer B, Andersen JT, et al. Neonatal Fc receptor for IgG (FcRn) regulates cross-presentation of IgG immune complexes by CD8–CD11b+ dendritic cells. *Proc Natl Acad Sci USA* 2011;**108**(24):9927–32.
98. Mi W, Wanjie S, Lo ST, Gan Z, Pickl-Herk B, Ober RJ, et al. Targeting the neonatal fc receptor for antigen delivery using engineered Fc fragments. *J Immunol* 2008;**181**(11):7550–61.
99. Qiao SW, Kobayashi K, Johansen FE, Sollid LM, Andersen JT, Milford E, et al. Dependence of antibody-mediated presentation of antigen on FcRn. *Proc Natl Acad Sci USA* 2008;**105**(27):9337–42.

100. Heijnen IA, Van Vugt MJ, Fanger NA, Graziano RF, de Wit TP, Hofhuis FM, et al. Antigen targeting to myeloid-specific human Fc gamma RI/CD64 triggers enhanced antibody responses in transgenic mice. *J Clin Invest* 1996;**97**(2):331–8.
101. Sauer-Eriksson AE, Kleywegt GJ, Uhlen M, Jones TA. Crystal structure of the C2 fragment of streptococcal protein G in complex with the Fc domain of human IgG. *Structure* 1995;**3**(3):265–78.
102. Deisenhofer J. Crystallographic refinement and atomic models of a human Fc fragment and its complex with fragment B of protein A from *Staphylococcus aureus* at 2.9- and 2.8-A resolution. *Biochemistry* 1981;**20**(9):2361–70.
103. Jefferis R, Lund J, Pound JD. IgG-Fc-mediated effector functions: molecular definition of interaction sites for effector ligands and the role of glycosylation. *Immunol Rev* 1998;**163**:59–76.
104. Bjorck L, Kronvall G. Purification and some properties of streptococcal protein G, a novel IgG-binding reagent. *J Immunol* 1984;**133**(2):969–74.
105. Stone GC, Sjobring U, Bjorck L, Sjoquist J, Barber CV, Nardella FA. The Fc binding site for streptococcal protein G is in the C gamma 2–C gamma 3 interface region of IgG and is related to the sites that bind staphylococcal protein A and human rheumatoid factors. *J Immunol* 1989;**143**(2):565–70.
106. Van LE, Frangione B, Recht B, Franklin EC. Staphylococcal protein A and human IgG subclasses and allotypes. *Scand J Immunol* 1982;**15**(3):275–8.
107. Lian LY, Barsukov IL, Derrick JP, Roberts GC. Mapping the interactions between streptococcal protein G and the Fab fragment of IgG in solution. *Nat Struct Biol* 1994;**1**(6):355–7.
108. Derrick JP, Wigley DB. The third IgG-binding domain from streptococcal protein G. An analysis by x-ray crystallography of the structure alone and in a complex with Fab. *J Mol Biol* 1994;**243**(5):906–18.
109. Perosa F, Luccarelli G, Dammacco F. Absence of streptococcal protein G (PG)-specific determinant in the Fab region of human IgG2. *Clin Exp Immunol* 1997;**109**(2):272–8.
110. Silverman GJ. B-cell superantigens. *Immunol Today* 1997;**18**(8):379–86.
111. Berkowska MA, Driessen GJ, Bikos V, Grosserichter-Wagener C, Stamatopoulos K, Cerutti A, et al. Human memory B cells originate from three distinct germinal center-dependent and -independent maturation pathways. *Blood* 2011;**118**(8):2150–8.
112. Pan Q, Hammarstrom L. Molecular basis of IgG subclass deficiency. *Immunol Rev* 2000;**178**:99–110.
113. Vlug A, Nieuwenhuys EJ, van Eijk RV, Geertzen HG, van Houte AJ. Nephelometric measurements of human IgG subclasses and their reference ranges. *Ann Biol Clin (Paris)* 1994;**52**(7–8):561–7.
114. Ferrante A, Beard LJ, Feldman RG. IgG subclass distribution of antibodies to bacterial and viral antigens. *Pediatr Infect Dis J* 1990;**9**(8 Suppl.):S16–24.
115. Jefferis R, Kumararatne DS. Selective IgG subclass deficiency: quantification and clinical relevance. *Clin Exp Immunol* 1990;**81**(3):357–67.
116. Siber GR, Schur PH, Aisenberg AC, Weitzman SA, Schiffman G. Correlation between serum IgG-2 concentrations and the antibody response to bacterial polysaccharide antigens. *N Engl J Med* 1980;**303**(4):178–82.
117. Barrett DJ, Ayoub EM. IgG2 subclass restriction of antibody to pneumococcal polysaccharides. *Clin Exp Immunol* 1986;**63**(1):127–34.
118. Schauer U, Stemberg F, Rieger CH, Buttner W, Borte M, Schubert S, et al. Levels of antibodies specific to tetanus toxoid, *Haemophilus influenzae* type b, and pneumococcal capsular polysaccharide in healthy children and adults. *Clin Diagn Lab Immunol* 2003;**10**(2):202–7.
119. Hammarstrom L, Smith CI. IgG2 deficiency in a healthy blood donor. Concomitant lack of IgG2, IgA and IgE immunoglobulins and specific anti-carbohydrate antibodies. *Clin Exp Immunol* 1983;**51**(3):600–4.
120. Kuijpers TW, Weening RS, Out TA. IgG subclass deficiencies and recurrent pyogenic infections, unresponsiveness against bacterial polysaccharide antigens. *Allergol Immunopathol (Madr)* 1992;**20**(1):28–34.
121. von GS, Smith DF, Cummings RD, Riedel S, Miescher S, Schaub A, et al. Intravenous immunoglobulin contains a broad repertoire of anticarbohydrate antibodies that is not restricted to the IgG2 subclass. *J Allergy Clin Immunol* 2009;**123**(6):1268–76.
122. Hassan MS, Islam KB, Hammarstrom L, Smith CI. Regulation of C gamma 3 expression. Role of switch in the allotype-associated variation of human serum IgG3 levels. *J Immunol* 1992;**148**(8):2555–62.
123. Brezski RJ, Jordan RE. Cleavage of IgGs by proteases associated with invasive diseases: an evasion tactic against host immunity? *MAbs* 2010;**2**(3):212–20.
124. Soderstrom T, Enskog A, Samuelsson BE, Cedergren B. Immunoglobulin subclass (IgG3) restriction of anti-P and anti-Pk antibodies in patients of the rare p blood group. *J Immunol* 1985;**134**(1):1–3.
125. Aalberse RC, van der Gaag R, van Leeuwen J. Serologic aspects of IgG4 antibodies. I. Prolonged immunization results in an IgG4-restricted response. *J Immunol* 1983;**130**:722–6.
126. Aalberse RC, Dieges PH, Knul-Bretlova V, Vooren P, Aalbers M, van LJ. IgG4 as a blocking antibody. *Clin Rev Allergy* 1983;**1**(2):289–302.

127. Nouri-Aria KT, Wachholz PA, Francis JN, Jacobson MR, Walker SM, Wilcock LK, et al. Grass pollen immunotherapy induces mucosal and peripheral IL-10 responses and blocking IgG activity. *J Immunol* 2004;**172**(5):3252–9.
128. Aalberse RC, Stapel SO, Schuurman J, Rispens T. Immunoglobulin G4: an odd antibody. *Clin Exp Allergy* 2009;**39**(4):469–77.
129. Jutel M, Akdis CA. Immunological mechanisms of allergen-specific immunotherapy. *Allergy* 2011;**66**(6):725–32.
130. van Helden PM, van den Berg HM, Gouw SC, Kaijen PH, Zuurveld MG, Mauser-Bunschoten EP, et al. IgG subclasses of anti-FVIII antibodies during immune tolerance induction in patients with hemophilia A. *Br J Haematol* 2008;**142**(4):644–52.
131. Andersen BR, Terry WD. Gamma G4 globulin Ab causing inhibition of clotting factor VIII. *Nature* 1968;**217**:174.
132. Iizuka A, Nagao T. Analysis of IgG heavy chain subclasses of alloantibodies to factor IX by crossed immunoelectrophoresis of factor IX using the intermediate gel technique. *Br J Haematol* 1983;**53**(4):687–8.
133. Hart MH, de VH, Wouters D, Wolbink GJ, Killestein J, de Groot ER, et al. Differential effect of drug interference in immunogenicity assays. *J Immunol Methods* 2011;**372**(1–2):196–203.
134. Ottesen EA, Skvaril F, Tripathy SP, Poindexter RW, Hussain R. Prominence of IgG4 in the IgG antibody response to human filariasis. *J Immunol* 1985; **134**(4):2707–12.
135. Adjobimey T, Hoerauf A. Induction of immunoglobulin G4 in human filariasis: an indicator of immunoregulation. *Ann Trop Med Parasitol* 2010;**104**(6):455–64.
136. Kurniawan A, Yazdanbakhsh M, van RR, Aalberse R, Selkirk ME, Partono F, et al. Differential expression of IgE and IgG4 specific antibody responses in asymptomatic and chronic human filariasis. *J Immunol* 1993;**150**(9):3941–50.
137. Sah RP, Chari ST. Serologic issues in IgG4-related systemic disease and autoimmune pancreatitis. *Curr Opin Rheumatol* 2011;**23**(1):108–13.
138. Yamamoto M, Tabeya T, Naishiro Y, Yajima H, Ishigami K, Shimizu Y, et al. Value of serum IgG4 in the diagnosis of IgG4-related disease and in differentiation from rheumatic diseases and other diseases. *Mod Rheumatol* 2012;**22**(3):419–25.
139. Oganesyan V, Gao C, Shirinian L, Wu H, Dall'Acqua WF. Structural characterization of a human Fc fragment engineered for lack of effector functions. *Acta Crystallogr D Biol Crystallogr* 2008;**64**(Pt. 6):700–4.
140. An Z, Forrest G, Moore R, Cukan M, Haytko P, Huang L, et al. IgG2m4, an engineered antibody isotype with reduced Fc function. *MAbs* 2009;**1**(6):572–9.
141. Salfeld JG. Isotype selection in antibody engineering. *Nat Biotechnol* 2007;**25**(12):1369–72.
142. Mueller JP, Giannoni MA, Hartman SL, Elliott EA, Squinto SP, Matis LA, et al. Humanized porcine VCAM-specific monoclonal antibodies with chimeric IgG2/G4 constant regions block human leukocyte binding to porcine endothelial cells. *Mol Immunol* 1997;**34**(6):441–52.
143. Ghevaert C, Wilcox DA, Fang J, Armour KL, Clark MR, Ouwehand WH, et al. Developing recombinant HPA-1a-specific antibodies with abrogated Fcgamma receptor binding for the treatment of fetomaternal alloimmune thrombocytopenia. *J Clin Invest* 2008;**118**(8):2929–38.
144. Dall'Acqua WF, Woods RM, Ward ES, Palaszynski SR, Patel NK, Brewah YA, et al. Increasing the affinity of a human IgG1 for the neonatal Fc receptor: biological consequences. *J Immunol* 2002;**169**(9):5171–80.
145. Ward ES, Zhou J, Ghetie V, Ober RJ. Evidence to support the cellular mechanism involved in serum IgG homeostasis in humans. *Int Immunol* 2003;**15**(2):187–95.
146. Patel DA, Puig-Canto A, Challa DK, Montoyo HP, Ober RJ, Ward ES. Neonatal Fc receptor blockade by Fc engineering ameliorates arthritis in a murine model. *J Immunol* 2011;**187**(2):1015–22.
147. Jaggi JS, Carrasquillo JA, Seshan SV, Zanzonico P, Henke E, Nagel A, et al. Improved tumor imaging and therapy via i.v. IgG-mediated time-sequential modulation of neonatal Fc receptor. *J Clin Invest* 2007;**117**(9):2422–30.
148. Materials and methods are available as supporting material on ScienceOnline.com.
149. Broug E, Bland-Ward PA, Powell J, Johnson KS. Fab–arm exchange. *Nat Biotechnol* 2010;**28**(2):123–5.
150. Labrijn AF, Buijsse AO, van den Bremer ET, Verwilligen AY, Bleeker WK, Thorpe SJ, et al. Therapeutic IgG4 antibodies engage in Fab–arm exchange with endogenous human IgG4 *in vivo*. *Nat Biotechnol* 2009;**27**(8):767–71.
151. Stubenrauch K, Wessels U, Regula JT, Kettenberger H, Schleypen J, Kohnert U. Impact of molecular processing in the hinge region of therapeutic IgG4 antibodies on disposition profiles in cynomolgus monkeys. *Drug Metab Dispos* 2010;**38**(1):84–91.

CHAPTER

10

Antibody Glycosylation

*Xiaojie Yu, Kavitha Baruah, Christopher N. Scanlan and Max Crispin**

Oxford Glycobiology Institute, Department of Biochemistry, University of Oxford, Oxford, United Kingdom

The antibody Fc region is posttranslationally modified by *N*-linked glycosylation. In immunoglobulin G (IgG), the processing of the glycans is restricted by the presence of extensive interaction with the protein surface. The resulting set of antibody glycoforms exhibit a range of effector functions. In this chapter, we outline the impact of glycosylation on the immune function of antibodies and discuss the implications for monoclonal antibody and intravenous immunoglobulin therapies.

HUMAN ANTIBODY: AN OVERVIEW OF STRUCTURE AND FUNCTION

Immunoglobulins (Igs), also called antibodies, are an important component of the human immune system. The multiple isotypes of antibodies differ between different animal species, varying from seven in horses to only one in rabbits. Human antibodies are classified into five categories based on their distinct structure, function, and location: IgA, IgD, IgE, IgG, and IgM, of which IgG is the most investigated and thus most well characterized to date.[1,2] IgG is a relatively large glycoprotein with an overall Y-shaped structure comprised of two heavy chains, each approximately 50 kDa, and two light chains, each approximately 25 kDa. Together, the heavy and light chains form three distinctive regions: the antigen binding region (Fab), the crystallizable region (Fc), and the hinge region. Fab binds a specific antigen, and Fc bridges the innate and adaptive immunity by binding to Fc receptors (FcRs) as well as components of the complement system. The hinge region serves to link the Fab and Fc regions. There are two well-established functions for antibodies in the immune system. First, they bind to antigens, such as foreign pathogens, to form an immune complex to neutralize their pathogenicity. Second, the Fc region of the immune complex can bind to FcRs or complement components to clear pathogens and trigger both innate and adaptive immune responses.

Different antibody isotypes, which mediate distinct functions, are produced at different stages of an immune response under different stimulatory milieus, via a regulated isotype

* Corresponding Author

switching mechanism in B cells.[3] By default, B cells produce IgM without previous exposure to an antigen. IgM circulates in the human serum at about 1 to 2.5 mg/mL, and its typical pentameric form is a potent activator of the complement pathway.[4] IgG represents the most abundant isotype in human serum, circulating at around 12 mg/mL, and is the main isotype produced in response to active vaccination.[4] IgE is known to bind large pathogens such as parasites and is responsible for causing hypersensitivity, including the commonly known allergic reactions.[4,5] IgA is present in human serum at about 2.5 mg/mL in its monomeric form and is predominately dimeric on the mucosal surfaces, which prevents antigens such as bacteria from breaching the mucosal system.[6,7] IgD is an ancient antibody preserved in most jawed vertebrates; however, its precise function remains unclear due to a lack of investigation.[8]

HUMAN IgG Fc STRUCTURE AND FUNCTION

Human IgG Fc has a well-defined horseshoe structure and mediates a range of effector functions, including antibody-dependent cellular cytotoxicity (ADCC), phagocytosis, complement-dependent cytotoxicity (CDC), and IgG recycling, as well as recently described antiinflammatory activity.[4,9,10,108] The Cγ2 and Cγ3 domains from each heavy chain form two interchain disulfide bonds between the two Cγ2 domains. An *N*-linked glycan is attached to the Asn297 at the Cγ2 domain, which has been shown to influence the openness of the horseshoe structure (Figure 10.1) and Fc affinity for the FcγRs and C1q.

Human IgGs are further divided into four subclasses called IgG_1, IgG_2, IgG_3, and IgG_4, according to their relative abundance in serum. Each IgG subclass is elicited by different antigens. For example, IgG_2 is mainly induced by carbohydrate antigens. Moreover, IgG_4 is typically induced by prolonged immunization with protein antigens. The hinge region of each subclass has notable differences in flexibility due to length and amino acid composition. IgG_1 and IgG_3 have approximately the same level of flexibility despite the fact that IgG_3 has many more residues at the hinge, include 21 prolines, restricting its flexibility. The IgG_2 hinge lacks a glycine residue, which reduces its relative

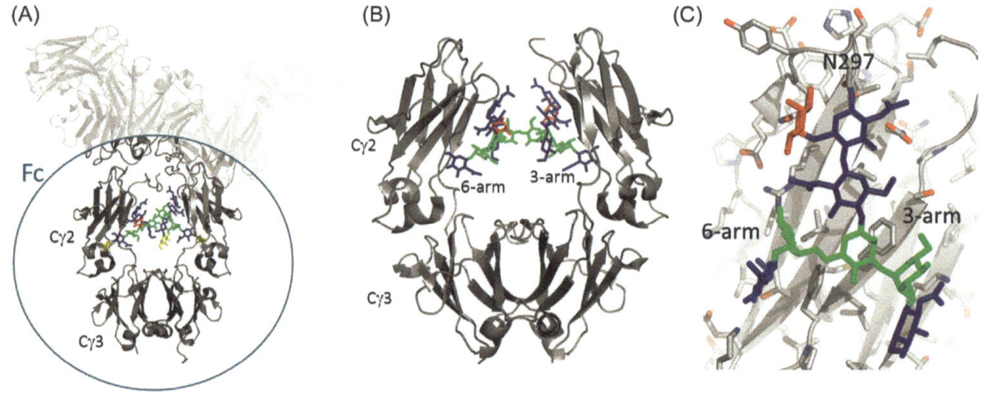

FIGURE 10.1 **Crystal structure of IgG.** (A) Crystal structure of an intact IgG_1 monoclonal antibody, b12 (PDB 1HZH).[85] The highlighted region corresponds to the Fc domain. (B) Crystal structure of IgG_1 Fc (PDB 3AVE).[63] (C) Structure of an *N*-linked glycan at Asn297 packing against the protein moiety of the Cγ2 domain (PDB 3AVE; chain A). Protein is displayed in gray, and glycans are displayed as colored sticks (red, fucose; blue, *N*-acetylglucosamine; green, mannose).

flexibility. IgG_4 has a key residue difference upstream of the second cysteine that normally forms the interchain disulfide bond, which is thought to account for the lack of interchain disulfide bonds for IgG_4 and provides a basis for bispecific IgG_4 generation.[11] In summary, the degree of flexibility of each subclass conferred by the hinge region is as follows: $IgG_1 = IgG_3 > IgG_2 > IgG_4$.

IgG Fc mediates antibody effector functions by binding to diverse Fc receptors on cell surfaces. These well-established receptors include FcγRs, the complement molecule C1q, and FcRn. Recently, a specific C-type lectin, DC-SIGN, has been proposed to bind to a natural population of IgG Fc capable of mediating antiinflammatory signaling,[12,13] although a direct interaction has not been supported in a biophysical study using recombinant tertrameric DC-SIGN and glycan-engineered antibodies.[14] FcγRs are type 1 single-pass transmembrane proteins; so far six human FcγRs have been cloned: FcγRIa, FcγRIIa, FcγRIIb, FcγRIIc, FcγRIIIa, and FcγRIIIb.[15] Moreover, they are classified as either activatory or inhibitory, depending on whether their intracellular signaling components contain the immunoreceptor tyrosine-based activation motif (ITAM) (FcγRIa, FcγRIIa, FcγRIIc, and FcγRIIIa) or the immunoreceptor tyrosine-based inhibition motif (ITIM) (FcγRIIb). FcγRIIIb is a glycosylphosphatidylinositol (GPI)-anchored receptor expressed on neutrophils. Various immune cells express multiple classes of FcγRs; for example, myeloid-derived dendritic cells and macrophages are found to express all classes of FcγRs except FcγRIIIb, in contrast to B cells and natural killer (NK) cells, which express only FcγRIIb or FcγRIIIa, respectively. The extracellular regions of FcγRs have conserved structures. Available crystal structures of FcγRs demonstrate that they have two Ig-like extracellular domains named the D1 and D2 regions.[16] Each domain is comprised of five-stranded and three-stranded β-sheets. The crystal structure of the Fc–FcγRIIIa complex shows that the interdomain angle of FcγRIIIa opens by about 10 degrees upon Fc binding. Concomitantly, Fc adopts an asymmetric opening of the horseshoe structure between the Cγ2 domains at the N-terminal tip. The Cγ2 domains and the lower hinge region of Fc form the binding site for FcγRs. Based on the structure, a high-resolution scanning of the IgG_1 Fc region has been carried out to determine the residues essential for Fc–FcγR interaction.[17] As expected due to their homologous extracellular regions, a conserved set of Fc amino acids affected binding to all FcγRs. In addition, some Fc residues were found to modulate Fc binding to only selective FcγRs, establishing a basis for selective FcγR targeting by protein engineering.

HUMAN IgG Fc GLYCOSYLATION

All human immunoglobulins are glycosylated, albeit to varying extents. IgG glycosylation accounts for 2 to 3% of total IgG molecular weight, which is relatively low compared with the 12 to 14% for IgM, IgD, and IgE. IgG Fc has a conserved *N*-linked glycosylation site at Asn297 across all subclasses. On the other hand, sequence analysis shows that only about 20% of human IgG Fab regions are glycosylated. Moreover, these *N*-linked glycosylation consensus sequences on Fab result from somatic mutations, indicating that Fab *N*-linked glycosylation is positively selected.[18,19] Indeed, most Fab *N*-linked glycosylation is shown to occur on exposed loop regions and has been reported to significantly influence antigen binding.[4] Total human serum IgG exhibits mainly biantennary, complex-type glycans, of which the neutral glycoforms represent about 86%, with agalactosylated, monogalactosylated, and digalactosylated glycoforms accounting for 25%, 35%, and 20%, respectively. Sialylated structures account for the remaining 20% (Figure 10.2). Moreover, about 30% of

IgG glycan have bisecting GlcNAc attached to the β-mannose, and between 80 and 92% of IgG glycan are core-fucosylated.[4,18,22,23] The Fc and Fab glycans differ significantly in their levels of terminal sialylation at their reducing end. As much as 80% of Fab glycan can be sialylated in contrast to about 10% of Fc glycan. A summary of human serum IgG glycosylation is presented in Figure 10.2. Interestingly, the presence of large multi-antennary IgG glycans such as triantennary glycans have not been reported in healthy people, even on the exposed Fab glycosylation sites. In contrast, other glycoproteins such as fetuin and FcγRs have been shown to contain a fair amount of triantennary and tetraantennary oligosaccharides on their solvent-exposed glycosylation sites.[24,25] This indicates that the glycosylation sites on the Fab region are not sufficiently exposed, B cells lack the enzymes required for generating multi-antennary oligosaccharide, or mechanisms may exist for specifically tuning IgG glycosylation.

The lack of terminal processing of the Fc glycan may be due to limited access of Golgi-resident glycosyltransferases as a result of limited glycan flexibility imposed by the unusually prolific glycan–protein interactions in the Fc region (Figure 10.1). The crystal structures of Fc show that the two opposing Fc glycans are positioned in the Fc horseshoe structure in

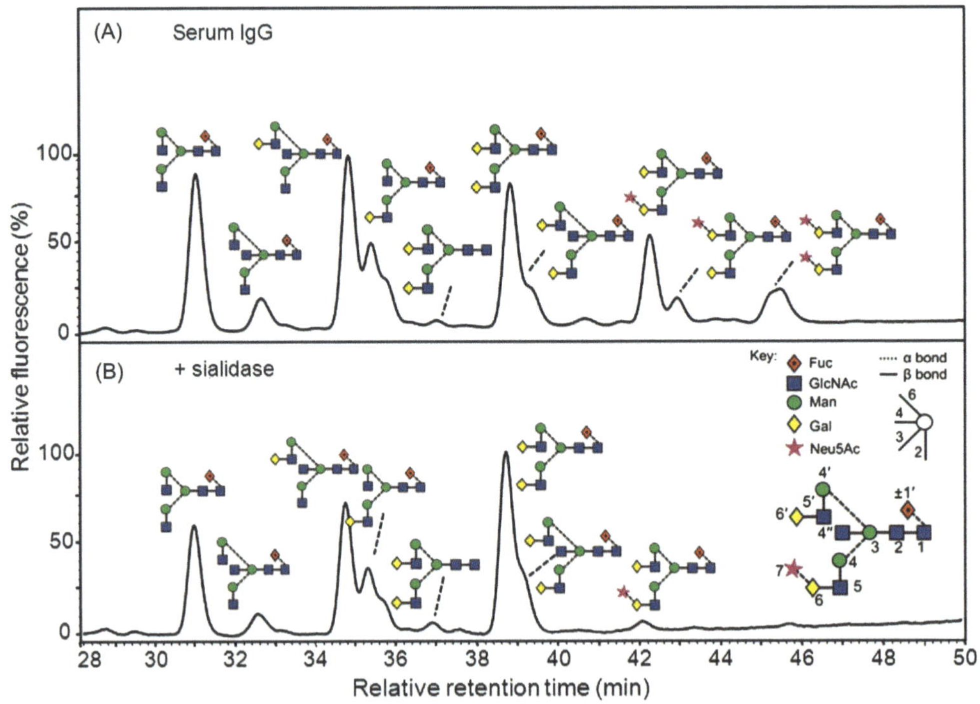

FIGURE 10.2 **Glycosylation of human serum IgG.** Normal-phase high-performance liquid chromatography of human serum IgG *N*-linked glycan fluorescently labeled with 2-aminobenzoic acid. (A) Total glycan pool. (B) Glycan profile following sialidase digestion. The symbolic representation of glycans follows that of Harvey et al.,[44] with residues in both the schematic diagrams and molecular graphics following the color scheme of the Centre for Functional Glycomics.[17] A labeled monosialylated glycan is shown to illustrate the residue labeling scheme adopted in this text. The scheme follows that of Vliegenthart et al.,[99] with the additional modifications of **7** and **7′** for sialic acid and **1′** for α1→6–linked core fucose.[31] HPLC profiles are reproduced from Yu et al.[108]

a precisely defined fashion. Each glycan lies close to a patch of amino acid residues on the Cγ2 domain, forming a number of non-covalent interactions dominated by hydrophobic and electrostatic interactions. A ladder of four hydrophobic residues, Phe241, Phe243, Val262, and V264, form CH–π interactions with the hexose rings of the core heptasaccharide and the GlcNAc on the 6-arm (Figure 10.1C). In addition, Glu265 and Arg301 form electrostatic interactions with sugar residues at the reducing end of the oligosaccharide.[30] These interactions collectively limit the Fc glycan flexibility and may result in reduced terminal galactosylation and sialylation. Moreover, this glycan immobility is also reflected in the fact that the entire oligosaccharide of the agalactosylated glycoform shows well-defined electron density in Fc domain crystal structures. Abolition of these Fc glycan–protein interactions, realized by mutating the residues along the hydrophobic ladder into alanine, significantly increased Fc terminal glycan galactosylation and sialylation.[30] In addition to the interaction between the hydrophobic ladder and the core pentasaccharide, the terminal galactose on the 6-arm has been shown to interact with the Fc protein backbone to further restrict Fc glycan flexibility. The 6-arm Fc glycan has been shown to exhibit flexibility similar to that of the Fc protein backbone,[31] while some have reported that the galactose on the 3-arm is more mobile than the Fc backbone.[32] In addition, recent NMR data show that the 6-arm has both bound and free states from the protein backbone, giving access to terminal glycosyltransferases.[33] In contrast, terminal sialylation does not influence Fc glycan flexibility.[34]

ROLE OF IgG Fc GLYCOSYLATION IN Fc STRUCTURE

The limited Fc terminal glycan processing was shown to be due to restricted access of Golgi-resident glycosyltransferases as a result of limited glycan flexibility imposed by the unusually prolific glycan–protein interaction at the Cγ2 region.[4] Early crystal structures of Fc show that the twin Fc glycans are positioned in the Fc horseshoe structure in a precisely defined fashion.[21,27,35] Each glycan lies close to a number of amino acid residues on the Cγ2 domain to which the glycan is attached, forming a number of non-covalent interactions dominated by hydrophobic and electrostatic interactions.[21,36] Moreover, the extent of twin Fc terminal glycan processing has been shown to regulate the distance between the two opposing Cγ2 domains. The successive removal of monosaccharide residues from the reducing end of Fc glycan by exoglycosidases narrows the gap between the two Cγ2 domains, while the Cγ3 domains remain unaffected.[35–37] Removal of the two terminal GlcNAc residues and the core mannoses further decreases the distance between the Cγ2 domains and lowers the Fc melting temperature, an indication of structural instability.[58,66] The impact of the Fc glycoform on Fc effector functions is discussed further below.

Crystal structures of a series of Fc glycoforms have been obtained over the years, including $Man_9GlcNAc_2$,[39] hybrid,[27] $Gal_2GlcNAc_2Man_3GlcNAc_2Fuc$,[84] $GlcNAc_2Man_3GlcNAc_2Fuc$,[21] $Man_3GlcNAc_2Fuc$,[36] $ManGlcNAc_2Fuc$,[36] and deglycosylated Fc.[36] These structures capture Fc glycoforms at different stages of glycan biogenesis, from the early oligomannose structures to the mature complex type glycans, and provide insights into the differential Fc glycan–protein packings. A comparison of these structures reveals that, regardless of the glycoform, interactions between the core pentassacharide ($Man_3GlcNAc_2$) and the Fc protein backbone are conserved.[27] One of the major changes in protein–glycan packing during Fc glycan biogenesis occurs during the transition from hybrid type to complex type. During this transition, the GlcNAc**5′** is transferred to the 6-arm core mannose (Man**4**) by the GnTII, which allows the formation of stacking interaction between the GlcNAc**5′** and the hydrophobic residue Phe243.[27] This stacking interaction has been shown to increase Fc stability while suppressing subsequent enzymatic processing of Fc glycan.[27,41]

Apart from Phe243, which only forms significant protein–glycan interactions in complex-type Fc glycoforms, a series of hydrophobic residues comprised of Phe241, Val262, and Val264 readily forms CH–π interactions with the core pentasaccharide, regardless of the Fc glycoform.[21,30] Together, Phe241, Phe243, Val262, and Val264, in close three-dimensional proximity, form a ladder of hydrophobic residues crucial for maintaining Fc protein–glycan interactions. In addition to the hydrophobic interactions, significant electrostatic interactions occur between the positively charged Glu265 and Arg301 residues and the hydroxyl groups projecting from sugar hexoses at the reducing end of the oligosaccharide.[21,30] These hydrophobic and electrostatic interactions collectively limit Fc glycan flexibility and result in reduced terminal galactosylation and sialylation due to restricted access of Golgi-resident glycosyltransferases. Abolition of these Fc glycan–protein interactions, realized by the mutagenesis of the hydrophobic and charged residues, dramatically increased Fc terminal glycan galactosylation and sialylation, accompanied by decreased Fc-mediated cytotoxicity.[30,42–44] Several potential mechanisms have been proposed to explain this decreased Fc effector function. One possibility is that the increased Fc terminal glycan processing, particularly terminal sialylation, could alter the Fc tertiary structure to result in decreased FcγR binding. Moreover, it could be due to the putatively increased Fc glycan flexibility, as a result of reduced Fc protein–glycan interactions. In addition, a decreased glycosylation site occupancy, as observed in the hydrophobic mutants,[30] could lead to a larger fraction of aglycosylated Fc, which is known to have decreased effector functions.[17,45]

Besides the interaction between the Fc hydrophobic ladder and the core pentasaccharide of the Fc glycan, terminal galactoses have been shown to interact with the Fc protein backbone and further restrict Fc glycan flexibility. The 6-arm of Fc glycan has been shown to exhibit mobility similar to that of the Fc protein backbone,[31] an indication of the 6-arm glycan immobility. Some have reported that the Gal**6** on the 3-arm is more mobile than the Fc backbone.[32] Consistently, removal of the Gal**6′** significantly increases Fc glycan flexibility.[31] More recent NMR data show that the 6-arm of Fc glycan has both bound and free states from the protein backbone,[34] potentially permitting access to terminal glycosyltransferases. Additionally, terminal sialylation does not influence Fc glycan flexibility.[33]

ACTIVITIES OF IgG GLYCOFORMS

Deglycosylation

The Fc glycan has been shown to be essential for maintaining Fc structural stability.[27,36,37,46] As a result, deglycosylation abrogates Fc binding to all FcγRs apart from FcγRIa, which retains a tenfold decrease in binding compared to the wild type.[45,47] For example, when the Fc glycan is cleaved by the bacterial EndoS, leaving only one GlcNAc attached to Asn297, Fc binding for FcγRIIIa is abolished.[48] Moreover, mutations at the *N*-linked glycosylation site, which leads to the generation of aglycosylated Fc, abolishes Fc binding to all FcγRs.[45] On the other hand, combinations of mutations have been shown to be able to restore aglycosylated Fc binding to selective FcγRs, including FcγRIa, FcγRIIa, and FcγRIIb, albeit to a varying extent.[45] The minimal Fc glycan required for Fc structural stability and effector function measured by FcγRI-mediated superoxide assay is found to be the core trisaccharide.[37]

Core Fucosylation

The α1,6-linked core fucose attached to Fc glycan has been established to exclusively reduce Fc binding affinity for activatory FcγRIIIa.[49,50] Defucosylation of Fc glycan increases the affinity of Fc binding affinity for FcγRIIIa by about 27-fold.[50] A comparison of the crystal structures of the fucosylated Fc–FcγRIIIa complex and defucosylated Fc–FcγRIIIa structures gives a molecular explanation for this altered affinity.[49,50] The structures showed for the first time that the *N*-glycan attached to the Asn162 of FcγRIIIa interacts directly with the core pentasaccharide of the Fc glycan. Moreover, defucosylated Fc glycan interacts more favorably with the Asn162 glycan of FcγRIIIa than its fucosylated counterpart, thus explaining the reduced affinity of fucosylated glycans (Figure 10.3). Defucosylated IgG Fc has been shown to have enhanced ADCC activities.[52–55]

Natural human serum IgG Fc glycan has a fucosylation level of between 80 and 92%; however, the *in vitro* expressed recombinant IgG has a relatively high fucosylation level of over 90%,[53] indicating that the fucosylation level could be a regulatory mechanism for antibody activity. While elevations in the serum levels of fucosylated IgG were observed in association with fetal maternal allotype thrombocytopenia, natural variations in the levels of fucosylated serum IgG in healthy or immune compromised conditions have not been reported to date.[56]

Terminal Galactosylation

Terminal galactosylated Fcs account for about 63% of all Fc glycoforms[23] and have been shown to affect Fc affinity for FcγRs. For example, hypergalactosylation of Fc terminal glycan has been shown to increase Fc affinity for FcγRIIIa

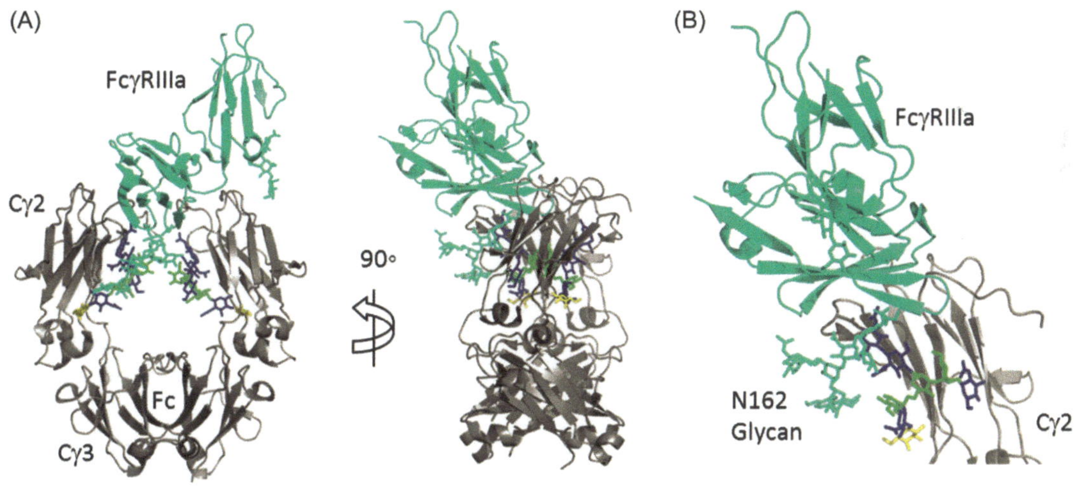

FIGURE 10.3 (A) Crystal structure of glycosylated FcγRIIIa in complex with afucosylated IgG_1 Fc (PDB 3AY4).[34,67] (B) Close-up view of glycan–glycan interactions. The receptor is shown in cyan and the IgG Fc is shown in gray. Glycans are shown as sticks, and the Fc glycans are colored according to Figure 10.2.

by threefold, presumably due to increased structural rigidity of the Fc Cγ2 domains.[57] In contrast, other reports suggest that hypogalactosylated Fc has increased affinity for FcγRs.[58] The level of Fc galactosylation has been shown to change with age,[59] and agalactosylation is found to be associated with inflammatory conditions such as rheumatoid arthritis.[58] Patients with rheumatoid arthritis have been found to have elevated levels of agalactosylated serum IgG glycans;[60] these patients showed an increase of 117% in serum agalactosylated IgG glycoform compared with the controls.[60] Further examination revealed that the IgG Fc is hypogalactosylated, whereas the Fab galactosylation level remained normal.[23] A similar study found that an increase in IgG agalactosyl glycoform is also present in a small number of other inflammatory diseases, including tuberculosis and Crohn's disease.[61] Interestingly, pregnant women affected by rheumatoid arthritis, who normally experience pregnancy-induced disease remission, show increased IgG galactosylation before reverting back to hypogalactosylation after giving birth.[62] The cellular mechanism behind this increased agalactosylated IgG level has been found to be due to lower galactosyltransferase activity in B cells;[63,64] however, this does not fully explain the selective agalactosylation of the Fc region. A suggested proinflammatory mechanism of rheumatoid arthritis, mediated by the agalactosylated glycoform, involves the binding of a cluster of agalactosylated Fc glycoform to the mannose-binding lectin, which subsequently activates the alternative complement pathway and leads to inflammation.[65] In contrast to its proinflammatory roles, a more recent study reveals an antiinflammatory pathway that requires Fc galactosylation. In this newly proposed antiinflammatory pathway, an immune complex formed by IgG_1 with a high level of Fc galactosylation promotes the association of inhibitory FcγRIIb and Dectin-1, a C-type lectin, and subsequently triggers an inhibitory signaling cascade.[66]

Terminal Sialylation

Terminal sialylation occurs in about 10% of Fc glycan[9,46] and, regardless of linkage type, has been shown to decrease Fc binding affinity for FcγRIIIa,[67] FcγRIIb, and the murine FcγRIIII by at least tenfold.[68] This decreased binding affinity correlates with decreased *in vivo* activities of hypersialylated monoclonal antibodies.[68] Although the crystal structure of sialylated Fc glycoform is unavailable, it has been speculated that the addition of a bulky sialic acid residue at the glycan terminus might impact the structure of the hinge that has been shown to affect FcγRs binding.[67,69] IgG Fc terminal glycan sialylation is regulated by the immune system. For example, active immunization was found to decrease the level of IgG Fc sialylation by 40%, an effect restricted to IgG but not IgM.[68] Moreover, a proinflammatory milieu during immunization favors the generation of antigen-specific IgG with lower Fc sialylation and *vice versa*.[70] However, this immunization-mediated decrease in antigen specific IgG Fc sialylation, observed in mouse models, does not seem to translate into human trials.[71] In addition to modulating Fc binding to FcγRs, Fc sialylation, in an α2,6-linkage-specific manner, has been shown to exert antiinflammatory properties in both mice and humans.[68,72,73] In fact, the α2,6-sialylated Fc fraction has been determined to be the active component of intravenous immunoglobulin (IVIg) therapy,[68] a common therapeutic used for treating a range of autoimmune conditions.[74] Moreover, recombinant hyper-α2,6-sialylated IgG Fc, at a tenfold-less dose, has been shown to recapitulate the therapeutic effect of IVIg in autoimmune mouse models.[72] On the other hand, this sialic acid-dependent antiinflammatory effect has not been reproducible in some mouse models.[75,76] This discrepancy could be explained by the different methods for enriching sialylated IVIg, or by the fact that different mouse strains react differently to IVIg treatment.

Terminal Mannose

High mannose glycoforms form a small fraction of total Fc glycoforms. High mannose glycoforms, including $Man_5GlcNAc_2$, generated using the GnTI-deficient HEK293S cell line, and $Man_9GlcNAc_2$, generated using the α-mannosidase inhibitor kifunesine, have been shown to increase Fc affinity for FcγRIIIa and decrease Fc affinity for FcγRIIb compared with Fc with biantennary complex glycans.[77,78] The increased affinity for FcγRIIIa is mainly attributed to the lack of core fucose at these oligomannose structures,[77] which is known to increase Fc affinity for FcγRIIIa.[49] In addition, $Man_9GlcNAc_2$ has been shown to perturb the quaternary organization of the Fc, but the impact of this on receptor binding has yet to be determined.[39] In addition to affecting FcγR binding, oligomannose glycoforms have been shown to increase Fc clearance rates,[79,80] possibly through mannose binding receptors on cell surfaces. On the other hand, some report the faster clearance of the oligomannose Fc to be due to the trimming of the oligomannose by serum mannosidases, an effect recapitulated by incubating oligomannose glycoform in human serum.[81] Studies using radiolabeled antibodies show that oligomannose glycoforms have clearance rates similar to those of other glycoforms; however, terminal mannose and terminal galactose increase the amount of Fc catabolized in the liver.[82]

Complement Activation

Fc glycosylation has been shown to be essential for effective binding to C1q and complement activation.[37,47,83] Different glycoforms exhibit different affinity for C1q and different efficacy in activating complement dependent cytotoxicity.[77] Specifically, complex type glycoforms, regardless of their fucosylation status, activate the complement cascade more efficiently than the hybrid or oligomannose glycoforms.[77] Moreover, increased terminal galactosylation has been found to increase C1q binding.[84] Furthermore, increased terminal sialylation and/or glycan flexibility might impair Fc affinity for C1q. The Fc glycan forms extensive hydrophobic and electrostatic interactions with the Fc protein backbone.[30,44,53] When this hydrophobic interaction is disrupted by mutating one of the hydrophobic residues, a significant increase in terminal galactosylation and sialylation was observed.[30,44] The increased terminal processing was accompanied by decreased Fc affinity for the C1q and consequently reduced Fc mediated complement activation.[30] However, generating the same hydrophobic F243A mutant in murine IgG_{2a} did not result in any difference in binding activity to C1q or complement activation compared to the wild type.[85] These contradictory results might be explained by the different IgG species and the different sialic acid species, Neu5Ac or Neu5Gc, present on Fc terminal glycan. Further investigation is needed to confirm the influence of increased glycan flexibility and terminal sialylation on Fc binding to C1q.

Besides directly influencing Fc binding to C1q, the Fc terminal GlcNAc has been shown *in vitro* to bind the mannose binding protein to indirectly activate the alternative complement cascade, a mechanism proposed to explain the inflammatory rheumatoid arthritis associated with decreased Fc terminal glycan galacosylation.[86,87] The physiological significance of this pathway is, however, less clear.

GLYCAN ENGINEERING OF ANTIBODIES

Given the importance of glycosylation for Fc function, the modification of *N*-linked glycosylation of IgG Fc has become a major focus for antibody engineering.[53,109] The most common mammalian expressions systems used to produce recombinant antibodies are the CHO, NS0, and Sp2/0 cell lines. Glycosylation profiles of recombinant antibodies produced in these expression systems are characterized by predominantly fucosylated biantennary complex-type glycans similar to serum IgG. However, all of these cell lines show lower levels of galactosylation than serum IgG Fc.[88] NS0 and Sp2/0 cell lines are of murine origin and often contain glycans bearing α1→3-linked galactose residues that are unusual in humans and have led to hypersensitivity reactions in patients.[89]

These differences in glycosylation profiles of CHO, NS0, and Sp2/0 cell lines and more recent studies on enhanced effector functions of defucosylated antibodies have led to a greater focus on the production of recombinant antibodies with homogenous glycoforms.

Manipulations of the *N*-linked glycosylation pathway can yield unnatural Fc glycoforms with modified effector functions. Antibodies with oligomannose-type, hybrid-type, and defucosylated complex-type glycans have been shown to display differential binding to FcγRIIIa and varying levels of ADCC.[52,77] Defucosylation of antibodies has been associated with the greatest increase in ADCC. To date, no correlation between core fucosylation and increase in CDC has been reported; however, differences in terminal glycan residues of IgG Fc have been associated with differences in CDC activity. While mapping of amino acid residues on IgG Fc crucial for C1q binding has been reported,[83] there are currently no reported studies on the structural implications of IgG Fc glycosylation on Fc-C1q binding. Differences in ADCC and CDC activity of fucosylated and defucosylated IgG antibodies of all subclasses have again shown the potent effect of defucosylation on ADCC.[90] These differences in IgG Fc effector functions with variations in Fc glycosylation are summarized in Table 10.1. Reduced binding affinity to FcγRIIIa for terminal sialylated IgG Fc has also been reported previously;[67,68] however, no direct correlation between ADCC or CDC activity and Fc sialylation is known to date.

One of the first reported glycoengineered cell lines was generated to overexpress *N*-acetylglucosaminyltransferase III (GnT III), the Golgi enzyme responsible for the addition of a bisecting GlcNAc residue to the central β mannose of the Fc glycan. Recombinant

TABLE 10.1 Glycoforms of Human IgG Fc and Their Associated Effector Functions and Affinity for FcγRIIIa and C1q

IgG Fc Glycoform	FcγRIIIa (V158)	C1q	FcRn	ADCC	CDC
Complex type (+Fuc)	+++	+++	+++	+++	++++
Complex type (−Fuc)	++++++	+++	+++	+++++	++++
Hybrid type (+Fuc)	++	++	+++	+	++++
Hybrid type (−Fuc)	++++	+++	+++	+++++	++++
Degalactosylated (−Fuc)	++++	+++	nd	+++	nd
Degalactosylated (+Fuc)	+++	nd	nd	+	nd
Galactosylated (−Fuc)	++++	nd	nd	+++	nd
$Man_5GlcNAc_2$	++++	+	+	++++	+++
$Man_9GlcNAc_2$	+++++	++	++++	++++	+++

Source: Data based on Forthal et al.,[35] Kanda et al.,[54] Niwa et al.,[72] and Shinkawa et al.[93]

Note: Fucosylated and defucosylated Fc glycoforms are shown as +/− Fuc. Data not determined is shown as nd.

antibodies produced in this cell line displayed enhanced ADCC.[93] It was later discovered that the presence of bisecting GlcNAc residues inhibits core fucosylation and was responsible for the enhanced effector function.[92] Ferrara et al.[94] further engineered GnT III for improved localization and along with overexpression of Golgi α mannosidase II enzyme, produced recombinant antibodies with hybrid- or complex-type defucosylated glycans. This study led to the development of GA-101, a glycoengineered CD20 specific antibody that is now in Phase II clinical trials for non-Hodgkin lymphoma[95] and is being evaluated in Phase III studies in chronic lymphocytic leukemia. CHO cell lines lacking expression of α1→6 fucosyltransferase are also being used to produce defucosylated recombinant antibodies with enhanced ADCC function.[96] MEDI-563 is one such non-fucosylated antibody that has reached clinical testing.[97] Besides mammalian expression systems, extensively glyco-engineered strains of *Pichia pastoris*, *Lemna*, *Nicotiana benthamiana*, and moss have also been used to improve yields and lower the cost of production of recombinant antibodies.[52,53,98]

ENDOGLYCOSIDASES IN IMMUNE EVASION AND THERAPEUTICS

Removal of the *N*-linked glycan at Asn297 of the IgG Fc domains leads to loss of antibody effector functions and impaired complement activation.[99] Recombinant antibodies expressed in bacteria or designed with mutations at the Asn297 *N*-linked glycosylation site at the Fc domain are aglycosylated and unable to trigger ADCC and inflammation. Such aglycosylated antibodies are particularly suited in a therapeutic setting where the mode of action of the recombinant antibody is through high-affinity binding to target antigen and Fc-mediated effector functions are unnecessary or may be detrimental.

Deglycosylation of antibodies by bacterial endoglycosidases serves as an important strategy for immune evasion.[100,107] Endoglycosidases are a class of enzymes that cleave the GlcNAc β1→4GlcNAc linkage in the chitobiose core of *N*-linked glycans. EndoS is one such endoglycosidase secreted by the Gram-positive pathogenic bacteria *Streptococcus pyogenes*. It exhibits a surprising specificity for native glycosylated IgG.[100] EndoS can successfully hydrolyze *N*-linked glycans from all four subclasses of IgG and leads to loss of antibody effector functions and complement activation.[101]

This unique property has been further used to treat autoimmune disease phenotypes in animal models. EndoS treatment of mice models of systemic lupus erythematosus led to significantly prolonged life and reduced disease.[102] Further, treatment of healthy rabbits with low doses of EndoS led to no toxicity and minimal production of anti-EndoS antibodies. EndoS is currently being studied as a potential therapeutic for autoimmune diseases in humans.[103]

A further application of IgG-specific endoglycosidases is in the boosting of monoclonal antibody effector functions.[48] At physiological antibody concentrations, the FcγRs of effector cells are largely saturated by serum IgG. A consequence of this saturation is that large amounts of therapeutic antibody are required to achieve cell killing. It is also likely that monoclonal antibody therapies that rely on immune-recruitment through their Fc domains are only effective against high-copy antigens. The problem of competing serum IgG can be solved by the deglycosylation of serum IgG with EndoS, while the monoclonal antibody is engineered to be resistant to the hydrolase, for example, by expressing the antibody with bisecting GlcNAc or as hybrid- or oligomannose-type glycans.[104] This technique has a significant impact on receptor binding by the monoclonal antibody and may find utility in broadening the therapeutic impact of monoclonal antibodies.

VARIATIONS OF ANTIBODY GLYCOSYLATION IN DISEASE

Variations in the glycosylation profile of serum IgG have been correlated with age, pregnancy, and several inflammatory diseases.[59,62,105] Levels of agalactosylated and bisected GlcNAc-containing Fc glycans increase with age.[23,59,60] Similarly, sialylation of IgG decreases with age.[106] Elevated levels of agalactosylated Fc glycoforms have been observed in patients with rheumatoid arthritis.[60] Early studies suggested that agalactosylated antibodies may play a causative role in inflammatory disease pathology.[65,86] However, elevated levels of agalactosylated antibodies in several other inflammatory conditions have since been reported,[23] and it now appears that agalactosylation may in fact be a consequence of inflammation.

Terminal sialylation of IgG Fc has been shown to lead to potent antiinflammatory effects,[68] and sialylated IgG Fc has been shown to be the active antiinflammatory component of intravenous immunoglobulin therapy.[72] Specifically, IgG Fc containing terminal $\alpha 2 \rightarrow 6$-linked sialic acid residues confers enhanced antiinflammatory activity in both mouse models of thrombocytopenia and *in vitro* ADCC assays.[72]

While the exact mechanism for this activity is still not completely clear,[14] recent evidence showed that mouse IgG Fc with sialylated Fc binds to SIGNR1, a mouse homolog of the human dendritic cell lectin DC-SIGN. Blockade of Fc-SIGNR1 binding or genetic deletion of SIGNR1 expression led to loss of antiinflammatory properties of sialylated Fc.[13]

CONCLUSION AND PERSPECTIVES

Antibody glycosylation has important consequences on antibody effector functions both within the natural repertoire of immunoglobulin glycoforms and on antibody-based therapeutics. In the case of IVIg therapy, understanding the mode of action on the molecular level and the role of glycosylation will guide the development of recombinant alternatives to the human-derived material in current use and may provide routes to increased efficacy. Engineering glycosylation is a well-established route to enhance the *in vivo* efficacy of many therapeutic monoclonal antibodies. Exploration of the selective deglycosylation of competing serum IgG offers a route to the further enhancement of this important class of therapeutic agent.

References

1. Amzel LM, Poljak RJ. Three-dimensional structure of immunoglobulins. *Annu Rev Biochem* 1979;**48**:961–97.
2. Davies DR, Metzger H. Structural basis of antibody function. *Annu Rev Immunol* 1983;**1**:87–117.
3. Stavnezer J, Guikema JE, et al. Mechanism and regulation of class switch recombination. *Annu Rev Immunol* 2008;**26**:261–92.
4. Arnold JN, Wormald MR, et al. The impact of glycosylation on the biological function and structure of human immunoglobulins. *Annu Rev Immunol* 2007;**25**:21–50.
5. Gould HJ, Sutton BJ, et al. The biology of IGE and the basis of allergic disease. *Annu Rev Immunol* 2003;**21**:579–628.
6. Gonzalez-Quintela A, Alende R, et al. Serum levels of immunoglobulins (IgG, IgA, IgM) in a general adult population and their relationship with alcohol consumption, smoking and common metabolic abnormalities. *Clin Exp Immunol* 2008;**151**(1):42–50.
7. Monteiro RC, Van De Winkel JG. IgA Fc receptors. *Annu Rev Immunol* 2003;**21**:177–204.
8. Chen K, Cerutti A. The function and regulation of immunoglobulin D. *Curr Opin Immunol* 2011;**23**(3):345–52.
9. Nimmerjahn F, Ravetch JV. Anti-inflammatory actions of intravenous immunoglobulin. *Annu Rev Immunol* 2008;**26**:513–33.
10. Samuelsson A, Towers TL, et al. Anti-inflammatory activity of IVIG mediated through the inhibitory Fc receptor. *Science* 2001;**291**(5503):484–6.
11. Aalberse RC, Schuurman J. IgG4 breaking the rules. *Immunology* 2002;**105**(1):9–19.
12. Anthony RM, Kobayashi T, et al. Intravenous gammaglobulin suppresses inflammation through a novel T(H)2 pathway. *Nature* 2011;**475**:110–3.

13. Anthony RM, Wermeling F, et al. Identification of a receptor required for the anti-inflammatory activity of IVIG. *Proc Natl Acad Sci USA* 2008;**105**(50):19571–8.
14. Yu X, Vasiljevic S, et al. Dissecting the molecular mechanism of IVIg therapy: the interaction between serum IgG and DC-SIGN is independent of antibody glycoform or Fc domain. *J Mol Biol* 2013 doi: 10.1016/j.jmb.2013.02.006. [Epub ahead of print].
15. Ravetch JV, Bolland S. IgG Fc receptors. *Annu Rev Immunol* 2001;**19**:275–90.
16. Woof JM, Burton DR. Human antibody–Fc receptor interactions illuminated by crystal structures. *Nat Rev Immunol* 2004;**4**(2):89–99.
17. Shields RL, Namenuk AK, et al. High resolution mapping of the binding site on human IgG1 for Fc gamma RI, Fc gamma RII, Fc gamma RIII, and FcRn and design of IgG1 variants with improved binding to the Fc gamma R. *J Biol Chem* 2001;**276**(9):6591–604.
18. Jefferis R. Glycosylation of recombinant antibody therapeutics. *Biotechnol Prog* 2005;**21**(1):11–16.
19. Jefferis R. Antibody therapeutics: isotype and glycoform selection. *Expert Opin Biol Ther* 2007;**7**(9):1401–13.
20. Saphire EO, Stanfield RL, et al. Contrasting IgG structures reveal extreme asymmetry and flexibility. *J Mol Biol* 2002;**319**(1):9–18.
21. Matsumiya S, Yamaguchi Y, et al. Structural comparison of fucosylated and nonfucosylated Fc fragments of human immunoglobulin G1. *J Mol Biol* 2007;**368**(3):767–79.
22. Guile GR, Rudd PM, et al. A rapid high-resolution high-performance liquid chromatographic method for separating glycan mixtures and analyzing oligosaccharide profiles. *Anal Biochem* 1996;**240**(2):210–26.
23. Holland M, Yagi H, et al. Differential glycosylation of polyclonal IgG, IgG-Fc and IgG-Fab isolated from the sera of patients with ANCA-associated systemic vasculitis. *Biochim Biophys Acta* 2006;**1760**(4):669–77.
24. Shibata-Koyama M, Iida S, et al. The *N*-linked oligosaccharide at Fc gamma RIIIa Asn-45: an inhibitory element for high Fc gamma RIIIa binding affinity to IgG glycoforms lacking core fucosylation. *Glycobiology* 2009;**19**(2):126–34.
25. Takasaki S, Kobata A. Asparagine-linked sugar chains of fetuin: occurrence of tetrasialyl triantennary sugar chains containing the Gal beta 1—3GlcNAc sequence. *Biochemistry* 1986;**25**(19):5709–15.
26. Harvey DJ, Merry AH, et al. Proposal for a standard system for drawing structural diagrams of *N*- and *O*-linked carbohydrates and related compounds. *Proteomics* 2009;**9**(15):3796–801.
27. Bowden TA, Baruah K, et al. Chemical and structural analysis of an antibody folding intermediate trapped during glycan biosynthesis. *J Am Chem Soc* 2012;**134**(42):17554–63.
28. Vliegenthart JFG, Dorland L, et al. High-resolution 1H nuclear magnetic resonance spectroscopy as a tool in the structural analysis of carbohydrates related to glycoproteins. *Adv Carbohydr Chem Biochem* 1983;**41**:209–374.
29. Dwek RA, Lellouch AC, et al. Glycobiology: 'the function of sugar in the IgG molecule.' *J Anat* 1995;**187**(Pt 2):279–92.
30. Lund J, Takahashi N, et al. Multiple interactions of IgG with its core oligosaccharide can modulate recognition by complement and human Fc gamma receptor I and influence the synthesis of its oligosaccharide chains. *J Immunol* 1996;**157**(11):4963–9.
31. Wormald MR, Rudd PM, et al. Variations in oligosaccharide–protein interactions in immunoglobulin G determine the site-specific glycosylation profiles and modulate the dynamic motion of the Fc oligosaccharides. *Biochemistry* 1997;**36**(6):1370–80.
32. Yamaguchi Y, Kato K, et al. Dynamics of the carbohydrate chains attached to the Fc portion of immunoglobulin G as studied by NMR spectroscopy assisted by selective ^{13}C labeling of the glycans. *J Biomol NMR* 1998;**12**(3):385–94.
33. Barb AW, Meng L, et al. NMR characterization of immunoglobulin G Fc glycan motion on enzymatic sialylation. *Biochemistry* 2012;**51**(22):4618–26.
34. Barb AW, Prestegard JH. NMR analysis demonstrates immunoglobulin G *N*-glycans are accessible and dynamic. *Nat Chem Biol* 2011;**7**(3):147–53.
35. Scanlan CN, Burton DR, et al. Making autoantibodies safe. *Proc Natl Acad Sci USA* 2008;**105**(11):4081–2.
36. Krapp S, Mimura Y, et al. Structural analysis of human IgG-Fc glycoforms reveals a correlation between glycosylation and structural integrity. *J Mol Biol* 2003;**325**(5):979–89.
37. Mimura Y, Church S, et al. The influence of glycosylation on the thermal stability and effector function expression of human IgG1-Fc: properties of a series of truncated glycoforms. *Mol Immunol* 2000;**37**(12–13):697–706.
38. Mimura Y, Ghirlando R, et al. The molecular specificity of IgG-Fc interactions with Fc gamma receptors. *Adv Exp Med Biol* 2001;**495**:49–53.
39. Crispin M, Bowden TA, et al. Carbohydrate and domain architecture of an immature antibody glycoform exhibiting enhanced effector functions. *J Mol Biol* 2009;**387**(5):1061–6.
40. Saphire EO, Parren PW, et al. Crystal structure of a neutralizing human IGG against HIV-1: a template for vaccine design. *Science* 2001;**293**(5532):1155–9.
41. Butler M, Quelhas D, et al. Detailed glycan analysis of serum glycoproteins of patients with congenital disorders of glycosylation indicates the specific defective glycan processing step and provides an insight into pathogenesis. *Glycobiology* 2003;**13**(9):601–22.

42. Jassal R, Jenkins N, et al. Sialylation of human IgG-Fc carbohydrate by transfected rat alpha2,6-sialyltransferase. *Biochem Biophys Res Commun* 2001;**286**(2):243–9.
43. Stewart R, Thom G, et al. A variant human IgG1-Fc mediates improved ADCC. *Protein Eng Des Sel* 2011;**24**(9):671–8.
44. Voynov V, Chennamsetty N, et al. Dynamic fluctuations of protein–carbohydrate interactions promote protein aggregation. *PLoS One* 2009;**4**(12):e8425.
45. Sazinsky SL, Ott RG, et al. Aglycosylated immunoglobulin G1 variants productively engage activating Fc receptors. *Proc Natl Acad Sci USA* 2008;**105**(51):20167–72.
46. Borrok MJ, Jung ST, et al. Revisiting the role of glycosylation in the structure of human IgG Fc. *ACS Chem Biol* 2012;**7**(9):1596–602.
47. Nose M, Wigzell H. Biological significance of carbohydrate chains on monoclonal antibodies. *Proc Natl Acad Sci USA* 1983;**80**(21):6632–6.
48. Baruah K, Bowden TA, et al. Selective deactivation of serum IgG: a general strategy for the enhancement of monoclonal antibody receptor interactions. *J Mol Biol* 2012;**420**(1–2):1–7.
49. Ferrara C, Grau S, et al. Unique carbohydrate–carbohydrate interactions are required for high affinity binding between Fc{gamma}RIII and antibodies lacking core fucose. *Proc Natl Acad Sci USA* 2011;**108**(31):12669–74.
50. Ferrara C, Stuart F, et al. The carbohydrate at FcgammaRIIIa Asn-162. An element required for high affinity binding to non-fucosylated IgG glycoforms. *J Biol Chem* 2006;**281**(8):5032–6.
51. Mizushima T, Yagi H, et al. Structural basis for improved efficacy of therapeutic antibodies on defucosylation of their Fc glycans. *Genes Cells* 2011;**16**(11):1071–80.
52. Forthal DN, Gach JS, et al. Fc-glycosylation influences Fcgamma receptor binding and cell-mediated anti-HIV activity of monoclonal antibody 2G12. *J Immunol* 2010;**185**(11):6876–82.
53. Jefferis R. Glycosylation as a strategy to improve antibody-based therapeutics. *Nat Rev Drug Discov* 2009;**8**(3):226–34.
54. Mori K, Iida S, et al. Non-fucosylated therapeutic antibodies: the next generation of therapeutic antibodies. *Cytotechnology* 2007;**55**(2–3):109–14.
55. Satoh M, Iida S, et al. Non-fucosylated therapeutic antibodies as next-generation therapeutic antibodies. *Expert Opin Biol Ther* 2006;**6**(11):1161–73.
56. Wuhrer M, Porcelijn L, et al. Regulated glycosylation patterns of IgG during alloimmune responses against human platelet antigens. *J Proteome Res* 2009;**8**(2):450–6.
57. Houde D, Peng Y, et al. Post-translational modifications differentially affect IgG1 conformation and receptor binding. *Mol Cell Proteomics* 2010;**9**(8):1716–28.
58. Rademacher TW, Williams P, et al. Agalactosyl glycoforms of IgG autoantibodies are pathogenic. *Proc Natl Acad Sci USA* 1994;**91**(13):6123–7.
59. Parekh R, Roitt I, et al. Age-related galactosylation of the *N*-linked oligosaccharides of human serum IgG. *J Exp Med* 1988;**167**(5):1731–6.
60. Parekh RB, Dwek RA, et al. Association of rheumatoid arthritis and primary osteoarthritis with changes in the glycosylation pattern of total serum IgG. *Nature* 1985;**316**(6027):452–7.
61. Parekh R, Isenberg D, et al. A comparative analysis of disease-associated changes in the galactosylation of serum IgG. *J Autoimmun* 1989;**2**(2):101–14.
62. Rook GA, Steele J, et al. Changes in IgG glycoform levels are associated with remission of arthritis during pregnancy. *J Autoimmun* 1991;**4**(5):779–94.
63. Alavi A, Axford J. Beta 1,4-galactosyltransferase variations in rheumatoid arthritis. *Adv Exp Med Biol* 1995;**376**:185–92.
64. Axford JS, Mackenzie L, et al. Reduced B-cell galactosyltransferase activity in rheumatoid arthritis. *Lancet* 1987;**2**(8574):1486–8.
65. Garred P, Madsen HO, et al. Two edged role of mannose binding lectin in rheumatoid arthritis: a cross sectional study. *J Rheumatol* 2000;**27**(1):26–34.
66. Karsten CM, Pandey MK, et al. Anti-inflammatory activity of IgG1 mediated by Fc galactosylation and association of FcgammaRIIB and dectin-1. *Nat Med* 2012;**18**(9):1401–6.
67. Scallon BJ, Tam SH, et al. Higher levels of sialylated Fc glycans in immunoglobulin G molecules can adversely impact functionality. *Mol Immunol* 2007;**44**(7):1524–34.
68. Kaneko Y, Nimmerjahn F, et al. Anti-inflammatory activity of immunoglobulin G resulting from Fc sialylation. *Science* 2006;**313**(5787):670–3.
69. Dall'Acqua WF, Cook KE, et al. Modulation of the effector functions of a human IgG1 through engineering of its hinge region. *J Immunol* 2006;**177**(2):1129–38.
70. Oefner CM, Winkler A, et al. Tolerance induction with T cell-dependent protein antigens induces regulatory sialylated IgGs. *J Allergy Clin Immunol* 2012;**129**(6):1647–55.
71. Selman MH, de Jong SE, et al. Changes in antigen-specific IgG1 Fc N-glycosylation upon influenza and tetanus vaccination. *Mol Cell Proteomics* 2012;**11**(4) M111.014563.
72. Anthony RM, Nimmerjahn F, et al. Recapitulation of IVIG anti-inflammatory activity with a recombinant IgG Fc. *Science* 2008;**320**(5874):373–6.
73. Debre M, Bonnet MC, et al. Infusion of Fc gamma fragments for treatment of children with acute immune thrombocytopenic purpura. *Lancet* 1993;**342**(8877):945–9.

74. Gelfand EW. Intravenous immune globulin in autoimmune and inflammatory diseases. *N Engl J Med* 2012;**367**(21):2015–25.
75. Leontyev D, Katsman Y, et al. Sialylation-independent mechanism involved in the amelioration of murine immune thrombocytopenia using intravenous gammaglobulin. *Transfusion* 2012;**52**(8):1799–805.
76. Ramakrishna C, Newo AN, et al. Passively administered pooled human immunoglobulins exert IL-10 dependent anti-inflammatory effects that protect against fatal HSV encephalitis. *PLoS Pathog* 2011;**7**(6):e1002071.
77. Kanda Y, Yamada T, et al. Comparison of biological activity among nonfucosylated therapeutic IgG1 antibodies with three different *N*-linked Fc oligosaccharides: the high-mannose, hybrid, and complex types. *Glycobiology* 2007;**17**(1):104–18.
78. Zou G, Ochiai H, et al. Chemoenzymatic synthesis and Fcgamma receptor binding of homogeneous glycoforms of antibody Fc domain. Presence of a bisecting sugar moiety enhances the affinity of Fc to FcgammaIIIa receptor. *J Am Chem Soc* 2011;**133**(46):18975–91.
79. Goetze AM, Liu YD, et al. High-mannose glycans on the Fc region of therapeutic IgG antibodies increase serum clearance in humans. *Glycobiology* 2011;**21**(7):949–59.
80. Millward TA, Heitzmann M, et al. Effect of constant and variable domain glycosylation on pharmacokinetics of therapeutic antibodies in mice. *Biologicals* 2008;**36**(1):41–7.
81. Chen X, Liu YD, et al. The effect of Fc glycan forms on human IgG2 antibody clearance in humans. *Glycobiology* 2009;**19**(3):240–9.
82. Wright A, Sato Y, et al. *In vivo* trafficking and catabolism of IgG1 antibodies with Fc associated carbohydrates of differing structure. *Glycobiology* 2000;**10**(12):1347–55.
83. Duncan AR, Winter G. The binding site for C1q on IgG. *Nature* 1988;**332**(6166):738–40.
84. Hodoniczky J, Zheng YZ, et al. Control of recombinant monoclonal antibody effector functions by Fc *N*-glycan remodeling *in vitro*. *Biotechnol Prog* 2005;**21**(6):1644–52.
85. Baudino L, Shinohara Y, et al. Crucial role of aspartic acid at position 265 in the CH2 domain for murine IgG2a and IgG2b Fc-associated effector functions. *J Immunol* 2008;**181**(9):6664–9.
86. Malhotra R, Wormald MR, et al. Glycosylation changes of IgG associated with rheumatoid arthritis can activate complement via the mannose-binding protein. *Nat Med* 1995;**1**(3):237–43.
87. Raju TS. Terminal sugars of Fc glycans influence antibody effector functions of IgGs. *Curr Opin Immunol* 2008;**20**(4):471–8.
88. Birch JR, Racher AJ. Antibody production. *Adv Drug Deliv Rev* 2006;**58**(5–6):671–85.
89. Chung CH, Mirakhur B, et al. Cetuximab-induced anaphylaxis and IgE specific for galactose-alpha-1,3-galactose. *N Engl J Med* 2008;**358**(11):1109–17.
90. Niwa R, Natsume A, et al. IgG subclass-independent improvement of antibody-dependent cellular cytotoxicity by fucose removal from Asn297-linked oligosaccharides. *J Immunol Methods* 2005;**306**(1–2):151–60.
91. Kanda Y, Yamane-Ohnuki N, et al. Comparison of cell lines for stable production of fucose-negative antibodies with enhanced ADCC. *Biotechnol Bioeng* 2006;**94**(4):680–8.
92. Shinkawa T, Nakamura K, et al. The absence of fucose but not the presence of galactose or bisecting *N*-acetylglucosamine of human IgG1 complex-type oligosaccharides shows the critical role of enhancing antibody-dependent cellular cytotoxicity. *J Biol Chem* 2003;**278**(5):3466–73.
93. Umana P, Jean-Mairet J, et al. Engineered glycoforms of an antineuroblastoma IgG1 with optimized antibody-dependent cellular cytotoxic activity. *Nat Biotech* 1999;**17**(2):176–80.
94. Ferrara C, Brünker P, et al. Modulation of therapeutic antibody effector functions by glycosylation engineering: influence of Golgi enzyme localization domain and co-expression of heterologous β1, 4-*N*-acetylglucosaminyltransferase III and Golgi α-mannosidase II. *Biotechnol Bioeng* 2006;**93**(5):851–61.
95. Mössner E, Brünker P, et al. Increasing the efficacy of CD20 antibody therapy through the engineering of a new type II anti-CD20 antibody with enhanced direct and immune effector cell-mediated B-cell cytotoxicity. *Blood* 2010;**115**(22):4393–402.
96. Yamane-Ohnuki N, Kinoshita S, et al. Establishment of FUT8 knockout Chinese hamster ovary cells: an ideal host cell line for producing completely defucosylated antibodies with enhanced antibody-dependent cellular cytotoxicity. *Biotechnol Bioeng* 2004;**87**(5):614–22.
97. Chan AC, Carter PJ. Therapeutic antibodies for autoimmunity and inflammation. *Nat Rev Immunol* 2010;**10**(5):301–16.
98. Li H, Sethuraman N, et al. Optimization of humanized IgGs in glycoengineered *Pichia pastoris*. *Nat Biotech* 2006;**24**(2):210–5.
99. Walker MR, Lund J, et al. Aglycosylation of human IgG1 and IgG3 monoclonal antibodies can eliminate recognition by human cells expressing Fc gamma RI and/or Fc gamma RII receptors. *Biochem J* 1989;**259**(2):347–53.
100. Collin M, Olsen A. Effect of SpeB and EndoS from *Streptococcus pyogenes* on human immunoglobulins. *Infect Immun* 2001;**69**(11):7187–9.

101. Allhorn M, Olin AI, et al. Human IgC/FcγR interactions are modulated by streptococcal IgG glycan hydrolysis. *PLoS One* 2008;**3**:1.
102. Albert H, Collin M, et al. *In vivo* enzymatic modulation of IgG glycosylation inhibits autoimmune disease in an IgG subclass-dependent manner. *Proc Natl Acad Sci USA* 2008;**105**(39):15005–9.
103. Collin M, Shannon O, et al. IgG glycan hydrolysis by a bacterial enzyme as a therapy against autoimmune conditions. *Proc Natl Acad Sci USA* 2008;**105**(11):4265–70.
104. Goodfellow JJ, Baruah K, et al. An endoglycosidase with alternative glycan specificity allows broadened glycoprotein remodelling. *J Am Chem Soc* 2012;**134**(19):8030–3.
105. van de Geijn FE, Wuhrer M, et al. Immunoglobulin G galactosylation and sialylation are associated with pregnancy-induced improvement of rheumatoid arthritis and the postpartum flare: results from a large prospective cohort study. *Arthritis Res Ther* 2009;**11**(6):R193.
106. Knezevic A, Gornik O, et al. Effects of aging, body mass index, plasma lipid profiles, and smoking on human plasma *N*-glycans. *Glycobiology* 2010;**20**(8):959–69.
107. Collin M, Olsen A. EndoS, a novel secreted protein from *Streptococcus pyogenes* with endoglycosidase activity on human IgG. *EMBO J* 2001;**20**(12):3046–55.
108. Forthal DN, Landucci G, et al. IgG2 inhibits HIV-1 internalization by monocytes, and IgG subclass binding is affected by gp120 glycosylation. *AIDS* 2011;**25**(17):2099–104.
109. Jefferis R. Recombinant antibody therapeutics: the impact of glycosylation on mechanisms of action. *Trends Pharmacol Sci* 2009;**30**(7):356–62.

CHAPTER

11

Activating and Inhibitory FcγRs in Autoimmune Disorders

Falk Nimmerjahn

Institute of Genetics, Department of Biology, University of Erlangen-Nürnberg, Erlangen, Germany

INTRODUCTION

Arthritis, multiple sclerosis (MS), autoimmune diabetes, and systemic lupus erythematosus (SLE) are autoimmune diseases that affect millions of people worldwide and require continuous medical attention. Linkage and association studies have established that several genetic and non-genetic factors contribute to the development of disease.[1] The importance of the adaptive and innate arms of the immune system in these processes is highlighted by the fact that immunosuppression is an effective treatment for these diseases.[2] Systemic immune suppression, however, renders the patient more susceptible to infections, and treatment has to be stopped during an acute infection, leading to the reoccurrence of autoimmune symptoms. Thus, more specific approaches to eliminate self-reactive cells might have fewer side-effects. Indeed, depletion of B cells has shown promising results for autoimmune diseases such as SLE.[2,3] Research in mouse models that recapitulate the human disease phenotypes has led to important insights into the mechanisms that cause an uncontrolled immune response and destruction of self tissues. A normal immune response is characterized by a delicate balance of activating and inhibitory signals that will determine the strength of the following response.[4] It must be strong and long lasting enough to eliminate foreign pathogens or malignant cells but controlled and specific enough to avoid damage to non-infected or healthy tissues. Several control mechanisms prevent autoreactive or overwhelming immune responses, and potentially harmful cells can be deleted or inactivated at central or peripheral checkpoints. During early B-cell development in the bone marrow, for example, cells expressing self-reactive receptors are eliminated by mechanisms such as receptor editing, deletion, or anergy.[5–7] It is widely accepted, however, that this process is incomplete and self-reactive cells can escape into the periphery; in addition, autoreactive B cells can be generated *de novo* in the periphery during the germinal center reaction.[8,9] Therefore, other checkpoints must be in place continuously preventing the accumulation and activation of autoreactive cells. In particular, B cells that secrete class-switched self-reactive antibodies that can trigger inflammatory effector functions have to be tightly regulated.[10,11]

Gene deletion studies in mice have identified the important role of negative regulatory proteins, such as CD5, CD22, CD72, PD-1, CTLA-4, and the inhibitory FcγRIIB (CD32B), which control signals triggered by activating receptors, thus setting a threshold for immune cell activation. Lack of these proteins results in autoimmune phenotypes and uncontrolled immune responses.[12–17] The hallmark of this protein family is the presence of an immunoreceptor tyrosine-based inhibitory motif (ITIM).[18] The Fc receptor (FcR) system has become a paradigm for such simultaneous triggering of activating and inhibitory signals, and several proteins of this family have been suggested to be associated with the incidence or severity of human autoimmune disorders, which will be the focus of this review. Besides the Fc receptor family, other players of the innate and adaptive immune system have been associated with autoimmune disorders in mice and humans, which has been reviewed elsewhere.[19,20]

Research over the last years has established that FcRs are central players in several processes that, if not tightly regulated, can lead to the appearance of autoreactive antibodies or autoimmune phenotypes.[21,22] These range from a failure to delete or prevent the expansion of self-reactive B cells to maintaining dendritic cells in an immature and tolerizing state; in addition, the rapid clearance of potential autoantigens such as apoptotic cells by macrophages is important to prevent the initiation of autoimmune processes.[23]

A QUESTION OF BALANCE: CO-EXPRESSION OF ACTIVATING AND INHIBITORY Fc RECEPTORS

The family of Fc receptors is well conserved among different species,[11] although the human family is the most numerous due to gene duplication and diversification processes.[24] To date, FcRs for all antibody isotypes have been identified, however, this chapter concentrates on the FcRs for IgG, the FcγRs. Generally, Fc receptors can be divided into two classes: the activating and the inhibitory FcRs. Most activating receptors cannot signal autonomously and have to associate with additional adaptor molecules to be functional. A notable exception to this rule is human FcγRIIA, which can transmit activating signals by itself. Therefore, a functional FcR consists of a ligand-binding α-domain associated with signaling adaptor molecules containing immunoreceptor tyrosine-based activation motifs (ITAMs). Depending on the cell type, the associated signaling adaptor molecules vary. Whereas in the majority of cells, such as monocytes, macrophages, neutrophils, and dendritic cells, FcRs are associated with the common gamma chain (γ-chain), in human natural killer (NK) cells FcRs are found in combination with the zeta chain (ζ-chain). In addition to the signaling function, these molecules are important for cell surface expression of the respective α-chains. Animals deficient in the γ-chain lack the cell surface expression of all activating Fcγ-receptors and several other non-FcR-related proteins such as PIR-A and NK cell cytotoxicity receptors.[22,25] As expected, these animals were demonstrated to have significant defects in antibody-dependent effector cell responses.[26–30] The inhibitory receptor is a single-chain molecule that contains an immunoreceptor tyrosine-based inhibitory motif (ITIM) in its cytosolic tail.[18]

Humans have eight genes that encode Fcγ receptors (FcγRIA/IB/IC, FcγRIIA/B/C, and FcγRIIIA/B), located on chromosome 1. The majority of other species, including the mouse, have four different classes of IgG Fc receptors that correspond to their human counterparts: FcγRI (CD64), FcγRII (CD32), FcγRIII (CD16), and FcγRIV. FcγRIV is an activating Fc receptor with intermediate affinity ($10^7 M^{-1}$) and restricted subclass specificity. Based on its sequence similarity the mouse could be considered as a homolog to human FcγRIIIA.[31–33] Whereas FcγRI displays high affinity for the antibody constant region (10^8 to $10^9 M^{-1}$), FcγRIIB and FcγRIII have a much lower affinity ($\sim 10^6 M^{-1}$).[34,35] The low-affinity Fc receptor genes are clustered in close proximity to each other in syntenic regions on chromosome 1 in humans, chimpanzees, and mice. In contrast, the high-affinity FcγRI is located on chromosome 3 in mice and chromosome 1 in humans and chimpanzees.[11] This Fcγ receptor complexity is mirrored by the existence of several IgG isotypes that show differential binding to FcγRs. In the mouse, the high-affinity FcγRI exclusively binds IgG_{2a}, the medium-affinity FcγRIV binds IgG_{2a} and IgG_{2b}, and the low-affinity receptors FcγRIIB and FcγRIII bind IgG_1, IgG_{2a}, and IgG_{2b}.[11] In humans, IgG_1 and IgG_3 bind better to FcRs than IgG_2 or IgG_4. However, due to the presence of multiple FcR alleles that influence the antibody–FcR interaction, the situation is more complex.[10] As will be discussed later, some of these alleles show a significant association with autoimmune diseases, which allows us to draw some conclusions about the role of antibody–FcR interactions in these disorders.

ESTABLISHING THE THRESHOLD FOR CELL ACTIVATION: ACTIVATING AND INHIBITORY Fc RECEPTOR SIGNALING

As indicated, activating and inhibitory FcRs are co-expressed on the same cell. Thus, immune complex (IC) binding will result in simultaneous triggering of activating and inhibitory signaling pathways (Figure 11.1). Factors that determine whether this co-engagement results in cell activation or inhibition are the relative affinities of the antibody isotype to specific FcRs, the expression level of activating and inhibitory Fc-receptors, and the cytokine environment, which can influence their relative expression levels.[11] Moreover, differential antibody glycosylation during an inflammatory response can influence the antibody–FcR interaction and thus regulate antibody activity in mice and humans.[36] Effector responses controlled by these opposing signals most prominently include degranulation of mast cells and neutrophils, release of cytotoxic mediators and inflammatory cytokines by macrophages, antibody-dependent cellular cytotoxicity (ADCC), dendritic cell (DC) activation, phagocytosis, and antigen presentation.[22]

SIGNALING PATHWAYS OF ACTIVATING Fc RECEPTORS

The affinity of the majority of activating Fc receptors for monomeric antibodies is not sufficient for stable binding and induction of signaling. High-affinity receptors, such as FcγRI and FcεRI, can associate with monomeric IgG or IgE antibodies, but activating signals are only triggered upon replacement of bound IgG by immune complexes (in the case of FcγRI) or upon allergen binding and concomitant cross-linking of cell surface-bound IgE.[37,38] Ligands that bind with low affinity cannot trigger sustained receptor aggregation and might even behave as antagonists.[39] FcR aggregation by ICs induces a relocation into cell membrane subdomains called lipid rafts that are enriched in signaling molecules such as SRC protein kinases (Figure 11.1A).[40] Tyrosine residues in the ITAM motif of the γ-chain then become phosphorylated by SRC kinases, creating SH2 docking sites for the subsequent recruitment of SYK kinases. Depending on cell type and the receptor in question, different members of the SRC family kinases, such as LYN, HCK or LCK, are involved in phosphorylation of the γ-chain (Figure 11.1A). This enables members of the SYK family kinases to bind and to recruit and phosphorylate a number of downstream

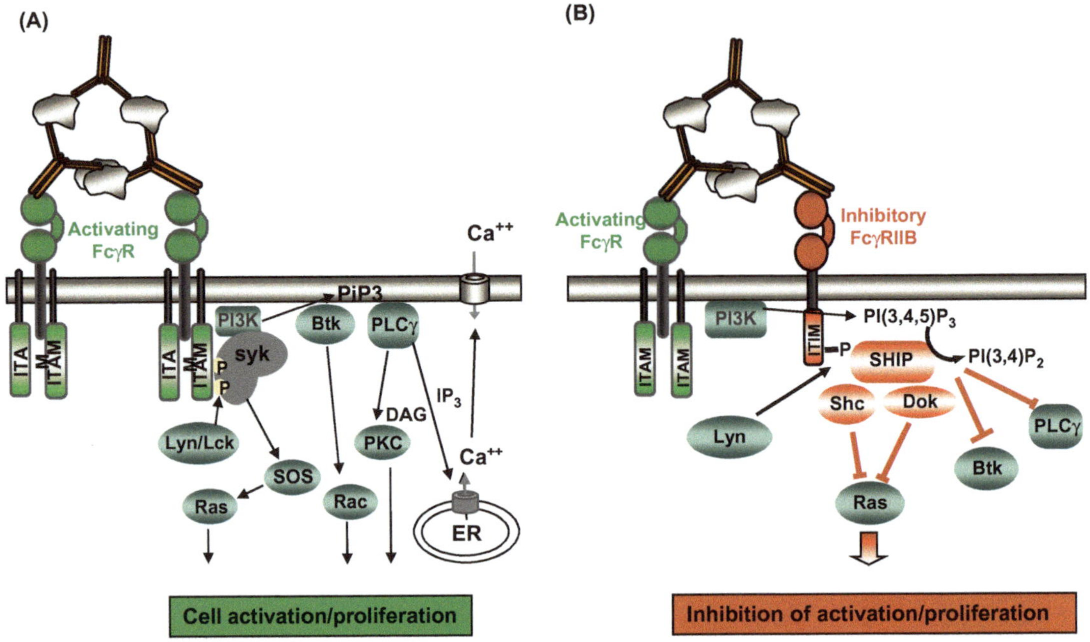

FIGURE 11.1 **Signaling pathways of activating and inhibitory Fc receptors.** (A) Immune complex-triggered cross-linking of activating FcRs induces phosphorylation of the ITAM motif by members of the SRC-kinase family, resulting in activation of downstream signaling events and cell activation. (B) Simultaneous triggering of the inhibitory FcR interferes with cell activation by recruitment of the phosphatase SHIP and inhibition of activating signaling pathways. The strength of activating versus inhibitory signals triggered by immune complexes is determined by the affinity of individual antibody isotypes to activating and inhibitory FcRs and other factors such as the cytokine environment (see text for details).

targets, including the linker for the activation of T cells (LAT), multi-molecular adaptor complexes, and members of the Btk and Tec family kinases.[41–43] Important downstream events triggered by SYK-mediated activation of phosphatidylinositol 3-kinase (PI3-K) and phospholipase-Cγ (PLCγ) are sustained calcium release and protein kinase C (PKC) activation. Moreover, the Ras–Raf–MAPK pathway becomes activated through Sos present in the multimolecular adaptor complex.[22,44]

INHIBITORY SIGNALING PATHWAYS

Depending on the cell type, alternatively spliced forms of the inhibitory Fc receptor FcγRIIB have been described that have a differential capacity to endocytose bound ICs (termed FcγRIIB-1 and FcγRIIB-2). FcγRIIB-1 is expressed on B cells, whereas the endocytic FcγRIIB-2 shows a myeloid expression pattern.[44] All of these splice forms, however, contain the ITIM motif and trigger inhibitory signaling pathways. On B cells, FcγRIIB regulates activating signals transmitted by the B-cell receptor (BCR), whereas on mast cells, neutrophils, or macrophages it balances activating signals triggered by Fcε- or Fcγ-receptors.[22,44] Upon co-aggregation with its activating counterpart, Lyn phosphorylates the ITIM, which leads to recruitment of SHIP (SH2 domain-containing inositol 5′-phosphatase). SHIP activation leads to enhanced hydrolysis of phosphatidylinositol intermediates and thereby interferes with the membrane recruitment of BTK and PLCγ, resulting in inhibition of ITAM signaling-mediated calcium release and downstream effector functions (Figure 11.1B).[45,46] Moreover, tyrosine phosphorylated SHIP can bind to Shc and Dok, thereby inhibiting activation of the Ras pathway and ultimately cell proliferation. A third ITIM- and SHIP-independent signaling pathway has been described for the cross-linking of FcγRIIB on B cells without concomitant activating signals by the BCR. This leads to B-cell apoptosis via Abl-family-kinase-dependent pathways.[47,48] Although the *in vivo* relevance of this pathway remains to be established, this situation may arise during the germinal center reaction when somatic hypermutation generates BCRs that lose specificity for their cognate antigen retained in the form of ICs on follicular dendritic cells and on plasma cells, which downregulate BCR expression while simultaneously upregulating FcγRIIB.[49] Thus, FcγRIIB has been suggested to be important for maintaining tolerance.

DISTURBING THE THRESHOLD: HORROR AUTOTOXICUS

There are several ways in which balanced signaling through activating and inhibitory FcR pairs might be perturbed, ranging from aberrant expression of Fc receptors to allelic variants of activating receptors that have a differential affinity for certain antibody isotypes.[10,11,50] Most of our current knowledge stems from gene deletion studies, autoimmune models in mice, and indirect data from human autoimmune patients. Loss or inactivation of FcRs in humans has only been described for the high-affinity FcγRI and FcγRIIIB. Whereas FcγRI deficiency had no apparent impact on health, a significant amount of individuals who lost FcγRIIIB expression had autoimmune disorders.[51–54] As activating and inhibitory FcR pairs are expressed on a variety of cell types, the resulting phenotypes are a complex mixture of impaired responses at several stages throughout the adaptive and innate immune response. The following paragraphs summarize these phenotypes with respect to the affected cell types and the molecular changes resulting in impaired FcR-dependent responses.

CHANGING THE EXPRESSION LEVEL OF THE INHIBITORY RECEPTOR ON B CELLS

FcγRIIB, together with other negative regulatory proteins such as CD22 or CD72, regulates activating signals triggered by the B-cell receptor, thus setting a threshold for B-cell activation.[45,55,56] Loss of FcγRIIB was therefore predicted to result in uncontrolled B-cell activation. This was confirmed by the generation of FcγRIIB-deficient mice that spontaneously develop a lupus-like disease characterized by the production of autoantibodies and premature death due to severe glomerulonephritis.[12,16,57] This autoimmune phenotype is strain dependent; C57BL/6 but not Balb/c mice develop autoimmune disease, suggesting that other epistatic modifiers are involved in disease susceptibility and severity.[58] Supporting this notion, Balb/c mice doubly deficient in programmed death 1 (PD-1) and FcγRIIB developed autoimmune hydronephrosis, whereas mice only deficient in one of these inhibitory proteins did not.[59] Moreover, Balb/c FcγRIIB knockout mice showed enhanced disease phenotypes in a model of pristane-induced lupus.[60] In addition, Balb/c mice have been suggested to be more efficient in silencing autoreactive heavy chains by receptor editing than C57Bl/6 mice, making the latter strain more permissive for the development of autoimmunity.[61,62]

Although genetic deletion of FcγRIIB results in loss of inhibitory signaling on a variety of cell types, there is evidence that the appearance of autoantibodies is a B-cell autonomous phenomenon. Autoimmune-prone mouse strains such as NZB, NOD, BXSB, and MRL express reduced levels of FcγRIIB on activated and germinal-center B cells due to a polymorphism in the FcγRIIB promoter.[63–66] Moreover, FcγRIIB bone marrow chimeras expressing normal levels of the inhibitory receptor on radiation-resistant cells but lacking FcγRIIB on B cells develop autoantibodies and disease.[12] In contrast, restoring FcγRIIB function prevented the development of autoantibodies in autoimmune-prone mouse strains.[67,68] Another important issue is understanding at which stage of B-cell development FcγRIIB regulates tolerance. As indicated, autoreactive B cells can be generated throughout B-cell development.[6] There is accumulating evidence that FcγRIIB mediates its function during late stages of B-cell maturation in mice and humans, thus representing a distal checkpoint.[61,69,70] By using a mouse strain in which the endogenous Ig locus has been replaced with an autoreactive heavy chain, it was shown that the absence of FcγRIIB resulted in the accumulation of IgG-positive autoreactive plasma cells.[61] FcγRIIB deficiency neither impacted early events in the bone marrow such as receptor editing nor prevented the development of IgM-positive, autoreactive B cells. After class switching to IgG, however, FcγRIIB was essential in preventing the expansion of autoreactive B cells and their maturation into plasma cells. Taking into account the considerably higher pathogenic potential of IgG compared to IgM antibody isotypes, this relatively late stage of FcγRIIB-mediated negative regulation might be sufficient to prevent the initiation of severe autoreactive processes. Thus, FcγRIIB might serve as the final barrier to control class-switched autoreactive B cells that would otherwise induce tissue pathology by secretion of large amounts of pathogenic antibodies.

The most important question is whether data obtained in murine model systems are helpful in explaining the development of human autoimmune disease. Analysis of human autoimmune patient cohorts indicates that this is the case, and that some of the underlying mechanisms of aberrant FcγRIIB expression are quite similar in humans and mice; for example, polymorphisms in the human FcγRIIB promoter have been linked to the development of SLE.[69,71,72] The strongest association was found with a polymorphism that leads to decreased binding of the transcription factor AP-1, resulting in reduced surface expression of FcγRIIB on activated B cells of human lupus patients.[69] Other studies showed that memory B cells of SLE patients and humans with chronic inflammatory demyelinating polyneuropathy (CIDP) failed to upregulate FcγRIIB expression on memory B cells, and this lower expression level was correlated with a reduced threshold for B cell activation,[70,73] consistent with a previous study describing that B cells from lupus patients showed enhanced triggering of activating signaling pathways after B-cell receptor stimulation.[74] Such quantitative assessments of FcγRIIB expression were complicated until the recent development of a novel antibody specific for the human inhibitory FcγRIIB.[75] It will be of interest to determine the mechanism of this aberrant expression and if any of the known FcγRIIB polymorphisms are involved in this phenotype. Using a humanized mouse model, in which immunodeficient mouse strains were reconstituted with hematopoetic stem cells from donors carrying a functionally impaired FcγRIIB variant (FcgRIIB-I232T), it was demonstrated that the humoral immune system developing in these animals was characterized by higher levels of memory B and plasma cells and by a loss of humoral tolerance.[76] In this allele, exchange of a nonpolar isoleucine residue in the transmembrane domain (amino acid 232) for a threonine results in impaired recruitment to lipid rafts and thus exclusion from productive signaling.[77–79] The results of these studies are in agreement with data obtained in murine model systems identifying FcγRIIB as a checkpoint during late stages of B cell development. Indeed, this allelic

TABLE 11.1 Human Fc Receptor Alleles Associated with Systemic Lupus Erythematosus (SLE)

Fc Receptor	Disease Association	Population	Mechanism	Refs.
FcγRIIB	SLE incidence	Caucasian	Promoter polymorphism (impaired transcription factor binding)	McGaha et al.,[69] Su et al.[71,72]
		African-American	Decreased expression on memory cells	Mackay et al.[70]
		Asian, Caucasian	Allelic variant (FcγRIIB^{232T}) excluded from lipid rafts	Li et al.,[77] Floto et al.,[78] Kono et al.,[79] Siriboonrit et al.,[80] Chu et al.,[81] Kyogoku et al.,[82] Tsuchiya et al.,[83] Willcocks et al.[84]
FcγRIIA	SLE incidence/severity	African-American, Brazilian, German, Korean, Hispanic, Thai	Low-affinity 131 R allele	Siriboonrit et al.,[80] Bazilio et al.,[137] Dijstelbloem et al.,[139] Gelmetti et al.,[140] Manger et al.,[142] Salmon et al.,[144] Yun et al.,[147] Zuniga et al.,[148] Lee et al.[155]
FcγRIIIA	SLE incidence/severity	Caucasian, Dutch, Korean	Low-affinity158 F allele	Dijstelbloem et al.,[138] Koene et al.,[141] Seligman et al.,[145] Salmon et al.[156]
FcγRIIIB	SLE incidence/severity	Thai, Spanish, Japanese	Low-affinity NA2 allele	Siriboonrit et al.,[80] Gonzalez-Escribano et al.,[149] Hatta et al.[150]

variant of FcγRIIB has been associated with human SLE and arthritis in several Asian and European populations (Table 11.1).[80–84] This represents a novel mechanism of impaired FcγRIIB function and is unique to humans; however, the great disparities among different human populations and ethnicities highlight the importance of genetic background and other susceptibility factors for the development of autoimmune disease (Table 11.1). For example, the decreased expression of FcγRIIB on memory cells of SLE patients was overrepresented in the African-American population.[70]

FcγRIIB AS A REGULATOR OF DENDRITIC CELL ACTIVITY

Dendritic cells (DCs) have long been recognized as central mediators that, depending on their activation state, determine whether an adaptive immune response or tolerance is induced.[85] Several groups have shown that cross-linking of FcRs on DCs by immune complexes results in cell activation and cross-presentation of endocytosed antigen on MHC class I molecules to CD8+ cytotoxic T cells.[86–89] As low levels of ICs are constantly present in the serum, FcγRIIB might be crucial in preventing spontaneous activation of DCs. Indeed, blocking FcγRIIB on human dendritic cells was sufficient to induce DC maturation by serum immune complexes. Besides upregulation of costimulatory molecules, these DCs were more potent in generating and activating antigen-specific T cells,[75,90] as described before for mouse DCs deficient in FcγRIIB expression.[91] Although beneficial for immunotherapeutic or vaccination approaches, this suggests that a slight deregulation of FcγRIIB expression might result in the initiation of autoreactive processes. It will be of great interest to determine if FcR-mediated uptake of immune complexes containing autoantigens by DCs plays a role in autoimmune diseases that depend on the priming of autoreactive T cells. In addition, expression of the inhibitory receptor on DCs present in epithelia has been implicated in establishing tolerance to airborne and food allergens.[92]

Whereas the essential role of dendritic cells in regulating T-cell responses is well accepted, it has only recently become clear that DCs are also important for the B-cell response.[93–95] Unlike in macrophages, which rapidly degrade phagocytosed material, antigen taken up by DCs is degraded more slowly and therefore is present in an intact form for prolonged times.[96] This might allow antigen transport from the periphery to lymphoid organs where it can be presented to B cells. DC–B-cell interactions have been observed *in vivo* and it has been suggested that these interactions are important for the generation of IgG responses *in vitro* and *in vivo*.[95] The role of FcγRIIB in this process is that ICs taken up via FcγRIIB are inefficiently degraded and recycled for cell surface presentation to B cells. In contrast, uptake via FcγRIII results in a faster degradation of the antigen.[93] The importance of this novel function of FcγRIIB for human or murine autoimmune diseases remains to be established.

THE ROLE OF FcγRIIB IN THE EFFERENT RESPONSE: CONTROLLING INNATE IMMUNE EFFECTOR CELL ACTIVATION

Besides its regulatory role on B cells and DCs in the afferent response, FcγRIIB is an important modulator of inflammatory effector cells such as mast cells, neutrophils, and macrophages during the efferent phase of an immune response.[22] On these cell types, FcγRIIB is co-expressed with activating Fc receptors of varying affinities and isotype specificities and negatively regulates signals delivered by these receptors. Lack of FcγRIIB leads to elevated IC-mediated inflammation and phagocytosis as demonstrated by an enhanced Arthus reaction, systemic anaphylaxis, anti-GBM glomerulonephritis, immunothrombocytopenia, hemolytic anemia, collagen-induced arthritis, and IgG-mediated clearance of pathogens and tumor cells.[11,21] On allergic effector cells such as mast cells and basophils, FcγRIIB regulates activating signals triggered by cross-linking FcεRI, resulting in enhanced IgE-mediated anaphylaxis and heightened sensitivity to allergic rhinitis.[97] Moreover, FcγRIIB deficiency renders otherwise resistant mouse strains susceptible to the development of certain forms of collagen-induced arthritis.[98] As described for human autoimmune disease in some of these models both increased autoantibody production due to FcγRIIB deficiency on B cells and heightened effector cell responses are likely to contribute to the observed phenotype.

Another long known observation is that IgG_{2a} and IgG_{2b} antibodies trigger stronger effector responses than IgG_1 or IgG_3 in passive antibody transfer models.[99–107] Similarly, in highly pathogenic autoimmune models such as the accelerated nephrotoxic nephritis model, the pathogenic autoantibodies are of the IgG_{2b} isotype.[108] In human SLE patients, IgG_1, IgG_3, and, to a lesser extent, IgG_2 anti-DNA antibodies dominate in the serum, whereas all subclasses can be found in kidney biopsies.[109–112]

The molecular mechanism of differential antibody isotype activity was addressed recently.[104] It was shown that the differences in affinity of different IgG isotypes for activating and inhibitory Fc receptors might explain this phenomenon.[33,104] By measuring the affinities of all antibody isotypes for the various FcRs and dividing the affinities of antibody isotypes for activating FcRs by the affinity for the inhibitory receptor a so-called A/I ratio was established which predicted antibody activity *in vivo*.[11,104] Thus, IgG_1 (which only binds to the FcγRIII/FcγRIIB pair) has a lower affinity for the activating than for the inhibitory FcR (A/I ratio<<1), resulting in lower activity. In contrast, IgG_{2a} and IgG_{2b} have 20- to 40-fold higher affinity for the activating FcγRIV than for FcγRIII/FcγRIIB, which results in preferential triggering of FcγRIV and a lower degree of negative regulation by the inhibitory Fc receptor. As will be discussed below, other factors such as cytokines or differential antibody glycosylation can affect this ratio. In humans, the presence of different activating FcR alleles that have differential affinities for certain human antibody isotypes might result in a similar situation, thus changing the A/I ratio and antibody activity.

THE ACTIVATING Fc RECEPTORS IN THE EFFERENT RESPONSE

In contrast to the inhibitory FcγRIIB, expression of activating Fc receptors is limited to DCs and innate immune effector cells such as mast cells, basophils, monocytes, macrophages, neutrophils, and NK cells. There is considerable heterogeneity in the expression of specific activating FcRs. In the mouse, macrophages express all activating FcRs (I, III, and IV), DCs mainly express FcγRI and III, neutrophils express FcγRIII and IV, and NK cells express FcγRIII. Genetic inactivation of all activating FcRs by deletion of the common γ-chain in mice results in abrogated or heavily impaired immune complex or allergen-mediated responses, such as antibody-dependent cellular cytotoxicity (ADCC), release of inflammatory mediators, cytokine release, and phagocytosis of immune complexes.[11,29] As several activating Fc receptors are co-expressed on the same cell, subsequent deletion of the individual ligand-binding α-chains was crucial in elucidating the role of the individual Fc receptors in the activity of different antibody isotypes. Identifying the receptor and cell type responsible for tissue pathology in autoimmune diseases might allow development of more specific therapeutic interventions. Consistent with its *in vitro* isotype binding profile, activating FcγRIII was essential for IgG_1-mediated effector functions in a variety of models, such as arthritis, glomerulonephritis, IgG-dependent anaphylaxis, IgG-mediated hemolytic anemia, and immunothrombocytopenia (ITP).[33,100,104,113–117]

In contrast, IgG_{2b} activity was not impaired in FcγRIII or FcγRI knockout mice but was almost completely abrogated in mice injected with an FcγRIV-blocking antibody in passive and active models of antibody-mediated inflammation, including models of immunothrombocytopenia (ITP) and nephrotoxic nephritis (NTN).[100,101,104,108,118] In the NTN model, mice are injected with a sheep hyperimmune serum specific for murine glomerular basement membranes (GBMs). To enhance disease development, mice are pre-immunized with sheep serum, which results in an IgG_{2b}-dominated antibody response.[108] After injection of the sheep anti-GBM serum, many animals die within 8 to 10 days due to severe inflammation and kidney failure. In the presence of an FcγRIV-blocking antibody, however, animals did not develop fatal glomerulonephritis. Despite C3 deposition in the kidneys, the observed pathology was fully dependent on activating FcRs as observed before.[26,28,119–121] Similar results were obtained in a model of autoantibody-induced skin blistering disease, in which skin detachment and blister formation induced by collagen-type VII-specific antibodies were completely abrogated in FcγRIV-deficient mice.[122] This suggests that identification and blocking of the responsible activating FcRs in human autoimmune disease might be a promising therapeutic intervention.

Similar to IgG_{2b}, IgG_{2a} antibody activity was greatly impaired in mice with blocked FcγRIV activity in models of antibody-mediated clearance of platelets, B cells, or tumor cells and neither deficiency in members of the complement cascade nor deficiency in FcγRI or FcγRIII had a significant effect on antibody activity.[101,104,107,123] Depending on the model system, the amount of ICs, and effector cell type, FcγRI and FcγRIII variably contributed to IgG_{2a} activity.[100,124–126] For example, in a model of autoimmune hemolytic anemia (AIHA), which, in contrast to the ITP model, requires higher antibody doses and several days to develop a maximal response, FcγRIII was significantly involved in mediating IgG_{2a} activity;[100] in addition, the complement component C3 enhanced IgG_{2b} and IgG_3 activity.[127] Regarding the role of FcγRIII in this model, it was recently demonstrated that C5a, a strong inflammatory mediator, induces upregulation of FcγRIII which is important for the development of AIHA.[128,129] Further, generation of C5a occurred independently of the classical and alternative complement pathways and was triggered in an FcR-dependent fashion.[128,130] Taken together, this demonstrates the influence of the effector cell type and the cytokine milieu on the cellular FcR expression pattern, which will be discussed in greater detail later.

In humans, low-affinity FcγRs bind better to IgG_1 and IgG_3 than to IgG_2 or IgG_4. However, certain FcγRIIA and IIIA alleles show increased binding to human antibody isotypes.[10] For example, the $Fc\gamma RIIA^{131H}$ allele binds IgG_2 approximately tenfold better than FcγRIIA with arginine at that position ($Fc\gamma RIIA^{131R}$). Similarly, human $Fc\gamma RIIIA^{158V}$ has a higher affinity for IgG_1 and IgG_3 than its 158F counterpart.[10] This selectively higher affinity of the activating FcR increases the A/I ratio and predicts that cytotoxic antibodies show a higher activity in such individuals. Indeed, cancer patients with the $Fc\gamma RIIIA^{158V}$ allele responded better to antibody therapy.[131–133] In autoimmune patients, the $Fc\gamma RIIIA^{158V}$ allele was linked to more severe arthritis in Caucasians.[134,135] In the majority of studies, however, the low-affinity alleles have been identified as risk factors for the development or severity of autoimmune disease. Several studies have found an association between low-affinity $Fc\gamma RIIIA^{158F}$ and $Fc\gamma RIIA^{131R}$ alleles and the incidence and severity of lupus nephritis and arthritis.[80,136–148] In addition, the low-affinity allele of human FcγRIIIB (FcγRIIIB-NA2) has been associated with SLE.[80,149,150] Alternatively, a low-copy-number polymorphism of this gene was associated with glomerulonephritis in humans and rats.[151] The results of these various studies suggest a model in which FcRs on macrophages or neutrophils might be involved in clearance of ICs containing potential autoantigens under non-inflammatory conditions, thereby preventing the initiation of autoimmune responses. Data from other model systems indicate that inefficient or delayed clearance of apoptotic cells can lead to the loss of tolerance and is associated with autoimmune diseases such as SLE.[23,152–154]

As described for FcγRIIB, a strong heterogeneity exists between different ethnicities and populations. For example, studies in African-American, Brazilian, German, and Thai populations have found significant associations between the $Fc\gamma RIIA^{131R}$ allele and SLE disease susceptibility or severity of nephritis.[80,137,139,140,142,144,147,148,155] Moreover, several studies in Caucasian, Dutch, and Korean populations have found associations between the $Fc\gamma RIIIA^{158F}$ allele and disease susceptibility and severity.[138,141,145,156] In addition, some studies found a connection between the FcγRIIIB-NA2 allele and SLE in Thai, Spanish, and Japanese populations.[80,149,150] In contrast, the $Fc\gamma RIIA^{131R}$ allele was not increased in SLE or nephritis in African-Caribbean, British, Dutch, Greek, Hispanic, Korean, and Spanish populations.[138,141,145,150,156–160] Similarly, studies in Chinese, German, and African-American populations found no associations between either the $Fc\gamma RIIIA^{158F}$ or the FcγRIIIB-NA2 allele.[80,138,142,149,155,161,162]

EXOGENOUS FACTORS MODULATING THE BALANCE: CYTOKINES AND SUGAR

Several studies have addressed the impact of cytokines on Fc receptor expression. Frequently, cytokines regulate expression of the associated signaling adaptors (β- and γ-chains) which leads to a concomitant change in α-chain expression, as shown for transforming growth factor β (TGF-β), IL-4, and IL-10.[163,164] Moreover, inflammatory cytokines/mediators, such as TNF-α, C5a, or LPS, tend to upregulate activating receptors such as Fcα, Fcε, and Fcγ receptors, whereas TH-2 cytokines such as TGF-β, IL-4, and IL-10 seem to decrease expression (Figure 11.2).[33,164,165] These effects can be cell type specific, as IL-4 upregulates the inhibitory FcγRIIB on myeloid cells but has the opposite effect on activated B cells.[166]

The outcome of cytokine-mediated changes in activating and inhibitory expression might vary depending on the differential regulation of IgG isotypes by the inhibitory Fc receptor. Thus, IgG_{2a} and to a lesser degree IgG_{2b} antibodies might be insensitive to elevated FcγRIIB expression, relative to the severe impairment of IgG_1 activity. During antibody-mediated inflammation, however, the steady-state ratios change in favor of the activating Fc receptors as the release of inflammatory mediators, such as IFN-γ and C5a, can upregulate

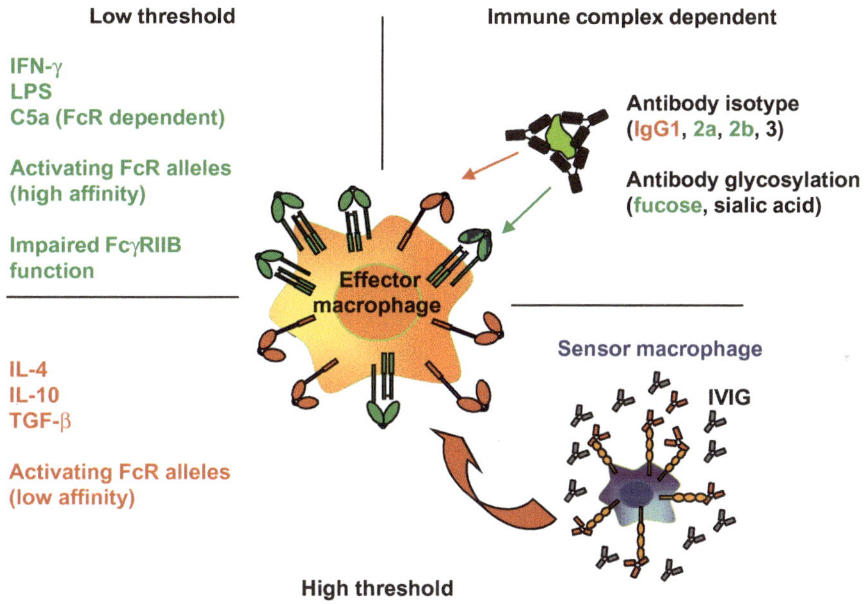

FIGURE 11.2 **Factors that influence FcR-dependent effector cell activation.** Factors that shift the balance toward cell activation or inhibition are shown in green or red, respectively. Inflammatory cytokines/mediators such as IFN-γ, LPS, or C5a upregulate activating FcRs (shown in green), result in a lower threshold for cell activation. In addition, allelic variants of activating and inhibitory receptors that influence antibody binding or FcR function might have similar effects. A higher threshold for cell activation is induced by antiinflammatory cytokines or therapeutics such as IVIG that upregulate the inhibitory FcγRIIB (shown in red). In addition, activating FcR alleles with low affinity for antibody isotypes will trigger activating signaling pathways less efficiently. Moreover, the composition of ICs with respect to antibody isotype and antibody glycosylation pattern determines if activating or inhibitory signals will dominate.

activating Fcγ receptors and at the same time reduce FcγRIIB expression levels.[167,168] Under these circumstances, autoreactive IgG_1 antibodies are capable of triggering severe damage. In fact, the regulation of FcR expression by cytokines is coupled with the regulation of isotypes by these same cytokines: TH-1 cytokines such as IFN-γ induce class switching to IgG_{2a}, TH-2-type cytokines (IL-4) induce class switching to IgG1, and TGF-β induces switching to IgG_{2b}.[169,170] Because these cytokines also influence Fc receptor expression, the pathogenicity of an autoimmune response will be determined by both cytokine-mediated regulation of class-switching and changes in expression levels of the responsible activating vs. inhibitory Fc receptors (Figure 11.2). This dual regulation might allow the development of new therapeutic strategies to treat autoimmune disease.

Another factor that can influence the interaction of antibodies with cellular FcRs is the sugar moiety attached to the asparagine residue at position 297 in the antibody Fc fragment. Deletion of this sugar side-chain results in loss of FcR binding.[171] In addition, this core sugar structure contains variable amounts of branching and terminal sugar residues such as *N*-acetylglucosamine, fucose, galactose, and sialic acid. The presence or absence of these terminal or branching sugar residues can significantly influence antibody–FcR interactions. Thus, antibodies without fucose bind approximately tenfold stronger to mouse activating FcγRIV and human FcγRIIIA.[172–174] In contrast, high levels of terminal sialic acid residues impair antibody binding to FcRs,[36] and there is evidence that antibody sialylation levels differ during an immune response. Antibodies from human arthritis patients and autoimmune mouse strains such as MRL/lpr have reduced amounts of terminal sialic acid and galactose and were found to be more pathogenic.[175–178] Similarly, murine serum IgG antibodies had reduced amounts of sialic acid after induction of nephrotoxic nephritis.[36] Taken together, these studies indicate that antibody sialylation represents another mechanism regulating antibody activity, and manipulating antibody sialylation levels *in vivo* might be a promising strategy to decrease autoantibody associated pathogenicity.

REGAINING THE BALANCE: THERAPEUTIC INTERVENTIONS THAT MODULATE FcR EXPRESSION

The most important question is how this information might be used to develop strategies that restore a balanced immune response and stop autoimmune processes. Regarding the lower expression level or functional impairment of the inhibitory receptor on B cells in SLE, one approach would be to restore FcγRIIB expression by gene transfer. This approach was recently tested in autoimmune prone mouse strains such as NZM, BXSB, and FcγRIIB knockout mice.[68] These animals had strongly reduced levels of autoantibodies and did not develop glomerulonephritis. Highlighting the threshold nature of autoimmunity, restoration of FcγRIIB expression on approximately 40% of peripheral B cells was sufficient to prevent the development of autoantibodies and autoimmune disease.[22,67,68]

Instead of gene transfer one could manipulate the expression level of activating and inhibitory receptors with antiinflammatory drugs. The successful use of high-dose intravenous immunoglobulin (IVIG) for the treatment of several autoimmune diseases provides an excellent example of the validity of this approach.

Currently, IVIG is used to alleviate autoimmune symptoms in SLE, Kawaski disease, and multiple sclerosis.[179] IVIG consists of the pooled serum IgG fraction of thousands of human donors and has to be given at high doses to obtain its beneficial antiinflammatory activity. Immunotherapeutic studies in mice and humans have shown that the Fc portion of IVIG antibodies is responsible for its activity.[108,113,180,181] Although several mechanisms of IVIG action have been proposed,[179,182–185] mounting evidence suggests that terminal sialic acid residues attached to the IgG sugar moiety, the inhibitory FcγRIIB, and SignR1/DC-Sign may be critical for the antiinflammatory activity of IVIG. Thus, IVIG infusion upregulated FcγRIIB expression on effector macrophages in mice and humans, resulted in a heightened threshold for cell activation (Figure 11.2). In addition, IVIG induced a significant reduction of the triggering activating FcγRIV in the NTN model, thus strongly modulating the balance of activating and inhibitory receptors.[73,108] Indeed, it was shown that a novel TH2 cytokine pathway may be responsible for this change in inhibitory and activatory FcgR expression.[186] A more detailed description of this novel antiinflammatory pathway can be found in Chapter 16 in this volume.

Consistently, adoptive transfer of DCs engineered to produce high levels of IL-4 blocked active arthritis in mice.[187,188] Besides modifying FcR expression levels, this would also skew the antibody response to IgG_1 rather than IgG_{2a} and IgG_{2b}, resulting in a more strict regulation by the inhibitory receptor. Moreover, IL-4 inhibits the TH-1 cytokines IL-2 and IFN-γ, thus suppressing inflammatory macrophage activation.

Whereas these previous approaches predominantly interfere with the effector phase of an autoimmune response, an alternative strategy would target DCs and thus block the initiation phase. Efficient work by the groups of Nussenzweig and Steinman suggests that targeting antigens to immature DCs *in vivo* results in the induction of tolerance.[85] Antigen targeting is achieved by genetic fusion to a DEC-205-specific antibody that selectively recognizes DCs. To prevent activation of DCs by cross-linking activating FcRs this antibody contains a mutation that abrogates FcR binding. With the current development of antibodies with preferential binding to activating or inhibitory FcRs one could generate a DEC-205 antibody that specifically engages FcγRIIB to deliver a strong tolerogenic signal and block the priming of autoreactive cells.

CONCLUSIONS

Research over the last years has provided important insights into the regulation of cell activation by cellular Fc receptors. Disturbing the threshold set by co-expression of activating and inhibitory FcRs results in an uncontrolled immune response, ultimately leading to the loss of tolerance and initiation of autoimmune pathology (Figure 11.2). The inhibitory FcγRIIB represents a distal checkpoint during B-cell development and regulates the expansion of autoreactive memory or plasma cells in mice and humans. In addition, it controls the activation of innate immune effector cells, including neutrophils, mast cells, and macrophages. Restoring FcγRIIB expression might be a promising strategy to interfere with self-destructive processes both in the initiation and effector phases of an autoimmune response. Despite disparate results between different human populations, the analysis of autoimmune patients has demonstrated that low-affinity allelic variants of activating FcRs are frequently associated with the severity or incidence of autoimmune diseases, suggesting that impaired removal of ICs by FcRs contributes to disease development. Finally, the antibody–FcR interaction is significantly influenced by the antibody glycosylation pattern. Autoimmune patients and mice with active autoimmune disease have antibodies with a lower level of terminal galactose and sialic acid, which enhances the interaction with cellular FcRs. Thus, influencing antibody glycosylation might be another strategy to interfere with autoimmune pathology.

Acknowledgments

This work was supported by grants from the German Research Foundation (DFG), the CAVD network within the Bill and Melinda Gates Foundation, and the Bavarian Genome Research Network. I apologize to all colleagues whose important work was not directly cited due to limitations of space. These references can be found in the numerous review articles referred to in this article.

References

1. Tsao BP. The genetics of human systemic lupus erythematosus. *Trends Immunol* 2003;**24**(11):595–602.
2. Bussel J. Treatment of immune thrombocytopenic purpura in adults. *Semin Hematol* 2006;**43**(3 Suppl. 5) S3–10; discussion S8–9.
3. Martin F, Chan AC. B cell immunobiology in disease: evolving concepts from the clinic. *Annu Rev Immunol* 2006;**24**:467–96.
4. Lanier LL. Face off—the interplay between activating and inhibitory immune receptors. *Curr Opin Immunol* 2001;**13**(3):326–31.
5. Goodnow CC, Sprent J, de St Groth BF, Vinuesa CG. Cellular and genetic mechanisms of self tolerance and autoimmunity. *Nature* 2005;**435**(7042):590–7.
6. Grimaldi CM, Hicks R, Diamond B. B cell selection and susceptibility to autoimmunity. *J Immunol* 2005;**174**(4):1775–81.
7. Meffre E, Casellas R, Nussenzweig MC. Antibody regulation of B cell development. *Nat Immunol* 2000;**1**(5):379–85.
8. Bona CA, Stevenson FK. B cells producing pathogenic autoantibodies. In: Honjo T, Alt FW, Neuberger MS, editors. *Molecular Biology of B Cells*. Boston: Elsevier; 2004. p. 381–402.
9. Ray SK, Putterman C, Diamond B. Pathogenic autoantibodies are routinely generated during the response to foreign antigen: a paradigm for autoimmune disease. *Proc Natl Acad Sci USA* 1996;**93**(5):2019–24.
10. Dijstelbloem HM, van de Winkel JG, Kallenberg CG. Inflammation in autoimmunity: receptors for IgG revisited. *Trends Immunol* 2001;**22**(9):510–6.
11. Nimmerjahn F, Ravetch JV. Fcgamma receptors: old friends and new family members. *Immunity* 2006;**24**(1):19–28.
12. Bolland S, Ravetch JV. Spontaneous autoimmune disease in Fc(gamma)RIIB-deficient mice results from strain-specific epistasis. *Immunity* 2000;**13**(2):277–85.
13. Nishimura H, Nose M, Hiai H, Minato N, Honjo T. Development of lupus-like autoimmune diseases by disruption of the PD-1 gene encoding an ITIM motif-carrying immunoreceptor. *Immunity* 1999;**11**(2):141–51.
14. O'Keefe TL, Williams GT, Batista FD, Neuberger MS. Deficiency in CD22, a B cell-specific inhibitory receptor, is sufficient to predispose to development of high affinity autoantibodies. *J Exp Med* 1999;**189**(8):1307–13.
15. Penninger JM, Timms E, Shahinian A, Jezo-Bremond A, Nishina H, Ionescu J, et al. Alloreactive gamma delta thymocytes utilize distinct costimulatory signals from peripheral T cells. *J Immunol* 1995;**155**(8):3847–55.
16. Takai T, Ono M, Hikida M, Ohmori H, Ravetch JV. Augmented humoral and anaphylactic responses in Fc gamma RII-deficient mice. *Nature* 1996;**379**(6563):346–9.
17. Tivol EA, Borriello F, Schweitzer AN, Lynch WP, Bluestone JA, Sharpe AH, et al. Loss of CTLA-4 leads to massive lymphoproliferation and fatal multiorgan tissue destruction, revealing a critical negative regulatory role of CTLA-4. *Immunity* 1995;**3**(5):541–7.
18. Ravetch JV, Lanier LL. Immune inhibitory receptors. *Science* 2000;**290**(5489):84–9.
19. Carroll MC. The complement system in regulation of adaptive immunity. *Nat Immunol* 2004;**5**(10):981–6.
20. Nguyen C, Limaye N, Wakeland EK. Susceptibility genes in the pathogenesis of murine lupus. *Arthritis Res* 2002;**4**(Suppl. 3):S255–63.
21. Takai T. Roles of Fc receptors in autoimmunity. *Nat Rev Immunol* 2002;**2**(8):580–92.
22. Ravetch JV. Fc receptors. In: Paul WE, editor. *Fundamental Immunology* 5th ed. Philadelphia: Lippincott-Raven; 2003. p. 685–700.
23. Hanayama R, Tanaka M, Miyasaka K, Aozasa K, Koike M, Uchiyama Y, et al. Autoimmune disease and impaired uptake of apoptotic cells in MFG-E8-deficient mice. *Science* 2004;**304**(5674):1147–50.
24. Qiu WQ, de Bruin D, Brownstein BH, Pearse R, Ravetch JV. Organization of the human and mouse low-affinity Fc gamma R genes: duplication and recombination. *Science* 1990;**248**(4956):732–5.
25. Moretta A, Bottino C, Vitale M, Pende D, Cantoni C, Mingari MC, et al. Activating receptors and coreceptors involved in human natural killer cell-mediated cytolysis. *Annu Rev Immunol* 2001;**19**:197–223.
26. Clynes R, Ravetch JV. Cytotoxic antibodies trigger inflammation through Fc receptors. *Immunity* 1995;**3**(1):21–6.
27. Park SY, Ueda S, Ohno H, Hamano Y, Tanaka M, Shiratori T, et al. Resistance of Fc receptor-deficient mice to fatal glomerulonephritis. *J Clin Invest* 1998;**102**(6):1229–38.
28. Sylvestre DL, Ravetch JV. Fc receptors initiate the Arthus reaction: redefining the inflammatory cascade. *Science* 1994;**265**(5175):1095–8.
29. Takai T, Li M, Sylvestre D, Clynes R, Ravetch JV. FcR gamma chain deletion results in pleiotrophic effector cell defects. *Cell* 1994;**76**(3):519–29.

30. Zhang M, Zhang Z, Garmestani K, Goldman CK, Ravetch JV, Brechbiel MW, et al. Activating Fc receptors are required for antitumor efficacy of the antibodies directed toward CD25 in a murine model of adult T-cell leukemia. *Cancer Res* 2004;**64**(16):5825–9.
31. Davis RS, Dennis Jr G, Odom MR, Gibson AW, Kimberly RP, Burrows PD, et al. Fc receptor homologs: newest members of a remarkably diverse Fc receptor gene family. *Immunol Rev* 2002;**190**:123–36.
32. Mechetina LV, Najakshin AM, Alabyev BY, Chikaev NA, Taranin AV. Identification of CD16-2, a novel mouse receptor homologous to CD16/Fc gamma RIII. *Immunogenetics* 2002;**54**(7):463–8.
33. Nimmerjahn F, Bruhns P, Horiuchi K, Ravetch JV. FcgammaRIV: a novel FcR with distinct IgG subclass specificity. *Immunity* 2005;**23**(1):41–51.
34. Hulett MD, Hogarth PM. Molecular basis of Fc receptor function. *Adv Immunol* 1994;**57**:1–127.
35. Ravetch JV, Kinet JP. Fc receptors. *Annu Rev Immunol.* 1991;**9**:457–92.
36. Kaneko Y, Nimmerjahn F, Ravetch JV. Anti-inflammatory activity of immunoglobulin G resulting from Fc sialylation. *Science* 2006;**313**(5787):670–3.
37. Galli SJ, Kalesnikoff J, Grimbaldeston MA, Piliponsky AM, Williams CM, Tsai M. Mast cells as "tunable" effector and immunoregulatory cells: recent advances. *Annu Rev Immunol* 2005;**23**:749–86.
38. Gould HJ, Sutton BJ, Beavil AJ, Beavil RL, McCloskey N, Coker HA, et al. The biology of IGE and the basis of allergic disease. *Annu Rev Immunol* 2003;**21**:579–628.
39. Torigoe C, Inman JK, Metzger H. An unusual mechanism for ligand antagonism. *Science* 1998;**281**(5376):568–72.
40. Lang ML, Shen L, Wade WF. Gamma-chain dependent recruitment of tyrosine kinases to membrane rafts by the human IgA receptor Fc alpha R. *J Immunol* 1999;**163**(10):5391–8.
41. Gulle H, Samstag A, Eibl MM, Wolf HM. Physical and functional association of Fc alpha R with protein tyrosine kinase Lyn. *Blood* 1998;**91**(2):383–91.
42. Launay P, Grossetete B, Arcos-Fajardo M, Gaudin E, Torres SP, Beaudoin L, et al. Fcalpha receptor (CD89) mediates the development of immunoglobulin A (IgA) nephropathy (Berger's disease). Evidence for pathogenic soluble receptor–Iga complexes in patients and CD89 transgenic mice. *J Exp Med* 2000;**191**(11):1999–2009.
43. Park RK, Izadi KD, Deo YM, Durden DL. Role of Src in the modulation of multiple adaptor proteins in FcalphaRI oxidant signaling. *Blood* 1999;**94**(6):2112–20.
44. Daeron M. Fc receptor biology. *Annu Rev Immunol.* 1997;**15**:203–34.
45. Bolland S, Ravetch JV. Inhibitory pathways triggered by ITIM-containing receptors. *Adv Immunol* 1999;**72**:149–77.
46. Daeron M, Lesourne R. Negative signaling in Fc receptor complexes. *Adv Immunol* 2006;**89**:39–86.
47. Pearse RN, Kawabe T, Bolland S, Guinamard R, Kurosaki T, Ravetch JV. SHIP recruitment attenuates Fc gamma RIIB-induced B cell apoptosis. *Immunity* 1999;**10**(6):753–60.
48. Tzeng SJ, Bolland S, Inabe K, Kurosaki T, Pierce SK. The B cell inhibitory Fc receptor triggers apoptosis by a novel c-Abl-family kinase dependent pathway. *J Biol Chem* 2005;**22**:22.
49. Xiang Z, Cutler AJ, Brownlie RJ, Fairfax K, Lawlor KE, Severinson E, et al. FcgammaRIIb controls bone marrow plasma cell persistence and apoptosis. *Nat Immunol* 2007;**8**(4):419–29.
50. Wijngaarden S, van de Winkel JG, Jacobs KM, Bijlsma JW, Lafeber FP, van Roon JA. A shift in the balance of inhibitory and activating Fcgamma receptors on monocytes toward the inhibitory Fcgamma receptor IIb is associated with prevention of monocyte activation in rheumatoid arthritis. *Arthritis Rheum* 2004;**50**(12):3878–87.
51. de Haas M, Kleijer M, van Zwieten R, Roos D, von dem Borne AE. Neutrophil Fc gamma RIIIb deficiency, nature, and clinical consequences: a study of 21 individuals from 14 families. *Blood* 1995;**86**(6):2403–13.
52. Clark MR, Liu L, Clarkson SB, Ory PA, Goldstein IM. An abnormality of the gene that encodes neutrophil Fc receptor III in a patient with systemic lupus erythematosus. *J Clin Invest* 1990;**86**(1):341–6.
53. Huizinga TW, Kuijpers RW, Kleijer M, Schulpen TW, Cuypers HT, Roos D, et al. Maternal genomic neutrophil FcRIII deficiency leading to neonatal isoimmune neutropenia. *Blood* 1990;**76**(10):1927–32.
54. van de Winkel JG, de Wit TP, Ernst LK, Capel PJ, Ceuppens JL. Molecular basis for a familial defect in phagocyte expression of IgG receptor I (CD64). *J Immunol* 1995;**154**(6):2896–903.
55. Nitschke L, Tsubata T. Molecular interactions regulate BCR signal inhibition by CD22 and CD72. *Trends Immunol* 2004;**25**(10):543–50.
56. Ravetch JV, Bolland S. IgG Fc receptors. *Annu Rev Immunol.* 2001;**19**:275–90.
57. Boross P, Arandhara VL, Martin-Ramirez J, Santiago-Raber ML, Carlucci F, Flierman R, et al. The inhibiting Fc receptor for IgG, FcgammaRIIB, is a modifier of autoimmune susceptibility. *J Immunol* 2011;**187**(3):1304–13.
58. Bolland S, Yim YS, Tus K, Wakeland EK, Ravetch JV. Genetic modifiers of systemic lupus erythematosus in FcgammaRIIB(−/−) mice. *J Exp Med* 2002;**195**(9):1167–74.
59. Okazaki T, Otaka Y, Wang J, Hiai H, Takai T, Ravetch JV, et al. Hydronephrosis associated with antiurothelial and antinuclear autoantibodies in

BALB/c-Fcgr2b−/−Pdcd1−/− mice. *J Exp Med* 2005;**202**(12):1643–8.
60. Clynes R, Calvani N, Croker BP, Richards HB. Modulation of the immune response in pristane-induced lupus by expression of activation and inhibitory Fc receptors. *Clin Exp Immunol* 2005;**141**(2):230–7.
61. Fukuyama H, Nimmerjahn F, Ravetch JV. The inhibitory Fcgamma receptor modulates autoimmunity by limiting the accumulation of immunoglobulin G+ anti-DNA plasma cells. *Nat Immunol* 2005;**6**(1):99–106.
62. Witsch EJ, Cao H, Fukuyama H, Weigert M. Light chain editing generates polyreactive antibodies in chronic graft-versus-host reaction. *J Exp Med* 2006;**203**(7):1761–72.
63. Jiang Y, Hirose S, Abe M, Sanokawa-Akakura R, Ohtsuji M, Mi X, et al. Polymorphisms in IgG Fc receptor IIB regulatory regions associated with autoimmune susceptibility. *Immunogenetics* 2000;**51**(6):429–35.
64. Jiang Y, Hirose S, Sanokawa-Akakura R, Abe M, Mi X, Li N, et al. Genetically determined aberrant down-regulation of FcgammaRIIB1 in germinal center B cells associated with hyper-IgG and IgG autoantibodies in murine systemic lupus erythematosus. *Int Immunol* 1999;**11**(10):1685–91.
65. Pritchard NR, Cutler AJ, Uribe S, Chadban SJ, Morley BJ, Smith KG. Autoimmune-prone mice share a promoter haplotype associated with reduced expression and function of the Fc receptor FcgammaRII. *Curr Biol* 2000;**10**(4):227–30.
66. Xiu Y, Nakamura K, Abe M, Li N, Wen XS, Jiang Y, et al. Transcriptional regulation of Fcgr2b gene by polymorphic promoter region and its contribution to humoral immune responses. *J Immunol* 2002;**169**(8):4340–6.
67. Brownlie RJ, Lawlor KE, Niederer HA, Cutler AJ, Xiang Z, Clatworthy MR, et al. Distinct cell-specific control of autoimmunity and infection by FcgammaRIIb. *J Exp Med* 2008;**205**(4):883–95.
68. McGaha TL, Sorrentino B, Ravetch JV. Restoration of tolerance in lupus by targeted inhibitory receptor expression. *Science* 2005;**307**(5709):590–3.
69. Blank MC, Stefanescu RN, Masuda E, Marti F, King PD, Redecha PB, et al. Decreased transcription of the human *Fcgr2b* gene mediated by the C343 G/C promoter polymorphism and association with systemic lupus erythematosus. *Hum Genet* 2005;**117**(2–3):220–7.
70. Mackay M, Stanevsky A, Wang T, Aranow C, Li M, Koenig S, et al. Selective dysregulation of the Fc{gamma}IIB receptor on memory B cells in SLE. *J Exp Med* 2006;**203**(9):2157–64.
71. Su K, Li X, Edberg JC, Wu J, Ferguson P, Kimberly RP. A promoter haplotype of the immunoreceptor tyrosine-based inhibitory motif-bearing FcgammaRIIb alters receptor expression and associates with autoimmunity. II. Differential binding of GATA4 and Yin-Yang1 transcription factors and correlated receptor expression and function. *J Immunol* 2004;**172**(11):7192–9.
72. Su K, Wu J, Edberg JC, Li X, Ferguson P, Cooper GS, et al. A promoter haplotype of the immunoreceptor tyrosine-based inhibitory motif-bearing FcgammaRIIb alters receptor expression and associates with autoimmunity. I. Regulatory FCGR2B polymorphisms and their association with systemic lupus erythematosus. *J Immunol* 2004;**172**(11):7186–91.
73. Tackenberg B, Jelcic I, Baerenwaldt A, Oertel WH, Sommer N, Nimmerjahn F, et al. Impaired inhibitory Fc gamma receptor IIB expression on B cells in chronic inflammatory demyelinating polyneuropathy. *Proc Natl Acad Sci USA* 2009;**106**(12):4788–92.
74. Enyedy EJ, Mitchell JP, Nambiar MP, Tsokos GC. Defective FcgammaRIIb1 signaling contributes to enhanced calcium response in B cells from patients with systemic lupus erythematosus. *Clin Immunol* 2001;**101**(2):130–5.
75. Boruchov AM, Heller G, Veri MC, Bonvini E, Ravetch JV, Young JW. Activating and inhibitory IgG Fc receptors on human DCs mediate opposing functions. *J Clin Invest* 2005;**15**:15.
76. Baerenwaldt A, Lux A, Danzer H, Spriewald BM, Ullrich E, Heidkamp G, et al. Fcgamma receptor IIB (FcgammaRIIB) maintains humoral tolerance in the human immune system *in vivo*. *Proc Natl Acad Sci USA* 2011;**108**(46):18772–7.
77. Li X, Wu J, Carter RH, Edberg JC, Su K, Cooper GS, et al. A novel polymorphism in the Fcgamma receptor IIB (CD32B) transmembrane region alters receptor signaling. *Arthritis Rheum* 2003;**48**(11):3242–52.
78. Floto RA, Clatworthy MR, Heilbronn KR, Rosner DR, MacAry PA, Rankin A, et al. Loss of function of a lupus-associated FcgammaRIIb polymorphism through exclusion from lipid rafts. *Nat Med* 2005;**11**(10):1056–8.
79. Kono H, Kyogoku C, Suzuki T, Tsuchiya N, Honda H, Yamamoto K, et al. FcgammaRIIB Ile232Thr transmembrane polymorphism associated with human systemic lupus erythematosus decreases affinity to lipid rafts and attenuates inhibitory effects on B cell receptor signaling. *Hum Mol Genet* 2005;**14**(19):2881–92.
80. Siriboonrit U, Tsuchiya N, Sirikong M, Kyogoku C, Bejrachandra S, Suthipinittharm P, et al. Association of Fcgamma receptor IIb and IIIb polymorphisms with susceptibility to systemic lupus erythematosus in Thais. *Tissue Antigens* 2003;**61**(5):374–83.
81. Chu ZT, Tsuchiya N, Kyogoku C, Ohashi J, Qian YP, Xu SB, et al. Association of Fcgamma receptor

IIb polymorphism with susceptibility to systemic lupus erythematosus in Chinese: a common susceptibility gene in the Asian populations. *Tissue Antigens* 2004;**63**(1):21–7.
82. Kyogoku C, Dijstelbloem HM, Tsuchiya N, Hatta Y, Kato H, Yamaguchi A, et al. Fcgamma receptor gene polymorphisms in Japanese patients with systemic lupus erythematosus: contribution of FCGR2B to genetic susceptibility. *Arthritis Rheum* 2002;**46**(5):1242–54.
83. Tsuchiya N, Kyogoku C. Role of Fc gamma receptor IIb polymorphism in the genetic background of systemic lupus erythematosus: insights from Asia. *Autoimmunity* 2005;**38**(5):347–52.
84. Willcocks LC, Carr EJ, Niederer HA, Rayner TF, Williams TN, Yang W, et al. A defunctioning polymorphism in FCGR2B is associated with protection against malaria but susceptibility to systemic lupus erythematosus. *Proc Natl Acad Sci USA* 2010;**107**(17):7881–5.
85. Steinman RM, Hawiger D, Liu K, Bonifaz L, Bonnyay D, Mahnke K, et al. Dendritic cell function *in vivo* during the steady state: a role in peripheral tolerance. *Ann NY Acad Sci* 2003;**987**:15–25.
86. Dhodapkar KM, Krasovsky J, Williamson B, Dhodapkar MV. Antitumor monoclonal antibodies enhance cross-presentation of cellular antigens and the generation of myeloma-specific killer T cells by dendritic cells. *J Exp Med* 2002;**195**(1):125–33.
87. Groh V, Li YQ, Cioca D, Hunder NN, Wang W, Riddell SR, et al. Efficient cross-priming of tumor antigen-specific T cells by dendritic cells sensitized with diverse anti-MICA opsonized tumor cells. *Proc Natl Acad Sci USA* 2005;**102**(18):6461–6.
88. Rafiq K, Bergtold A, Clynes R. Immune complex-mediated antigen presentation induces tumor immunity. *J Clin Invest* 2002;**110**(1):71–9.
89. Regnault A, Lankar D, Lacabanne V, Rodriguez A, Thery C, Rescigno M, et al. Fcgamma receptor-mediated induction of dendritic cell maturation and major histocompatibility complex class I-restricted antigen presentation after immune complex internalization. *J Exp Med* 1999;**189**(2):371–80.
90. Dhodapkar KM, Kaufman JL, Ehlers M, Banerjee DK, Bonvini E, Koenig S, et al. Selective blockade of inhibitory Fcgamma receptor enables human dendritic cell maturation with IL-12p70 production and immunity to antibody-coated tumor cells. *Proc Natl Acad Sci USA* 2005;**102**(8):2910–5.
91. Kalergis AM, Ravetch JV. Inducing tumor immunity through the selective engagement of activating Fcgamma receptors on dendritic cells. *J Exp Med* 2002;**195**(12):1653–9.
92. Samsom JN, van Berkel LA, van Helvoort JM, Unger WW, Jansen W, Thepen T, et al. Fc gamma RIIB regulates nasal and oral tolerance: a role for dendritic cells. *J Immunol* 2005;**174**(9):5279–87.
93. Bergtold A, Desai DD, Gavhane A, Clynes R. Cell surface recycling of internalized antigen permits dendritic cell priming of B cells. *Immunity* 2005;**23**(5):503–14.
94. Kushnir N, Liu L, MacPherson GG. Dendritic cells and resting B cells form clusters *in vitro* and *in vivo*: T cell independence, partial LFA-1 dependence, and regulation by cross-linking surface molecules. *J Immunol* 1998;**160**(4):1774–81.
95. Wykes M, Pombo A, Jenkins C, MacPherson GG. Dendritic cells interact directly with naive B lymphocytes to transfer antigen and initiate class switching in a primary T-dependent response. *J Immunol* 1998;**161**(3):1313–9.
96. Delamarre L, Pack M, Chang H, Mellman I, Trombetta ES. Differential lysosomal proteolysis in antigen-presenting cells determines antigen fate. *Science* 2005;**307**(5715):1630–4.
97. Kraft S, Novak N. Fc receptors as determinants of allergic reactions. *Trends Immunol* 2006;**27**(2):88–95.
98. Yuasa T, Kubo S, Yoshino T, Ujike A, Matsumura K, Ono M, et al. Deletion of fcgamma receptor IIB renders H-2(b) mice susceptible to collagen-induced arthritis. *J Exp Med* 1999;**189**(1):187–94.
99. Coutelier JP, van der Logt JT, Heessen FW, Warnier G, Van Snick J. IgG2a restriction of murine antibodies elicited by viral infections. *J Exp Med* 1987;**165**(1):64–9.
100. Fossati-Jimack L, Ioan-Facsinay A, Reininger L, Chicheportiche Y, Watanabe N, Saito T, et al. Markedly different pathogenicity of four immunoglobulin G isotype-switch variants of an antierythrocyte autoantibody is based on their capacity to interact *in vivo* with the low-affinity Fcgamma receptor III. *J Exp Med* 2000;**191**(8):1293–302.
101. Hamaguchi Y, Xiu Y, Komura K, Nimmerjahn F, Tedder TF. Antibody isotype-specific engagement of Fcgamma receptors regulates B lymphocyte depletion during CD20 immunotherapy. *J Exp Med* 2006;**203**(3):743–53.
102. Kipps TJ, Parham P, Punt J, Herzenberg LA. Importance of immunoglobulin isotype in human antibody-dependent, cell-mediated cytotoxicity directed by murine monoclonal antibodies. *J Exp Med* 1985;**161**(1):1–17.
103. Markine-Goriaynoff D, Coutelier JP. Increased efficacy of the immunoglobulin G2a subclass in antibody-mediated protection against lactate dehydrogenase-elevating virus-induced polioencephalomyelitis revealed with switch mutants. *J Virol* 2002;**76**(1):432–5.

104. Nimmerjahn F, Ravetch JV. Divergent immunoglobulin g subclass activity through selective Fc receptor binding. *Science* 2005;**310**(5753):1510–2.
105. Schlageter AM, Kozel TR. Opsonization of *Cryptococcus neoformans* by a family of isotype-switch variant antibodies specific for the capsular polysaccharide. *Infect Immun* 1990;**58**(6):1914–8.
106. Taborda CP, Rivera J, Zaragoza O, Casadevall A. More is not necessarily better: prozone-like effects in passive immunization with IgG. *J Immunol* 2003;**170**(7):3621–30.
107. Uchida J, Hamaguchi Y, Oliver JA, Ravetch JV, Poe JC, Haas KM, et al. The innate mononuclear phagocyte network depletes B lymphocytes through Fc receptor-dependent mechanisms during anti-CD20 antibody immunotherapy. *J Exp Med* 2004;**199**(12):1659–69.
108. Kaneko Y, Nimmerjahn F, Madaio MP, Ravetch JV. Pathology and protection in nephrotoxic nephritis is determined by selective engagement of specific Fc receptors. *J Exp Med* 2006;**203**(3):789–97.
109. Bijl M, Dijstelbloem HM, Oost WW, Bootsma H, Derksen RH, Aten J, et al. IgG subclass distribution of autoantibodies differs between renal and extra-renal relapses in patients with systemic lupus erythematosus. *Rheumatology (Oxford)* 2002;**41**(1):62–7.
110. Imai H, Hamai K, Komatsuda A, Ohtani H, Miura AB. IgG subclasses in patients with membranoproliferative glomerulonephritis, membranous nephropathy, and lupus nephritis. *Kidney Int* 1997;**51**(1):270–6.
111. Winkler TH, Henschel TA, Kalies I, Baenkler HW, Skvaril F, Kalden JR. Constant isotype pattern of anti-dsDNA antibodies in patients with systemic lupus erythematosus. *Clin Exp Immunol* 1988;**72**(3):434–9.
112. Loizou S, Cofiner C, Weetman AP, Walport MJ. Immunoglobulin class and IgG subclass distribution of anticardiolipin antibodies in patients with systemic lupus erythematosus and associated disorders. *Clin Exp Immunol* 1992;**90**(3):434–9.
113. Bruhns P, Samuelsson A, Pollard JW, Ravetch JV. Colony-stimulating factor-1-dependent macrophages are responsible for IVIG protection in antibody-induced autoimmune disease. *Immunity* 2003;**18**(4):573–81.
114. Hazenbos WL, Gessner JE, Hofhuis FM, Kuipers H, Meyer D, Heijnen IA, et al. Impaired IgG-dependent anaphylaxis and Arthus reaction in Fc gamma RIII (CD16) deficient mice. *Immunity* 1996;**5**(2):181–8.
115. Hazenbos WL, Heijnen IA, Meyer D, Hofhuis FM, Renardel de Lavalette CR, Schmidt RE, et al. Murine IgG1 complexes trigger immune effector functions predominantly via Fc gamma RIII (CD16). *J Immunol* 1998;**161**(6):3026–32.
116. Ji H, Ohmura K, Mahmood U, Lee DM, Hofhuis FM, Boackle SA, et al. Arthritis critically dependent on innate immune system players. *Immunity* 2002;**16**(2):157–68.
117. Meyer D, Schiller C, Westermann J, Izui S, Hazenbos WL, Verbeek JS, et al. FcgammaRIII (CD16)-deficient mice show IgG isotype-dependent protection to experimental autoimmune hemolytic anemia. *Blood* 1998;**92**(11):3997–4002.
118. Biburger M, Aschermann S, Schwab I, Lux A, Albert H, Danzer H, et al. Monocyte subsets responsible for immunoglobulin G-dependent effector functions *in vivo*. *Immunity* 2011;**35**(6):932–44.
119. Clynes R, Dumitru C, Ravetch JV. Uncoupling of immune complex formation and kidney damage in autoimmune glomerulonephritis. *Science* 1998;**279**(5353):1052–4.
120. Clynes R, Maizes JS, Guinamard R, Ono M, Takai T, Ravetch JV. Modulation of immune complex-induced inflammation *in vivo* by the coordinate expression of activation and inhibitory Fc receptors. *J Exp Med* 1999;**189**(1):179–85.
121. Sylvestre D, Clynes R, Ma M, Warren H, Carroll MC, Ravetch JV. Immunoglobulin G-mediated inflammatory responses develop normally in complement-deficient mice. *J Exp Med* 1996;**184**(6):2385–92.
122. Kasperkiewicz M, Nimmerjahn F, Wende S, Hirose M, Iwata H, Jonkman MF, et al. Genetic identification and functional validation of FcgammaRIV as key molecule in autoantibody-induced tissue injury. *J Pathol* 2012;**228**(1):8–19.
123. Beers SA, Chan CH, James S, French RR, Attfield KE, Brennan CM, et al. Type II (tositumomab) anti-CD20 monoclonal antibody out performs type I (rituximab-like) reagents in B-cell depletion regardless of complement activation. *Blood* 2008;**112**(10):4170–7.
124. Barnes N, Gavin AL, Tan PS, Mottram P, Koentgen F, Hogarth PM. FcgammaRI-deficient mice show multiple alterations to inflammatory and immune responses. *Immunity* 2002;**16**(3):379–89.
125. Bevaart L, Jansen MJ, van Vugt MJ, Verbeek JS, van de Winkel JG, Leusen JH. The high-affinity IgG receptor, FcgammaRI, plays a central role in antibody therapy of experimental melanoma. *Cancer Res* 2006;**66**(3):1261–4.
126. Ioan-Facsinay A, de Kimpe SJ, Hellwig SM, van Lent PL, Hofhuis FM, van Ojik HH, et al. FcgammaRI (CD64) contributes substantially to severity of arthritis, hypersensitivity responses, and protection from bacterial infection. *Immunity* 2002;**16**(3):391–402.
127. Azeredo da Silveira S, Kikuchi S, Fossati-Jimack L, Moll T, Saito T, Verbeek JS, et al. Complement activation selectively potentiates the pathogenicity of the

IgG2b and IgG3 isotypes of a high affinity anti-erythrocyte autoantibody. *J Exp Med* 2002;**195**(6):665–72.
128. Kumar V, Ali SR, Konrad S, Zwirner J, Verbeek JS, Schmidt RE, et al. Cell-derived anaphylatoxins as key mediators of antibody-dependent type II autoimmunity in mice. *J Clin Invest* 2006;**116**(2):512–20.
129. Schmidt RE, Gessner JE. Fc receptors and their interaction with complement in autoimmunity. *Immunol Lett* 2005;**100**(1):56–67.
130. Mihai S, Nimmerjahn F. The role of Fc receptors and complement in autoimmunity. *Autoimmun Rev* 2012 Nov 29.
131. Cartron G, Dacheux L, Salles G, Solal-Celigny P, Bardos P, Colombat P, et al. Therapeutic activity of humanized anti-CD20 monoclonal antibody and polymorphism in IgG Fc receptor FcgammaRIIIa gene. *Blood* 2002;**99**(3):754–8.
132. Weng WK, Czerwinski D, Timmerman J, Hsu FJ, Levy R. Clinical outcome of lymphoma patients after idiotype vaccination is correlated with humoral immune response and immunoglobulin G Fc receptor genotype. *J Clin Oncol* 2004;**22**(23):4717–24.
133. Weng WK, Levy R. Two immunoglobulin G fragment C receptor polymorphisms independently predict response to rituximab in patients with follicular lymphoma. *J Clin Oncol* 2003;**21**(21):3940–7.
134. Morgan AW, Griffiths B, Ponchel F, Montague BM, Ali M, Gardner PP, et al. Fcgamma receptor type IIIA is associated with rheumatoid arthritis in two distinct ethnic groups. *Arthritis Rheum* 2000;**43**(10):2328–34.
135. Morgan AW, Keyte VH, Babbage SJ, Robinson JI, Ponchel F, Barrett JH, et al. FcgammaRIIIA-158V and rheumatoid arthritis: a confirmation study. *Rheumatology (Oxford)* 2003;**42**(4):528–33.
136. Magnusson V, Johanneson B, Lima G, Odeberg J, Alarcon-Segovia D, Alarcon-Riquelme ME. Both risk alleles for FcgammaRIIA and FcgammaRIIIA are susceptibility factors for SLE: a unifying hypothesis. *Genes Immun* 2004;**5**(2):130–7.
137. Bazilio AP, Viana VS, Toledo R, Woronik V, Bonfa E, Monteiro RC. Fc gamma RIIa polymorphism: a susceptibility factor for immune complex-mediated lupus nephritis in Brazilian patients. *Nephrol Dial Transplant* 2004;**19**(6):1427–31.
138. Dijstelbloem HM, Bijl M, Fijnheer R, Scheepers RH, Oost WW, Jansen MD, et al. Fcgamma receptor polymorphisms in systemic lupus erythematosus: association with disease and *in vivo* clearance of immune complexes. *Arthritis Rheum* 2000;**43**(12):2793–800.
139. Dijstelbloem HM, Hepkema BG, Kallenberg CG, van der Linden MW, Keijsers V, Huizinga TW, et al. The R-H polymorphism of FCgamma receptor IIa as a risk factor for systemic lupus erythematosus is independent of single-nucleotide polymorphisms in the interleukin-10 gene promoter. *Arthritis Rheum* 2002;**46**(4):1125–6.
140. Gelmetti AP, Freitas AC, Woronik V, Barros RT, Bonfa E, Monteiro RC. Polymorphism of the FcgammaRIIalpha IgG receptor in patients with lupus nephritis and glomerulopathy. *J Rheumatol* 2006;**33**(3):523–30.
141. Koene HR, Kleijer M, Swaak AJ, Sullivan KE, Bijl M, Petri MA, et al. The Fc gammaRIIIA-158F allele is a risk factor for systemic lupus erythematosus. *Arthritis Rheum* 1998;**41**(10):1813–8.
142. Manger K, Repp R, Jansen M, Geisselbrecht M, Wassmuth R, Westerdaal NA, et al. Fcgamma receptor IIa, IIIa, and IIIb polymorphisms in German patients with systemic lupus erythematosus: association with clinical symptoms. *Ann Rheum Dis* 2002;**61**(9):786–92.
143. Nieto A, Caliz R, Pascual M, Mataran L, Garcia S, Martin J. Involvement of Fcgamma receptor IIIA genotypes in susceptibility to rheumatoid arthritis. *Arthritis Rheum* 2000;**43**(4):735–9.
144. Salmon JE, Millard S, Schachter LA, Arnett FC, Ginzler EM, Gourley MF, et al. Fc gamma RIIA alleles are heritable risk factors for lupus nephritis in African Americans. *J Clin Invest* 1996;**97**(5):1348–54.
145. Seligman VA, Suarez C, Lum R, Inda SE, Lin D, Li H, et al. The Fcgamma receptor IIIA-158F allele is a major risk factor for the development of lupus nephritis among Caucasians but not non-Caucasians. *Arthritis Rheum* 2001;**44**(3):618–25.
146. Tanaka Y, Suzuki Y, Tsuge T, Kanamaru Y, Horikoshi S, Monteiro RC, et al. FcgammaRIIa-131R allele and FcgammaRIIIa-176V/V genotype are risk factors for progression of IgA nephropathy. *Nephrol Dial Transplant* 2005;**20**(11):2439–45.
147. Yun HR, Koh HK, Kim SS, Chung WT, Kim DW, Hong KP, et al. FcgammaRIIa/IIIa polymorphism and its association with clinical manifestations in Korean lupus patients. *Lupus* 2001;**10**(7):466–72.
148. Zuniga R, Ng S, Peterson MG, Reveille JD, Baethge BA, Alarcon GS, et al. Low-binding alleles of Fcgamma receptor types IIA and IIIA are inherited independently and are associated with systemic lupus erythematosus in Hispanic patients. *Arthritis Rheum* 2001;**44**(2):361–7.
149. Gonzalez-Escribano MF, Aguilar F, Sanchez-Roman J, Nunez-Roldan A. FcgammaRIIA, FcgammaRIIIA and FcgammaRIIIB polymorphisms in Spanish patients with systemic lupus erythematosus. *Eur J Immunogenet* 2002;**29**(4):301–6.
150. Hatta Y, Tsuchiya N, Ohashi J, Matsushita M, Fujiwara K, Hagiwara K, et al. Association of Fc gamma receptor IIIB, but not of Fc gamma receptor

IIA and IIIA polymorphisms with systemic lupus erythematosus in Japanese. *Genes Immun* 1999;**1**(1):53–60.
151. Aitman TJ, Dong R, Vyse TJ, Norsworthy PJ, Johnson MD, Smith J, et al. Copy number polymorphism in Fcgr3 predisposes to glomerulonephritis in rats and humans. *Nature* 2006;**439**(7078):851–5.
152. Davies KA, Peters AM, Beynon HL, Walport MJ. Immune complex processing in patients with systemic lupus erythematosus. *In vivo* imaging and clearance studies. *J Clin Invest* 1992;**90**(5):2075–83.
153. Herrmann M, Voll RE, Zoller OM, Hagenhofer M, Ponner BB, Kalden JR. Impaired phagocytosis of apoptotic cell material by monocyte-derived macrophages from patients with systemic lupus erythematosus. *Arthritis Rheum* 1998;**41**(7):1241–50.
154. Potter PK, Cortes-Hernandez J, Quartier P, Botto M, Walport MJ. Lupus-prone mice have an abnormal response to thioglycolate and an impaired clearance of apoptotic cells. *J Immunol* 2003;**170**(6):3223–32.
155. Lee HS, Chung YH, Kim TG, Kim TH, Jun JB, Jung S, et al. Independent association of HLA-DR and FCgamma receptor polymorphisms in Korean patients with systemic lupus erythematosus. *Rheumatology (Oxford)* 2003;**42**(12):1501–7.
156. Salmon JE, Ng S, Yoo DH, Kim TH, Kim SY, Song GG. Altered distribution of Fcgamma receptor IIIA alleles in a cohort of Korean patients with lupus nephritis. *Arthritis Rheum* 1999;**42**(4):818–9.
157. Villarreal J, Crosdale D, Ollier W, Hajeer A, Thomson W, Ordi J, et al. Mannose binding lectin and FcgammaRIIa (CD32) polymorphism in Spanish systemic lupus erythematosus patients. *Rheumatology (Oxford)* 2001;**40**(9):1009–12.
158. Botto M, Theodoridis E, Thompson EM, Beynon HL, Briggs D, Isenberg DA, et al. Fc gamma RIIa polymorphism in systemic lupus erythematosus (SLE): no association with disease. *Clin Exp Immunol* 1996;**104**(2):264–8.
159. Smyth LJ, Snowden N, Carthy D, Papasteriades C, Hajeer A, Ollier WE. Fc gamma RIIa polymorphism in systemic lupus erythematosus. *Ann Rheum Dis* 1997;**56**(12):744–6.
160. Yap SN, Phipps ME, Manivasagar M, Tan SY, Bosco JJ. Human Fc gamma receptor IIA (FcgammaRIIA) genotyping and association with systemic lupus erythematosus (SLE) in Chinese and Malays in Malaysia. *Lupus* 1999;**8**(4):305–10.
161. Oh M, Petri MA, Kim NA, Sullivan KE. Frequency of the Fc gamma RIIIA-158F allele in African American patients with systemic lupus erythematosus. *J Rheumatol* 1999;**26**(7):1486–9.
162. Yap SN, Phipps ME, Manivasagar M, Bosco JJ. Fc gamma receptor IIIB-NA gene frequencies in patients with systemic lupus erythematosus and healthy individuals of Malay and Chinese ethnicity. *Immunol Lett* 1999;**68**(2–3):295–300.
163. Gillespie SR, DeMartino RR, Zhu J, Chong HJ, Ramirez C, Shelburne CP, et al. IL-10 inhibits Fc epsilon RI expression in mouse mast cells. *J Immunol* 2004;**172**(5):3181–8.
164. Tridandapani S, Wardrop R, Baran CP, Wang Y, Opalek JM, Caligiuri MA, et al. TGF-beta 1 suppresses myeloid Fc gamma receptor function by regulating the expression and function of the common gamma-subunit. *J Immunol* 2003;**170**(9):4572–7.
165. Otten MA, van Egmond M. The Fc receptor for IgA (FcalphaRI, CD89). *Immunol Lett* 2004;**92**(1–2):23–31.
166. Rudge EU, Cutler AJ, Pritchard NR, Smith KG. Interleukin 4 reduces expression of inhibitory receptors on B cells and abolishes CD22 and Fc gamma RII-mediated B cell suppression. *J Exp Med* 2002;**195**(8):1079–85.
167. Guyre PM, Morganelli PM, Miller R. Recombinant immune interferon increases immunoglobulin G Fc receptors on cultured human mononuclear phagocytes. *J Clin Invest* 1983;**72**(1):393–7.
168. Shushakova N, Skokowa J, Schulman J, Baumann U, Zwirner J, Schmidt RE, et al. C5a anaphylatoxin is a major regulator of activating versus inhibitory FcgammaRs in immune complex-induced lung disease. *J Clin Invest* 2002;**110**(12):1823–30.
169. Coffman RL, Savelkoul HF, Lebman DA. Cytokine regulation of immunoglobulin isotype switching and expression. *Semin Immunol* 1989;**1**(1):55–63.
170. Finkelman FD, Holmes J, Katona IM, Urban Jr JF, Beckmann MP, Park LS, et al. Lymphokine control of *in vivo* immunoglobulin isotype selection. *Annu Rev Immunol* 1990;**8**:303–33.
171. Shields RL, Namenuk AK, Hong K, Meng YG, Rae J, Briggs J, et al. High resolution mapping of the binding site on human IgG1 for Fc gamma RI, Fc gamma RII, Fc gamma RIII, and FcRn and design of IgG1 variants with improved binding to the Fc gamma R. *J Biol Chem* 2001;**276**(9):6591–604.
172. Okazaki A, Shoji-Hosaka E, Nakamura K, Wakitani M, Uchida K, Kakita S, et al. Fucose depletion from human IgG1 oligosaccharide enhances binding enthalpy and association rate between IgG1 and FcgammaRIIIa. *J Mol Biol* 2004;**336**(5):1239–49.
173. Shields RL, Lai J, Keck R, O'Connell LY, Hong K, Meng YG, et al. Lack of fucose on human IgG1 *N*-linked oligosaccharide improves binding to human

Fcgamma RIII and antibody-dependent cellular toxicity. *J Biol Chem* 2002;**277**(30):26733–40.

174. Shinkawa T, Nakamura K, Yamane N, Shoji-Hosaka E, Kanda Y, Sakurada M, et al. The absence of fucose but not the presence of galactose or bisecting *N*-acetylglucosamine of human IgG1 complex-type oligosaccharides shows the critical role of enhancing antibody-dependent cellular cytotoxicity. *J Biol Chem* 2003;**278**(5):3466–73.
175. Bond A, Cooke A, Hay FC. Glycosylation of IgG, immune complexes and IgG subclasses in the MRL-lpr/lpr mouse model of rheumatoid arthritis. *Eur J Immunol* 1990;**20**(10):2229–33.
176. Matsumoto A, Shikata K, Takeuchi F, Kojima N, Mizuochi T. Autoantibody activity of IgG rheumatoid factor increases with decreasing levels of galactosylation and sialylation. *J Biochem (Tokyo)* 2000;**128**(4):621–8.
177. Mizuochi T, Hamako J, Nose M, Titani K. Structural changes in the oligosaccharide chains of IgG in autoimmune MRL/Mp-lpr/lpr mice. *J Immunol* 1990;**145**(6):1794–8.
178. Rademacher TW, Williams P, Dwek RA. Agalactosyl glycoforms of IgG autoantibodies are pathogenic. *Proc Natl Acad Sci USA* 1994;**91**(13):6123–7.
179. Sherer Y, Shoenfeld Y. Intravenous immunoglobulin for immunomodulation of systemic lupus erythematosus. *Autoimmun Rev* 2006;**5**(2):153–5.
180. Debre M, Bonnet MC, Fridman WH, Carosella E, Philippe N, Reinert P, et al. Infusion of Fc gamma fragments for treatment of children with acute immune thrombocytopenic purpura. *Lancet* 1993;**342**(8877):945–9.
181. Samuelsson A, Towers TL, Ravetch JV. Anti-inflammatory activity of IVIG mediated through the inhibitory Fc receptor. *Science* 2001;**291**(5503):484–6.
182. Schwab I, Nimmerjahn F. Intravenous immunoglobulin therapy: how does IgG modulate the immune system?. *Nat Rev Immunol* 2013;**13**(3):176–89.
183. Bayry J, Negi VS, Kaveri SV. Intravenous immunoglobulin therapy in rheumatic diseases. *Nat Rev Rheumatol* 2011;**7**(6):349–59.
184. Imbach P. Treatment of immune thrombocytopenia with intravenous immunoglobulin and insights for other diseases. A historical review. *Swiss Med Wkly* 2012;**142**:w13593.
185. Negi VS, Elluru S, Siberil S, Graff-Dubois S, Mouthon L, Kazatchkine MD, et al. Intravenous immunoglobulin: an update on the clinical use and mechanisms of action. *J Clin Immunol* 2007;**27**(3):233–45.
186. Anthony RM, Kobayashi T, Wermeling F, Ravetch JV. Intravenous gammaglobulin suppresses inflammation through a novel T(H)2 pathway. *Nature* 2011;**475**(7354):110–3.
187. Kim SH, Kim S, Evans CH, Ghivizzani SC, Oligino T, Robbins PD. Effective treatment of established murine collagen-induced arthritis by systemic administration of dendritic cells genetically modified to express IL-4. *J Immunol* 2001;**166**(5):3499–505.
188. Morita Y, Yang J, Gupta R, Shimizu K, Shelden EA, Endres J, et al. Dendritic cells genetically engineered to express IL-4 inhibit murine collagen-induced arthritis. *J Clin Invest* 2001;**107**(10):1275–84.

CHAPTER

12

Fcγ Receptor Polymorphisms and Susceptibility to Infection

Menna R. Clatworthy

Cambridge Institute for Medical Research and Department of Medicine, University of Cambridge School of Clinical Medicine, Cambridge, UK; Laboratory of Systems Biology, National Institute of Allergy and Infectious Diseases, National Institutes of Health, Bethesda, Maryland

INTRODUCTION

The role of the immune system is to recognize and destroy pathogens while minimizing damage to the host. In mammals, this is characterized by an immediate "innate" response involving inflammation and the activation of complement and phagocytes. This is followed by an "acquired" antigen-specific response mediated by T and B lymphocytes and characterized by immunological memory which augments future responses to the antigen. Humoral or antibody-mediated immunity contributes to both innate and adaptive responses. Antibodies are synthesized by terminally differentiated B cells (plasma cells) and are comprised of a variable region that binds antigen and a constant (Fc) region, which may activate complement components or bind to immune cells via specific receptors. Antibodies contribute to protection against all types of pathogens including viruses, bacteria, fungi, and multicellular parasites. Patients with hypogammaglobulinemia are more susceptible to infections, particularly by organisms such as *Streptococcus*, *Haemophilus*, *Neisseria*, *Staphylococcus*, and *Giardia*.[1] The protective effects of the antibody are mediated via direct and indirect effector mechanisms. Antibodies may directly neutralize bacterial toxins (for example, diphtheria toxin) and viruses or directly block cellular invasion (for example, erythrocyte invasion by *Plasmodium falciparum*[2]). Indirect effects include pathogen opsonization, which increases uptake of extracellular bacteria by phagocytes and enhances complement activation, and the induction of antibody-dependent cell-mediated cytotoxicity (ADCC), providing protection against intracellular and multicellular organisms.[3] The indirect effector functions of an antibody require engagement with cell surface Fc receptors, which are expressed by immune cells and are specific for the antibody isotype; for example, Fcγ receptors (FcγRs) bind IgG, Fcε receptors bind IgE, etc. During the course of a humoral response, a naïve B-cell receptor (BCR) undergoes a number of changes, including the type of heavy chain utilized (class switching from IgM to other isotypes, frequently IgG) and in the affinity of the variable region for antigen, via somatic hypermutation. Thus, IgG antibodies are usually potent humoral effectors, are a characteristic feature of a memory response, and form the majority of circulating antibodies. The importance of IgG is reflected in the fact that the family of Fc receptors required for its recognition by immune cells (FcγRs) play a critical role in defense against a number of infections. FcγRs may be activating or inhibitory.[4] Activating FcγR cross-linking by antibody-opsonized pathogen results in pathogen clearance by the effector mechanisms described previously. This powerful system leads to the release of proinflammatory cytokines and other potentially harmful immune mediators and requires tight regulation, a critical function of the inhibitory FcγR, FcγRIIB. It is therefore unsurprising that, in humans, genetic variation in both activating and inhibitory FcγRs that alter expression or function have been associated with susceptibility to both infection and autoimmunity.[5] This chapter reviews the structure and function of the polymorphisms present in low-affinity FcγR and discusses all of the data available relating to FcγRs and their role in defense against infection, including bacteria, viruses, and parasites.

THE Fcγ RECEPTOR FAMILY GENES

Humans and mice have orthologous FcγRs and, in both species, most of the corresponding genes are clustered in close proximity to each other in syntenic regions on chromosome 1.[6] In mice, four IgG FcRs have been described, three activating receptors—FcγRI (CD64), FcγRIII (CD16), and FcγRIV—and a single inhibitory receptor, FcγRIIB (CD32). In humans, the receptor family includes FcγRI (CD64), FcγRIIA (CD32A), FcγRIIB (CD32B, the inhibitory receptor), FcγRIIIA (CD16A), and FcγRIIIB (CD16B). Many FcR genes are thought to have arisen from gene duplication and diversification processes, thus *FCGR* genes have high sequence homology.[7–9] Humans have three genes in the *FCGR1* family (*FCGR1A, FCGR1B,* and *FCGR1C*), as well as *FCGR2A, FCGR2B, FCGR2C* and *FCGR3A* and *FCGR3B*. These genes have a number of single nucleotide polymorphisms (SNPs), and there is also copy number variation (CNV) in *FCGR2C, FCGR3A,* and *FCGR3B*. The combination of gene duplication, multiple common SNPs, and CNVs is characteristic of regions involved in immune regulation. The generation of such genetic diversity is likely to increase the probability of successful defense against pathogens and has been described at other loci of immunological importance such as the MHC and killer cell immunoglobulin-like receptor loci.[10]

All Fcγ receptors are glycoproteins with a ligand-binding α-subunit consisting of two (FcγRII and FcγIII) or three (FcγRI, FcγRII, and FcγIII) C2-type extracellular immunoglobulin domains. Fcγ receptors show a high degree of sequence identity in their extracellular portion (50 to 96%) but differ in their cytoplasmic domains.[4,11] FcγRIIB (in human and mouse) contains an immunoreceptor tyrosine-based inhibitory motif (ITIM) in its cytoplasmic domain, whereas human FcγRIIA and FcγRIIC contain immunoreceptor tyrosine-based activating motifs (ITAMs) in their intracellular domain. Human FcγRIIIB does not have an intracellular domain but is secured in the cell membrane by a glycosylphosphatidylinositol (GPI) anchor and is thought to signal through association with complement receptor 3,[12] FcγRIIA,[13] or lipid rafts.[14] The remaining Fcγ receptors (both mouse and human) exist as dimers consisting of the ligand-binding α-chain and a signal-transducing γ-chain, known as the Fc receptor common γ-chain.[11]

FcγRI binds monomeric IgG with high affinity. In contrast, FcγRII, FcγRIII, and FcγRIV are low-affinity receptors that bind only immune-complexed IgG.[6,11] Despite the low affinity of these receptors for monomeric IgG, cells that express multiple FcγRs have a high avidity for a pathogen opsonized with multiple IgG molecules.[15]

IgG molecules are glycosylated in the CH2 domain, and these sugar moieties are critical for Fc binding.[16] Heterogeneity in CH2 glycans may alter binding affinity to FcγR; for example, the presence of a terminal sialic acid on the glycan is associated with a 10-fold reduction in FcγR affinity.[17,18] FcγR also bind pentraxins, a family of innate immune mediators that includes the acute-phase proteins serum amyloid P (SAP)[19] and C-reactive protein (CRP).[20] Both SAP and CRP recognize various pathogens, including bacteria, fungi, and yeast, and they have similar functions to antibody in that they can both activate complement via C1q[11] and interact with FcγR.[20,21] Thus, FcγR plays a role in early, innate immune responses as well as later, humoral responses.

FcγR DISTRIBUTION AND FUNCTION

FcγRs are expressed widely on immune cells, including neutrophils, monocytes, macrophages, dendritic cells (DCs), mast cells, and natural killer cells, but the type of FcγRs expressed differs between cell types. The inhibitory receptor FcγRIIB is the only FcγR expressed on B cells and functions to downregulate BCR-mediated activation by immune-complexed antigen. Broadly speaking, ligation of activating FcγRs on myeloid cells results in processes that promote pathogen clearance such as ADCC, degranulation of cytotoxic cells, phagocytosis, and the release of cytokines and other inflammatory mediators. In DCs, activating FcγR ligation promotes maturation and immunogenic antigen presentation. FcγRIIB inhibits all of these processes and therefore acts as a critical regulator of immune complex-mediated immune activation.

The ratio of activating FcγR binding affinity to FcγRIIB binding affinity of an IgG molecule has been called the *activating/inhibitory (A/I) ratio* and is a measure of the efficacy of IgG in mediating effector responses.[22] In mice, these A/I ratios differ by several orders of magnitude between IgG subclasses. IgG_1 has the lowest A/I ratio at 0.1, suggesting that the activity of this isotype is strongly influenced by the inhibitory receptor FcγRIIB, while IgG_{2a}, with an A/I of 70, is much less regulated by FcγRIIB. In humans, the polymorphisms in *FCGR2A*, *FCGR3A*, and *FCGR3B* that affect IgG binding will also impact the A/I ratio. The A/I ratio will also be influenced by the relative expression of activating to inhibitory FcγR on the surface of a given cell. Thus, factors that preferentially reduce or increase the expression of either the activating or inhibitory FcγR will modulate the A/I ratio and thus the activation threshold. A number of cytokines have been shown to influence FcγR expression; for example, in human monocytes, interferon-γ (IFN-γ), a Th1 cytokine, induces the expression of FcγRI and FcγRIIA,[23,24] and Th2 cytokines such as IL-4 increase the expression of inhibitory FcγRIIB while downregulating all classes of activating FcγR.[23]

GENETIC VARIATION IN HUMAN FcγRs

Activating FcγRs

FcγRIIA

FcγRIIA is a single chain receptor, unique to humans, containing an ITAM in its cytoplasmic tail. It is the most broadly distributed FcγR, being found on monocytes, macrophages, platelets, and neutrophils and also in a soluble form

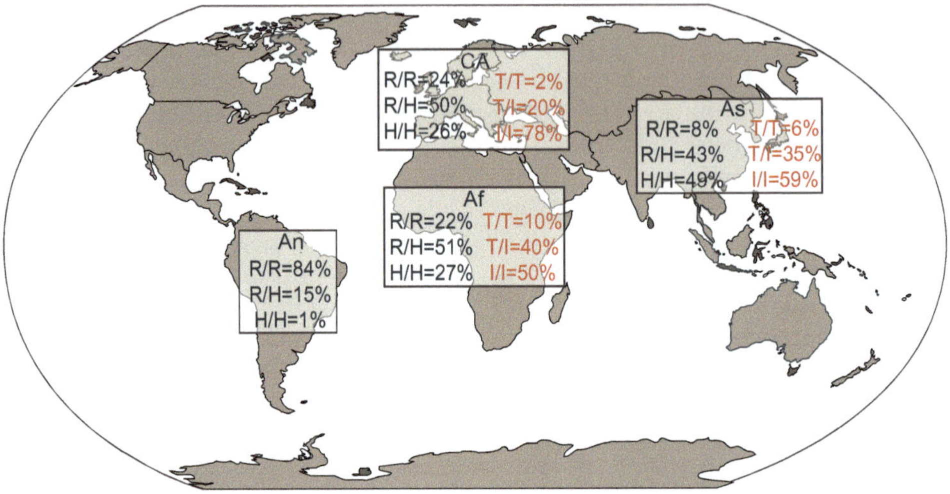

FIGURE 12.1 **Frequency of FcγRIIA-H131R and FcγRIIB-I232T genotypes.** World map showing the frequency of *FCGR2A* (black) and *FCGR2B* (red) polymorphisms in Caucasian (CA), African (Af), Asian (As), and Native American (An) populations. Data represent the mean frequency across available studies. *(Based on Lehrnbecher et al.,[28] Kuwano et al.,[29] and Willcocks.[37])*

(FcγRIIA2).[25] A G>A point mutation in *FCGR2A* (rs1801274) has been identified that results in an arginine (R) to histidine (H) amino acid substitution at position 131. FcγRIIA is the only FcγR that significantly binds IgG_2, and the rs1801274 SNP significantly affects this binding. FcγRIIA-H131 has a greater affinity for IgG_2 and IgG_3 than FγRIIA-R131, which barely binds this isotype.[26] In contrast, FcγRIIA-H131 binds CRP poorly compared with FcγRIIA-R131.[27] The allelic frequencies of the FcγRIIA polymorphisms vary significantly between different populations (summarized in Lehrnbecher et al.[28] and Figure 12.1). In Southeast Asian populations, the frequency of the FcγRIIA-R/R131 genotype is low (8% average across multiple studies[28]). In contrast, 84% of Amazonian Indians were found to have the FcγRIIA-R/R131 genotype.[29] This variation in frequency has most likely arisen due to different selection pressures encountered by individuals within geographically distinct populations. It is therefore of relevance that FcγRIIA polymorphisms have been associated with susceptibility or resistance to a number of pathogens.

FcγRIIIA

FcγRIIIA is expressed on NK cells, monocytes, and macrophages.[30] The major polymorphism in *FCGR3A* is a point mutation (T>G) at nucleotide 559 (rs396991), which results in either a valine (V158) or phenylalanine (F158) at amino acid position 158. These alleles are also co-dominantly expressed, and, as for FcγRIIA, the change in an amino acid in the extracellular domain of the receptor results in altered binding to its principle ligands. It has been shown that the FcγRIIIA-V158 allele has a higher affinity for IgG_1 and IgG_3 and can also interact with IgG_4. Functionally, IgG-induced NK cell activity is increased in FcγRIIIA-V/V158 homozygotes compared with FcγRIIIA-F/F158 individuals.[31] Again, there is geographical variation in the frequency of alleles, the FcγRIIIA-V/V genotype being most common in China and least common in the United States.[28,32]

FcγRIIIB

FcγRIIIB is a GPI-linked protein expressed exclusively on neutrophils, although it can be induced on eosinophils.[30] FcγRIIIB can be released from the surface of neutrophils upon activation.[33] Two isoforms of FcγRIIIB exist, varying in their expression of the neutrophil antigen (NA). The genes differ by five nucleotides (141, 147, 227, 277, and 349) within exon 3, resulting in a four amino acid substitution in its membrane-distal immunoglobulin-like extracellular domain and giving rise to two polymorphic forms. These are termed FγRIIIB-NA1 and FcγRIIIB-NA2 (also known as HNA1a and HNA1b, respectively).[34] Due to differential glycosylation (the NA-1 isoform has four N-linked glycosylation sites, whereas the NA2 isoform has six sites), they vary in their interaction with IgG in that FcγRIIIB-NA1 has a higher affinity for IgG_1 and IgG_3 and can mediate phagocytosis of IgG_1/IgG_3-complexed particles.[35] An additional, rarer polymorphism, FcγRIIIB-SH(HNA1c), has been identified that differs from NA2 by only one base substitution at nucleotide 266, resulting in an alanine to aspartate substitution at amino acid 78.[34] About 0.1% of central Europeans do not express FcγRIIIB on neutrophils (NA_{null} phenotype) due to deletion of *FCGRIIIB* and part of *FCGRIIC*. The frequency of the FcγRIIIB polymorphism has been studied in a number of populations worldwide and shows considerable geographic variation. Homozygosity for the low-affinity allele NA2 is more common in Indian and African American individuals (55 and 54%, respectively), compared with Caucasian populations (11 to 43%), and is lowest in Native Americans (9%).[28,29]

Inhibitory FcγRs

Seven non-synonymous SNPs have been identified in the human *FCGR2B* gene, but only one of these occurs at significant frequency;[36,37] rs1050501 in exon 5 of *FCGR2B* encodes a C>T transition at nucleotide 695, resulting in threonine replacing isoleucine at position 232 in the transmembrane domain of the receptor. This causes the variant receptor, FcγRIIB-232T, to be excluded from lipid rafts, preventing interaction with activating receptors.[38,39] Monocyte-derived macrophages from individuals homozygous for the polymorphism have an increased phagocytic capacity when challenged with IgG-opsonized immune complexes, and B cells show heightened activation and proliferation when both the BCR and FcγRIIB are ligated.[38] The minor allele frequency of $Fc\gamma RIIB^{T232}$ is subject to considerable ethnic variation and is lower in Caucasians (0.10) than East Africans (0.25)[40] or Southeast Asians (0.22 to 0.25)[32,36,41,42] (Figure 12.1). Two *FCGR2B* promoter haplotypes have been described: the common –386G/–120T and less common –386C/–120A.[43] The 386C/–120A variant has been shown in one study to result in increased binding of the transcription factors GATA4 and Yin-Yang 1 to the promoter regulation[43] and in increased expression of FcγRIIB on monocytes, neutrophils, and myeloid DCs,[44] whereas, another study showed that –386C/C homozygosity reduced the transcription and surface expression levels of FcγRIIB in peripheral B cells compared to –386G/G.[45] Given these conflicting results, the functional significance of these promoter polymorphisms is unclear.

FcγRs AND INFECTION: EVIDENCE BASE

Although there are difference in FcγRs between mice and humans, studies in murine models of infection have provided an invaluable insight into the role of FcγRs in defense against infection. Knock-out mice are available for the common γ-chain (required for FcγRI and FcγRIII signaling), FcγRI, FcγRIII, and FcγRIIB, and where available the data for these knockouts will be considered. In humans, studies have been hampered by technical difficulties. CNVs in a number of *FCGR* loci, combined with the high sequence homology between the two *FCGR3* genes and the three *FCGR2* genes, have made the locus challenging to study. Few SNPs in this locus have been included in genome-wide association studies (GWAS), as the genotyping complexity has led to a lack of Hardy–Weinberg equilibrium in control samples and non-Mendelian inheritance in trios.[46] Furthermore, candidate gene studies of polymorphisms in the *FCGR* locus have often given conflicting results, which may be due to genotyping methodology and/or small sample size; however, the available evidence from human genetic and functional studies will be discussed.

FcγRs AND DEFENSE AGAINST INFECTION

Bacteria

Streptococcus Pneumoniae

Streptococcus pneumoniae is a Gram-positive, encapsulated diplococcus and an important human pathogen. *S. pneumoniae* may colonize the nasopharynx in some individuals and can subsequently cause pneumonia, bacteremia, peritonitis, and meningitis. Invasive pneumococcal disease results in significant morbidity and mortality worldwide, killing around 5 million people annually. The main defense against *S. pneumoniae* is provided by anti-capsular polysaccharide and anti-cell wall phosphocholine antibodies that bind pneumococci and mediate FcγR-dependent phagocytosis by neutrophils and macrophages.[47,48]

In humans, IgG_2-deficiency predisposes to streptococcal infection, thus IgG_2 is thought to play an important role in the immune response to this bacterium. Because IgG_2 is a relatively inefficient activator of complement, binding to FcγRIIA is likely to be important in the immune response to streptococci, particularly Fc-dependent phagocytosis. The FcγRIIA isoform, FcγRIIA-H131, is the only human FcγR capable of effectively binding complexed IgG_2. *In vitro*, neutrophils from donors homozygous for FcγRIIA-H131 have a higher phagocytic capacity for IgG-opsonized *Streptococcus pneumoniae* than neutrophils from FcγRIIA-R/R131 donors.[49]

The genetic studies published to date on FcγR polymorphisms and pneumococcal disease are summarized in Table 12.1. Most early studies demonstrated an association between FcγRIIA-R/R131 homozygosity and susceptibility to invasive pneumococcal disease[50–54] and more severe sepsis in community-acquired pneumonia.[55] However, a recent, much larger study showed no difference in the frequency of FcγRIIA-H/R131 genotype between patients with pneumococcal pneumonia and controls and found a significantly higher frequency of FCGR2A-H/H131 in patients with bacteremic pneumococcal community-acquired pneumonia than in those without bacteremia.[56] In this study, multivariate analysis was performed to adjust for known risk factors such as age and chronic disease. These conflicting results may reflect the generation of spurious data due to small sample size in some studies, although it is possible that the results reflect true associations and that in some patient groups the FcγRIIA-R/R131 genotype confers risk whilst in others the FcγRIIA-H/H131 genotype increases susceptibility to pneumococcus. The studies did not control for pneumococcal vaccination, and children tend to generate increased IgG_2 in response to immunization. Many of the studies implicating the FcγRIIA-R/R131 genotype were performed in children, where the IgG_2–FcγRIIA interaction may be of central importance in mediating protection against pneumonia, and the presence of the low-affinity FcγRIIA-R131 receptor may be a significant disadvantage. In contrast, the data in adults indicate an association of the high-affinity FcγRIIA-H131 variant, with a different clinical phenotype, bacteremia, rather than pneumonia. Thus, it may be that CRP–FcγRIIA interactions are more important in localizing pneumococcus to the lung, and

TABLE 12.1 FcγRIIA-H131R (rs1801274) and Susceptibility to Pneumococcal Disease

Study	*N* (Cases and Controls)	Finding	Population
FcγRIIA-R/R131 associated with susceptibility			
Yee et al.[51]	*Cases:* 70 patients with pneumococcal pneumonia (42 bacteremic, 28 non-bacteremic) *Controls:* 136	50% of patients with bacteremic pneumococcal pneumonia were homozygous for FcγRIIA-R/R131 compared with 28% with non-bacteremic pneumococcal pneumonia and 29% of uninfected controls ($p < 0.05$).	U.S.
Yuan et al.[52]	*Cases:* 63 children with pneumococcal sepsis *Controls:* 20 healthy children and 57 adult blood donors	The frequency of homozygosity for FcγRIIA-R/R131 in patients was significantly higher than in the healthy random donor population (43% vs. 21%; $p < 0.05$).	Australian
Yuan et al.[54]	*Cases:* 89 children with pneumococcal sepsis *Controls:* 409	FcγRIIA-R/R131 genotype was significantly higher in cases (39% vs. 21%; OR, 2.5; $p < 0.001$; 95% CI, 1.4–4).	Australian
Endeman et al.[55]	*Cases:* 200 patients with community-acquired pneumonia *Controls:* 313	No difference between cases and controls *but* FcγRIIA-R/R131 genotype was found more frequently in patients with severe sepsis and invasive pneumococcal disease (OR, 2.55; $p < 0.01$; 95% CI, 1.30–5.00).	Dutch
No difference in FcγRIIA SNP between cases and controls			
Moens et al.[53]	*Cases:* 55 Caucasian patients with invasive pneumococcal disease *Controls:* 100 Caucasians	No difference in the frequency of FcγRIIA-H/R131 genotypes between cases and controls was observed.	Belgian
Endeman et al.[55]	*Cases:* 200 patients with community-acquired pneumonia *Controls:* 313	No difference between cases and controls was observed, but there were differences between case subsets (see above).	Dutch
Sole-Violan et al.[56]	*Cases:* 1262 patients with pneumococcal community-acquired pneumonia; 319 with confirmed pneumococcus *Controls:* 1224	No difference between cases and controls was observed, but there were differences between case subsets (see below).	Spanish
FcγRIIA-H/H131 associated with bacteremia			
Sole-Violan et al.[56]	*Cases:* 1262 patients with pneumococcal community-acquired pneumonia; 319 with confirmed pneumococcus *Controls:* 1224	No difference between cases and controls were observed, but patients with bacteremia had significantly higher frequencies of FcγRIIA-H/H131 than those without bacteremia (OR, 2.9; p=0.00016; 95% CI, 1.58–5.3).	Spanish

this interaction is known to be reduced in the FcγRIIA-H131.[27] In favor of this explanation is the observation that a polymorphism in the CRP gene has been associated with mortality in patients with pneumococcal bacteremia.[57] However, data from a murine model suggest that the CRP–FcγRIIA interaction is not critical for the protective effects of human CRP against

Streptococcus pneumoniae.[48] Another possible explanation for increased mortality in individuals with the high-affinity FcγRIIA-H131 may be increased proinflammatory cytokine release and subsequent systemic inflammatory response. In support of this, in the study by Sole-Violan et al.[56] the bacteremic group in which the FcγRIIA-H131 allele was over-represented had more severe disease, including organ failure, which would likely be associated with a systemic inflammatory response. This explanation would also be in keeping with the studies performed in FcγRIIB-deficient mice showing that the inhibitory receptor modulates susceptibility to septic shock in animals previously vaccinated with Pneumovax®[58] (see later discussion).

Pneumococcus is likely to be a powerful evolutionary selection pressure, since much of the mortality burden associated with it is concentrated in infants. The frequency of the FcγRIIA-R/H alleles is almost equal in Caucasian and African populations (Figure 12.1), supporting the idea that both alleles confer risk to certain aspects of disease.

Murine studies of FcγR and *Streptococcus pneumoniae* have been limited to those examining the role of the inhibitory receptor FcγRIIB. *In vitro*, FcγRIIB-deficient murine macrophages demonstrate enhanced uptake of opsonized bacteria compared with control cells. *In vivo*, FcγRIIB–/– mice are protected against infection with *Streptococcus pneumonia*.[58] Conversely, mice with transgenic overexpression of FcγRIIB on macrophages are more susceptible to pneumococcal peritonitis and pneumonia.[59] However, the inhibitory receptor FcγRIIB plays a more complex role; although unimmunized FcγRIIB-deficient mice are less susceptible to pneumococcal infection, following immunization and the generation of antibody these mice become more susceptible to subsequent challenge with high-dose pneumococcus. This increased mortality is associated with a robust rise in systemic proinflammatory cytokines[58] and suggests a role for FcγRIIB in balancing efficient pathogen clearance with the cytokine-mediated consequences of sepsis.

In vitro studies utilizing human primary monocyte-derived macrophages demonstrated an increase in phagocytosis of antibody-opsonized *Streptococcus pneumonia* by macrophages obtained from individuals expressing the polymorphic form of *FCGR2B*, FcγRIIB-232T.[38] As yet, no genetic studies have been published examining the effect of this SNP on susceptibility to pneumococcal disease. However, data from *in vivo* studies with the FcγRIIB-deficient mice and the human *in vitro* data would predict a reduced susceptibility to initial infection in individuals homozygous for the FcγRIIB-232T SNP, but perhaps an increased susceptibility to septic shock in those with high anti-pneumococcal antibody titers.

Staphylococcus Aureus

Staphylococcus aureus is a Gram-positive, facultative anaerobe that is frequently found as part of the colonizing skin flora. *S. aureus* can cause minor skin infections, as well as life-threatening pneumonia, meningitis, toxic shock syndrome, and septicemia. Studies of activatory FcγR-deficient mice do not indicate a significant role in protection against *S. aureus*. Deficiency of the Fc receptor γ-chain did not affect susceptibility to staphylococcal septicemia or arthritis, and bacterial load was equivalent in wild-type and γ-chain-deficient mice.[60] In contrast to the data generated in the activatory FcγR-deficient mice, FcγRIIB deficiency increased uptake of opsonized bacteria by phagocytes, and FcγRIIB knockout mice showed reduced susceptibility to staphylococcal bacteremia.[60] Phagocytosis assays in human neutrophils homozygous for FcγRIIIB-NA2 demonstrated a lower IgG_1-mediated phagocytosis of *S. aureus* while PMNs from FcγRIIA-R131 were virtually incapable of phagocytosing *S. aureus* opsonized with IgG_2 antibodies[61,62] (as observed for IgG_2-opsonized *Streptococcus pneumoniae*). These data indicate that the activatory FcγR SNPs are likely to affect susceptibility to disease, despite the negative data generated from mouse models. However, no case-control studies have been performed to date in patients with staphylococcal disease examining the effects of either activatory or inhibitory FcγR SNPs.

Haemophilus Influenzae

Haemophilus influenzae is a Gram-negative, encapsulated bacterium that can cause pneumonia and meningitis. *In vitro* studies utilizing human neutrophils demonstrated a reduction in phagocytosis in cells isolated from individuals with the FcγRIIA-R/R131 genotype.[61] Endeman and colleagues[55] investigated the FcγRIIA-R/H131 SNP in 201 patients with community-acquired pneumonia. Of these, 14 patients were found to have *H. influenza*, and the FcγRIIA-R/R131 genotype was found more frequently in this subset compared with controls (50% of cases versus 27% of controls, $p \leq 0.01$).

Neisseria Meningitidis

Neisseria meningitidis is a Gram-negative, encapsulated bacterium that is a commensal organism in up to 10% of healthy individuals, but in a minority of cases it may cause invasive meningococcal disease, manifesting as meningitis or septicemia.[63] The host response to meningococcal infection begins with the production of antibody in response to colonization, facilitating FcR-mediated uptake of bacteria by phagocytes.[63] As with *Streptococcus pneumoniae*, IgG_2 is important in defense against *N. meningitidis*, and neutrophils with the FcγRIIA-R/R131 genotype phagocytose IgG_2-opsonized *N. meningitidis* less effectively than those with FcγRIIA-H/H131.[64,65] In a small retrospective study of 24 Dutch children who had survived fulminate meningococcal septic shock, 44% were homozygous for FcγRIIA-R131 polymorphism compared with 23% of controls.[64] However, in a Norwegian case-control study and an additional Dutch study, no association with incidence or severity of meningococcal disease was identified.[66,67] Some studies have found associations of FcγRIIA-R/R131 with meningococcal disease only in older individuals.[68–70] Of note, van der Pol and colleagues[66] demonstrated that, although there were no differences in FcγRIIA-R/H131 frequencies between cases and controls, FcγRIIA-R131 was more common in patients with meningococcal meningitis and FcγRIIA-H131 more common in those with sepsis. These differences may reflect the variation in presentation of meningococcal disease with age (younger patients tend to present with meningitis and older ones with sepsis) and the relative importance of IgG_2–FcγRIIA versus CRP–FcγRIIA interactions in defense against infection in these patient subsets, or indeed in different clinical presentations, as discussed for *S. pneumoniae*. Alternatively, the high-affinity IgG_2–FcγRIIA interaction in patients with FcγRIIA-H131 may result in bacterial clearance at the expense of increased cytokine release and septic shock.

Bordatella Pertussis

Bordatella pertussis is a Gram-negative, aerobic coccobacillus that is the principle cause of whooping cough, a disease with significant mortality in infants under the age of one year. *In vitro* studies using human neutrophils have shown the importance of FcγRIIA and FcγRIIIB in efficient phagocytosis of IgG-opsonized *B. pertussis* through the triggering of a respiratory burst that results in bacterial killing.[71] Murine studies utilizing FcγRI-, Fcγ-chain-, and FcγRIII-deficient mice have confirmed the importance of FcγRI and FcγRIII in mediating protection to *B. pertussis in vivo*.[72,73] No available data are currently available on the effects of human *FCGR* polymorphisms on disease susceptibility.

Periodontitis

Periodontitis is a major cause of tooth loss in adults, resulting from both the direct effect of periodontopathic Gram-negative bacteria on the gums and the host inflammatory response. The disease is characterized by the production of very high concentrations of serum antibodies reactive with a limited number of periodontal disease pathogens, and serum concentrations of IgG_2 are particularly elevated.[74] Associations between FcγR polymorphisms and susceptibility to periodontitis have been investigated in a number of small studies in Caucasian, Asian, and African American populations.[75–79] These studies suggest that polymorphisms in the FcγR-encoding genes related to aggressive periodontitis risk are different among ethnic populations, which may reflect differences in the frequencies of mouth commensal bacteria. Larger studies, however, are needed to validate these findings.

A recent meta-analysis of activating *FCGR* SNPs examined published data from 17 studies involving 1685 cases and 1570 controls.[80] The FcγRIIIB-NA2/NA2 polymorphism was associated with both aggressive (per-allele OR, 2.005; 95% CI, 1.044–3.851) and chronic periodontitis (OR, 1.397; 95% CI, 1.039–1.878). There was a weak association between the FcγRIIA-H131R polymorphism and aggressive periodontitis in Asians (R versus H allele OR, 1.579; 95% CI, 1.025–2.432). In contrast, no relationship was identified between FcγRIIIA-F158V and periodontal disease.

Polymorphisms in the inhibitory receptor FcγRIIB have been assessed in Japanese patients with aggressive peridontitis and chronic peridonitis.[78] The FcγRIIB-232T allele was found with increased frequency in patients with aggressive peridontitis compared with healthy controls ($p = 0.006$). An SNP within intron 4 of the *FCGR2B* gene (nt 646-184A/G) was also found to vary significantly between study groups, with enrichment of nt 646-184A allele in patients with chronic peridontitis compared with controls.

Viral Infections

Dengue Fever

Dengue viruses belong to the family Flaviviridae, genus *Flavivirus*, and are transmitted to humans by mosquitoes. Dengue fever is an acute viral infection characterized by fever, rash, headache, myalgia, and arthralgia. Occasionally, dengue fever progresses to dengue shock syndrome (DSS), a potentially life-threatening illness associated with increased vascular permeability, hemorrhage, and shock.[81] Epidemiological studies show that severe complications of dengue viral infections, such as DSS, are more commonly observed during secondary infections compared with primary infections, suggesting that the presence of circulating dengue-specific antibodies constitutes a risk factor for DSS.[82] DSS can occur in primary infections, but this is more unusual and tends to affect infants born to dengue antibody-positive mothers;[81] in these infants, higher antibody levels correlate with more severe disease.[83] *In vitro*, dengue-specific IgG can enhance viral entry and infection of cells, a phenomenon referred to as *antibody-dependent enhancement*,[81,84] and this effect is mediated by both FcγRI and FcγRIIA.[85,86] In contrast, ligation of FcγRIIB inhibits antibody-dependent enhancement of dengue virus infection.[87] Two case-control studies have been performed examining FcγR SNPs in dengue fever. One study in 352 Vietnamese patients with DSS and 251 controls found a lower frequency of FcγRIIA-R131 homozygotes in the patient group, suggesting that this genotype may be protective, perhaps because the weaker binding affinity reduces viral entry into cells.[88] This protective effect of FcγRIIA-R/R131 was replicated in a more recent Cuban study.[89] The effects of other FcγR polymorphisms have not been assessed.

Polio

Poliovirus is an RNA virus that in 90% of individuals is entirely asymptomatic. In fewer than 1% of cases, however, the virus enters the central nervous system, preferentially infecting and destroying motor neurons, leading to muscle weakness and acute flaccid paralysis.[90] Poliovirus enters susceptible cells through a specific poliovirus receptor but can also be taken up by FcγR,[91] and FcγRs have been found to be expressed on both microglia and perivascular macrophages.[92] IgG_3 is the main antibody subtype produced in response to poliovirus in humans,[93] and, although FcγRI is the receptor with the highest affinity for IgG_3, of the low-affinity FcγRs FcγRIIIa-V/V158 predominates. A Norwegian study of patients who contracted poliomyelitis in the 1950–1954 epidemic found the FcγRIIA-V/V158 genotype was under-represented in patients with a history of acute poliomyelitis, suggesting that V/V homozygous individuals might have increased binding and clearance of antibody-opsonized poliovirus and therefore be protected against disease.[94]

Human Herpesvirus 8

Kaposi's sarcoma is the most common malignant condition associated with HIV infection. It is thought that, in its early stages, Kaposi's sarcoma is an angioproliferative, inflammatory lesion induced by infection with human herpesvirus 8 (HHV-8). The immunopathogenesis of Kaposi's sarcoma involves the activation of lymphocytes, resulting in the production of proinflammatory cytokines and angiogenic factors.[95] NK cells are important in mediating antibody-dependent cellular cytotoxicity of both virally infected and malignant cells, as their absence increases the severity of HHV-8 infections.[96] FcγRIIIA is expressed on NK cells, and two studies have found that the higher binding FcγRIIIA-V/V158 genotype is associated with the development of Kaposi's sarcoma in individuals with HIV.[28,97] Thus, more avid binding of antibody to FcγRIIIA-V/V158 could lead to an increase in cytokine production, driving inflammation and angiogenesis.

Influenza Virus

Influenza virus is an RNA virus of the Orthomyxoviridae family that can give rise to severe pulmonary disease and intermittently causes widespread pandemics. Antibodies are important for the prevention of influenza infection through neutralization of free infective particles,[98] and there is also some evidence that antibody–FcγR interactions may facilitate destruction of virus-infected cells; Fcγ-chain-deficient mice are more susceptible to influenza virus infection, with reduced macrophage phagocytosis and NK ADCC.[99] There are currently no studies in humans that have assessed the importance of *FCGR* polymorphisms in influenza infection.

Human Immunodeficiency Virus

Human immunodeficiency virus (HIV)/acquired immune deficiency syndrome (AIDS) has become a leading cause of mortality worldwide and the main cause of death in sub-Saharan Africa. HIV-1 is a retrovirus that invades cells via CD4, a cell surface receptor found predominantly on T-helper lymphocytes. Antibodies are important in host response to HIV infection, and IgG antibody subclasses differ in their ability to neutralize HIV-1 and inhibit HIV–cell fusion, with IgG_1 and IgG_3 being more efficient than IgG_2.[100] The role of FcγR in HIV infection is unclear, but *in vitro* studies suggest that FcγR on monocytes, when cross-linked with IgG antibody–virus immune complexes, allow viral entry and activation of HIV gene transcription.[101,102]

Surprising results have come from studies characterizing the role of FcγR polymorphisms or changes in expression in the context of HIV infection. The FcγRIIIA-V/V158 polymorphism was found to have no effect on disease progression in one study,[97] whereas in more recent studies this high-affinity allele was correlated with rapid progression, lack of antiviral control,[103] and increased risk of infection in a vaccinated population,[104] which may be the first clinical evidence of antibody-dependent enhancement in HIV. It is thought that the detrimental effect of this receptor in association studies conducted on infected subjects may be due to increased inflammation, contributing to chronic dysregulation of the immune system and disease progression. In contrast, the *FCGR2* allele with high affinity for IgG_2 and improved affinity for IgG_3 has been found to be protective against progression in adults[97] but associated with perinatal infection.[105] Finally, because these polymorphisms may affect risk of infection and risk of progression in different ways, whether recruitment of FcγR activity is beneficial or detrimental may depend on the stage of infection. Inflammatory and cytolytic processes may have protective effects in blocking infection but also contribute to chronic inflammation and immune exhaustion, resulting in accelerated progression after infection. Indeed, ADCC and antibody-dependent cellular viral inhibition have been associated with both infection and protection in HIV vaccine trials.[106,107] Discrepancies such as this are not easily resolved, but it is hoped that continued study will generate a consensus on both the role of IgG and FcγR in HIV.

Parasites

Malaria

Malarial parasites are the cause of significant morbidity and mortality in many tropical countries, particularly in sub-Saharan Africa, resulting in more than 300 million clinical cases and approximately 3 million deaths per year.[108] The disease is caused by intracellular, protozoan parasites of the genus *Plasmodium* and is transmitted by the bite of an infected female *Anopheles* mosquito. Human malaria is caused by one of four species of *Plasmodium*: *falciparum*, *vivax*, *malariae*, and *ovale*.[109] The vast majority of severe malarial cases and deaths are caused by *P. falciparum*, which is endemic in most of sub-Saharan Africa. The *P. falciparum* life cycle includes a non-pathogenic, asymptomatic extra-erythrocyte stage, which is followed by the invasion of mature erythrocytes by infective merozoites. These form multiple mature schizonts within red blood cells, which finally rupture and release their progeny.[110] Unless restrained by an immune response or by antimalarial drugs, blood parasitemia increases exponentially until all available erythrocytes are infected and death is inevitable. Inflammatory mediators have been repeatedly implicated in the severity of disease, giving rise to the belief that severe malaria may be in part immune mediated.[111]

The importance of antibody in the immune response to the erythrocytic stages of malaria has been demonstrated by the protective effects wrought by the passive transfer of immune IgG to naïve recipients in murine[112] and non-human primate[113] malarial models and in humans.[114] In humans, the predominant protective antibody isotypes in malaria are IgG_1 and IgG_3,[115] which are thought to opsonize merozoites or infected erythrocytes and enhance their clearance by macrophages and neutrophils.[116–118] In a murine malarial model, *Plasmodium bergei* XAT, γ-chain-deficient mice showed reduced antibody-mediated phagocytosis and increased susceptibility to infection.[119]

Case-control studies performed in humans with malaria that have given conflicting results are summarized in Table 12.2. Some have shown that the low-affinity FcγRIIA-R131 is associated with protection from some aspects of malarial disease; in Kenyan and Gambian children, the FcγRIIA-R/R131 genotype was associated with protection against severe malaria.[120,121] A subsequent study of 493 Kenyan children with acute malaria showed that homozygotes for the FcγRIIA-R131 allele were protective against high-density

TABLE 12.2 FcγRIIA- H131R(rs1801274) and Susceptibility to Malaria

Study	*N* (Cases and Controls)	Finding	Population
FcγRIIA-R131 protective			
Shi et al.[120]	*Cases:* 97 infants with high-density parasitemia (>30% routine blood smears +ve) *Controls:* 85 infants with low-density parasitemia (<8% routine blood smears +ve)	Infants with FcγRIIA-R/R131 were associated with protection from high-density *P. falciparum* infection compared with infants with the FcγRIIA-H/R131 genotype (OR, 0.278; $p = .0021$).	West Kenyan
Cooke et al.[121]	*Cases:* 333 children (ages 0–10 years) with mild malaria; 524 with severe malaria (cerebral malaria ± severe anemia ± hypoglycemia) *Controls:* 558 children ages 0–10 years	FcγRIIA-H/H131 was significantly associated with severe malaria (OR, 1.40; $p = 0.034$); more significantly in children<5 years old (OR, 1.50; $p = 0.021$). FcγRIIA-R/R131 was *not* associated with protection from severe malaria.	Gambian
Ouma et al.[122]	*Cases:* 451 children<4 years old: 151 with mild, 141 with moderate, and 159 with severe malarial anemia *Controls:* 38 uncomplicated malaria	Relative to FcγRIIA-H/R131, FcγRIIA-R/R131 was significantly associated with protection against high-density parasitemia (OR, 0.58; $p = 0.02$).	Western Kenyan
FcγRIIA-H131 protective			
Nasr et al.[123]	*Cases:* 115 patients with severe malaria, 85 with mild malaria. *Controls:* 56 malaria-free subjects	FcγRIIA-R/R131 was significantly higher in severe malaria compared with patients with mild malaria (OR, 2.05; $p = 0.04$). FcγRIIA-H/H131 was associated with mild malaria adjusted (OR, 0.28; $p = 0.01$).	Sudanese
Sinha et al.[124]	*Cases:* 54 with non-severe malaria; 63 with severe malaria Controls: 92 matched subjects	FcγRIIA-H/H131 was associated with protection from malaria; frequency of H/H131 = 41.3% in controls vs. 20.3% in non-severe malaria ($p = 0.001$) and 20.6% in severe malaria ($p = 0.002$).	Indian
Schuldt et al.[125]	*Cases:* 1591 with severe anemia; 562 with cerebral malaria; 497 with other malaria complications *Controls:* 2027 matched healthy controls	FcγRIIA-R/R131 was associated with severe malaria collectively (OR, 1.20; $p = 0.021$) and, after stratification for phenotypes, with severe anemia (OR, 1.33; $p = 0.009$), but not with cerebral malaria (OR, 1.04; $p = 0.733$).	Ghanan
FcγRIIA-H/H131/FcγRIIIB-NA2/NA2 associated with susceptibility			
Omi et al.[126]	*Cases:* 107 patients with cerebral malaria; 157 with non-cerebral severe malaria *Controls:* 202 with mild malaria	FcγRIIA-131H/H,FcγRIIIB-NA2 haplotype was associated with cerebral malaria (OR, 1.85; $p = 0.012$). No association was found if individual polymorphisms were considered in isolation.	Thai
Ouma et al.[127]	*Cases:* 230 patients with severe malarial anemia (Hb <6.0 g/dL); 298 with non-severe malarial anemia (Hb >6.0 g/dL)	FcγRIIA-131H/FcγRIIIB-NA2 haplotype increased susceptibility to severe malarial anemia (RR, 1.47). FcγRIIA-131H/FcγRIIIB-NA1 was haplotype associated with reduced risk of severe malarial anemia (RR, 0.65) and all-cause mortality.	Kenyan

parasitemia, but no effect was seen on severe malarial anemia.[122]

In contrast, a number of studies implicate the low-affinity FcγRIIA-R/R131 with susceptibility rather than protection; in a Sudanese population, the frequency of the FcγRIIA-R/R131 genotype was significantly higher in those with severe malaria. Levels of IgG_1 and IgG_3 antibodies were higher in the mild malaria compared with the severe malaria. The lowest risk of severe malaria was seen with where high levels of IgG_3 antibodies were combined with the FcγRIIA-H/H131 genotype.[123] Subsequent studies have also shown a protective effect of the FcγRIIA-H/H131 genotype against severe malaria.[124] A large Ghanaian study demonstrated that FcγRIIA-R/R131 was associated with severe malaria collectively and, in particular, with severe anemia (OR, 1.33; $p = 0.009$) but not with cerebral malaria (OR, 1.04; $p = 0.733$).[125]

Other studies have demonstrated that particular haplotypes of FcγRIIA-H/R131/FcγRIIIB-NA rather than individual alleles determine susceptibility to malaria. In Northwest Thailand, the FcγRIIA-131H/H genotype in combination with the FcγRIIIB-NA2 allele was associated with susceptibility to cerebral malaria.[126] Similarly, a more recent Kenyan study demonstrated that individuals with the FcγRIIA-131H/FcγRIIIB-NA2 haplotype had increased susceptibility to severe malarial anemia (RR, 1.47).[127] In contrast, the FcγRIIA-131H/FcγRIIIB-NA1 haplotype was associated with reduced risk of severe malarial anemia (RR, 0.65) and all-cause mortality.[127]

The discrepancies in results between studies may reflect differences in the ethnic background of the populations studied. There may be other genes that differ between these populations which significantly alter outcomes and confound the effect of the *FCGRA* polymorphism. In addition, the patients included in the studies (e.g., children versus adults) and the control groups (e.g., healthy controls versus those with mild malarial disease) were also different, which may confound results. Finally, as is the case for protection against bacterial infections, it may be that the relative importance of FcγRIIA binding to IgG_2 versus CRP differs in the different clinical manifestations of disease. Of possible relevance to this is the observation of differences in the frequency of a CRP gene SNP between malaria-susceptible and -resistant ethnic groups in Mali and the Sudan.[128]

The effects of the inhibitory receptor SNP on malarial susceptibility appears relatively straightforward. FcγRIIB-deficient mice are resistant to *Plasmodium chabaudi chabaudi*, a model of the erythrocytic stage of human malarial infection,[40] and to *Plasmodium bergei ANKA*, a model of cerebral malaria.[129] In humans, FcγRIIB-T232 increases phagocytosis of antibody-opsonized, *P. falciparum*-parasitized erythrocytes by monocyte-derived macrophages *in vitro*.[40] A large study in two cohorts has shown that homozygosity for the FcγRIIB-T232 is associated with substantial protection against severe malaria in Kenyan children.[37] Several mechanisms may contribute to this protective effect, including increased phagocytosis, malarial-specific antibody titers, and TNF production.[40,130,131]

The high mortality rate associated with malarial infection has resulted in its recognition as the strongest known force for evolutionary selection in the recent history of the human genome.[132] The most well-recognized examples of this are the retention of sickle cell and thalassemia traits. In Kenyan children from the coastal region of Kilifi, heterozygous and homozygous alpha thalassemia confers a protective effect against malarial infection.[133] FcγRIIB-T232 has a protective effect of similar magnitude to heterozygous alpha thalassemia,[37] and thus could explain the higher frequency of FcγRIIB-T232 in Africans and Southeast Asians. This might provide the first example of an immune polymorphism predisposing to polygenic autoimmunity, selected and retained by virtue of its protective effect in malaria infection, thus providing an explanation for the ethnic differences seen in the frequency of autoimmune susceptibility.

Brugia Malayi

There is also evidence to support an important role for activatory FcγR in defense against parasitic infection. B-cell-deficient mice injected with *Brugia malayi* retained significant numbers of live microfilariae in their blood in comparison to wild type mice.[134] Treatment of these mice with hyperimmune serum within the first week of infection reduced the number of microfilariae seen. FcγR-deficient mice also had higher levels of microfilariae following infection, suggesting that FcγRs are mediating the protective effects of antibody, probably via ADCC.[134]

CONCLUSIONS

Activating FcγRs play a key role in the humoral response to infection, mediating many important IgG effector functions that favor pathogen clearance. The inhibitory receptor FcγRIIB acts to counterbalance the effects of activating FcγR ligation and perhaps the ligation of other immune receptors.[135] Thus, SNPs that alter IgG binding or function of either activating or inhibitory FcγRs can lead to differing levels of immune activation that might favor pathogen clearance or might have deleterious effects if an excessive immune response occurs (Figure 12.2). Pathogens exert a powerful

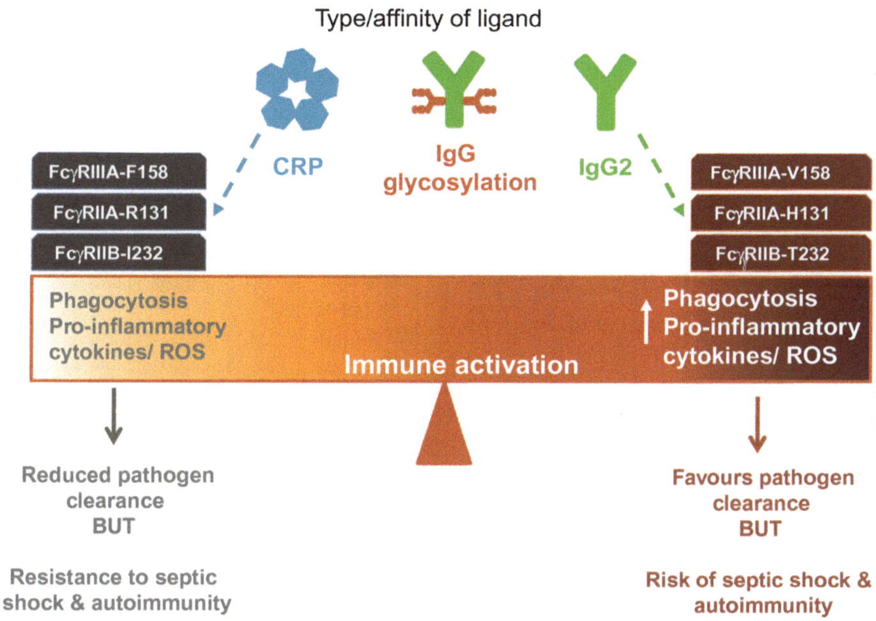

FIGURE 12.2 **FCGR SNPs and ligands determine net level of IgG-mediated immune activation.** The level of immune activation generated following encounter of an IgG-opsonized pathogen will vary depending on a variety of factors: (A) The principle antibody isotype generated and its relative affinity for FcγR isoforms; for example, IgG_2 binds FcγRIIA-H131 with high affinity but has minimal binding to FcγRIIA-R131. (B) The glycosylation of IgG; for example, the presence of a terminal sialic acid on the Fc glycan reduces binding to FcγRs. (C) FcγR–CRP interactions; FcγRIIA-R131 binds CRP with higher affinity than FcγRIIA-H131. In addition, different FCGR SNPs may favor immune activation; for example, the FcγRIIB-T232 SNP results in significantly reduced inhibitory receptor function. The interaction of all of these factors will determine whether the immune response generated results in pathogen clearance or development of the unwanted effects of immune activation, such as susceptibility to septic shock or autoimmunity.

selective pressure on immune polymorphisms, and it is likely that the interaction between microbes and human FcγRs has had significant effects on the frequency of *FCGR* SNPs in different populations. Some of these SNPs may have beneficial effects on pathogen clearance, but they may also be associated with increased immune responses to self-antigen and to autoimmunity. Although much progress has been made in understanding how genetic variation in *FCGRs* can affect susceptibility to infection, there are still many areas of uncertainty. In particular, larger studies are needed to characterize genetic variation (SNPs and CNV) across the entire *FCGR* locus so that interactions between variants in the different FcγRs can be defined. Major future challenges are not only to acquire these large, comprehensive genetic datasets but also to marry this information to detailed clinical and phenotypic data, so that the subtleties of FcγR function in infection can be properly delineated. Such studies will provide critical information for the important field of vaccine design.

Acknowledgments and Funding

Financial support for the author was provided by a Wellcome Trust Intermediate Fellowship.

References

1. Ballow M. Primary immunodeficiency disorders: antibody deficiency. *J Allergy Clin Immunol* 2002;**109**(4):581–91.
2. Guevara Patino JA, Holder AA, McBride JS, Blackman MJ. Antibodies that inhibit malaria merozoite surface protein-1 processing and erythrocyte invasion are blocked by naturally acquired human antibodies. *J Exp Med* 1997;**186**(10):1689–99.
3. Ravetch JV, Clynes RA. Divergent roles for Fc receptors and complement *in vivo*. *Annu Rev Immunol* 1998;**16**:421–32.
4. Ravetch JV, Bolland S. IgG Fc receptors. *Annu Rev Immunol* 2001;**19**:275–90.
5. Smith KG, Clatworthy MR. FcγRIIB in autoimmunity and infection: evolutionary and therapeutic implications. *Nat Rev Immunol* 2010;**10**(5):328–43.
6. Nimmerjahn F, Ravetch JV. Fcγ receptors: old friends and new family members. *Immunity* 2006;**24**(1):19–28.
7. Warmerdam PA, Nabben NM, van de Graaf SA, van de Winkel JG, Capel PJ. The human low affinity immunoglobulin G Fc receptor IIC gene is a result of an unequal crossover event. *J Biol Chem* 1993;**268**(10):7346–9.
8. Qiu WQ, de Bruin D, Brownstein BH, Pearse R, Ravetch JV. Organization of the human and mouse low-affinity Fc gamma R genes: duplication and recombination. *Science* 1990;**248**(4956):732–5.
9. Hughes AL. Gene duplication and recombination in the evolution of mammalian Fc receptors. *J Mol Evol* 1996;**43**(1):4–10.
10. Traherne JA, Martin M, Ward R, Ohashi M, Pellett F, Gladman D, et al. Mechanisms of copy number variation and hybrid gene formation in the KIR immune gene complex. *Hum Mol Genet* 2009;**19**(5):737–51.
11. Ravetch JV, Kinet JP. Fc receptors. *Annu Rev Immunol* 1991;**9**:457–92.
12. Galon J, Gauchat JF, Mazieres N, Spagnoli R, Storkus W, Lotze M, et al. Soluble Fcgamma receptor type III (FcgammaRIII, CD16) triggers cell activation through interaction with complement receptors. *J Immunol* 1996;**157**(3):1184–92.
13. Chuang FY, Sassaroli M, Unkeless JC. Convergence of Fcγ receptor IIA and Fcγ receptor IIIB signaling pathways in human neutrophils. *J Immunol* 2000;**164**(1):350–60.
14. Fernandes MJ, Rollet-Labelle E, Pare G, Marois S, Tremblay ML, Teillaud JL, et al. CD16b associates with high-density, detergent-resistant membranes in human neutrophils. *Biochem J* 2006;**393**(Pt. 1):351–9.
15. Nimmerjahn F, Ravetch JV. Fcgamma receptors as regulators of immune responses. *Nat Rev Immunol* 2008;**8**(1):34–47.
16. Radaev S, Motyka S, Fridman WH, Sautes-Fridman C, Sun PD. The structure of a human type III Fcgamma receptor in complex with Fc. *J Biol Chem* 2001;**276**(19):16469–77.
17. Ferrara C, Stuart F, Sondermann P, Brunker P, Umana P. The carbohydrate at FcgammaRIIIa Asn-162. An element required for high affinity binding to non-fucosylated IgG glycoforms. *J Biol Chem* 2006;**281**(8):5032–6.
18. Lux A, Nimmerjahn F. Impact of differential glycosylation on IgG activity. *Adv Exp Med Biol*. **780**: 113–124.
19. Bharadwaj D, Mold C, Markham E, Du Clos TW. Serum amyloid P component binds to Fc gamma receptors and opsonizes particles for phagocytosis. *J Immunol* 2001;**166**(11):6735–41.
20. Bharadwaj D, Stein MP, Volzer M, Mold C, Du Clos TW. The major receptor for C-reactive protein on leukocytes is Fcgamma receptor II. *J Exp Med* 1999;**190**(4):585–90.
21. Lu J, Marnell LL, Marjon KD, Mold C, Du Clos TW, Sun PD. Structural recognition and functional activation of FcgammaR by innate pentraxins. *Nature* 2008;**456**(7224):989–92.

22. Nimmerjahn F, Ravetch JV. Divergent immunoglobulin g subclass activity through selective Fc receptor binding. *Science* 2005;**310**(5753):1510–2.
23. Pricop L, Redecha P, Teillaud JL, Frey J, Fridman WH, Sautes-Fridman C, et al. Differential modulation of stimulatory and inhibitory Fcγ receptors on human monocytes by Th1 and Th2 cytokines. *J Immunol* 2001;**166**(1):531–7.
24. Grattage LP, McKenzie IF, Hogarth PM. Effects of PMA, cytokines and dexamethasone on the expression of cell surface Fc receptors and mRNA in U937 cells. *Immunol Cell Biol* 1992;**70**(Pt. 2):97–105.
25. van de Winkel JG, Capel PJ. Human IgG Fc receptor heterogeneity: molecular aspects and clinical implications. *Immunol Today* 1993;**14**(5):215–21.
26. Parren PW, Warmerdam PA, Boeije LC, Arts J, Westerdaal NA, Vlug A, et al. On the interaction of IgG subclasses with the low affinity Fc gamma RIIa (CD32) on human monocytes, neutrophils, and platelets. Analysis of a functional polymorphism to human IgG2. *J Clin Invest* 1992;**90**(4):1537–46.
27. Stein MP, Edberg JC, Kimberly RP, Mangan EK, Bharadwaj D, Mold C, et al. C-reactive protein binding to FcgammaRIIa on human monocytes and neutrophils is allele-specific. *J Clin Invest* 2000;**105**(3):369–76.
28. Lehrnbecher T, Foster CB, Zhu S, Leitman SF, Goldin LR, Huppi K, et al. Variant genotypes of the low-affinity Fcγ receptors in two control populations and a review of low-affinity Fcγ receptor polymorphisms in control and disease populations. *Blood* 1999;**94**(12):4220–32.
29. Kuwano ST, Bordin JO, Chiba AK, Mello AB, Figueiredo MS, Vieira-Filho JP, et al. Allelic polymorphisms of human Fcgamma receptor IIa and Fcgamma receptor IIIB among distinct groups in Brazil. *Transfusion* 2000;**40**(11):1388–92.
30. Ravetch JV, Perussia B. Alternative membrane forms of Fc gamma RIII(CD16) on human natural killer cells and neutrophils. Cell type-specific expression of two genes that differ in single nucleotide substitutions. *J Exp Med* 1989;**170**(2):481–97.
31. Wu J, Edberg JC, Redecha PB, Bansal V, Guyre PM, Coleman K, et al. A novel polymorphism of FcgammaRIIIa (CD16) alters receptor function and predisposes to autoimmune disease. *J Clin Invest* 1997;**100**(5):1059–70.
32. Chu ZT, Tsuchiya N, Kyogoku C, Ohashi J, Qian YP, Xu SB, et al. Association of Fcgamma receptor IIB polymorphism with susceptibility to systemic lupus erythematosus in Chinese: a common susceptibility gene in the Asian populations. *Tissue Antigens* 2004;**63**(1):21–7.
33. Huizinga TW, de Haas M, van Oers MH, Kleijer M, Vile H, van der Wouw PA, et al. The plasma concentration of soluble Fc-gamma RIII is related to production of neutrophils. *Br J Haematol* 1994;**87**(3):459–63.
34. Bux J, Stein EL, Bierling P, Fromont P, Clay M, Stroncek D, et al. Characterization of a new alloantigen (SH) on the human neutrophil Fcγ receptor IIIB. *Blood* 1997;**89**(3):1027–34.
35. Salmon JE, Millard SS, Brogle NL, Kimberly RP. Fc gamma receptor IIIB enhances Fc gamma receptor IIa function in an oxidant-dependent and allele-sensitive manner. *J Clin Invest* 1995;**95**(6):2877–85.
36. Kyogoku C, Dijstelbloem HM, Tsuchiya N, Hatta Y, Kato H, Yamaguchi A, et al. Fcgamma receptor gene polymorphisms in Japanese patients with systemic lupus erythematosus: contribution of FCGR2B to genetic susceptibility. *Arthritis Rheum* 2002;**46**(5):1242–54.
37. Willcocks LC, Carr EJ, Niederer HA, Rayner TF, Williams TN, Yang W, et al. A defunctioning polymorphism in FCGR2B is associated with protection against malaria but susceptibility to systemic lupus erythematosus. *Proc Natl Acad Sci USA* 2010;**107**(17):7881–5.
38. Floto RA, Clatworthy MR, Heilbronn KR, Rosner DR, MacAry PA, Rankin A, et al. Loss of function of a lupus-associated FcgammaRIIB polymorphism through exclusion from lipid rafts. *Nat Med* 2005;**11**(10):1056–8.
39. Kono H, Kyogoku C, Suzuki T, Tsuchiya N, Honda H, Yamamoto K, et al. FcγRIIB Ile232Thr transmembrane polymorphism associated with human systemic lupus erythematosus decreases affinity to lipid rafts and attenuates inhibitory effects on B cell receptor signaling. *Hum Mol Genet* 2005;**14**(19):2881–92.
40. Clatworthy MR, Willcocks L, Urban B, Langhorne J, Williams TN, Peshu N, et al. Systemic lupus erythematosus-associated defects in the inhibitory receptor FcgammaRIIB reduce susceptibility to malaria. *Proc Natl Acad Sci USA* 2007;**104**(17):7169–74.
41. Chen JY, Wang CM, Ma CC, Luo SF, Edberg JC, Kimberly RP, et al. Association of a transmembrane polymorphism of Fcgamma receptor IIB (FCGR2B) with systemic lupus erythematosus in Taiwanese patients. *Arthritis Rheum* 2006;**54**(12):3908–17.
42. Siriboonrit U, Tsuchiya N, Sirikong M, Kyogoku C, Bejrachandra S, Suthipinittharm P, et al. Association of Fcgamma receptor IIB and IIIB polymorphisms with susceptibility to systemic lupus erythematosus in Thais. *Tissue Antigens* 2003;**61**(5):374–83.
43. Su K, Wu J, Edberg JC, Li X, Ferguson P, Cooper GS, et al. A promoter haplotype of the immunoreceptor tyrosine-based inhibitory motif-bearing FcgammaRIIB alters receptor expression and associates with autoimmunity. I. Regulatory FCGR2B polymorphisms and their association with systemic lupus erythematosus. *J Immunol* 2004;**172**(11):7186–91.

44. Su K, Yang H, Li X, Gibson AW, Cafardi JM, Zhou T, et al. Expression profile of FcgammaRIIB on leukocytes and its dysregulation in systemic lupus erythematosus. *J Immunol* 2007;**178**(5):3272–80.
45. Blank MC, Stefanescu RN, Masuda E, Marti F, King PD, Redecha PB, et al. Decreased transcription of the human FCGR2B gene mediated by the 343 G/C promoter polymorphism and association with systemic lupus erythematosus. *Hum Genet* 2005;**117**(2–3):220–7.
46. Estivill X, Armengol L. Copy number variants and common disorders: filling the gaps and exploring complexity in genome-wide association studies. *PLoS Genet* 2007;**3**(10):1787–99.
47. Briles DE, Nahm M, Schroer K, Davie J, Baker P, Kearney J, et al. Antiphosphocholine antibodies found in normal mouse serum are protective against intravenous infection with type 3 *Streptococcus pneumoniae*. *J Exp Med* 1981;**153**(3):694–705.
48. Mold C, Rodic-Polic B, Du Clos TW. Protection from *Streptococcus pneumoniae* infection by C-reactive protein and natural antibody requires complement but not Fc gamma receptors. *J Immunol* 2002;**168**(12):6375–81.
49. Rodriguez ME, van der Pol WL, Sanders LA, van de Winkel JG. Crucial role of FcgammaRIIa (CD32) in assessment of functional anti-*Streptococcus pneumoniae* antibody activity in human sera. *J Infect Dis* 1999;**179**(2):423–33.
50. Yee AM, Ng SC, Sobel RE, Salmon JE. Fc gammaRIIA polymorphism as a risk factor for invasive pneumococcal infections in systemic lupus erythematosus. *Arthritis Rheum* 1997;**40**(6):1180–2.
51. Yee AM, Phan HM, Zuniga R, Salmon JE, Musher DM. Association between FcgammaRIIa-R131 allotype and bacteremic pneumococcal pneumonia. *Clin Infect Dis* 2000;**30**(1):25–8.
52. Yuan FF, Wong M, Pererva N, Keating J, Davis AR, Bryant JA, et al. FcgammaRIIA polymorphisms in *Streptococcus pneumoniae* infection. *Immunol Cell Biol* 2003;**81**(3):192–5.
53. Moens L, Van Hoeyveld E, Verhaegen J, De Boeck K, Peetermans WE, Bossuyt X. Fcgamma-receptor IIA genotype and invasive pneumococcal infection. *Clin Immunol* 2006;**118**(1):20–3.
54. Yuan FF, Marks K, Wong M, Watson S, de Leon E, McIntyre PB, et al. Clinical relevance of TLR2, TLR4, CD14 and FcgammaRIIA gene polymorphisms in *Streptococcus pneumoniae* infection. *Immunol Cell Biol* 2008;**86**(3):268–70.
55. Endeman H, Cornips MC, Grutters JC, van den Bosch JM, Ruven HJ, van Velzen-Blad H, et al. The Fcγ receptor IIA-R/R131 genotype is associated with severe sepsis in community-acquired pneumonia. *Clin Vaccine Immunol* 2009;**16**(7):1087–90.
56. Sole-Violan J, Garcia-Laorden MI, Marcos-Ramos JA, de Castro FR, Rajas O, Borderias L, et al. The Fcγ receptor IIA-H/H131 genotype is associated with bacteremia in pneumococcal community-acquired pneumonia. *Crit Care Med* 2011;**39**(6):1388–93.
57. Eklund C, Huttunen R, Syrjanen J, Laine J, Vuento R, Hurme M. Polymorphism of the C-reactive protein gene is associated with mortality in bacteraemia. *Scand J Infect Dis* 2006;**38**(11–12):1069–73.
58. Clatworthy MR, Smith KG. FcγRIIB balances efficient pathogen clearance and the cytokine-mediated consequences of sepsis. *J Exp Med* 2004;**199**(5):717–23.
59. Brownlie RJ, Lawlor KE, Niederer HA, Cutler AJ, Xiang Z, Clatworthy MR, et al. Distinct cell-specific control of autoimmunity and infection by FcgammaRIIB. *J Exp Med* 2008;**205**(4):883–95.
60. Gjertsson I, Kleinau S, Tarkowski A. The impact of Fcgamma receptors on Staphylococcus aureus infection. *Microb Pathog* 2002;**33**(4):145–52.
61. Bredius RG, de Vries CE, Troelstra A, van Alphen L, Weening RS, van de Winkel JG, et al. Phagocytosis of *Staphylococcus aureus* and *Haemophilus influenzae* type B opsonized with polyclonal human IgG1 and IgG2 antibodies. Functional hFc gamma RIIa polymorphism to IgG2. *J Immunol* 1993;**151**(3):1463–72.
62. Bredius RG, Fijen CA, De Haas M, Kuijper EJ, Weening RS, Van de Winkel JG, et al. Role of neutrophil Fc gamma RIIa (CD32) and Fc gamma RIIIB (CD16) polymorphic forms in phagocytosis of human IgG1- and IgG3-opsonized bacteria and erythrocytes. *Immunology* 1994;**83**(4):624–30.
63. Pathan N, Faust SN, Levin M. Pathophysiology of meningococcal meningitis and septicaemia. *Arch Dis Child* 2003;**88**(7):601–7.
64. Bredius RG, Derkx BH, Fijen CA, de Wit TP, de Haas M, Weening RS, et al. Fc gamma receptor IIa (CD32) polymorphism in fulminant meningococcal septic shock in children. *J Infect Dis* 1994;**170**(4):848–53.
65. Fijen CA, Bredius RG, Kuijper EJ, Out TA, De Haas M, De Wit AP, et al. The role of Fcγ receptor polymorphisms and C3 in the immune defence against *Neisseria meningitidis* in complement-deficient individuals. *Clin Exp Immunol* 2000;**120**(2):338–45.
66. van der Pol WL, Huizinga TW, Vidarsson G, van der Linden MW, Jansen MD, Keijsers V, et al. Relevance of Fcγ receptor and interleukin-10 polymorphisms for meningococcal disease. *J Infect Dis* 2001;**184**(12):1548–55.
67. Smith I, Vedeler C, Halstensen A. FcγRIIa and FcγRIIIB polymorphisms were not associated with meningococcal disease in Western Norway. *Epidemiol Infect* 2003;**130**(2):193–9.
68. Platonov AE, Shipulin GA, Vershinina IV, Dankert J, van de Winkel JG, Kuijper EJ. Association of human Fc

gamma RIIa (CD32) polymorphism with susceptibility to and severity of meningococcal disease. *Clin Infect Dis* 1998;**27**(4):746–50.
69. Domingo P, Muniz-Diaz E, Baraldes MA, Arilla M, Barquet N, Pericas R, et al. Associations between Fc gamma receptor IIA polymorphisms and the risk and prognosis of meningococcal disease. *Am J Med* 2002;**112**(1):19–25.
70. Domingo P, Muniz-Diaz E, Baraldes MA, Arilla M, Barquet N, Pericas R, et al. Relevance of genetically determined host factors to the prognosis of meningococcal disease. *Eur J Clin Microbiol Infect Dis* 2004;**23**(8):634–7.
71. Rodriguez ME, Hellwig SM, Hozbor DF, Leusen J, van der Pol WL, van de Winkel JG. Fc receptor-mediated immunity against *Bordetella pertussis*. *J Immunol* 2001;**167**(11):6545–51.
72. Hellwig SM, van Oirschot HF, Hazenbos WL, van Spriel AB, Mooi FR, van De Winkel JG. Targeting to Fcγ receptors, but not CR3 (CD11b/CD18), increases clearance of *Bordetella pertussis*. *J Infect Dis* 2001;**183**(6):871–9.
73. Ioan-Facsinay A, de Kimpe SJ, Hellwig SM, van Lent PL, Hofhuis FM, van Ojik HH, et al. FcγRI (CD64) contributes substantially to severity of arthritis, hypersensitivity responses, and protection from bacterial infection. *Immunity* 2002;**16**(3):391–402.
74. Schenkein H.A., Barbour S.E., Tew J.G. Cytokines and inflammatory factors regulating immunoglobulin production in aggressive periodontitis. Periodontol 2000. 2007; **45**: 113–127.
75. Loos BG, Leppers-Van de Straat FG, Van de Winkel JG, Van der Velden U. Fcγ receptor polymorphisms in relation to periodontitis. *J Clin Periodontol* 2003;**30**(7):595–602.
76. Chung HY, Lu HC, Chen WL, Lu CT, Yang YH, Tsai CC. Gm (23) allotypes and Fcγ receptor genotypes as risk factors for various forms of periodontitis. *J Clin Periodontol* 2003;**30**(11):954–60.
77. Kobayashi T, van der Pol WL, van de Winkel JG, Hara K, Sugita N, Westerdaal NA, et al. Relevance of IgG receptor IIIB (CD16) polymorphism to handling of *Porphyromonas gingivalis*: implications for the pathogenesis of adult periodontitis. *J Periodontal Res* 2000;**35**(2):65–73.
78. Yasuda K, Sugita N, Kobayashi T, Yamamoto K, Yoshie H. FcgammaRIIB gene polymorphisms in Japanese periodontitis patients. *Genes Immun* 2003;**4**(8):541–6.
79. Wolf DL, Neiderud AM, Hinckley K, Dahlen G, van de Winkel JG, Papapanou PN. Fcgamma receptor polymorphisms and periodontal status: a prospective follow-up study. *J Clin Periodontol* 2006;**33**(10):691–8.
80. Dimou NL, Nikolopoulos GK, Hamodrakas SJ, Bagos PG. Fcgamma receptor polymorphisms and their association with periodontal disease: a meta-analysis. *J Clin Periodontol* 2010;**37**(3):255–65.
81. Halstead SB. Pathogenesis of dengue: challenges to molecular biology. *Science* 1988;**239**(4839):476–81.
82. Burke DS, Nisalak A, Johnson DE, Scott RM. A prospective study of dengue infections in Bangkok. *Am J Trop Med Hyg* 1988;**38**(1):172–80.
83. Kliks SC, Nimmanitya S, Nisalak A, Burke DS. Evidence that maternal dengue antibodies are important in the development of dengue hemorrhagic fever in infants. *Am J Trop Med Hyg* 1988;**38**(2):411–9.
84. Thein S, Aung MM, Shwe TN, Aye M, Zaw A, Aye K, et al. Risk factors in dengue shock syndrome. *Am J Trop Med Hyg* 1997;**56**(5):566–72.
85. Littaua R, Kurane I, Ennis FA. Human IgG Fc receptor II mediates antibody-dependent enhancement of dengue virus infection. *J Immunol* 1990;**144**(8):3183–6.
86. Moi ML, Lim CK, Takasaki T, Kurane I. Involvement of the Fc gamma receptor IIA cytoplasmic domain in antibody-dependent enhancement of dengue virus infection. *J Gen Virol* 2010;**91**(Pt. 1):103–11.
87. Chan KR, Zhang SL, Tan HC, Chan YK, Chow A, Lim AP, et al. Ligation of Fc gamma receptor IIB inhibits antibody-dependent enhancement of dengue virus infection. *Proc Natl Acad Sci USA* 2011;**108**(30):12479–84.
88. Loke H, Bethell D, Phuong CX, Day N, White N, Farrar J, et al. Susceptibility to dengue hemorrhagic fever in Vietnam: evidence of an association with variation in the vitamin D receptor and Fc gamma receptor IIa genes. *Am J Trop Med Hyg* 2002;**67**(1):102–6.
89. Garcia G, Sierra B, Perez AB, Aguirre E, Rosado I, Gonzalez N, et al. Asymptomatic dengue infection in a Cuban population confirms the protective role of the RR variant of the FcγRIIa polymorphism. *Am J Trop Med Hyg* 2010;**82**(6):1153–6.
90. Blondel B, Duncan G, Couderc T, Delpeyroux F, Pavio N, Colbere-Garapin F. Molecular aspects of poliovirus biology with a special focus on the interactions with nerve cells. *J Neurovirol* 1998;**4**(1):1–26.
91. Arita M, Horie H, Nomoto A. Interaction of poliovirus with its receptor affords a high level of infectivity to the virion in poliovirus infections mediated by the Fc receptor. *J Virol* 1999;**73**(2):1066–74.
92. Ulvestad E, Williams K, Vedeler C, Antel J, Nyland H, Mork S, et al. Reactive microglia in multiple sclerosis lesions have an increased expression of receptors for the Fc part of IgG. *J Neurol Sci* 1994;**121**(2):125–31.
93. Beck OE. Distribution of virus antibody activity among human IgG subclasses. *Clin Exp Immunol* 1981;**43**(3):626–32.
94. Rekand T, Langeland N, Aarli JA, Vedeler CA. Fcγ receptor IIIA polymorphism as a risk factor for acute poliomyelitis. *J Infect Dis* 2002;**186**(12):1840–3.

95. Schalling M, Ekman M, Kaaya EE, Linde A, Biberfeld P. A role for a new herpes virus (KSHV) in different forms of Kaposi's sarcoma. *Nat Med* 1995;**1**(7):707–8.
96. Jawahar S, Moody C, Chan M, Finberg R, Geha R, Chatila T. Natural killer (NK) cell deficiency associated with an epitope-deficient Fc receptor type IIIA (CD16-II). *Clin Exp Immunol* 1996;**103**(3):408–13.
97. Forthal DN, Landucci G, Bream J, Jacobson LP, Phan TB, Montoya B. FcγRIIa genotype predicts progression of HIV infection. *J Immunol* 2007;**179**(11):7916–23.
98. Bachmann MF, Zinkernagel RM. Neutralizing antiviral B cell responses. *Annu Rev Immunol* 1997;**15**:235–70.
99. Huber VC, Lynch JM, Bucher DJ, Le J, Metzger DW. Fc receptor-mediated phagocytosis makes a significant contribution to clearance of influenza virus infections. *J Immunol* 2001;**166**(12):7381–8.
100. Scharf O, Golding H, King LR, Eller N, Frazier D, Golding B, et al. Immunoglobulin G3 from polyclonal human immunodeficiency virus (HIV) immune globulin is more potent than other subclasses in neutralizing HIV type 1. *J Virol* 2001;**75**(14):6558–65.
101. Takeda A, Tuazon CU, Ennis FA. Antibody-enhanced infection by HIV-1 via Fc receptor-mediated entry. *Science* 1988;**242**(4878):580–3.
102. Tsitsikov EN, Fuleihan R, McIntosh K, Scholl PR, Geha RS. Cross-linking of Fc gamma receptors activates HIV-1 long terminal repeat-driven transcription in human monocytes. *Int Immunol* 1995;**7**(10):1665–70.
103. Poonia B, Kijak GH, Pauza CD. High affinity allele for the gene of FCGR3A is risk factor for HIV infection and progression. *PLoS One* 2010;**5**(12):e15562.
104. Forthal DN, Gabriel EE, Wang A, Landucci G, Phan TB. Association of Fcγ receptor IIIa genotype with the rate of HIV infection after gp120 vaccination. *Blood* 2012;**120**(14):2836–42.
105. Brouwer KC, Lal RB, Mirel LB, Yang C, van Eijk AM, Ayisi J, et al. Polymorphism of Fc receptor IIa for IgG in infants is associated with susceptibility to perinatal HIV-1 infection. *AIDS* 2004;**18**(8):1187–94.
106. Forthal DN, Gilbert PB, Landucci G, Phan T. Recombinant gp120 vaccine-induced antibodies inhibit clinical strains of HIV-1 in the presence of Fc receptor-bearing effector cells and correlate inversely with HIV infection rate. *J Immunol* 2007;**178**(10):6596–603.
107. Haynes B.F. Case-control study of the RV144 trial for immune correlates: the analysis and way forward. AIDS Vaccine Conference, September 12–15, 2011, Bangkok, Thailand.
108. Breman JG, Alilio MS, Mills A. Conquering the intolerable burden of malaria: what's new, what's needed: a summary. *Am J Trop Med Hyg* 2004;**71**(2 Suppl.):1–15.
109. Stevenson MM, Riley EM. Innate immunity to malaria. *Nat Rev Immunol* 2004;**4**(3):169–80.
110. Malaguarnera L, Musumeci S. The immune response to *Plasmodium falciparum* malaria. *Lancet Infect Dis* 2002;**2**(8):472–8.
111. Hunt NH, Grau GE. Cytokines: accelerators and brakes in the pathogenesis of cerebral malaria. *Trends Immunol* 2003;**24**(9):491–9.
112. Majarian WR, Daly TM, Weidanz WP, Long CA. Passive immunization against murine malaria with an IgG3 monoclonal antibody. *J Immunol* 1984;**132**(6):3131–7.
113. Fandeur T, Dubois P, Gysin J, Dedet JP, da Silva LP. *In vitro* and *in vivo* studies on protective and inhibitory antibodies against *Plasmodium falciparum* in the Saimiri monkey. *J Immunol* 1984;**132**(1):432–7.
114. McGregor IA. The passive transfer of human malarial immunity. *Am J Trop Med Hyg* 1964;**13**(Suppl):S237–9.
115. Bouharoun-Tayoun H, Druilhe P. *Plasmodium falciparum* malaria: evidence for an isotype imbalance which may be responsible for delayed acquisition of protective immunity. *Infect Immun* 1992;**60**(4):1473–81.
116. Taylor AM, Day NP, Sinh DX, Loc PP, Mai TT, Chau TT, et al. Reactive nitrogen intermediates and outcome in severe adult malaria. *Trans R Soc Trop Med Hyg* 1998;**92**(2):170–5.
117. Taylor RR, Allen SJ, Greenwood BM, Riley EM. IgG3 antibodies to *Plasmodium falciparum* merozoite surface protein 2 (MSP2): increasing prevalence with age and association with clinical immunity to malaria. *Am J Trop Med Hyg* 1998;**58**(4):406–13.
118. Ndungu FM, Bull PC, Ross A, Lowe BS, Kabiru E, Marsh K. Naturally acquired immunoglobulin (Ig)G subclass antibodies to crude asexual *Plasmodium falciparum* lysates: evidence for association with protection for IgG1 and disease for IgG2. *Parasite Immunol* 2002;**24**(2):77–82.
119. Yoneto T, Waki S, Takai T, Tagawa Y, Iwakura Y, Mizuguchi J, et al. A critical role of Fc receptor-mediated antibody-dependent phagocytosis in the host resistance to blood-stage *Plasmodium berghei* XAT infection. *J Immunol* 2001;**166**(10):6236–41.
120. Shi YP, Nahlen BL, Kariuki S, Urdahl KB, McElroy PD, Roberts JM, et al. Fcγ receptor IIa (CD32) polymorphism is associated with protection of infants against high-density *Plasmodium falciparum* infection. VII. Asembo Bay Cohort Project. *J Infect Dis* 2001;**184**(1):107–11.
121. Cooke GS, Aucan C, Walley AJ, Segal S, Greenwood BM, Kwiatkowski DP, et al. Association of Fcgamma receptor IIa (CD32) polymorphism with severe malaria in West Africa. *Am J Trop Med Hyg* 2003;**69**(6):565–8.
122. Ouma C, Keller CC, Opondo DA, Were T, Otieno RO, Otieno MF, et al. Association of FC gamma receptor IIA (CD32) polymorphism with malarial anemia and high-density parasitemia in infants and young children. *Am J Trop Med Hyg* 2006;**74**(4):573–7.

123. Nasr A, Iriemenam NC, Troye-Blomberg M, Giha HA, Balogun HA, Osman OF, et al. Fc gamma receptor IIa (CD32) polymorphism and antibody responses to asexual blood-stage antigens of *Plasmodium falciparum* malaria in Sudanese patients. *Scand J Immunol* 2007;**66**(1):87–96.
124. Sinha S, Mishra SK, Sharma S, Patibandla PK, Mallick PK, Sharma SK, et al. Polymorphisms of TNF-enhancer and gene for FcγRIIa correlate with the severity of falciparum malaria in the ethnically diverse Indian population. *Malar J* 2008;**7**:13.
125. Schuldt K, Esser C, Evans J, May J, Timmann C, Ehmen C, et al. FCGR2A functional genetic variant associated with susceptibility to severe malarial anaemia in Ghanaian children. *J Med Genet* 2010;**47**(7):471–5.
126. Omi K, Ohashi J, Patarapotikul J, Hananantachai H, Naka I, Looareesuwan S, et al. Fcγ receptor IIA and IIIB polymorphisms are associated with susceptibility to cerebral malaria. *Parasitol Int* 2002;**51**(4):361–6.
127. Ouma C, Davenport GC, Garcia S, Kempaiah P, Chaudhary A, Were T, et al. Functional haplotypes of Fc gamma (Fcγ) receptor (FcγRIIA and FcγRIIIB) predict risk to repeated episodes of severe malarial anemia and mortality in Kenyan children. *Hum Genet* 2012;**131**(2):289–99.
128. Israelsson E, Ekstrom M, Nasr A, Dolo A, Kearsley S, Arambepola G, et al. Marked differences in CRP genotype frequencies between the Fulani and sympatric ethnic groups in Africa. *Malar J* 2009;**8**:136.
129. Waisberg M, Tarasenko T, Vickers BK, Scott BL, Willcocks LC, Molina-Cruz A, et al. Genetic susceptibility to systemic lupus erythematosus protects against cerebral malaria in mice. *Proc Natl Acad Sci USA* 2011;**108**(3):1122–7.
130. Kumaratilake LM, Rathjen DA, Mack P, Widmer F, Prasertsiriroj V, Ferrante A. A synthetic tumor necrosis factor-alpha agonist peptide enhances human polymorphonuclear leukocyte-mediated killing of *Plasmodium falciparum in vitro* and suppresses *Plasmodium chabaudi* infection in mice. *J Clin Invest* 1995;**95**(5):2315–23.
131. Muniz-Junqueira MI, dos Santos-Neto LL, Tosta CE. Influence of tumor necrosis factor-alpha on the ability of monocytes and lymphocytes to destroy intraerythrocytic *Plasmodium falciparum in vitro*. *Cell Immunol* 2001;**208**(2):73–9.
132. Kwiatkowski DP. How malaria has affected the human genome and what human genetics can teach us about malaria. *Am J Hum Genet* 2005;**77**(2):171–92.
133. Williams TN, Wambua S, Uyoga S, Macharia A, Mwacharo JK, Newton CR, et al. Both heterozygous and homozygous alpha+ thalassemias protect against severe and fatal *Plasmodium falciparum* malaria on the coast of Kenya. *Blood* 2005;**106**(1):368–71.
134. Gray CA, Lawrence RA. A role for antibody and Fc receptor in the clearance of *Brugia malayi* microfilariae. *Eur J Immunol* 2002;**32**(4):1114–20.
135. Karsten CM, et al. Anti-inflammatory actvity of IgG1 mediated by Fc galactosylation and association of FcγRIIB and dectin-1. *Nat Med* 2012;**18**:1401–6.

CHAPTER

13

Role of IgG Fc Receptors in Monoclonal Antibody Therapy of Cancer

*Marije B. Overdijk, Sandra Verploegen, Wim K. Bleeker and Paul W.H.I. Parren**

Genmab, Utrecht, The Netherlands

MECHANISMS OF ACTION OF MONOCLONAL ANTIBODIES IN ONCOLOGY

Unmodified therapeutic monoclonal antibodies (mAbs) can achieve clinical effect by one or several potential direct or indirect mechanisms of action (MoAs), consistent with the activities of natural antibodies.[1] For oncology targets, direct, or Fab-domain-related effects are induced by binding of the mAb to its target via its antigen-binding site, resulting in ligand binding inhibition, receptor cross-linking, and/or internalization, which may lead to growth inhibition or apoptosis (Figure 13.1). Indirect, or Fc-domain-related effects are mediated by the antibody constant regions (Fc) and may result in the antibody-mediated effector functions, which include complement-dependent cytotoxicity (CDC), antibody-dependent cellular cytotoxicity (ADCC), and antibody-dependent cellular phagocytosis (ADCP) (Figure 13.1). Indeed, the first publication of mAb therapy in a human dates back to 1980 and describes treatment of a patient with non-Hodgkin's lymphoma (NHL), in which a murine IgG directed against a unique tumor-associated antigen induced adherence of the patient's tumor cells to macrophages and tumor cell lysis via CDC.[1,2] This study demonstrated for the first time that tumor cell depletion with a mAb could occur with minimal toxicity in humans and might employ tumor-killing mechanisms including CDC and cell clearance via the reticuloendothelial system. It was rapidly followed by others (see text below), giving rise to a growing class of approved therapeutics, as well as to more recent efforts to expand upon the natural activities of antibodies.

* Corresponding Author

DEVELOPMENT OF THERAPEUTIC MONOCLONAL ANTIBODIES FOR THE TREATMENT OF CANCER

Since their introduction into the clinic, therapeutic antibodies have continuously evolved in terms of species origin, isotype, and MoA,

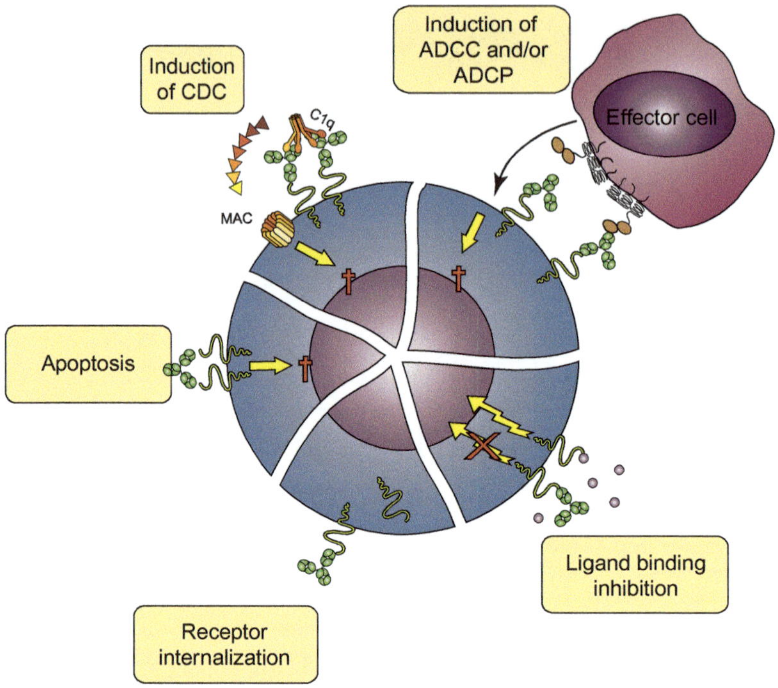

FIGURE 13.1 **Possible therapeutic antibody mechanisms of action.** MoA of therapeutic antibodies can be divided in Fab-domain-related effects and Fc-domain-related effects. Fab-domain or direct effects are represented by ligand binding inhibition, receptor internalization, and apoptosis. Fc-domain or indirect effects are represented by complement-dependent cytotoxicity, antibody-dependent cellular cytotoxicity (ADCC), and antibody-dependent cellular phagocytosis (ADCP).

as well as composition, including sequence and chemical modifications.[2,3] Initially, murine mAbs were developed, followed by the generation of chimeric and human(ized) mAbs. The principal drivers behind this evolution were the aim to reduce immunogenicity and to increase efficacy to permit serial administration and optimize interaction of the antibody Fc domain with the patient's innate immune system. Currently, most mAbs approved for human use are full-length, unmodified, human(ized) mAbs. The first antibody marketed for the treatment of cancer was rituximab, a chimeric IgG_1 CD20 mAb, in 1997. This was rapidly followed in 1998 by the approval of trastuzumab, a humanized IgG_1 against HER2. In 2006, panitumumab, the first mAb consisting solely of human antibody sequences, was approved. Panitumumab is a human IgG_2 mAb against epidermal growth factor receptor (EGFR) which was isolated via immunization of human antibody transgenic mice. Today, 10 unmodified mAbs are being used for the treatment of cancer (Figure 13.2), most often in conjunction with classical treatments such as radio- and chemotherapy, and hundreds more are at various stages of clinical and preclinical development.

Novel antibody formats to potentiate or optimize the activity of unmodified antibodies with the aim to increase clinical efficacy have been investigated for decades, but their development has only recently come of age. Among others, these formats include mAb–payload conjugates comprised of toxins or radioisotopes,[4] bispecific

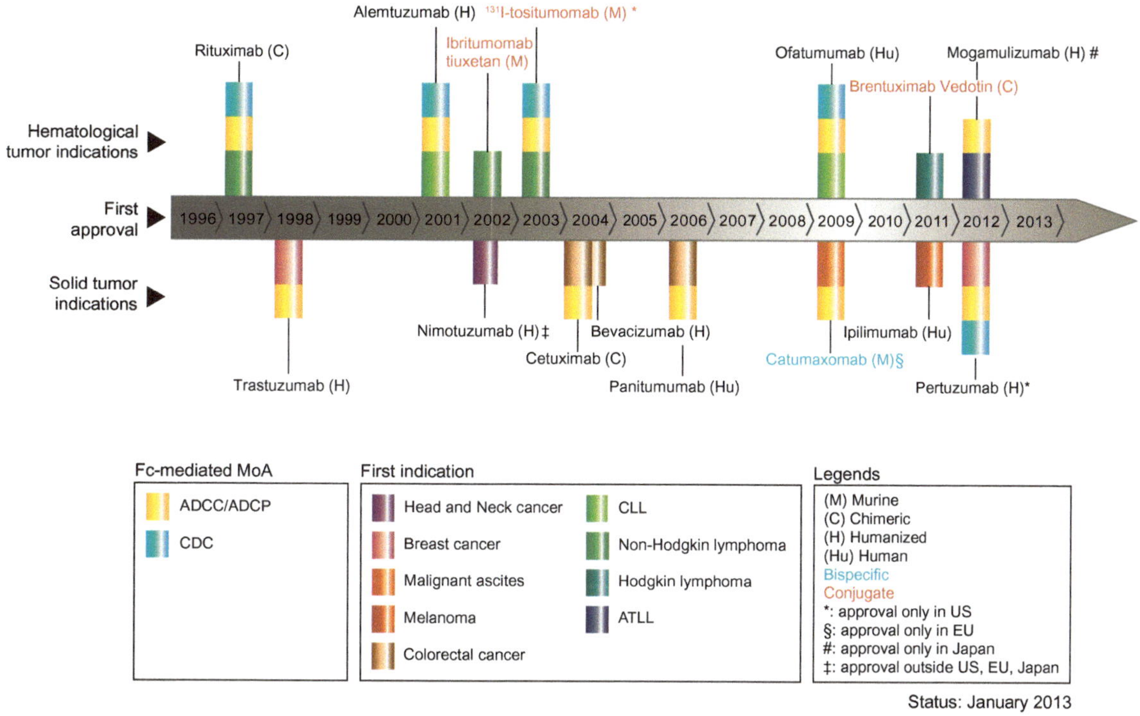

FIGURE 13.2 **mAbs currently approved for use in cancer therapy.** Therapeutic antibodies approved for use in cancer by the regulatory authorities are shown by their time of first registration. Note that nimotuzumab is only approved outside the United States, European Union, and Japan. Catumaxomab was only approved by the European Medicines Agency (EMA) for the treatment of malignant ascites. Mogamulizumab is thus far only approved by the Japanese authorities. Clinical trials for these three antibodies are currently underway in the other territories. The colors for the indications in the figure describe the first therapeutic area for which the antibodies were approved. The yellow and blue bars indicate whether the mAb is described to induce Fc-related effects as ADCC/ADCP or CDC, respectively. (Figure is adapted from Parren, P.W. and van de Winkel, J.G., *Curr. Opin. Immunol.*, **20**(4): 426–430, 2008; Reichert, J.M., *MAbs*, **4**(3): 413–415, 2012.)

mAbs,[5] and mAbs with enhanced immune effector function due to Fc-domain mutations or glycoengineering.[6,7] The first mAb–payload conjugate, gemtuzumab ozogamicin, an IgG_4 mAb against CD33 conjugated to the DNA-cleaving agent calicheamycin, was approved in 2000 but was subsequently withdrawn from the market in 2010 due to an unfavorable safety profile. Currently, there are three mAb–payload conjugates approved for treating cancer (Figure 13.2). The first two, ibritumomab tiuxetan and ^{131}I-tositumomab, are CD20 mAb–radioconjugates and have been available for human use for about a decade. The third is brentuximab vedotin, which is a CD30 mAb conjugated to the tubulin inhibitor auristatin, which was approved in the United States (2011) and European Union (2012) for the treatment of Hodgkin's lymphoma and anaplastic large-cell lymphoma (ALCL).

Mogamulizumab, an anti-CCR4 mAb, recently approved in Japan for the treatment of adult T-cell leukemia–lymphoma (ATLL), represents the first marketed effector-function enhanced mAb. NK cell-mediated ADCC for this antibody has been improved by decreased fucosylation of the Fc-domain-associated carbohydrate.[8,9] Mogamulizumab is being assessed in a number in clinical trials in the United States and European Union, along with other afucosylated mAbs such as the CD20 mAb obinutuzumab[10,11] and the CD19 mAb MEDI-551.[12,13]

Finally, bispecific mAbs, which combine the ability to bind two distinct epitopes or targets, are an area of high interest.[5] Most clinical validation has been generated for bispecific antibodies that can recruit a novel effector reservoir (i.e., T cells) for antibody-mediated tumor cell killing. The bispecific mAb catumaxomab, a murine IgG_{2a} anti-EpCAM/$rIgG_{2b}$ CD3 mAb approved for the treatment of malignant ascites (Figure 13.2), thus represents a novel, highly potent approach to recruit innate immune cells for cancer therapy.[14]

In the following sections, we will specifically address the MoAs of unmodified therapeutic mAbs in cancer, in both preclinical experiments and the clinical setting, with an emphasis on Fcγ receptor (FcγR)-mediated effector functions.

Fc-MEDIATED EFFECTOR FUNCTIONS, PRECLINICAL DATA

Evidence for the role of Fc-mediated effector functions, including CDC, ADCC, and ADCP, in the MoAs of therapeutic mAbs was first established in preclinical studies. CDC is induced by binding of C1q to the Fc domain, leading to deposition of C3b on the surface of Ab-coated tumor cells. The presence of C3b catalyzes formation of the C5–C9 membrane attack complex (MAC), resulting in tumor cell lysis. ADCC and ADCP are mediated by recognition of clustered antibody Fc-domains on tumor cells by specific FcγRs on immune-effector cells such as NK cells, macrophages, and neutrophils. The potency of a mAb to induce Fc-mediated effector functions depends on a number of factors, including the species origin, the isotype and subclass, the glycosylation profile, and the cognate epitope of the mAb.

In preclinical studies, rituximab,[15,16] ofatumumab (IgG_1 CD20 mAb),[17,18] and alemtuzumab (IgG_1 CD52 mAb)[19–21] were found to induce potent ADCC and CDC and they may also induce direct cell killing via apoptosis following receptor cross-linking. Trastuzumab (anti-HER2)[22,23] and cetuximab (anti-EGFR),[24] also of the IgG_1 isotype, can induce killing via ADCC and apoptosis. The IgG_1 isotype is highly effective in triggering ADCC via NK cells, which represent the principal effector cells in the peripheral blood mononuclear cell (PBMC) populations commonly used in *in vitro* ADCC assays. As human IgG_2 is not able to recruit NK cells,[25] panitumumab, a human IgG_2 mAb, was originally reported to induce ADCC poorly; however, panitumumab was later shown to be able to induce effective ADCC via myeloid cells (i.e., neutrophils and monocytes) with comparable efficacy to an IgG_1 mAb,[26] highlighting the subclass dependence of effector cell recruitment.

The role of Fc-mediated effector functions for immunotherapy was investigated in more detail using various Fc receptor knock-out mouse models. Clynes et al.[27] were the first to demonstrate a critical role for FcγR-mediated effector functions for antibody therapy by demonstrating loss of efficacy of trastuzumab and rituximab in common γ-chain knock-out mice ($FcR\gamma^{-/-}$, mice lacking expression of activating IgG Fc receptors). Their experiments therefore strongly suggest a critical role for ADCC in the MoAs of these mAbs, at least under the early treatment conditions employed in their study. Similarly, efficacy of alemtuzumab in a murine ATL model was lost in the $FcR\gamma^{-/-}$ mouse model. The authors suggested ADCC as the MoA, but argued that a role for FcγR-induced cross-linking leading to apoptosis could not be excluded.[28] The potential of apoptosis induction via FcγR-induced cross-linking was demonstrated by Wilson et al.[29] with a DR5-specific mAb. To settle this question for CD20 antibody therapy, de Haij et al.[30] developed a novel mouse model with normal expression of common γ-chain-associated FcγRs in which signal transduction and thereby ADCC were inactivated through an intracellular mutation in this γ-chain. These studies confirmed that ADCC indeed represents a critical MoA for rituximab and ofatumumab.

It is important to note, however, that timing of treatment as well as tumor load impact the importance of ADCC as an effector mechanism. Thus, Boross et al.[31] demonstrated that *in vivo* ADCC may be enhanced by concomitant complement activation through recognition of complement deposits by macrophage complement receptors. Interestingly, it was shown that whereas complement alone was sufficient to eliminate a low tumor burden, high tumor burdens required both active complement as well as activating FcγR. Also, Gong et al.[32] demonstrated a requirement of multiple effector mechanisms for optimal cell depletion. Thus, a CD20 mAb rapidly cleared circulating B cells in a human CD20 transgenic mouse model via monocytes and macrophages, whereas depletion of resident B cells within the marginal zone compartment required both CDC and ADCC. Finally, our own study employing EGFR-specific mAbs suggests that ADCC induction can prevent tumor outgrowth or metastasis *in vivo*, but that ADCC alone, however, is not effective against established solid tumors.[33]

The studies above indicate an important role for FcγR-mediated effector functions in antibody therapy in which a major contribution of ADCC can be observed in early treatment, metastasis as well as against circulating cells. The engagement of ADCC alone appears to be inadequate in therapy of established tumors or resident cells, which appear to require the engagement of multiple effector mechanisms for treatment to be effective. An important question is whether these preclinical findings will be confirmed in the clinic.

ROLE FOR FcγR-MEDIATED EFFECTOR FUNCTIONS, CLINICAL DATA

Several studies have explored the potential role of FcγR-mediated effector functions as MoAs of trastuzumab in patients. ADCC of patient PBMCs and lymphoid cell infiltration into tumors were analyzed in a study in which trastuzumab was administered prior to surgery in patients with primary operable breast tumors overexpressing HER2. ADCC activity correlated with clinical response, and larger tumor lymphoid cell infiltrates were observed in responding compared to non-responding patients, suggesting that FcγR-mediated effector functions are beneficial in this setting. A study by Repka et al.[34] explored the potential of interleukin-2 (IL-2) treatment to enhance NK cell numbers, thereby increasing trastuzumab activity via NK cell-mediated ADCC. Patients receiving IL-2 indeed showed increased NK cell numbers, and combining IL-2 with trastuzumab resulted in enhanced ADCC of several breast cancer cell lines *ex vivo*. In a study of the potential role of different immune cells in the clinical response to trastuzumab Arnould et al.[35] demonstrated that in primary systemic therapy of HER2-positive primary breast cancer patients trastuzumab treatment influences the number and trafficking of various immune cells, including T and B lymphocytes and NK cells, into tumor infiltrates. The presence of increased numbers of NK cells, as well as the detection of cytotoxic proteins such as granzyme B, lends support to a role for NK cells in trastuzumab-induced tumor regression. Maréchal et al.[36] assessed the potential impact of intratumoral immune cells and efficacy of first-line cetuximab in combination with chemotherapy in metastatic colorectal cancer (M-CRC) patients. Although cetuximab treatment did not influence NK cell influx into the tumor compared to controls, if present, tumor-infiltrating NK cells were an independent

TABLE 13.1 Main FcγR Polymorphisms and Their Physiological Effects

Receptor family	Human genes	Variants	Effect
FcγRI (CD64)	FcγRIA	R92X	X92: undetectable expression of FcγRIA on phagocyte
FcγRII (CD32)	FcγRIIA	R131H	H131: higher affinity for IgG_2
	FcγRIIB	I232T	T232: lower affinity for lipid rafts/decreased inhibitory activity
	FcγRIIC	CNV	Gene copy number variation (CNV) resulting in higher or lower number of the receptor leading to an altered balance of activating and inhibitory FcγRs
FcγRIII (CD16)	FcγRIIIA	V158F	V158: higher affinity for IgG_1 and IgG_3; binds IgG_4
		CNV	CNV resulting in higher or lower number of the receptor leading to an altered balance of activating and inhibitory FcγRs
	FcγRIIIb	NA 1/2	NA 1: higher affinity for IgG_1 and IgG_3
		CNV	CNV resulting in higher or lower number of the receptor leading to an altered balance of activating and inhibitory FcγRs

Source: Adapted from Concetti, F. and Napolioni, V., *Recent Pat. Anticancer Drug Discov.*, **5**(3): 197–204, 2010.

predictor for progression-free survival (PFS) and objective response rate (ORR) in the cetuximab-treated group. Overall, these translational studies of trastuzumab- and cetuximab-treated patients suggest a role for FcγR-mediated effector functions, specifically NK-cell-mediated ADCC in clinical responses.

POLYMORPHISMS IN FcγRS

FcγRs are expressed by different immune cells and become activated upon aggregation by multivalent antigen–antibody complexes.[37] Functional polymorphisms in the coding regions of the different FcγRs impact the affinity for IgG. In addition, mutations that modulate the expression level of FcγR have been described (Table 13.1). In the field of therapeutic mAbs, many studies have focused on functional polymorphisms identified in FcγRII and FcγRIII. First, FcγRIIa, expressed by myeloid cells, platelets, a subset of T cells, and endothelial cells, harbors a functional polymorphism due to an arginine (R) to histidine (H) amino acid substitution at position 131 (FcγRIIa-131H),[38–40] which results in a higher binding affinity for complexed IgG_2 and IgG_3 compared to FcγRIIa-131R.[41] Second, FcγRIIb, expressed by B cells, monocytes, and macrophages, harbors a functional polymorphism resulting in an isoleucine (I) to threonine (T) amino acid substitution at position 232,[42] which impairs the association of FcγRIIb-232T with lipid rafts and attenuates its inhibitory effect.[43] Third, FcγRIIIa, expressed by NK cells, macrophages, a subset of monocytes, and a subset of T-cells, has a polymorphism with a phenylalanine (F) to valine (V) substitution at amino acid position 158,[44,45] which results in a higher binding affinity of FcγRIIIa-158V to complexed IgG_1, IgG_3, and IgG_4.[46] Finally, FcγRIIIb, expressed by neutrophils and eosinophils, bears the neutrophil antigen (NA) polymorphisms NA-1 or NA-2 in its membrane-distal Ig-like domain,[47] in which IgG_1- or IgG_3-opsonized particles are more efficiently ingested upon interaction with the FcγRIIIb–NA-1 allotype.[48] Bruhns et al.[49] studied the specificity and affinity of the individual FcγRs and their polymorphic variants for the four human IgG isotypes, confirming the findings described above. Interestingly, FcγR polymorphisms have been identified as genetic factors that may impact susceptibility to autoimmune or infectious diseases,[50] and they also correlated with the therapeutic efficacy of therapeutic mAbs, where FcγR-mediated effector functions are part of the *in vivo* MoA.

IMPACT OF FcγR POLYMORPHISMS ON mAb TREATMENT, PRECLINICAL *IN VITRO* DATA

Several *in vitro* studies have demonstrated the impact of FcγR polymorphisms on FcγR-mediated effector functions. We previously demonstrated that monocytes expressing only the FcγRIIA-131H allele support IgG_2 anti-CD3 induced T-cell proliferation efficiently, whereas monocytes homozygous for the FcγRIIA-131R allele do not.[51] For cetuximab it was found that ADCC against squamous cell carcinoma of head and neck (SCCHN) cells was significantly higher with NK cells homozygous or heterozygous for the high-affinity FcγRIIIA-158V allele than NK cells homozygous for the low-affinity FcγRIIIA-158F.[52,53] FcγRIIIa-158V was also related to significantly higher expression of NK activation markers CD69 and CD107a and significantly higher secretion levels of IFN-γ, MIP-1α, MIP-1β, RANTES, and TNF-α. Dall'Ozzo et al.[54] compared ADCC of rituximab-opsonized human Burkitt's lymphoma cells by NK cells. This study demonstrated that rituximab was about four times more potent in ADCC with NK cells homozygously expressing FcγRIIIa-158V. Comparable results were found for the CD20 mAb, ofatumumab.[18] For trastuzumab, ADCC efficacy of a human breast cancer cell line was significantly higher, with PBMCs expressing only FcγRIIIa-158V compared to 158F carriers;[55] no significant differences were found for FcγRIIa-131H versus 131R. These *in vitro* studies clearly demonstrate that FcγR polymorphisms, with an emphasis on the FcγRIIIa-158V/F polymorphism, may affect mAb efficacy and indicates that exploring the relationship between FcγR polymorphisms and clinical responses may provide additional evidence for the contributions of FcγR-mediated effector functions to mAb therapy.

IMPACT OF FcγR POLYMORPHISMS IN mAb TREATMENT, CLINICAL DATA

Studies on the correlation of FcγR polymorphisms with clinical outcome have been reported for four mAbs: rituximab, alemtuzumab, cetuximab, and trastuzumab. The findings of these studies are summarized in Table 13.2. The CD20 mAb, rituximab was the first therapeutic mAb for which the influence of the functional polymorphism in FcγRIIIa was studied. Cartron et al.[56] observed a significantly higher ORR in patients homozygous for FcγRIIIa-158V compared to FcγRIIIa-158F carriers, indicating a significant role for FcγRIIIa-mediated effector functions in the treatment of follicular lymphoma (FL) patients with rituximab. The FcγRIIIa-158F carriers nonetheless did show significant clinical responses to rituximab. This can be explained by the *in vitro* observation that a reduction in FcγR affinity reduces, but does not abrogate, ADCC, as well as the contribution of multiple additional MoA (such as CDC and apoptosis), as discussed above. Two other studies confirmed homozygous FcγRIIIa-158V expression to be associated with a higher clinical response to monotherapy with rituximab in FL.[57,58] Ghielmini et al.[59] observed that homozygosity for 158V correlated with significantly longer event-free survival (EFS) in FL patients compared to 158F carriers, although they did not see significantly enhanced ORR. Cornec et al.[57] analyzed response rates in association with genetic polymorphisms in low-grade NHL

TABLE 13.2 Impact of FcγR Polymorphisms on Clinical Outcome

Therapy	FcγR	*N*	*N* (polymorphism)	Indication	Clinical outcome: CR	ORR	EFS/PFS	OS	Refs.
Monotherapy									
Rituximab	FcγRIIIa	49	10 (158V/V)	FL	ND	+	+	ND	Cartron et al.[56]
	FcγRIIIa	101	15 (158V/V)	FL	ND	+	+	ND	Weng and Levy[58,62]
	FcγRIIa		21 (131H/H)		ND	+	+	ND	
	FcγRIIIa	30	6 (158V/V)	CLL	ND	–	ND	ND	Farag et al.[61]
	FcγRIIIa	58	10 (158V/V)	WM	ND	+	–	ND	Treon et al.[60]
	FcγRIIIa	171	32 (158V/V)	FL	ND	–	+	ND	Ghielmini et al.[59]
				MCL	ND	–	–	ND	
	FcγRIIb	101	15 (232I/T)	FL	ND	–	–	ND	Weng and Levy[62]
	FcγRIIIa	50	6 (158V/V)	FL/MZ	+	ND	ND	ND	Cornec et al.[57]
	FcγRIIa		13 (131H/H)		–	ND	ND	ND	
Alemtuzumab	FcγRIIIa	33	4 (158V/V)	CLL	ND	–	ND	ND	Lin et al.[72]
	FcγRIIa		6 (131H/H)		ND	–	ND	ND	
Cetuximab	FcγRIIIa	35	5 (158V/V)	M-CRC	ND	ND	–	–	Zhang et al.[74]
	FcγRIIa		9 (131H/H)		ND	ND	+	–	
Trastuzumab	FcγRIIIa	35	15 (158V/V)	MBC	ND	+/–	+/–	ND	Tamura et al.[78]
	FcγRIIa		15 (131H/H)		ND	+	+	ND	
Combination therapy									
R-CHOP	FcγRIIIa	113	53 (158V/V)	DLBCL	+	+	–	–	Kim et al.[64]
	FcγRIIa		60 (131H/H)		–	–	–	–	
	FcγRIIIa	94	18 (158V/V)	FL	–	–	–	ND	Carlotti et al.[70]
	FcγRIIa		30 (131H/H)		–	–	–	ND	
	FcγRIIIa	58	16 (158V/V)	DLBCL	–	ND	–	–	Mitrovic et al.[66]
	FcγRIIa		23 (131H/H)		–	ND	–	–	

R + chemo	FcγRIIa	55	11 (131H/H)	NHL	+	–	–	–	Paiva et al.[92]
R-FC	FcγRIIIa	210	20 (158V/V)	CLL	ND	–	–	–	Dornan et al.[71]
	FcγRIIa		54 (131H/H)		ND	–	–	–	
R-CHOP	FcγRIIIa	87	15 (158V/V)	DLBCL	–	ND	–	–	Fabisiewicz et al.[67]
	FcγRIIa		27 (131H/H)		–	ND	–	–	
	FcγRIIIa	263	76 (158V/V)	DLBCL	–	ND	–	–	Ahlgrimm et al.[68]
	FcγRIIa		111 (131H/H)		–	ND	–	–	
	FcγRIIIa	30	1 (158V/V)	FL	ND	ND	–	+	Persky et al.[65]
	FcγRIIa		9 (131H/H)		ND	ND	–	–	
Cetuximab + irinotecan	FcγRIIIa	69	10 (158V/V)	M-CRC	ND	–	+	–	Bibeau et al.[75]
	FcγRIIa		17 (131H/H)		ND	–	–	–	
Cetuximab + chemo	FcγRIIIa	44	31*(158V carrier)	M-CRC	ND	+/–	ND	ND	Rodríguez et al.[76]
	FcγRIIa		12 (131H/H)		ND	+	ND	ND	
Trastuzumab + chemotaxane	FcγRIIIa	54	11 (158V/V)	MBC	ND	+	+	ND	Musolino et al.[55]
	FcγRIIa		10 (131H/H)		ND	+/–	+/–	ND	
Trastuzumab + chemo	FcγRIIIa	15	7 (158V/V)	MBC	ND	–	ND	ND	Tamura et al.[78]
	FcγRIIa		7 (131H/H)		ND	+	ND	ND	

Abbreviations: N, number of patients; CR, complete response; ORR, objective response rate; EFS, event-free survival; PFS, progression-free survival; OS, overall survival; FL, follicular lymphoma; MZ, marginal-zone lymphoma; WM, Waldenström macroglobulinemia; CLL, chronic lymphatic leukemia; MCL, mantle-cell lymphoma; M-CRC, metastatic colorectal cancer; MBC, metastatic breast cancer; +, significant effect high-affinity polymorphism compared to the low-affinity polymorphism (158VV vs. 158FF, 131HH vs. 131RR, 232TT vs. 232II); –, no significant effect; +/–, a beneficial trend; ND, not determined; *, V carrier.

(FL and marginal-zone [MZ] lymphoma) and found that 158V homozygotes exhibited a significantly higher complete response rate (CR). Additionally, a correlation with the FcγRIIIa polymorphism was also demonstrated in Waldenström's macroglobulinemia (WM).[60] In WM patients the ORR was significantly higher in patients expressing only FcγRIIIa-158V, but this was not observed for PFS. However, the correlation between the FcγRIIIa polymorphism and response to rituximab has not been observed in all B-cell malignancies; for example, no correlation was found in chronic lymphocytic leukemia (CLL)[61] and mantle cell lymphoma (MCL).[59]

In addition to FcγRIIIa polymorphisms, the impact of the FcγRIIa polymorphisms has also been studied. *In vitro*, only very limited differences in IgG_1 binding to the polymorphic forms of FcγRIIa have been observed.[41] In patients, Weng and Levy[58,62] found that not only homozygous FcγRIIIa-158V expression but also homozygous expression of FcγRIIa-131H was associated with a higher ORR and PFS in rituximab treatment of FL. The question has been raised whether this association was due to a non-random association of the FcγRIIa-131H and FcγRIIIa-158V alleles, as may be caused by linkage disequilibrium, due to the close proximity of all FcγR genes on chromosome 1.[63] In view of this Weng and Levy[62] provided additional arguments that both polymorphisms independently correlate with response rates in a second study with an extended patient population and longer follow-up. However, the correlation between the FcγRIIa polymorphism and rituximab response rates in monotherapy was not confirmed by Cornec et al.[57] in a smaller study of FL/MZ patients, with CR as read-out. Altogether, the response to rituximab monotherapy therefore displays only a clear correlation with the FcγRIIIa polymorphism in FL, MZ, and WM, suggesting a role for FcγR-mediated effector functions in the *in vivo* MoA in Ab therapy of these diseases.

In standard-of-care cancer therapy, however, rituximab is most often used in combination with chemotherapy, resulting in a significantly enhanced response compared to either agent alone. Several studies have explored whether the enhanced efficacy in combination therapy is impacted by FcγR-mediated effector functions. Kim et al.[64] observed no correlation between the FcγRIIa polymorphism with response rate, whereas the FcγRIIIa polymorphism was found predictive for CR and ORR in treatment with rituximab in combination with cyclophosphamide/doxorubicin/vincristine/prednisone (R-CHOP) in patients with diffuse large B-cell lymphoma (DLBCL). However, the FcγRIIIa polymorphism was not predictive for event-free survival (EFS) or overall survival (OS), suggesting that FcγR-mediated effector functions are most important in initial responses. Also, Persky et al.[65] found the FcγRIIIa polymorphism to be predictive of survival in FL patients given treatments containing a CD20 antibody but not by treatment with chemotherapy alone. Conversely, in other studies, neither FcγRIIa nor FcγRIIIa polymorphisms influenced the EFS or OS to R-CHOP.[66,67,68] These results suggest that FcγR-mediated effects are not a dominant MoA in R-CHOP therapy in DLBCL. Boettcher et al.[69] and Carlotti et al.[70] also did not observe a correlation of CR, ORR, or PFS in FL patients treated with R-CHOP with FcγRIIa or FcγRIIIa polymorphisms. Dornan et al.[71] retrospectively analyzed FcγRIIa and FcγRIIIa polymorphisms of patients enrolled in a controlled randomized study of relapsed CLL, which were treated with either fludarabine and cyclophosphamide (FC) or rituximab plus FC (R-FC). Also in this study, neither the FcγRIIa nor the FcγRIIIa polymorphism significantly influenced ORR, PFS, or OS.

Overall, there seems to be a contrast between the convincing association of FcγRIIIa polymorphism and rituximab efficacy in monotherapy, and the limited correlation when rituximab is used in combination with chemotherapy.

These conflicting data may imply that FcγR-mediated responses are not the principal MoA when rituximab is used in combination with chemotherapy; however, the lack of a clear correlation may be due to the immunosuppressive effect of most chemotherapeutic drugs, causing effector cells to be less responsive to mAbs and thereby impacting FcγR-mediated effector functions. Also, chemotherapy enhances the efficacy of the treatment, which potentially results in a smaller difference in responses between high- and low-affinity polymorphic FcγR. Overall, therefore, for rituximab, the role of FcγR-mediated effector functions as suggested by FcγR polymorphisms have only been convincingly demonstrated for monotherapy in FL, MZ, and WM.

A correlation between FcγR polymorphisms and efficacy of alemtuzumab (CD52 mAb) treatment has been studied in CLL patients. Lin et al.[72] could not demonstrate a correlation between the FcγRIIa and FcγRIIIa polymorphisms and alemtuzumab ORR, similar to rituximab treatment in CLL. No further studies investigating the role of FcγR polymorphisms in combination with alemtuzumab treatment are available.

Cetuximab, an EGFR-targeting mAb used for the treatment of M-CRC, has been shown to induce ADCC *in vitro*.[73] In a small study of only 35 patients containing a limited number of homozygotes, Zhang et al.[74] explored whether FcγRIIa and FcγRIIIa polymorphisms could serve as molecular markers to predict cetuximab response, OS, and toxicity in M-CRC. Indeed, homozygous expression of FcγRIIa-131H correlated with a longer PFS after monotherapy with cetuximab in M-CRC. Unexpectedly, homozygotes for the high-affinity FcγRIIIa-158V demonstrated a shorter PFS compared to 158F carriers. In contrast, Bibeau et al.[75] demonstrated in a retrospective study comprised of 69 M-CRC patients, of whom 10 were 158V and 17 were 131H homozygotes, that FcγRIIIa-158V significantly improved PFS of patients treated with cetuximab in combination therapy with irinotecan. A recent study by Rodríguez et al.[76] of M-CRC patients treated with cetuximab combined with standard chemotherapy showed a significantly stronger ORR and a trend for a beneficial effect for FcγRIIa-131H and FcγRIIIa-158V carriers, respectively. Overall, therefore, patients appear to benefit from carrying the 158V and 131H polymorphisms in cetuximab treatment. The data available, however, are incomplete and this point therefore requires more study.

Finally, ADCC induction was demonstrated *in vitro* for the HER2 mAb trastuzumab.[35,77] Musolino et al.[55] investigated the potential role of FcγR-mediated effector functions in trastuzumab plus taxane treatment of HER2-positive metastatic breast cancer (MBC) patients. Indeed, patients homozygous for FcγRIIIa-158V, alone and in combination with the FcγRIIA-131HH genotype, showed significantly better ORR and PFS upon trastuzumab treatment. Tamura et al.[78] conducted a prospective study in MBC patients, treated either with trastuzumab monotherapy or trastuzumab plus taxane, to determine the predictive value of the FcγR polymorphisms. In both trastuzumab monotherapy and in combination with taxane, homozygosity for FcγRIIa-131H was significantly associated with a stronger anti-tumor response and a longer PFS. Patients homozygous for FcγRIIIa-158V showed only a favorable trend in PFS after trastuzumab monotherapy.

In summary, studies correlating FcγR polymorphisms with clinical response suggest a role for FcγR-mediated effector functions in mAb therapy. Results from monotherapy treatments in this respect are more clear cut than from antibody–chemotherapy combination regimens. The contribution also seems to be more pronounced in hematological tumors compared to solid tumors, although within the hematological tumors not all malignancies seem to have a similar sensitivity to FcγR-mediated effector functions. Differences for a particular mAb between indications may in addition be due to differences in target expression or expression of soluble forms of the target, differential expression of regulatory molecules, mutations downstream of the target, differences in the numbers of immune effector cells between patients, or differences between patient groups studied. There indeed some remarkable differences in results between similar studies, such as between studies on R-CHOP treatment of DLBCL patients. The study of Kim et al.[64] showed a significant benefit of the homozygous FcγRIIIA-158V genotype, while three other studies[66–68] did not reveal such a benefit. An important difference between these studies is that Kim et al. studied Asian DLBCL patients, in which the proportion of the FcγRIIIA-158VV genotype is much higher;[79] that is, 41.5% of the patients were homozygous for FcγRIIIa-158V in the study by Kim et al. versus only 27, 17, and 28% in the other three studies. Finally, factors such as small patient groups, the use of retrospective analysis, differences in treatment regimes, and differences in time for OS or ORR might also account for the observation that the beneficial effect of FcγR polymorphisms is more pronounced in some studies than in others.

OPPORTUNITIES TO ENHANCE FcγR-MEDIATED EFFECTOR FUNCTIONS

As already stated above, the impact of FcγR polymorphisms is most evident in mAb monotherapy compared to mAb combined with chemotherapy. However, in standard-of-care cancer therapy, most mAbs are used in combination with chemotherapy, which seems to reduce the contribution of FcγR-mediated effector functions to the overall therapeutic effect. Two strategies have been followed to take greater advantage of the benefit of FcγR-mediated effect, which include increasing the activation status of effector cells and modulating the strength of the antibody Fc–FcγR interaction.

Combination therapy with immune-modulatory drugs (IMiDs) impacts the activation status of effector cells. Lenalidomide is a structural analog of thalidomide with similar but more potent immune modulatory activities.[80] Its NK cell stimulatory properties suggest that lenalidomide could be highly effective in combination with therapeutic mAbs capable of inducing NK-cell-mediated ADCC, thereby enhancing efficacy of the mAb. Indeed, lenalidomide synergistically increased lysis of multiple myeloma (MM) cells by daratumumab, a human IgG_1 mAb targeting CD38, both in primary cultures of patient bone-marrow-derived mononuclear cells and in ADCC assays using PBMC from lenalidomide-treated patients.[81–83] Additionally, the impact of several undefined IMiDs was studied by Hayashi et al.[84] These IMiDs do not directly activate NK cells, but rather induce T cells to produce IL-2, which subsequently activates the NK cells. They demonstrated that ADCC induced by a chimeric CD20 mAb was enhanced with the IMiDs, again providing a preclinical rationale for the use of IMiDs in combination with mAb therapy. Chemotherapeutic taxane, which synergizes with trastuzumab, is described as inhibiting tumor growth and inducing immunosuppression of adaptive immunity, but also selectively increasing NK cell activity.[77,85] In combination studies with taxanes, immune effector functions are probably not the main MoA; however, the enhanced NK activity can likely contribute to an enhanced FcγR-mediated efficacy of the mAb.

A second strategy to enhance FcγR-mediated effector functions is to increase the affinity of the Fc-domain for FcγRs by Ab engineering, either via mutations in the Fc-domain or by changing the glycosylation of the Fc domain. Desjarlais and Lazar[6] provided an overview of the clinical stage of mAbs with improved effector functions. Several *in vitro* studies showed the effect of Fc engineering on binding to the different FcγR variants. Fc-domain single mutants S239D or I332E and the double and triple mutants S239D/I332E and S239D/I332E/A330L exhibited significantly higher affinities for FcγRIIIa-158F, even higher than the affinity of WT IgG_1 mAb for the FcγRIIIa-158V polymorphism.[86] XmAb5574, a CD19 IgG_1 mAb, contains the S239D and I332E mutations in the Fc domain which showed enhanced ADCC efficacy compared to its WT IgG_1 analog.[87] Pretreating NK cells with lenalidomide could enhance the ADCC efficacy of CD19 mAb XmAb5574 even more. Enhanced ADCC was also demonstrated for the glycoengineered CD20 mAb obinutuzumab, which bound more strongly to FcγRIIIa-158V and -158F,[88] resulting in increased ADCC activity.[10,89] Enhanced ADCC activity was also observed for MEDI 551, a CD19 mAb that is afucosylated by using a fucosyltransferase-deficient producer cell line.[12] The same technology was used for the generation of the afucosylated anti-CCR4 antibody mogamulizumab (KW-0761), which demonstrated positive results in a Phase II study for the treatment of ATLL[8,9] and was recently approved in Japan (Figure 13.2). Niwa et al.[90] demonstrated enhanced ADCC mediated by a low-fucose version of rituximab compared to rituximab. Low-fucose mAb displayed a three- to four-fold higher affinity to the homozygous FcγRIIIa-158F polymorphism than the WT IgG_1 for homozygous FcγRIIIa-158V, suggesting that this enhancement is achieved independently of the FcγRIIIa functional polymorphism. This result was confirmed by a study with a low-fucose mAb targeting EGFR.[91] However, this latter study also demonstrated that ADCC with polymorphonuclear cells (PMN) is less effective with defucosylated EGFR mAb than with the high-fucose form, which may have implications for therapeutic mAbs that recruit PMNs for their *in vivo* therapeutic effects.

FUTURE PERSPECTIVES

Overall, preclinical studies performed *in vitro* and *in vivo* have identified FcγR-mediated effector functions as important mechanisms for tumor cell killing. These findings have been translated to the clinic by studies that demonstrate positive correlations between clinical response and effector cell activation, or the influx of effector cells into tumors. The correlation of certain functional FcγR polymorphisms with clinical responses furthermore provides additional evidence for the role of FcγR-mediated effector functions in the clinical efficacy of unmodified mAbs. That said, it should be noted, however, that the impact of FcγR polymorphisms on clinical efficacy may be modulated by multiple factors such as target expression, indication, patient population, dosing regimen, effector cells availability, and concomitant therapy, resulting in more or less pronounced effects. Because of this variability, FcγR polymorphisms therefore currently do not seem to provide particularly useful predictive biomarkers for patient selection. The evidence for the impact of antibody–FcγR interactions in mAb therapy indicates that there may be room for further improvement of such therapies by optimizing mAb–FcγR interactions, as well as by strategies to effectively recruit, activate, or retain effector cell compartments.

References

1. Oldham RK, Dillman RO. Monoclonal antibodies in cancer therapy: 25 years of progress. *J Clin Oncol* 2008;**26**(11):1774–7.
2. Nadler LM, Stashenko P, Hardy R, Kaplan WD, Button LN, Kufe DW, et al. Serotherapy of a patient with a monoclonal antibody directed against a human lymphoma-associated antigen. *Cancer Res* 1980;**40**(9):3147–54.
3. Parren PW, van de Winkel JG. An integrated science-based approach to drug development. *Curr Opin Immunol* 2008;**20**(4):426–30.
4. FitzGerald DJ, Wayne AS, Kreitman RJ, Pastan I. Treatment of hematologic malignancies with

immunotoxins and antibody-drug conjugates. *Cancer Res* 2011;**71**(20):6300–9.

5. Muller D, Kontermann RE. Bispecific antibodies for cancer immunotherapy: current perspectives. *BioDrugs* 2010;**24**(2):89–98.
6. Desjarlais JR, Lazar GA. Modulation of antibody effector function. *Exp Cell Res* 2011;**317**(9):1278–85.
7. Labrijn AF, Aalberse RC, Schuurman J. When binding is enough: nonactivating antibody formats. *Curr Opin Immunol* 2008;**20**(4):479–85.
8. Ishida T, Joh T, Uike N, Yamamoto K, Utsunomiya A, Yoshida S, et al. Defucosylated Anti-CCR4 monoclonal antibody (KW-0761) for relapsed adult T-cell leukemia-lymphoma: a multicenter Phase II study. *J Clin Oncol* 2012;**30**(8):837–42.
9. Ishii T, Ishida T, Utsunomiya A, Inagaki A, Yano H, Komatsu H, et al. Defucosylated humanized anti-CCR4 monoclonal antibody KW-0761 as a novel immunotherapeutic agent for adult T-cell leukemia/lymphoma. *Clin Cancer Res* 2010;**16**(5):1520–31.
10. Mossner E, Brunker P, Moser S, Puntener U, Schmidt C, Herter S, et al. Increasing the efficacy of CD20 antibody therapy through the engineering of a new type II anti-CD20 antibody with enhanced direct and immune effector cell-mediated B-cell cytotoxicity. *Blood* 2010;**115**(22):4393–402.
11. Salles G, Morschhauser F, Lamy T, Milpied NJ, Thieblemont C, Tilly H, et al. Phase 1 study results of the type II glycoengineered humanized anti-CD20 monoclonal antibody obinutuzumab (GA101) in B-cell lymphoma patients. *Blood* 2012;**119**(22):5126–32.
12. Herbst R, Wang Y, Gallagher S, Mittereder N, Kuta E, Damschroder M, et al. B-cell depletion *in vitro* and *in vivo* with an afucosylated anti-CD19 antibody. *J Pharmacol Exp Ther* 2010;**335**(1):213–22.
13. Ward E, Mittereder N, Kuta E, Sims GP, Bowen MA, Dall'Acqua W, et al. A glycoengineered anti-CD19 antibody with potent antibody-dependent cellular cytotoxicity activity *in vitro* and lymphoma growth inhibition *in vivo*. *Br J Haematol* 2011;**155**(4):426–37.
14. Seimetz D. Novel monoclonal antibodies for cancer treatment: the trifunctional antibody catumaxomab (removab). *J Cancer* 2011;**2**:309–16.
15. Liu AY, Robinson RR, Murray Jr ED, Ledbetter JA, Hellstrom I, Hellstrom KE. Production of a mouse-human chimeric monoclonal antibody to CD20 with potent Fc-dependent biologic activity. *J Immunol* 1987;**139**(10):3521–6.
16. Golay J, Zaffaroni L, Vaccari T, Lazzari M, Borleri GM, Bernasconi S, et al. Biologic response of B lymphoma cells to anti-CD20 monoclonal antibody rituximab *in vitro*: CD55 and CD59 regulate complement-mediated cell lysis. *Blood* 2000;**95**(12):3900–8.
17. Pawluczkowycz AW, Beurskens FJ, Beum PV, Lindorfer MA, van de Winkel JG, Parren PW, et al. Binding of submaximal C1q promotes complement-dependent cytotoxicity (CDC) of B cells opsonized with anti-CD20 mAbs ofatumumab (OFA) or rituximab (RTX): considerably higher levels of CDC are induced by OFA than by RTX. *J Immunol* 2009;**183**(1):749–58.
18. Craigen JL, Mackus WJM, Engleberts P, Miller SR, Speller S, Chamberlain LC, et al. Ofatumumab, a human Mab targeting a membrane-proximal small-loop epitope on CD20, induces potent NK cell-mediated ADCC. *ASH Annu Meet Abstr* 2009;**114**(22):1725.
19. Crowe JS, Hall VS, Smith MA, Cooper HJ, Tite JP. Humanized monoclonal antibody CAMPATH-1H: myeloma cell expression of genomic constructs, nucleotide sequence of cDNA constructs and comparison of effector mechanisms of myeloma and Chinese hamster ovary cell-derived material. *Clin Exp Immunol* 1992;**87**(1):105–10.
20. Nuckel H, Frey UH, Roth A, Duhrsen U, Siffert W. Alemtuzumab induces enhanced apoptosis *in vitro* in B-cells from patients with chronic lymphocytic leukemia by antibody-dependent cellular cytotoxicity. *Eur J Pharmacol* 2005;**514**(2–3):217–24.
21. Siders WM, Shields J, Garron C, Hu Y, Boutin P, Shankara S, et al. Involvement of neutrophils and natural killer cells in the anti-tumor activity of alemtuzumab in xenograft tumor models. *Leuk Lymphoma* 2010;**51**(7):1293–304.
22. Sliwkowski MX, Lofgren JA, Lewis GD, Hotaling TE, Fendly BM, Fox JA. Nonclinical studies addressing the mechanism of action of trastuzumab (Herceptin). *Semin Oncol* 1999;**26**(4, Suppl. 12):60–70.
23. Spector NL, Blackwell KL. Understanding the mechanisms behind trastuzumab therapy for human epidermal growth factor receptor 2-positive breast cancer. *J Clin Oncol* 2009;**27**(34):5838–47.
24. Roda JM, Joshi T, Butchar JP, McAlees JW, Lehman A, Tridandapani S, et al. The activation of natural killer cell effector functions by cetuximab-coated, epidermal growth factor receptor positive tumor cells is enhanced by cytokines. *Clin Cancer Res* 2007;**13**(21):6419–28.
25. Bruggemann M, Williams GT, Bindon CI, Clark MR, Walker MR, Jefferis R, et al. Comparison of the effector functions of human immunoglobulins using a matched set of chimeric antibodies. *J Exp Med* 1987;**166**(5):1351–61.
26. Schneider-Merck T, Lammerts van Bueren JJ, Berger S, Rossen K, van Berkel PH, Derer S, et al. Human IgG2 antibodies against epidermal growth factor receptor effectively trigger antibody-dependent cellular cytotoxicity but, in contrast to IgG1, only by cells of myeloid lineage. *J Immunol* 2010;**184**(1):512–20.
27. Clynes RA, Towers TL, Presta LG, Ravetch JV. Inhibitory Fc receptors modulate *in vivo* cytoxicity against tumor targets. *Nat Med* 2000;**6**(4):443–6.
28. Zhang Z, Zhang M, Goldman CK, Ravetch JV, Waldmann TA. Effective therapy for a murine model

of adult T-cell leukemia with the humanized anti-CD52 monoclonal antibody, Campath-1H. *Cancer Res* 2003;**63**(19):6453–7.
29. Wilson NS, Yang B, Yang A, Loeser S, Marsters S, Lawrence D, et al. An Fcgamma receptor-dependent mechanism drives antibody-mediated target-receptor signaling in cancer cells. *Cancer Cell* 2011;**19**(1):101–13.
30. de Haij S, Jansen JH, Boross P, Beurskens FJ, Bakema JE, Bos DL, et al. *In vivo* cytotoxicity of type I CD20 antibodies critically depends on Fc receptor ITAM signaling. *Cancer Res* 2010;**70**(8):3209–17.
31. Boross P, Jansen JH, de Haij Beurskens FJ, van der Poel CE, Bevaart L, et al. The *in vivo* mechanism of action of CD20 monoclonal antibodies depends on local tumor burden. *Haematologica* 2011;**96**(12):1822–30.
32. Gong Q, Ou Q, Ye S, Lee WP, Cornelius J, Diehl L, et al. Importance of cellular microenvironment and circulatory dynamics in B cell immunotherapy. *J Immunol* 2005;**174**(2):817–26.
33. Overdijk MB, Verploegen S, van den Brakel JH, Lammerts van Bueren JJ, Vink T, van de Winkel JG, et al. Epidermal growth factor receptor (EGFR) antibody-induced antibody-dependent cellular cytotoxicity plays a prominent role in inhibiting tumorigenesis, even of tumor cells insensitive to EGFR signaling inhibition. *J Immunol* 2011;**187**(6):3383–90.
34. Repka T, Chiorean EG, Gay J, Herwig KE, Kohl VK, Yee D, et al. Trastuzumab and interleukin-2 in HER2-positive metastatic breast cancer: a pilot study. *Clin Cancer Res* 2003;**9**(7):2440–6.
35. Arnould L, Gelly M, Penault-Llorca F, Benoit L, Bonnetain F, Migeon C, et al. Trastuzumab-based treatment of HER2-positive breast cancer: an antibody-dependent cellular cytotoxicity mechanism?. *Br J Cancer* 2006;**94**(2):259–67.
36. Maréchal R, De Schutter J, Nagy N, Demetter P, Lemmers A, Deviere J, et al. Putative contribution of CD56 positive cells in cetuximab treatment efficacy in first-line metastatic colorectal cancer patients. *BMC Cancer* 2010;**10**:340.
37. Daeron M. Fc receptor biology. *Annu Rev Immunol* 1997;**15**:203–34.
38. Clark MR, Clarkson SB, Ory PA, Stollman N, Goldstein IM. Molecular basis for a polymorphism involving Fc receptor II on human monocytes. *J Immunol* 1989;**143**(5):1731–4.
39. Tax WJ, Willems HW, Reekers PP, Capel PJ, Koene RA. Polymorphism in mitogenic effect of IgG1 monoclonal antibodies against T3 antigen on human T cells. *Nature* 1983;**304**(5925):445–7.
40. Warmerdam PA, van de Winkel JG, Vlug A, Westerdaal NA, Capel PJ. A single amino acid in the second Ig-like domain of the human Fc gamma receptor II is critical for human IgG2 binding. *J Immunol* 1991;**147**(4):1338–43.
41. Parren PW, Warmerdam PA, Boeije LC, Arts J, Westerdaal NA, Vlug A, et al. On the interaction of IgG subclasses with the low affinity Fc gamma RIIa (CD32) on human monocytes, neutrophils, and platelets. Analysis of a functional polymorphism to human IgG2. *J Clin Invest* 1992;**90**(4):1537–46.
42. Kyogoku C, Dijstelbloem HM, Tsuchiya N, Hatta Y, Kato H, Yamaguchi A, et al. Fcgamma receptor gene polymorphisms in Japanese patients with systemic lupus erythematosus: contribution of FCGR2B to genetic susceptibility. *Arthritis Rheum* 2002;**46**(5):1242–54.
43. Kono H, Kyogoku C, Suzuki T, Tsuchiya N, Honda H, Yamamoto K, et al. FcgammaRIIB Ile232Thr transmembrane polymorphism associated with human systemic lupus erythematosus decreases affinity to lipid rafts and attenuates inhibitory effects on B cell receptor signaling. *Hum Mol Genet* 2005;**14**(19):2881–92.
44. Ravetch JV, Perussia B. Alternative membrane forms of Fc gamma RIII(CD16) on human natural killer cells and neutrophils. Cell type-specific expression of two genes that differ in single nucleotide substitutions. *J Exp Med* 1989;**170**(2):481–97.
45. Wu J, Edberg JC, Redecha PB, Bansal V, Guyre PM, Coleman K, et al. A novel polymorphism of FcgammaRIIIa (CD16) alters receptor function and predisposes to autoimmune disease. *J Clin Invest* 1997;**100**(5):1059–70.
46. Koene HR, Kleijer M, Algra J, Roos D, von dem Borne AE, de Haas M. Fc gammaRIIIa-158V/F polymorphism influences the binding of IgG by natural killer cell Fc gammaRIIIa, independently of the Fc gammaRIIIa-48L/R/H phenotype. *Blood* 1997;**90**(3):1109–14.
47. Huizinga TW, Kleijer M, Tetteroo PA, Roos D, von dem Borne AE. Biallelic neutrophil Na-antigen system is associated with a polymorphism on the phospho-inositol-linked Fc gamma receptor III (CD16). *Blood* 1990;**75**(1):213–7.
48. Salmon JE, Millard SS, Brogle NL, Kimberly RP. Fc gamma receptor IIIb enhances Fc gamma receptor IIa function in an oxidant-dependent and allele-sensitive manner. *J Clin Invest* 1995;**95**(6):2877–85.
49. Bruhns P, Iannascoli B, England P, Mancardi DA, Fernandez N, Jorieux S, et al. Specificity and affinity of human Fcgamma receptors and their polymorphic variants for human IgG subclasses. *Blood* 2009;**113**(16):3716–25.
50. van Sorge NM, van der Pol WL, van de Winkel JG. FcgammaR polymorphisms: implications for function, disease susceptibility and immunotherapy. *Tissue Antigens* 2003;**61**(3):189–202.
51. Parren PW, Warmerdam PA, Boeije LC, Capel PJ, van de Winkel JG, Aarden LA. Characterization of IgG FcR-mediated proliferation of human T cells induced by mouse and human anti-CD3 monoclonal antibodies.

Identification of a functional polymorphism to human IgG2 anti-CD3. *J Immunol* 1992;**148**(3):695–701.
52. Lopez-Albaitero A, Lee SC, Morgan S, Grandis JR, Gooding WE, Ferrone S, et al. Role of polymorphic Fc gamma receptor IIIa and EGFR expression level in cetuximab mediated, NK cell dependent *in vitro* cytotoxicity of head and neck squamous cell carcinoma cells. *Cancer Immunol Immunother* 2009;**58**(11):1853–64.
53. Taylor RJ, Chan SL, Wood A, Voskens CJ, Wolf JS, Lin W, et al. FcγRIIIa polymorphisms and cetuximab induced cytotoxicity in squamous cell carcinoma of the head and neck. *Cancer Immunol Immunother* 2009;**58**(7):997–1006.
54. Dall'Ozzo S, Tartas S, Paintaud G, Cartron G, Colombat P, Bardos P, et al. Rituximab-dependent cytotoxicity by natural killer cells: influence of FCGR3A polymorphism on the concentration-effect relationship. *Cancer Res* 2004;**64**(13):4664–9.
55. Musolino A, Naldi N, Bortesi B, Pezzuolo D, Capelletti M, Missale G, et al. Immunoglobulin G fragment C receptor polymorphisms and clinical efficacy of trastuzumab-based therapy in patients with HER-2/neu-positive metastatic breast cancer. *J Clin Oncol* 2008;**26**(11):1789–96.
56. Cartron G, Dacheux L, Salles G, Solal-Celigny P, Bardos P, Colombat P, et al. Therapeutic activity of humanized anti-CD20 monoclonal antibody and polymorphism in IgG Fc receptor FcgammaRIIIa gene. *Blood* 2002;**99**(3):754–8.
57. Cornec D, Tempescul A, Querellou S, Hutin P, Pers JO, Jamin C, et al. Identification of patients with indolent B cell lymphoma sensitive to rituximab monotherapy. *Ann Hematol* 2012;**91**(5):715–21.
58. Weng WK, Levy R. Two immunoglobulin G fragment C receptor polymorphisms independently predict response to rituximab in patients with follicular lymphoma. *J Clin Oncol* 2003;**21**(21):3940–7.
59. Ghielmini M, Rufibach K, Salles G, Leoncini-Franscini L, Leger-Falandry C, Cogliatti S, et al. Single agent rituximab in patients with follicular or mantle cell lymphoma: clinical and biological factors that are predictive of response and event-free survival as well as the effect of rituximab on the immune system: a study of the Swiss Group for Clinical Cancer Research (SAKK). *Ann Oncol* 2005;**16**(10):1675–82.
60. Treon SP, Hansen M, Branagan AR, Verselis S, Emmanouilides C, Kimby E, et al. Polymorphisms in FcγRIIIA (CD16) receptor expression are associated with clinical response to rituximab in Waldenstrom's macroglobulinemia. *J Clin Oncol* 2005;**23**(3):474–81.
61. Farag SS, Flinn IW, Modali R, Lehman TA, Young D, Byrd JC. FcγRIIIa and FcγRIIa polymorphisms do not predict response to rituximab in B-cell chronic lymphocytic leukemia. *Blood* 2004;**103**(4):1472–4.
62. Weng WK, Levy R. Genetic polymorphism of the inhibitory IgG Fc receptor FcgammaRIIb is not associated with clinical outcome in patients with follicular lymphoma treated with rituximab. *Leuk Lymphoma* 2009;**50**(5):723–7.
63. Lejeune J, Thibault G, Ternant D, Cartron G, Watier H, Ohresser M. Evidence for linkage disequilibrium between FcγRIIIa-V158F and FcγRIIa-H131R polymorphisms in white patients, and for an FcγRIIIa-restricted influence on the response to therapeutic antibodies. *J Clin Oncol* 2008;**26**(33):5489–91. Author reply 91–92.
64. Kim DH, Jung HD, Kim JG, Lee JJ, Yang DH, Park YH, et al. FCGR3A gene polymorphisms may correlate with response to frontline R-CHOP therapy for diffuse large B-cell lymphoma. *Blood* 2006;**108**(8):2720–5.
65. Persky DO, Dornan D, Goldman B, Braziel R, Fisher R, Leblanc M, et al. Fc gamma receptor 3a genotype predicts overall survival in follicular lymphoma patients treated on SWOG trials with combined monoclonal antibody plus chemotherapy but not chemotherapy alone. *Haematologica* 2012;**97**(6):937–42.
66. Mitrovic Z, Aurer I, Radman I, Ajdukovic R, Sertic J, Labar B. FCgammaRIIIA and FCgammaRIIA polymorphisms are not associated with response to rituximab and CHOP in patients with diffuse large B-cell lymphoma. *Haematologica* 2007;**92**(7):998–9.
67. Fabisiewicz A, Paszkiewicz-Kozik E, Osowiecki M, Walewski J, Siedlecki JA. FcγRIIA and FcγRIIIA polymorphisms do not influence survival and response to rituximab, cyclophosphamide, doxorubicin, vincristine, and prednisone immunochemotherapy in patients with diffuse large B-cell lymphoma. *Leuk Lymphoma* 2011;**52**(8):1604–6.
68. Ahlgrimm M, Pfreundschuh M, Kreuz M, Regitz E, Preuss KD, Bittenbring J. The impact of Fc-gamma receptor polymorphisms in elderly patients with diffuse large B-cell lymphoma treated with CHOP with or without rituximab. *Blood* 2011;**118**(17):4657–62.
69. Boettcher S, Pott C, Ritgen M, Hiddemann W, Unterhalt M, Kneba M. Evidence for Fcγ receptor IIIA-independent rituximab effector mechanisms in patients with follicular lymphoma treated with combined immuno-chemotherapy. *ASH Annu Meet Abstr* 2004;**104**(11):590.
70. Carlotti E, Palumbo GA, Oldani E, Tibullo D, Salmoiraghi S, Rossi A, et al. FcgammaRIIIA and FcgammaRIIA polymorphisms do not predict clinical outcome of follicular non-Hodgkin's lymphoma patients treated with sequential CHOP and rituximab. *Haematologica* 2007;**92**(8):1127–30.
71. Dornan D, Spleiss O, Yeh RF, Duchateau-Nguyen G, Dufour A, Zhi J, et al. Effect of FCGR2A and FCGR3A variants on CLL outcome. *Blood* 2010;**116**(20):4212–22.

72. Lin TS, Flinn IW, Modali R, Lehman TA, Webb J, Waymer S, et al. FCGR3A and FCGR2A polymorphisms may not correlate with response to alemtuzumab in chronic lymphocytic leukemia. *Blood* 2005;**105**(1):289–91.
73. Bier H, Hoffmann T, Haas I, van Lierop A. Anti-(epidermal growth factor) receptor monoclonal antibodies for the induction of antibody-dependent cell-mediated cytotoxicity against squamous cell carcinoma lines of the head and neck. *Cancer Immunol Immunother* 1998;**46**(3):167–73.
74. Zhang W, Gordon M, Schultheis AM, Yang DY, Nagashima F, Azuma M, et al. FCGR2A and FCGR3A polymorphisms associated with clinical outcome of epidermal growth factor receptor expressing metastatic colorectal cancer patients treated with single-agent cetuximab. *J Clin Oncol* 2007;**25**(24):3712–8.
75. Bibeau F, Lopez-Crapez E, Di Fiore F, Thezenas S, Ychou M, Blanchard F, et al. Impact of FcγRIIa-FcγRIIIa polymorphisms and KRAS mutations on the clinical outcome of patients with metastatic colorectal cancer treated with cetuximab plus irinotecan. *J Clin Oncol* 2009;**27**(7):1122–9.
76. Rodríguez J, Zarate R, Bandres E, Boni V, Hernandez A, Sola JJ, et al. Fc gamma receptor polymorphisms as predictive markers of cetuximab efficacy in epidermal growth factor receptor downstream-mutated metastatic colorectal cancer. *Eur J Cancer* 2012;**48**(12):1774–80.
77. Gennari R, Menard S, Fagnoni F, Ponchio L, Scelsi M, Tagliabue E, et al. Pilot study of the mechanism of action of preoperative trastuzumab in patients with primary operable breast tumors overexpressing HER2. *Clin Cancer Res* 2004;**10**(17):5650–5.
78. Tamura K, Shimizu C, Hojo T, Akashi-Tanaka S, Kinoshita T, Yonemori K, et al. FcγR2A and 3A polymorphisms predict clinical outcome of trastuzumab in both neoadjuvant and metastatic settings in patients with HER2-positive breast cancer. *Ann Oncol* 2011;**22**(6):1302–7.
79. Wang J, Feng J, Zhang L, Hu Y, Luan B, Yue W, et al. Distribution of variant genotypes of Fc gamma receptor IIIa in healthy Chinese population of Zhengzhou City. *J Huazhong Univ Sci Technolog Med Sci* 2003;**23**(3):239–41.
80. Armoiry X, Aulagner G, Facon T. Lenalidomide in the treatment of multiple myeloma: a review. *J Clin Pharm Ther* 2008;**33**(3):219–26.
81. de Weers M, Tai YT, van der Veer MS, Bakker JM, Vink T, Jacobs DC, et al. Daratumumab, a novel therapeutic human CD38 monoclonal antibody, induces killing of multiple myeloma and other hematological tumors. *J Immunol* 2011;**186**(3):1840–8.
82. van der Veer MS, de Weers M, van Kessel B, Bakker JM, Wittebol S, Parren PW, et al. Towards effective immunotherapy of myeloma: enhanced elimination of myeloma cells by combination of lenalidomide with the human CD38 monoclonal antibody daratumumab. *Haematologica* 2011;**96**(2):284–90.
83. van der Veer MS, de Weers M, van Kessel B, Bakker JM, Wittebol S, Parren PWHI, et al. The therapeutic human CD38 antibody daratumumab improves the anti-myeloma effect of newly emerging multi-drug therapies. *Blood Cancer J* 2011;**1**:e41.
84. Hayashi T, Hideshima T, Akiyama M, Podar K, Yasui H, Raje N, et al. Molecular mechanisms whereby immunomodulatory drugs activate natural killer cells: clinical application. *Br J Haematol* 2005;**128**(2):192–203.
85. Tsavaris N, Kosmas C, Vadiaka M, Kanelopoulos P, Boulamatsis D. Immune changes in patients with advanced breast cancer undergoing chemotherapy with taxanes. *Br J Cancer* 2002;**87**(1):21–7.
86. Lazar GA, Dang W, Karki S, Vafa O, Peng JS, Hyun L, et al. Engineered antibody Fc variants with enhanced effector function. *Proc Natl Acad Sci USA* 2006;**103**(11):4005–10.
87. Awan FT, Lapalombella R, Trotta R, Butchar JP, Yu B, Benson Jr DM, et al. CD19 targeting of chronic lymphocytic leukemia with a novel Fc-domain-engineered monoclonal antibody. *Blood* 2010;**115**(6):1204–13.
88. Ferrara C, Stuart F, Sondermann P, Brunker P, Umana P. The carbohydrate at FcgammaRIIIa Asn-162. An element required for high affinity binding to non-fucosylated IgG glycoforms. *J Biol Chem* 2006;**281**(8):5032–6.
89. Bologna L, Gotti E, Manganini M, Rambaldi A, Intermesoli T, Introna M, et al. Mechanism of action of type II, glycoengineered, anti-CD20 monoclonal antibody GA101 in B-chronic lymphocytic leukemia whole blood assays in comparison with rituximab and alemtuzumab. *J Immunol* 2011;**186**(6):3762–9.
90. Niwa R, Hatanaka S, Shoji-Hosaka E, Sakurada M, Kobayashi Y, Uehara A, et al. Enhancement of the antibody-dependent cellular cytotoxicity of low-fucose IgG1 is independent of FcγRIIIa functional polymorphism. *Clin Cancer Res* 2004;**10**(18, Pt. 1):6248–55.
91. Peipp M, Lammerts van Bueren JJ, Schneider-Merck T, Bleeker WW, Dechant M, Beyer T, et al. Antibody fucosylation differentially impacts cytotoxicity mediated by NK and PMN effector cells. *Blood* 2008;**112**(6):2390–9.
92. Paiva M, Marques H, Martins A, Ferreira P, Catarino R, Medeiros R. FcgammaRIIa polymorphism and clinical response to rituximab in non-Hodgkin lymphoma patients. *Cancer Genet Cytogenet* 2008;**183**(1):35–40.

CHAPTER

14

No Mechanism is an Island

Interactions Among Monoclonal Antibody Mechanisms of Action

George J. Weiner

University of Iowa, Iowa City

INTRODUCTION

In some B-cell malignancies, rituximab alone can induce high response rates and long-term remissions,[1,2] while in other clinical scenarios adding rituximab to chemotherapy enhances the complete response, long-term remission, and cure rate.[3,4] In some patients, rituximab therapy has little value, and in a large percentage of patients resistance to therapy develops. Although we understand the mechanisms that may contribute to the therapeutic effect of rituximab, we know little about why resistance develops. Understanding the mechanisms by which rituximab induces anti-tumor responses and how these mechanisms interact is central to our ability to improve on what is already a highly effective therapy. Such knowledge will help us to figure out why that therapy eventually fails in many patients, with results that may well be applicable to other mAb. Anti-cancer mAb mechanisms of action that are most likely to be important clinically include signaling on the malignant cell resulting in cell cycle arrest or induction of apoptosis, complement-dependent cytotoxicity (CDC), and antibody-dependent cellular cytotoxicity (ADCC). Outlined below is what is known and unknown about various mechanisms of action and how they interact, based on studies conducted *in vitro*, in animal models, and in clinical trials.

IN VITRO ANALYSIS

In vitro analysis has been extremely helpful in exploring the mechanisms of action of anti-cancer mAb; however, it is important to understand the limitations of such studies so the results can be interpreted in the correct perspective. *In vitro* studies of mAb mechanisms of action usually utilize cells that have been selected to grow rapidly *in vitro* and have given positive results in preliminary studies of the mechanism being tested. For example, in the case of rituximab, B-cell lines used most often in studies exploring the direct effect of signaling are relatively sensitive to signaling. Detection of signaling in response to rituximab often requires cross-linking of the rituximab with secondary antibodies. This artificially enhances the strength of the signal. It is unknown whether cross-linking serves to speed up and strengthen the physiological effect of signaling so it can be measured in a short assay, or if it provides such a strong signal that non-physiologic changes are induced that may not be relevant clinically.

Use of primary malignant cells for *in vitro* analysis has significant limitations. Primary cells obtained from lymph nodes require extensive manipulation, including mincing, filtering, and washing, before they can be evaluated. This obliterates the normal architecture of the microenvironment and alters their growth, viability, spontaneous signaling, and sensitivity to therapy. Chronic lymphocytic leukemia (CLL) cells obtained from peripheral blood require less manipulation than do lymphoma cells harvested from nodes, and the study of signaling in primary CLL cells (or circulating lymphoma cells) in response to rituximab[5] has fewer confusing artifacts than studies of signaling in primary lymphoma cells extracted from nodes. Nevertheless, CLL cells are taken out of their natural environment and are often cryopreserved and then thawed before analysis—a stress that could impact results.

In vitro assays of mAb mechanisms of action involve incubation times of minutes (when assessing for direct signaling) to hours (when evaluating for target cell cytotoxicity). This is based on technical considerations, not clinical relevance. Target cell lines often grow too quickly, and effector cells often die too quickly for longer assays to be informative. *In vivo* imaging studies demonstrate lymphocyte behavior changes within seconds of exposure to hypoxic conditions;[6] thus, manipulation of effector cells likely impacts their function *in vitro*, particularly for longer assays. On the other hand, tumors are exposed to mAb for weeks to months clinically, as opposed to just a few hours in the laboratory assays.

In vitro assays usually focus on one mechanism. Most studies of ADCC do not have functional complement, and studies of CDC do not include immune effector cells. Studies of signaling often lack both serum complement and cellular effectors. Thus, these analyses provide little information about interactions between mechanisms.

For all these reasons, *in vitro* analysis does not fully reflect what is happening in patients. Nevertheless, results from *in vitro* studies provide valuable information and have led to a better understanding of mAb mechanisms of action and their interactions. Perhaps most importantly, they have helped inform studies done in animal models and human subjects. What have we learned from *in vitro* studies of mechanisms of action? Anti-CD20 mAb alone can induce death of malignant B cells *in vitro*. Signaling mediated by cross-linking of CD20 is related to functional reorganization of CD20 into lipid rafts. The strength of this effect depends upon how the anti-CD20 mAb being used cross-links the target antigen[7] and the target cell line being studied.[8–11] Molecular changes induced by rituximab impact on a number of pathways involved in apoptosis and include inhibition of p38 mitogen-activated protein kinase, NF-κB, extracellular signal-regulated kinase 1/2 (ERK 1/2), and AKT. Development of *in vitro* resistance to rituximab is not associated with loss of CD20 or genetic changes in the CD20 molecule but has been found to be associated with down-stream changes in signaling.[12]

In vitro studies suggest synergy between rituximab and cytotoxic drugs.[13] Clones grown to be resistant to rituximab *in vitro* can also show resistance to chemotherapy, suggesting that the resistance to apoptosis induced by antibody signaling and cytotoxic drugs may be mediated by common pathways.[7] Demonstration of cross-resistance may be particularly important given the ongoing debate concerning the timing of treatment with antibodies and cytotoxic drugs in many patient populations.

Some, but not all, mAbs can mediate CDC. *In vitro* studies indicate this is related to a number of factors that pertain to the antigen, to the antibody, and to other characteristics of the target cell. Type I and type II anti-CD20 antibodies cross-link CD20 in different ways and have different abilities to fix complement. Type I antibodies such as rituximab cross-link between tetramers and fix complement well. In contrast, type II antibodies such as B1 do not cross-link between tetramer and fix complement poorly.[7,15] The expression of complement inhibitory molecules (CD55 and CD59) on malignant B cells correlates with the extent of *in vitro* lysis.[16–21] Complement-neutralizing proteins play a role in other malignancies, as well. Anti-HER2 antibodies can activate low levels of complement but induce limited CDC in part due to complement-neutralizing proteins on breast cancer cells.[22]

Studies exploring the impact of CDC use serum as a source of complement, which speaks to the importance of CDC in the circulation but tells us little about whether complement plays a role in the anti-tumor activity of rituximab or other mAb within lymph nodes or at other extravascular sites. When the levels of complement proteins in transudative pleural fluid and ascites as a surrogate for extravascular fluid were evaluated, the relative concentration of various complement components varied from protein to protein when these fluids were compared to serum. However, there was sufficient complement in these fluids to mediate CDC, although this CDC was not as robust as that seen when serum was used as a source of complement.[23] We still do not know whether CDC contributes to the clinical activity of rituximab in the extravascular, as well as intravascular, compartments.

In some cases, *in vitro* findings of CDC correlate with clinical observations, while in others they do not. Follicular B-cell lymphoma is more sensitive to rituximab clinically, and follicular lymphoma cells are more effectively lysed by complement *in vitro* when compared to cells from subjects with large-cell lymphoma or mantle-cell lymphoma.[24] On the other hand, the presence of complement-inhibiting proteins on the surface of CLL cells had no impact on the likelihood that patients would respond to rituximab therapy.[21]

MAbs can induce ADCC mediated by a variety of effector cells, including NK cells, granulocytes, and macrophages.[25–27] To trigger ADCC, antibody bound to the target cell interacts with Fcγ receptors (FcγRs) on the effector cells, triggering immune cell activation and death of the target cell.[28] *In vitro*, rituximab can induce ADCC of human lymphoma cell lines by human peripheral blood mononuclear cells;[16] however, *in vitro* detection of ADCC with rituximab and other antibodies often involves very high, non-physiologic effector-to-target cell ratios—often in the 25–50:1 range. Greater lysis is seen when immune effector cells are preactivated with cytokines such as IL-2 prior to the ADCC assay. Whether these manipulations serve to speed up ADCC so it can be measured in a 4-hour time frame or provide for killing via a mechanism that is not relevant clinically is not clear.

ANIMAL MODELS

Animal models can provide information on mAb mechanisms of action that reflect the impact of pharmacokinetics, biodistribution, the microenvironment, and toxicity not apparent *in vitro*; however, animal models also have significant limitations. Most models involve mice that have been inoculated with malignant cell lines grown *in vitro*. These grafts result in tumors that vary from clinical tumors with respect to growth kinetics, phenotype, infiltrating benign cells, and heterogeneity. Many models utilize xenografted human tumors and immune-compromised animals as hosts. Experimental conditions (tumor burden at time of therapy, dosing of therapy, etc) are usually selected with an eye toward enhancing the ability to detect a therapeutic response or study a particular mechanism of action. The mouse immune system, including antibody structure, IgG receptors, complement, etc., is different from that of the human. Each of these factors impacts our ability to apply results from animal models to our understanding of the relative clinical importance of various mAb mechanisms of action.

Analysis of the impact of mAb signaling in animal models carries the advantage of allowing for prolonged exposure of the malignant cells to mAb in a physiologic environment. Synergy has been observed in animal models of rituximab and chemotherapy,[29,30] and these studies have helped provide impetus for clinical evaluation of such combinations; however, they add little to our understanding of rituximab mechanisms of action as either single agents or in combination with chemotherapy.

A number of animal models suggest that the anti-tumor activity of rituximab is dependent, at least in part, on complement.[31,32] Depletion of cellular effectors in these models had no effect on the therapeutic response to mAb, while depletion of complement through the use of cobra venom factor abolished the therapeutic response. Many of these models, however, involved the use of rituximab (a chimeric humanized IgG) in mice—which would require interaction between a human IgG and murine target cells, murine complement and murine effector cells. In addition, the target cells in these models express low levels of complement inhibitor molecules. The demonstration that complement is important in this model does not necessarily mean it is important clinically. Complement activation was recently found to play a role in mAb-induced infusion toxicity in both a rodent model and non-human primates. Use of mAb modified to have a reduced ability to fix complement induced fewer infusion reactions. In the rodent model, this reduction in infusion reaction had little effect on anti-tumor activity.[33] These data support the contention that complement fixation contributes to infusion reactions. On the other hand, both clinical and animal model studies suggest that infusion reactions are not good predictors of a therapeutic response to mAb.

While CDC is the central mechanism of action in some animal models of mAb therapy, in others CDC appears to play a limited role and ADCC is most important.[34] Perhaps the strongest evidence for the importance of ADCC in animal models comes from the work of Clynes and colleagues[35] who found that mAb was effective in wild-type mice but not in mice lacking the common FcRγ chain. Furthermore, the anti-tumor effect of mAb therapy was enhanced in mice lacking FcγRIIb, which is an inhibitory receptor,[36] providing additional evidence that the interactions between the mAb and FcR are central to determining the efficacy of therapy. Other studies, including our own, have demonstrated that agents that enhance immune effector killing can also enhance the efficacy of mAb therapy.[34] Clinical trials exploring a similar strategy have led to results that are intriguing but less clear.[37–39]

CLINICAL TRIALS

Clinical trials and correlative assays represent the gold standard with respect to understanding various mAb mechanisms of action. On the other hand, the vast majority of clinical trials are designed to assess efficacy of therapy, not to understand mechanisms of action. Furthermore, there is a hesitancy to include rigorous correlative studies in large clinical trials because of the logistics and expense. As the name implies, correlative laboratory evaluation leads to a demonstration of a correlation rather than causation; such experiments are more often hypothesis generating than hypothesis testing.

Clinical trials point to all three major mechanisms of action as being clinically relevant. Intriguing data suggest that anti-CD20 therapy can result in regression of B-cell lymphoma in a manner that is not dependent on robust immune participation. The earliest such evidence comes from the first studies of radiolabeled anti-CD20 therapy. Subjects were preloaded with cold (unradiolabeled) murine mAb to improve biodistribution of the radiolabeled antibody. Unexpectedly, some subjects demonstrated shrinkage of lymphoma after the cold mAb but before the radiolabeled mAb was given.[40] The cold mAb used in this study was a murine IgG_{2a} (B1) with a relatively poor ability to interact with human Fc receptors or to fix human complement. Thus, an anti-CD20 mAb with limited interaction with the human immune system clearly had anti-tumor effects.

Rituximab has also been found to be effective in an acellular and relatively protein-free environment as demonstrated by the observation of anti-lymphoma effects when rituximab was injected directly into the cerebrospinal fluid in patients with central nervous system (CNS) lymphoma.[41] The lack of significant levels of complement or cells capable of mediating ADCC in the CNS would suggest a direct effect of rituximab on the malignant cells. On the other hand, a small study suggests that the therapeutic effect of CNS administration of rituximab can be augmented by concomitant injection of serum into the CNS as a source of complement.[42]

If one assumes that the primary mechanism of action of mAb therapy is lysis mediated by immune effector cells, then the overall concept that rituximab will enhance the efficacy of chemotherapy seems counterintuitive. However, clinical data in a variety of B-cell malignancies provide unequivocal evidence that rituximab and chemotherapy can work well together.[3,4,43,44] Together, these data suggest that direct signaling either induces apoptosis in chemo-sensitized cells or sensitizes the malignant cells to cytotoxic therapy when rituximab is given along with chemotherapy. An alternative explanation for the success of these regimens is that chemotherapy enhances the sensitivity of malignant B cells to immune mediated lysis; however, FcγRIIIA (CD16) and FcγRIIA (CD32) polymorphisms in follicular lymphoma patients treated with rituximab plus CHOP chemotherapy did not predict clinical outcome.[45]

Complement is activated during treatment with rituximab in some but not all patients.[46] Complement activation correlates with infusional toxicity[47] but not clinical response. CLL cells that remain after rituximab treatment have been found to have a higher surface expression of the complement inhibitor CD59 when compared to pretherapy expression of this marker.[48,49] This suggests selective elimination or trafficking out of the circulation of CLL cells expressing lower amounts of CD59 that might be more sensitive to CDC. However, no correlation has been found between expression of complement inhibitors and clinical response to rituximab treatment.[21]

Complement can also have immunosupresive effects. Clearance of apoptotic bodies by complement may impede development of an active immune response.[50,51] This could help explain a correlation between polymorphisms in the C1q component of complement (A versus G at position 276) and duration of response to single-agent rituximab.[52] In this study, subjects with a polymorphism associated with decreased protein expression had a better outcome.

Convincing evidence that ADCC is mechanistically involved in clinical response to rituximab therapy comes from correlative studies demonstrating an association between polymorphisms on CD16 (also known as FcγRIIIa) and clinical response to single-agent rituximab. CD16 homozygous for valine at 158 (VV) has a higher affinity for IgG_1 than does CD16 with phenylalanine at that position (VF or FF).[53] Patients with follicular lymphoma with the VV genotype have a better clinical response to rituximab than patients that are VF or FF.[54,55] The same polymorphism is also predictive of rituximab response in patients with Waldenström's macroglobulinemia.[56] We recently reported that subjects with the V genotype receiving their first dose of rituximab have activation of their circulating NK cells and clearance of those NK cells from circulation within 4 hours. Subjects who are FF did not have these changes.[57]

The convincing evidence that CD16 is important does not necessarily mean NK-cell activation and NK-cell-mediated ADCC is responsible. NK cells are activated and produce IFNγ when they come in contact with rituximab-coated target cells.[58] This IFNγ could have direct anti-tumor effects on the malignant cells or could activate other immune effector cells that could contribute to ADCC. Indeed, IFNγ is known to upregulate the high-affinity FcγI receptor (CD64) on granulocytes,[59] so IFNγ could enhance their ability to mediate ADCC. Alternatively, CD16 could serve to cross-link rituximab and enhance signaling that is independent of effector cell activation.

Follicular lymphoma patients homozygous for histidine at 131 (HH) on FcγRIIa also have an improved response to rituximab.[55] These data highlight the importance of Fc–FcγR interactions in the anti-tumor effects of rituximab and suggest that ADCC is a major mechanism of action. However, not all data indicate that these polymorphisms are clinically relevant. CD16 polymorphisms did not predict clinical response to rituximab in chronic lymphocytic leukemia (CLL) patients[60] or follicular lymphoma patients treated with rituximab plus CHOP.[45]

This strong, if indirect, evidence that the interaction between rituximab Fc and CD16 is important clinically has led to the development and clinical evaluation of novel strategies for enhancing target cell lysis by NK cells, including the addition to rituximab of immunostimulatory agents designed to activate NK cells[37,61] and development of anti-CD20 mAb with stronger affinity for CD16.[28,62] Thus far, none of these strategies has been unequivocally successful, but evaluation is ongoing.

INDIVIDUAL MECHANISMS OF ACTION

Where do we stand with respect to understanding the clinical significance of each of these mechanisms of action?

- *Signaling*—There is indirect but convincing evidence extending from *in vitro* analyses through clinical trial correlative studies of the signaling effects of rituximab on B cells, and that altered signaling can contribute to the anti-tumor activity of rituximab. The strongest such evidence is the clear demonstration in a large number of clinical trials that the combination of rituximab and cytotoxic chemotherapy is effective in a variety of B-cell malignancies. Many current clinical trials are evaluating novel approaches to combining rituximab with cytotoxic chemotherapy based on the synergistic effects of rituximab signaling and cytotoxic therapy.
- *Complement*—CDC can result in rapid cell death of rituximab-coated target cells *in vitro* and is a prime mechanism of action for mAb therapy in some animal models. There is considerable data suggesting that CDC occurs in patients after rituximab therapy and that complement fixation plays a role in infusion reactions. What is less clear is the degree to which CDC contributes to the clinical anti-tumor response to therapy. Most studies of CDC have been done in CLL and involve evaluation of the effect of therapy

on circulating cells. Very little is known about of the role of CDC in the extravascular compartment. Overall, the evidence that CDC contributes to the clinical efficacy of rituximab is strongest in CLL and is enough to encourage the clinical development of next-generation anti-CD20 mAb with an enhanced ability to fix complement.[63] Whether such approaches will be clinically superior to rituximab therapy remains to be seen.

- *Antibody-dependent cellular cytotoxicity—In vitro*, animal model, and correlative clinical studies all suggest that interaction of mAb Fc with CD16 contributes to the anti-tumor activity of single-agent rituximab. The most obvious interpretation of these findings is that immune effector cells such as NK cells are mediating ADCC of rituximab-coated target cells. Clinical trials comparing rituximab to next-generation anti-CD20 mAb that have an enhanced ability to bind to FcγR and activate NK cells will help us understand the clinical importance of ADCC in the anti-tumor activity of rituximab.

INTERACTING MECHANISMS

The discussion above focuses on each of the major mechanisms of action of rituximab in isolation, although it is clear that they do not act alone. There are clearly extensive interactions—both synergistic and antagonistic—between these mechanisms of action. A mechanism that may contribute to the anti-tumor activity of rituximab in one clinical scenario may inhibit the therapeutic response in another. Different mechanisms may contribute in different ways at different sites and times within an individual patient.

Many of these interactions revolve around the complex effects of complement, which go beyond traditional CDC. Complement can impact B-cell activation directly,[64] which could influence signaling. C3 has been shown to have a direct inhibitory effect on NK cell function,[65] which could influence ADCC. We found that the epitope to which C3b binds to IgG Fc is very close to the epitope on the IgG Fc that binds to CD16. Fixation of C3b by rituximab on the surface of the B cell is therefore blocking binding of CD16 to rituximab; thus, complement fixation by rituximab blocked NK-cell activation and ADCC.[66] Furthermore, depletion of complement enhanced the efficacy of mAb therapy in an animal model.[67]

Additionally, the presence of immune complexes on the surface of cells does not always lead to CDC. Taylor and colleagues[68,69] have demonstrated that monocytes and macrophages may "shave" rituximab–complement complexes off the surface of CLL cells, resulting in viable malignant cells that no longer express antigen on their surface. They also conducted studies suggesting that "immune exhaustion" can take place, where phagocytic cells are saturated and unable to clear circulating target cells coated with immune complexes.[70] Whether this phenomenon is limited to situations such as CLL, where a large number of opsonized cells circulate through the liver and spleen, or also takes place in the lymph nodes remains to be seen.

The dynamics of interaction between mechanisms are extremely complex and can be influenced by the microenvironment, saturation of receptors, host genetic polymorphisms, and possible exhaustion of proteins or cells vital for effective target cell destruction. Rituximab concentration, immune effector cell infiltration, FcR saturation, and complement depletion in the local micro-environment could all impact whether a given mechanism is important in a given patient at a given time. Mechanisms that are important in one setting may be less important in another, even in the same patient, at different times or locations.

CONCLUSION

MAb-mediated signaling, CDC, and ADCC all likely contribute to the anti-tumor activity of rituximab, and all likely interact. Given this complexity, how do we enhance the efficacy of what is an excellent, but not ideal, approach to therapy? *In vitro*, animal model, and clinical trial results all have contributed to our understanding of the mechanisms of action of rituximab and other mAbs and will continue to do so. This research has led to new rituximab-based combinations, novel schedules, and the design of the next generation of mAbs that are currently under evaluation. One approach in particular has been underutilized: Well-designed correlative studies should be included as a component of essentially all clinical trials to help us understand the importance of various mechanisms of action of rituximab in different settings. An enhanced understanding of mechanisms of action of rituximab could well be applicable beyond rituximab therapy and could help us make an outstanding therapy even better.

References

1. Maloney DG, Grillo-Lopez AJ, Bodkin DJ, White CA, Liles TM, Royston I, et al. IDEC-C2B8: results of a Phase I multiple-dose trial in patients with relapsed non-Hodgkin's lymphoma [see comments]. *J Clin Oncol* 1997;**15**(10):3266–74.
2. McLaughlin P, Grillo-Lopez AJ, Link BK, Levy R, Czuczman MS, Williams ME, et al. Rituximab chimeric anti-CD20 monoclonal antibody therapy for relapsed indolent lymphoma: half of patients respond to a four-dose treatment program. *J Clin Oncol* 1998;**16**(8):2825–33.
3. Habermann TM, Weller EA, Morrison VA, Gascoyne RD, Cassileth PA, Cohn JB, et al. Rituximab-CHOP versus CHOP alone or with maintenance rituximab in older patients with diffuse large B-cell lymphoma. *J Clin Oncol* 2006;**24**(19):3121–7.
4. Coiffier B, Lepage E, Briere J, Herbrecht R, Tilly H, Bouabdallah R, et al. CHOP chemotherapy plus rituximab compared with CHOP alone in elderly patients with diffuse large-B-cell lymphoma. *N Engl J Med* 2002;**346**(4):235–42.
5. Pedersen IM, Buhl AM, Klausen P, Geisler CH, Jurlander J. The chimeric anti-CD20 antibody rituximab induces apoptosis in B-cell chronic lymphocytic leukemia cells through a p38 mitogen activated protein-kinase-dependent mechanism. *Blood* 2002;**99**(4):1314–9.
6. Egeblad M, Ewald AJ, Askautrud HA, Truitt ML, Welm BE, Bainbridge E, et al. Visualizing stromal cell dynamics in different tumor microenvironments by spinning disk confocal microscopy. *Dis Model Mech* 2008; **1**(2–3):155–67. discussion 65.
7. Beers SA, Chan CH, James S, French RR, Attfield KE, Brennan CM, et al. Type II (tositumomab) anti-CD20 monoclonal antibody out performs type I (rituximab-like) reagents in B-cell depletion regardless of complement activation. *Blood* 2008;**112**(10):4170–7.
8. Shan D, Ledbetter JA, Press OW. Signaling events involved in anti-CD20-induced apoptosis of malignant human B cells. *Cancer Immunol Immunother* 2000;**48**(12):673–83.
9. Semac I, Palomba C, Kulangara K, Klages N, van Echten-Deckert G, Borisch B, et al. Anti-CD20 therapeutic antibody rituximab modifies the functional organization of rafts/microdomains of B lymphoma cells. *Cancer Res* 2003;**63**(2):534–40.
10. Jazirehi AR, Gan XH, De Vos S, Emmanouilides C, Bonavida B. Rituximab (anti-CD20) selectively modifies Bcl-xL and apoptosis protease activating factor-1 (Apaf-1) expression and sensitizes human non-Hodgkin's lymphoma B cell lines to paclitaxel-induced apoptosis. *Mol Cancer Ther* 2003;**2**(11):1183–93.
11. Bonavida B. Rituximab-induced inhibition of antiapoptotic cell survival pathways: implications in chemo/immunoresistance, rituximab unresponsiveness, prognostic and novel therapeutic interventions. *Oncogene* 2007;**26**(25):3629–36.
12. Czuczman MS, Olejniczak S, Gowda A, Kotowski A, Binder A, Kaur H, et al. Acquirement of rituximab resistance in lymphoma cell lines is associated with both global CD20 gene and protein down-regulation regulated at the pretranscriptional and posttranscriptional levels. *Clin Cancer Res* 2008;**14**(5):1561–70.
13. Emmanouilides C, Jazirehi AR, Bonavida B. Rituximab-mediated sensitization of B-non-Hodgkin's lymphoma (NHL) to cytotoxicity induced by paclitaxel, gemcitabine, and vinorelbine. *Cancer Biother Radiopharm* 2002;**17**(6):621–30.
14. Jazirehi AR, Vega MI, Bonavida B. Development of rituximab-resistant lymphoma clones with altered cell signaling and cross-resistance to chemotherapy. *Cancer Res* 2007;**67**(3):1270–81.
15. Teeling JL, Mackus WJ, Wiegman LJ, van den Brakel JH, Beers SA, French RR, et al. The biological activity of human CD20 monoclonal antibodies is linked to unique epitopes on CD20. *J Immunol* 2006;**177**(1):362–71.
16. Reff ME, Carner K, Chambers KS, Chinn PC, Leonard JE, Raab R, et al. Depletion of B cells *in vivo* by a chimeric mouse human monoclonal antibody to CD20. *Blood* 1994;**83**(2):435–45.

17. Flieger D, Renoth S, Beier I, Sauerbruch T, Schmidt-Wolf I. Mechanism of cytotoxicity induced by chimeric mouse human monoclonal antibody IDEC-C2B8 in CD20-expressing lymphoma cell lines. *Cell Immunol* 2000;**204**(1):55–63.
18. Golay J, Lazzari M, Facchinetti V, Bernasconi S, Borleri G, Barbui T, et al. CD20 levels determine the *in vitro* susceptibility to rituximab and complement of B-cell chronic lymphocytic leukemia: further regulation by CD55 and CD59. *Blood* 2001;**98**(12):3383–9.
19. Harjunpaa A, Junnikkala S, Meri S. Rituximab (anti-CD20) therapy of B-cell lymphomas: direct complement killing is superior to cellular effector mechanisms. *Scand J Immunol* 2000;**51**(6):634–41.
20. Bellosillo B, Villamor N, Lopez-Guillermo A, Marce S, Esteve J, Campo E, et al. Complement-mediated cell death induced by rituximab in B-cell lymphoproliferative disorders is mediated *in vitro* by a caspase-independent mechanism involving the generation of reactive oxygen species. *Blood* 2001;**98**(9):2771–7.
21. Weng WK, Levy R. Expression of complement inhibitors CD46, CD55, and CD59 on tumor cells does not predict clinical outcome after rituximab treatment in follicular non-Hodgkin lymphoma. *Blood* 2001;**98**(5):1352–7.
22. Jurianz K, Maslak S, Garcia-Schuler H, Fishelson Z, Kirschfink M. Neutralization of complement regulatory proteins augments lysis of breast carcinoma cells targeted with rhumAb anti-HER2. *Immunopharmacology* 1999;**42**(1–3):209–18.
23. Wang S-Y, Cagley J, Fritzinger D, Vogel C-W, John WS, Weiner GJ. Depletion of the C3 component of complement enhances the ability of rituximab-coated target cells to activate human NK cells and improves the efficacy of monoclonal antibody therapy in an *in vivo* model. *Blood* 2008;**114**(26):5322–30.
24. Manches O, Lui G, Chaperot L, Gressin R, Molens JP, Jacob MC, et al. *In vitro* mechanisms of action of rituximab on primary non-Hodgkin lymphomas. *Blood* 2003;**101**(3):949–54.
25. Stockmeyer B, Dechant M, van Egmond M, Tutt AL, Sundarapandiyan K, Graziano RF, et al. Triggering Fc alpha-receptor I (CD89) recruits neutrophils as effector cells for CD20-directed antibody therapy. *J Immunol* 2000;**165**(10):5954–61.
26. Dall'Ozzo S, Tartas S, Paintaud G, Cartron G, Colombat P, Bardos P, et al. Rituximab-dependent cytotoxicity by natural killer cells: influence of FCGR3A polymorphism on the concentration-effect relationship. *Cancer Res* 2004;**64**(13):4664–9.
27. Lefebvre ML, Krause SW, Salcedo M, Nardin A. *Ex vivo*-activated human macrophages kill chronic lymphocytic leukemia cells in the presence of rituximab: mechanism of antibody-dependent cellular cytotoxicity and impact of human serum. *J Immunother* 2006;**29**(4):388–97.
28. Bowles JA, Wang SY, Link BK, Allen B, Beuerlein G, Campbell MA, et al. Anti-CD20 monoclonal antibody with enhanced affinity for CD16 activates NK cells at lower concentrations and more effectively than rituximab. *Blood* 2006;**108**(8):2648–54.
29. Schliemann C, Palumbo A, Zuberbuhler K, Villa A, Kaspar M, Trachsel E, et al. Complete eradication of human B-cell lymphoma xenografts using rituximab in combination with the immunocytokine L19–IL2. *Blood* 2009;**113**(10):2275–83.
30. Mohammad RM, Aboukameel A, Nabha S, Ibrahim D, Al-Katib A. Rituximab, cyclophosphamide, dexamethasone (RCD) regimen induces cure in WSU-WM xenograft model and a partial remission in previously treated Waldenstrom's macroglobulinemia patient. *J Drug Target* 2002;**10**(5):405–10.
31. Di Gaetano N, Cittera E, Nota R, Vecchi A, Grieco V, Scanziani E, et al. Complement activation determines the therapeutic activity of rituximab *in vivo*. *J Immunol* 2003;**171**(3):1581–7.
32. Golay J, Cittera E, Di Gaetano N, Manganini M, Mosca M, Nebuloni M, et al. The role of complement in the therapeutic activity of rituximab in a murine B lymphoma model homing in lymph nodes. *Haematologica* 2006;**91**(2):176–83.
33. Tawara T, Hasegawa K, Sugiura Y, Harada K, Miura T, Hayashi S, et al. Complement activation plays a key role in antibody-induced infusion toxicity in monkeys and rats. *J Immunol* 2008;**180**(4):2294–8.
34. Wooldridge JE, Ballas Z, Krieg AM, Weiner GJ. Immunostimulatory oligodeoxynucleotides containing CpG motifs enhance the efficacy of monoclonal antibody therapy of lymphoma. *Blood* 1997;**89**(8):2994–8.
35. Clynes R, Takechi Y, Moroi Y, Houghton A, Ravetch JV. Fc receptors are required in passive and active immunity to melanoma. *Proc Natl Acad Sci USA* 1998;**95**(2):652–6.
36. Clynes RA, Towers TL, Presta LG, Ravetch JV. Inhibitory Fc receptors modulate *in vivo* cytoxicity against tumor targets. *Nat Med* 2000;**6**(4):443–6.
37. Leonard JP, Link BK, Emmanouilides C, Gregory SA, Weisdorf D, Andrey J, et al. Phase I trial of Toll-like receptor 9 agonist PF-3512676 with and following rituximab in patients with recurrent indolent and aggressive non-Hodgkin's lymphoma. *Clin Cancer Res* 2007;**13**(20):6168–74.
38. Sacchi S, Federico M, Vitolo U, Boccomini C, Vallisa D, Baldini L, et al. Clinical activity and safety of combination immunotherapy with IFN-alpha 2a and Rituximab in patients with relapsed low grade non-Hodgkin's lymphoma. *Haematologica* 2001;**86**(9):951–8.
39. McLaughlin P, Rodriguez MA, Reuben J, East K, Grimm E, Hagemeister FB, et al. Rituximab in

combination with GM–CSF for patients with recurrent indolent lymphoma. *Blood* 2001;**98**(Suppl. 11):2536. [abstract].

40. Kaminski MS, Zasadny KR, Francis IR, Milik AW, Ross CW, Moon SD, et al. Radioimmunotherapy of B-cell lymphoma with [^{131}I]anti-B1 (anti-CD20) antibody. *N Engl J Med* 1993;**329**(7):459–65.
41. Rubenstein JL, Fridlyand J, Abrey L, Shen A, Karch J, Wang E, et al. Phase I study of intraventricular administration of rituximab in patients with recurrent CNS and intraocular lymphoma. *J Clin Oncol* 2007;**25**(11):1350–6.
42. Takami A, Hayashi T, Kita D, Nishimura R, Asakura H, Nakao S. Treatment of primary central nervous system lymphoma with induction of complement-dependent cytotoxicity by intraventricular administration of autologous-serum-supplemented rituximab. *Cancer Sci* 2006;**97**(1):80–3.
43. Czuczman MS, Grillo-Lopez AJ, White CA, Saleh M, Gordon L, LoBuglio AF, et al. Treatment of patients with low-grade B-cell lymphoma with the combination of chimeric anti-CD20 monoclonal antibody and CHOP chemotherapy. *J Clin Oncol* 1999;**17**(1):268–76.
44. Keating MJ, O'Brien S, Albitar M, Lerner S, Plunkett W, Giles F, et al. Early results of a chemoimmunotherapy regimen of fludarabine, cyclophosphamide, and rituximab as initial therapy for chronic lymphocytic leukemia. *J Clin Oncol* 2005;**23**(18):4079–88.
45. Carlotti E, Palumbo GA, Oldani E, Tibullo D, Salmoiraghi S, Rossi A, et al. FcgammaRIIIA and FcgammaRIIA polymorphisms do not predict clinical outcome of follicular non-Hodgkin's lymphoma patients treated with sequential CHOP and rituximab. *Haematologica* 2007;**92**(8):1127–30.
46. Zhou X, Hu W, Qin X. The role of complement in the mechanism of action of rituximab for B-cell lymphoma: implications for therapy. *Oncologist* 2008;**13**(9):954–66.
47. van der Kolk LE, Grillo-Lopez AJ, Baars JW, Hack CE, van Oers MH. Complement activation plays a key role in the side-effects of rituximab treatment. *Br J Haematol* 2001;**115**(4):807–11.
48. Bannerji R, Kitada S, Flinn IW, Pearson M, Young D, Reed JC, et al. Apoptotic-regulatory and complement-protecting protein expression in chronic lymphocytic leukemia: relationship to *in vivo* rituximab resistance. *J Clin Oncol* 2003;**21**(8):1466–71.
49. Treon SP, Mitsiades C, Mitsiades N, Young G, Doss D, Schlossman R, et al. Tumor cell expression of CD59 is associated with resistance to CD20 serotherapy in patients with B-cell malignancies. *J Immunother* 2001;**24**(3):263–71.
50. Boackle SA. Complement and autoimmunity. *Biomed Pharmacother.* 2003;**57**(7):269–73.
51. Botto M, Walport MJ. C1q, autoimmunity and apoptosis. *Immunobiology* 2002;**205**(4–5):395–406.
52. Racila E, Link BK, Weng WK, Witzig TE, Ansell S, Maurer MJ, et al. A Polymorphism in the complement component C1qA correlates with prolonged response following rituximab therapy of follicular lymphoma. *Clin Cancer Res* 2008;**14**(20):6697–703.
53. Koene HR, Kleijer M, Algra J, Roos D, von dem Borne AE, de Haas M. FcγRIIIa-158V/F polymorphism influences the binding of IgG by natural killer cell FcγRIIIa, independently of the FcγRIIIa-48L/R/H phenotype. *Blood* 1997;**90**(3):1109–14.
54. Cartron G, Dacheux L, Salles G, Solal-Celigny P, Bardos P, Colombat P, et al. Therapeutic activity of humanized anti-CD20 monoclonal antibody and polymorphism in IgG Fc receptor FcγRIIIa gene. *Blood* 2002;**99**(3): 754–8.
55. Weng WK, Levy R. Two immunoglobulin G fragment C receptor polymorphisms independently predict response to rituximab in patients with follicular lymphoma. *J Clin Oncol* 2003;**21**(21):3940–7.
56. Treon SP, Hansen M, Branagan AR, Verselis S, Emmanouilides C, Kimby E, et al. Polymorphisms in FcγRIIIA (CD16) receptor expression are associated with clinical response to rituximab in Waldenstrom's macroglobulinemia. *J Clin Oncol* 2005;**23**(3):474–81.
57. Veeramani S, Wang SY, Dahle C, Blackwell S, Jacobus L, Knutson T, et al. Rituximab infusion induces NK activation in lymphoma patients with the high-affinity CD16 polymorphism. *Blood* 2011;**118**(12):3347–9.
58. Bowles JA, Weiner GJ. CD16 polymorphisms and NK activation induced by monoclonal antibody-coated target cells. *J Immunol Meth* 2005;**304**:88–99.
59. Hoffmeyer F, Witte K, Schmidt RE. The high-affinity FcγRI on PMN: regulation of expression and signal transduction. *Immunology* 1997;**92**(4):544–52.
60. Farag SS, Flinn IW, Modali R, Lehman TA, Young D, Byrd JC. FcγRIIIa and FcγRIIa polymorphisms do not predict response to rituximab in B-cell chronic lymphocytic leukemia. *Blood* 2004;**103**(4):1472–4.
61. Friedberg JW, Neuberg D, Gribben JG, Fisher DC, Canning C, Koval M, et al. Combination immunotherapy with rituximab and interleukin 2 in patients with relapsed or refractory follicular non-Hodgkin's lymphoma. *Br J Haematol* 2002;**117**(4):828–34.
62. Robak T. GA-101, a third-generation, humanized and glyco-engineered anti-CD20 mAb for the treatment of B-cell lymphoid malignancies. *Curr Opin Investig Drugs* 2009;**10**(6):588–96.
63. Pawluczkowycz AW, Beurskens FJ, Beum PV, Lindorfer MA, van de Winkel JG, Parren PW, et al. Binding of submaximal C1q promotes complement-dependent cytotoxicity (CDC) of B cells opsonized with anti-CD20 mAbs ofatumumab (OFA) or rituximab (RTX): considerably higher levels of CDC are induced by OFA than by RTX. *J Immunol* 2009;**183**(1):749–58.

64. Carroll MC. The complement system in B cell regulation. *Mol Immunol* 2004;**41**(2–3):141–6.
65. Charriaut C, Senik A, Kolb JP, Barel M, Frade R. Inhibition of *in vitro* natural killer activity by the third component of complement: role for the C3a fragment. *Proc Natl Acad Sci USA* 1982;**79**(19):6003–7.
66. Wang SY, Racila E, Taylor RP, Weiner GJ. NK-cell activation and antibody-dependent cellular cytotoxicity induced by rituximab-coated target cells is inhibited by the C3b component of complement. *Blood* 2008;**111**(3):1456–63.
67. Wang SY, Veeramani S, Racila E, Cagley J, Fritzinger DC, Vogel CW, et al. Depletion of the C3 component of complement enhances the ability of rituximab-coated target cells to activate human NK cells and improves the efficacy of monoclonal antibody therapy in an *in vivo* model. *Blood* 2009;**114**(26):5322–30.
68. Kennedy AD, Beum PV, Solga MD, DiLillo DJ, Lindorfer MA, Hess CE, et al. Rituximab infusion promotes rapid complement depletion and acute CD20 loss in chronic lymphocytic leukemia. *J Immunol* 2004;**172**(5):3280–8.
69. Beum PV, Lindorfer MA, Taylor RP. Within peripheral blood mononuclear cells, antibody-dependent cellular cytotoxicity of rituximab-opsonized Daudi cells is promoted by NK cells and inhibited by monocytes due to shaving. *J Immunol* 2008;**181**(4):2916–24.
70. Beurskens FJ, Lindorfer MA, Farooqui M, Beum PV, Engelberts P, Mackus WJ, et al. Exhaustion of cytotoxic effector systems may limit monoclonal antibody-based immunotherapy in cancer patients. *J Immunol* 2012;**188**(7):3532–41.

CHAPTER

15

Fc Receptor-Dependent Immunity

Joseph U. Igietseme[a,], Xiaoping Zhu[b] and Carolyn M. Black[c]*

[a]National Center for Emerging and Zoonotic Infectious Diseases, Centers for Disease Control and Prevention, Atlanta, Georgia; Department of Microbiology and Immunology, Morehouse School of Medicine, Atlanta, Georgia, [b]University of Maryland, College Park, Maryland, [c]National Center for Emerging and Zoonotic Infectious Diseases, Centers for Disease Control and Prevention, Atlanta, Georgia

Fc RECEPTORS AND SIGNALING MECHANISMS IN IMMUNE EFFECTOR CELLS

FcR Classes and Types

The mammalian FcRs are a highly conserved family of glycoproteins of the immunoglogulin (Ig) superfamily, which are expressed predominantly on a majority of innate immune cells, including monocytes, macrophages (Mϕs), dendritic cells (DCs), neutrophils, PMNs, basophils, mast cells, and eosinophils; B cells; follicular DCs; and some other tissues (mucosal epithelium, endothelium, and placenta), where they bind free or antigen-bound antibodies via the Fc portion to initiate diverse immunobiological processes, such as the functional activation of the cells, facilitation of antigen or cross-antigen presentation, and cytokine secretion.[1–3] There are distinct FcRs for the major antibody isotypes, which are designated as FcγR, FcεR, FcαR, FcμR, and FcδR (Table 15.1). Also, the neonatal FcR (FcRn) and the polymeric IgA receptor (pIgR) are respectively IgG- and IgA/IgM-binding and intracellular transport receptors that are expressed on mucosal epithelial cells lining the respiratory, gastrointestinal, and genital tracts. In addition, the FcRn is expressed on endothelial cells and the placenta. Although the precise biological functions of the recently identified FcR-like molecules (FcRLs) are not fully known, their differential expression by B-lineage cells and overexpression in some B-cell malignancies have suggested that they may play a role in pathogenesis of B cell disease.[3,4]

* Corresponding Author

Cellular Signaling Events Associated with FcRs

FcRs exist as high- or low-affinity receptors for binding the Fc portion of the different antibody ligands or the immune complexes. The binding initiates a signal transduction process

TABLE 15.1 Fc Receptors, Ligands, and Cellular Expression

FcRs Class/Type				
Human	**Mouse**	**Affinity for Ig**	**Ligands**	**Cellular Distribution**
FcγRI (CD64)	FcγRI (CD64)	High (Kd~10^{-9}M)	Monomeric IgG	Monocytes, Mϕs, PMNs, DCs
FcγRII (CD32a/c)	—	Low (Kd~10^{-7}M)	IC* IgG	PMNs, DCs, all monocytes, Mϕs, B cells
FcγRII B (CD32)	FcγRIIB (CD32)	Low (Kd~10^{-7}M)	IC* IgG	PMNs, DCs, all monocytes,Mϕs, B cells
FcγRIII (CD16a/b)	FcγRIII (CD16)	Low (Kd~10^{-6}M)	IC* IgG	PMNs, NK, all monocytes, Mϕs, DCs
—	FcγRIV	Low (Kd~10^{-7}M)	IC* IgG	PMNs, DCs, resident monocytes, Mϕs
FcεRI	—	High (Kd~10^{-10}M)	Monomeric IgE	Basophils, eosinophils, mast cells
FcεRII (CD23)	FcεRII (CD23)	Low (Kd~10^{-7}M)	IgE	Basophils, eosinophils, epithelial cells
FcαRI (CD89)		Low (Kd~10^{-6}M)	IgA	Myeloid cell lineages: PMNs, Mϕs, eosinophils, monocytes, interstitial DCs, Kupfer cells
Fcα/μR	Fcα/μR	High (Kd~10^{-8}M)	IgA/IgM	NK cells, B cells, Mϕs
FcδR	Same	?	IgD	B cells, T cells, other cells?
FcRn	FcRn	High (Kd~10^{-8}M)	IgG	Mucosal epithelium, Mϕsplacenta, endothelium, DCs
pIgR	pIgR	High (Kd~10^{-9}M)	IgA/IgM	Epithelium
FcRL	FcRL	Unknown	Unknown	B-cell lineage cells

**Immune complex.*

in the cells expressing the FcRs and results in expression of measurable immunobiological properties (i.e., phagocytosis, cytolysis, or cytokine secretion). FcRs whose engagement of the antibody ligands leads to cellular activation and expression of effector functions are called *activating FcRs* (e.g., FcγRI and FcγRIII, FcεRs, FcαRI), while those that suppress effectors are known as *inhibitory FcRs* (e.g., FcγRIIb and occasionally FcαRI). However, because most effector cells express both FcRs, balanced signaling through activating and inhibitory FcRs is required for the efficient regulation of the effector functions of antibodies through the various effector cells bearing the receptors.[5] Figure 15.1 shows the essential features of the activating and inhibitory FcRs, illustrated with FcγRIII and FcγRIIb, respectively.

For the activating FcRs, the signaling events for induction of cellular responses are similar to the action of the classic immunoreceptors such as B-cell receptors (BCRs) and T-cell

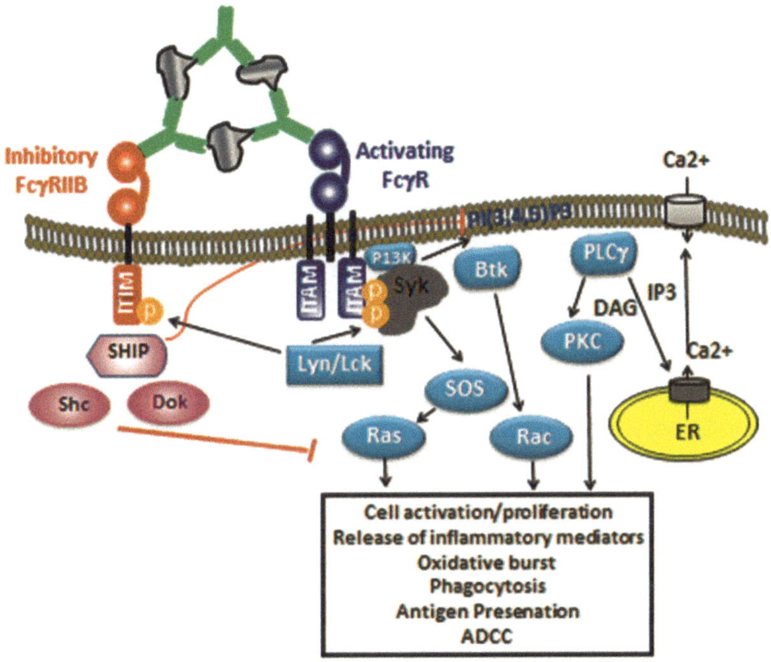

FIGURE 15.1 **Pathways for activating and inhibitory FcR signaling.** Immune complex (IC) binding to innate immune effector cells, such as monocytes, granulocytes, and macrophages, simultaneously triggers activating and inhibitory signaling pathways. Upon receptor cross-linking, Lyn phosphorylates both ITAM and ITIM in the cytoplasmic domain of the FcR common γ-chain and FcγRIIB, thereby initiating both signaling pathways. Red lines indicate points where inhibitory signaling pathways interfere with their activating counterparts. *(Modified from Nimmerjahn F, Ravetch* J. Adv Immunol *2007;**96**:179–204.)*

receptors (TCRs), in which the binding of the Fc portion of the antibody to FcRs propagates a signal transduction process, involving a series of kinase-mediated phosphorylation reactions, transcription factor activation, and induction of cellular responses. The cellular responses include degranulation, phagocytosis, endocytosis, antibody-dependent cell-mediated cytotoxicity (ADCC), release of inflammatory mediators, and the regulation of B-cell activation and antibody production. The molecular basis for the cellular signaling and response is the presence of immunoreceptor tyrosine-based activation motifs (ITAMs) on the receptor complex for mediating activating signals, either on the cytoplasmic tails of the receptors or on other molecules, such as common γ-chain, associated with them in the transmembrane and cytoplasmic regions.[6,7] First, FcR-binding leads to the phosphorylation of ITAM in the cytoplasmic region of the receptor by kinases of the Src family, which triggers the recruitment and activation of more sets of cytoplasmic protein tyrosine kinases, especially the SYK family kinases. Further action by these kinases results in the activation of various downstream targets, including the linker for activation of T cells (LAT), multimolecular adaptor complexes, and phosphoinositide-3-kinase (PI3K). PI3K generates phosphatidylinositol-3,4,5-triphosphate (PtdIns(3,4,5)P3), which creates membrane-docking sites for Bruton's tyrosine kinase

(BTK) and phospholipase Cγ (PLCγ). Second, activation of PLCγ leads to an increased intracellular calcium level and triggering of further downstream signaling events such as activation of the PKC and Ras pathways and extracellular signal-regulated kinases (ERK), JUN N-terminal kinase (JNK), and p38. The signaling events for FcR-mediated cell activation can also involve the Ras–Raf–MAPK (mitogen-activated protein kinase) pathway. The specificity and precision of the cellular effector function achieved (such as degranulation, phagocytosis, endocytosis, ADCC, or release of inflammatory mediators) may be determined by the antibody isotype, FcR type, and involvement of other signaling molecules.

The inhibitory FcγRIIb has the immunoreceptor tyrosine-based inhibitory motifs (ITIMs) in the cytoplasmic portion of the receptor.FcR engagement that triggers ITIM results in the recruitment of phosphatases such as SHIP (SH2-domain-containing inositol polyphosphate 5′ phosphatase) and SHP1 (SH2-domain-containing protein tyrosine phosphatase 1), which inhibit cell activation due to prevention of recruitment of BTK or PLCγ to the cell membrane, thereby diminishing downstream events such as the increase in intracellular calcium levels.

CONTRIBUTION OF FcR-MEDIATED IMMUNE EFFECTOR FUNCTIONS OF ANTIBODIES TO PROTECTIVE ACQUIRED IMMUNITY

Effectors of Adaptive or Acquired Immune Responses

The innate immune response is the first line of the mammalian body's defense against foreign insults, such as invading microbial pathogens or altered self-components as with tumor formation, and innate immune effectors also mobilize at all levels of host immune defense; however, the principal protective and immune defense mechanisms that form the basis of vaccine efficacy against microbial pathogens and tumors are the effectors of adaptive or acquired immune responses. The adaptive immune response has two forms: (1) The humoral immune response comprised of B cells and the antibodies secreted in response to antigenic activation; and (2) the T-cell-mediated immune response comprised principally of the antigen-specific and major histocompatibility complex (MHC)-restricted CD4 and CD8 T cells and their cytokines. Despite their distinct definitions, innate and adaptive immunity are biologically linked, as the innate immune response regulates adaptive immunity, especially at the afferent phase, and is often the source of nonspecific effectors that are mobilized and channeled by the specific elements of adaptive immune response to achieve protective immunity, including microbial clearance or tumor eradication.

The hallmarks of adaptive immune response include the exquisite specificity of the effector recognition of the inducing target resulting in its clearance and establishment of immunological memory that ensures an anamnestic response upon a re-encounter of the antigenic determinant. Microbial pathogens and tumors commonly elicit a mixed specific immune response comprised of the effectors of both arms of adaptive immunity (humoral and T-cell-mediated immunity) (Table 15.2). Vaccines against microbial pathogens and tumors depend on these effectors of humoral and T-cell-mediated immune (CMI) responses for their efficacy. Therefore, a better understanding of the relative contribution of the effectors of each arm of the adaptive immune response to protective immunity against specific microbes or tumors will aid vaccine design efforts to skew the response toward the desired

TABLE 15.2 Effectors of Adaptive Immunity against Microbial Pathogens and Tumors

Effectors	Mechanism of Antimicrobial and Anti-Tumor Action	Value in Protective Immunity Conferred by a Vaccine
CMI effectors: T cells (CD4 and CD8), activated macrophages, Th1 cytokines (e.g., IFN-γ, TNF-α, IL-2)	Activation of CTLs and destruction of infected or tumor cells; cytokine-activated antimicrobial processes in phagocytes and infected/tumor cells	Crucial for rapid microbial or tumor clearance and establishment of protective immunity
Humoral effectors: Antibodies (e.g., IgM, IgD, IgG1-4, IgA1-2, and IgE)	*Direct (FcR-independent) mechanisms:* Binding and neutralization of infectivity of microbes, virulence factors, or toxins *FcR-dependent mechanisms:* ADCC; activation of classical complement pathway; opsonization and enhancement of uptake, degradation, and/or processing of microbe/tumor antigens for rapid activation of CMI effectors	*Direct effect:* More effective against extracellular microbes than for strictly intracellular microbes *FcR-dependent effect:* Applied during reinfection and crucial for effective memory T-cell response *Application:* Can be used in passive immunotherapy, active immunotherapy as a delivery platform to boost T-cell immunity against intracellular microbial pathogens and tumors, and in drug delivery to target anti-tumor reagents

arm for optimal vaccine efficacy. However, the unfolding interdependence and mutual regulatory relationship between humoral and CMI[8–10] has resulted in a paradigm shift and the adoption of new strategies for designing better vaccines against microbial pathogens and tumors.

The Effectors of CMI

The principal effectors of CMI are cytotoxic T lymphocytes (CTLs), T-helper type-1 (Th1) cells, inflammatory cytokines such as interferon-gamma (IFN-γ) and tumor necrosis factor-alpha (TNF-α), activated macrophages, NK cells, and perhaps other less characterized immune cells and molecules. As an important effector mechanism of CMI, the MHC-restricted CTLs mediate antimicrobial or anti-tumor action via Fas-dependent and Fas-independent apoptosis or programmed cell death of infected or aberrant cells. Lysis of tumor cells curtails tumor progression; and lysis of infected cells limits the productive growth of intracellular microbes, exposing them to antibodies and other humoral factors, thereby ensuring either their neutralization or destruction and removal via other immune effector mechanisms. NK cells and macrophages exert antimicrobial and anti-tumor activity through recognition of target tumor or infected cells via immune complexes binding to FcRs on the effectors. Microbial or tumor destruction mechanisms by CTLs, NK cells, and macrophages include nucleic acid degradation by perforin and granzyme[11–13] and intracellular enzymatic degradation of phagocytized microbes, infected or tumor cells. In addition, apoptotic bodies containing tumor cells and dead or live microbes are rapidly scavenged by phagocytes. While both $CD4^+$ and $CD8^+$ CTLs exist, the $CD8^+$ T-cell subsets are the predominant CTLs *in vivo*. In addition, T cell (CD4 and CD8)-derived cytokines, especially IFN-γ and TNF-α, are crucial for anti-tumor defense and microbial clearance in humans and in experimental animals.[14–20] Barring microbial or tumor immune evasion mechanisms or host immunosuppression that limit immune responses, these CMI effectors are generally thought to contribute substantially to immunity against different categories of microbial pathogens and tumors.

The Immune Effector Functions of Antibodies: the FcR-Dependent and -Independent Functional Processes

The principal effectors of adaptive humoral immunity are the different classes and subclasses of antibodies: IgM, IgD, IgG_{1-4}, IgA1/2, and IgE. Structurally, antibodies are four-chain protein molecules (two identical heavy and two identical light chains), containing an antigen binding N-terminal region and an effector C-terminal domain. The molecules are evolutionarily conserved from lower vertebrates to mammals as host defense molecules, although different species exhibit certain differences. They are encoded by rearranged gene segments in B cells and are secreted upon antigenic stimulation via the B-cell receptor. In addition to the ontogenically predominant IgM (and IgD) during a primary antibody response to B-cell stimulation by the cognate antigen, T-cell help to B cells in the form of both direct cell-to-cell binding and cytokines such as IL-4/IL-5 are required for the isotype switching event that culminates in the expression and secretion of other antibody isotypes. Functionally, antibodies effect host defense against microbial pathogens (and probably or arguably tumors) by either directly binding to the antigenic determinants on microbes, or by an indirect mechanism involving the binding of the antibody–antigen complexes (known as immune complex, IC) to FcR-bearing effector cells such as NK cells, PMNs, and macrophages. These FcR-dependent and -independent effector functions of antibodies underlie their role in host defense and protective immunity, as well as the initiation of certain undesirable biological processes, including allergic reaction and inflammation that may lead to tissue damage.

FcR-Independent Functions of Antibodies

Direct antibody binding and neutralization of infectious agents are generally regarded as a major function of antibodies in host defense, and this action leads to microbial clearance or protective immunity. This action has the greatest impact on immunity against pathogens with prolonged extracellular existence, when compared to intracellular microbes,[7,21,22] although antibodies may be internalized into infected cells where they bind and neutralize microbes intracellularly, as well.[23–25] Protective antibodies effective against intracellular microbial pathogens including viruses appear to require high titers of the specific antibodies.[26] Other direct roles of antibodies in controlling microbial pathogens include toxin neutralization, an essential protective mechanism of vaccine-mediated resistance against diphtheria, tetanus, and pertussis toxins; receptor blocking, as with immunity against the malaria-causing protozoan parasite *Plasmodium falciparum*;[27,28] mucosal immunity by binding pathogens and preventing entry or restricting infection to mucosal compartments; and significant viral immunity through virus binding and inhibition of viral attachment, uncoating, assembly, and release, as well flagella binding and prevention of pathogen motility as with *Pseudomonas aeruginosa*.[29] Furthermore, although the effect of direct antibody binding to tumor cells on tumor clearance and immunity *in vivo* is unclear, such binding may likely target tumor cells to FcR-bearing cytolytic immune effector cells such as NK cells, neutrophils, and macrophages. Direct antibody binding via the intact microbial pathogen or toxic components and neutralization of infectivity or its pathologic manifestation is the immunotherapeutic basis of passive immunization. In addition, opsonization of enveloped microbes triggers the activation of the classical complement pathway leading to the formation of the membrane attack complex that culminates in microbial killing. The neutralization capacity of therapeutic anti-HIV and anti-toxin antibodies *in vitro* and *in vivo* has been attributed to FcR-mediated effector functions.[30,31]

FcR-Dependent Functions of Antibodies

The significance of FcR-mediated immunological processes in host defense is evident in the high susceptibility of persons with genetic deficiency or impairment in FcR-related signaling functions to major microbial pathogens and certain malignancies.[2] FcR-dependent effector functions of antibodies in protective immunity against microbial pathogens and tumors are achieved principally via several cellular processes resulting from the immune complex binding to FcRs on the effector cells (i.e., NK cells, macrophages, PMNs, and eosinophils) (Figure 15.2).[7] First, binding of ICs to inflammatory cells and monocytes also induces the release of IL-1β, IL-6, IL-8, IL-12, and GM–CSF. Thus, internalization of extracellular ICs of antibodies and microbial pathogens into effector cells via FcRs can activate the intracellular antimicrobial mechanisms of macrophages, as in protection against *Orientia tsutsugamushi* and *Ehrlichia chaffeensis*,[19,32] and induce the expression of proinflammatory cytokines such as IL-6 and TNF-α. Also, FcRs play a major role in immune phagocytosis of microbes by phagocytes such as PMNs and macrophages and triggering the induction of reactive oxygen and nitrogen species for intracellular killing of microbes.

Second, ADCC is an effective FcR-dependent mechanism for controlling intracellular microbial pathogens whose antigens expressed on the surface of infected cells are bound by specific antibodies. Also, the binding of tumor-associated antigens by specific antibodies can target tumor cells to FcR-bearing cytolytic immune effector cells such as NK cells and macrophages to effect killing via ADCC as well. In ADCC, the antibody provides the specificity of the target engagement by the killer cells; the concomitant activation of the killer cells and release of cytotoxic mediators such as granzyme-containing granules and stimulation of antimicrobial substances result in the lysis of infected or tumor cells, exposure of infectious agents to the neutralizing action of extracellular antibodies, microbial killing,[33] or limitation of tumor growth.

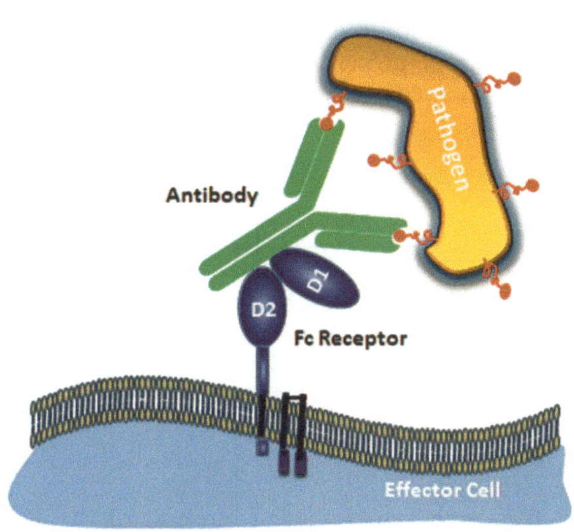

FIGURE 15.2 **Schematic illustration of Fc receptor interaction with an antibody-coated microbial pathogen.**

Third, in addition to the induction of cytokine production from effector cells, immune phagocytosis, and targeting of ICs for degradation, other functional consequences of Ab–FcR interactions include storage of ICs by follicular DCs in germinal centers of secondary lymphoid organs and the augmentation of MHC-restricted antigen presentation for CD4 and CD8 T-cell activation.[7–9,34] FcR-mediated modulation of antigen processing and presentation is a key role of antibodies in regulating T-cell response against intracellular microbial pathogens and possibly tumors; it involves enhancement of antigen uptake, processing, and presentation, as well as induction of adequate co-stimulation for rapid T-cell activation.[35]

THE IMMUNE EFFECTOR MECHANISMS OF FcR-DEPENDENT FUNCTIONAL PROCESSES AND THEIR APPLICATIONS IN IMMUNOTHERAPY AND IMMUNOMODULATION

FcR-Mediated Phagocytosis

This process entails the binding of the ICs to a critical number of FcRs and initiation of ITAM signaling,[36] which stimulates the cell to form membranous protrusions around the bound particles until a phagosome is formed within the cell. Other proteins contributing to this form of immune phagocytosis are the Rho family of proteins (i.e., Rac1 and Cdc42), which plays a key role in phagosome formation and its interaction with lysosomes, and the GTPase ARF6, which regulates actin assembly beneath the FcR-bound ICs, all leading to the rapid maturation into a phagolysosomal compartment containing activated proteolytic enzymes that degrade the engulfed particles. Microbial pathogens are rapidly degraded by this effective mechanism. Thus, infection by microbial particles whose antibodies are already present in the host as a result of prior immunization or previous infection (symptomatic or non-symptomatic) can stimulate FcR-mediated phagocytosis. As a strategic passive immunotherapy, the passive administration of specific antimicrobial antibodies can potentially clear the pathogen via FcR-mediated phagocytosis; however, other logistical considerations may prevent the regular use of this approach in the clinical setting. These considerations include the quantity of the pathogen-specific antibodies available, the effectiveness of available antibiotics against the pathogen, and the ability of the passively transferred antibodies to reach the site of infection.

ADCC and its Application in Immunotherapy

ADCC is an antibody targeting cytolytic action of the immune cells that involves FcR signaling. Thus, the binding of specific antibodies to either a tumor or microbial antigen on the surface of a cell targets the cell to an effector cell capable of ADCC, such as NK cells, PMNs, and macrophages. During ADCC, the signaling initiated by the FcR engagement of the Fc portion of an antibody bound to a target cell (tumor or infected cell or parasite) enhances the direct cell-to-cell contact between the effector and target cells; however, instead of phagocytosis, the interaction causes the release of cytolytic substances into the target cell that leads to DNA destruction and cell death by apoptosis. In the granule-dependent killing mechanism, several proteolytic enzymes called *granzymes* are delivered to the target cell through the immunological synapse between the effector and the target cells, activating a family of death-inducing proteases called *caspases*. Unlike CTLs, where the granules are synthesized only after specific antigenic stimulation, cytotoxic granules are formed in NK cells during development, such that NK cells are equipped to respond rapidly to the threat of tumorigenicity or infection if properly tagged by the specific antibodies. Two key components of the granules released during ADCC are perforin and granzymes. The role of perforin is apparently to form pores in the target cell membrane through which granzymes are introduced into the cell; the presence of perforin appears to be required for endosomal disruption that releases granzyme B into the cytosol of the target cell to induce apoptosis. In addition, nitric oxide and other reactive intermediates may be among the cytolytic substances released by effector cells

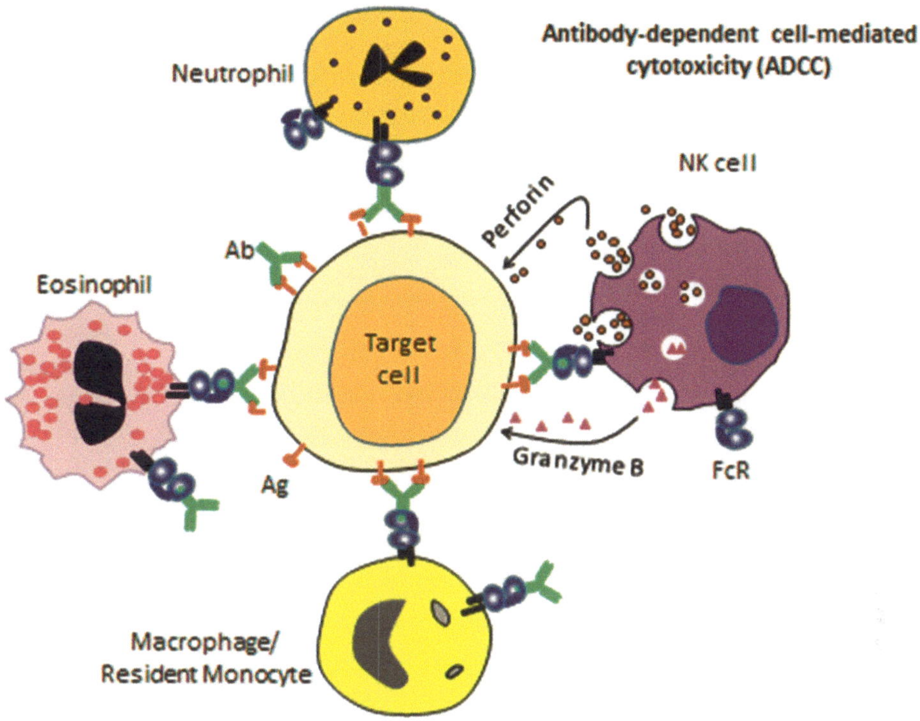

FIGURE 15.3 **ADCC by four major immune effector cells: macrophages/resident monocytes, NK cells, neutrophils, and eosinophils.** The target cell may either be microbe infected or a tumor cell that expresses the antigen recognized and bound by the antibody. Target cell killing is achieved by several cytolytic processes that also cause limitation of microbial or tumor growth.

such as macrophages and PMNs to cause the death of the target cell. Figure 15.3 shows the different forms of ADCC achieved following FcR engagement between an effector and an antibody-bound target cell.

Factors controlling ADCC may include the number of cross-linked Fc–FcR pairs between the effector and target cell; the potency of the killing machinery of the effector, which may depend on the intensity of FcR signaling; and the target cell type. It is important to realize that no MHC compatibility between killer and target cells is required for ADCC, although it appears cells are differentially susceptible to ADCC, such that not all cells will be killed, even when appropriately coated with antibodies. ADCC is relevant for immune action against intracellular microbial pathogens, such as virally infected cells, and tumor cells, provided the relevant antigens recognized by the antibodies are expressed on the cell surface. The immunotherapeutic applications of ADCC include the possibility that purified ADCC-competent effectors such as activated macrophages or NK cells can be transferred across MHC barriers from an immunocompetent donor to an immunocompromised recipient to effect killing of tumors or chronically infected target cells once specified by antibodies directed to their surface antigens. Also, passive transfer of designer antibodies against unique antigens expressed on the surface of tumors or infected cells can target the cells for ADCC by the host's resident effector cells. The clinical application and benefits of these therapeutic regimens are yet to be fully experimented on.

FcR-Mediated Regulation and Modulation of Adaptive Immune Responses and Application in Immunotherapy and Drug Delivery

The induction of cellular activation and secretion of proinflammatory cytokines such as TNF-α, IL-1-β, IL-6, and IL-8 upon IC cross-linking of FcR on different innate immune effector cells, including Mϕs and DCs, *in vitro* reflect the immunomodulatory capacity and immunoregulatory function of FcR signaling in shaping adaptive immune responses *in vivo*. In this respect, it has been established that the signaling events associated with exposure of DCs to ICs result in rapid DC maturation, increase the expression of co-stimulator molecules and IL-12 secretion, and facilitate the ability to stimulate an elevated primary T-cell response against the antibody-bound antigens. The rapid antigen processing may be associated with the activation of degradative enzymes and stimulation of the endosomal pathway during FcR signaling. In addition, some subsets of DCs acquire the capacity for cross-presentation of the exogenous antigen to activate $CD8^+$ T cells. Concomitant with the activation of these robust T-cell effectors, the central memory response induced by IC-pulsed DCs is apparently elevated as well,[33] since *in vivo* they induce potent protective immunity against intracellular pathogens such as *Chlamydia trachomatis* and *Leishmania* major.[37,38] The vital role for FcR-mediated augmentation of T-cell response against intracellular microbial pathogens *in vivo* has been demonstrated for *C. trachomatis*, *L. major*, *Mycobacterium tuberculosis*, and *Francisella tularensis*,[37–40] as well as *Cryptococcus neoformans*[41] and influenza virus immunity.[9,42] The profile of immune effectors induced by FcR targeting to DCs, with respect to the Th1/Th2 cytokine-based classification, may be dependent on the isotype and concentration of the antibody. In this respect, fusion of antigen to the Fc portion of the Th1-associated murine Ig2a antibody induced the required protective Th1 response against genital chlamydial infection and protection from infertility in mice.[37] Also, it has been suggested that FcR-mediated internalization of antigens into antigen-presenting cells (APCs) appears to target the antigens to the endolysosomal degradative pathway that enhances the processing and presentation of the antigen to T cells, thereby fostering immunity against T-cell-controlled pathogens, including *Legionella pneumophilia*, *Toxoplama gondii*, *C. trachomatis*, *Rickettsia conorii*, and the protozoan parasite *Encephalitozoon cuniculi*.[7] In addition, macrophages that phagocytized moderately IgG antibody-coated sheep red blood cells through the FcR-mediated signaling produced greater levels of IL-12 than SRBCs with higher densities of the antibody.[43] Furthermore, the acidic pH-dependent binding of IgG to FcRs may affect the antigen processing of ICs, thereby shaping presentation or cross-presentation, as recently reported with FcRn.[44,45] Additionally, the ability of FcR-mediated functions of antibodies to suppress immune responses[46,47] may be related to antibody isotypes, as well.

As summarized in Figure 15.4, the mechanism of immune augmentation following FcR delivery of antigen involves acceleration of the APC's antigen-capturing and internalization ability, enhancement of the antigen processing capacity through timely endosomal targeting to lysosome, upregulation of co-stimulatory molecules on the APC, and secretion of immunostimulatory cytokines, such as IL-1, CD40, and B7.1 (CD80), leading to a rapid and an augmented T-cell response. Stimulation of proteosomal and endosomal enzymes, IL-12

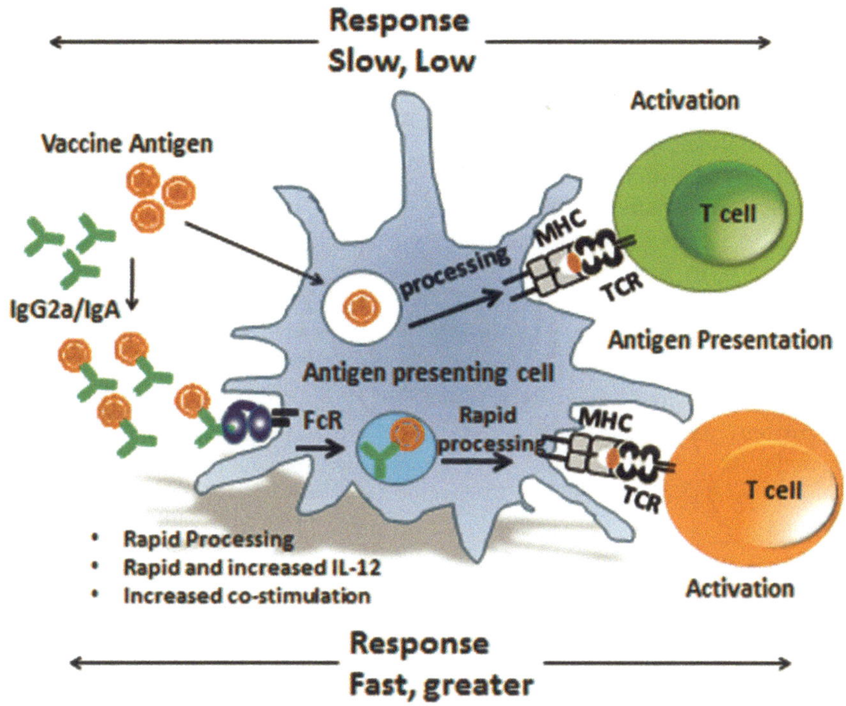

FIGURE 15.4 **Regulation of T-cell response by antibodies.** A schematic representation of the pathways for antigen handling by APC leading to T-cell activation. Antigen acquisition by pinocytosis and non-receptor-mediated endocytosis leads to a slow and low Th1 activation. On the other hand, antigen uptake by FcR-mediated endocytosis or phagocytosis leads to a fast and elevated T cell activation. *(Adapted from Igietseme JU, Eko FO, He Q, Black CM.* Expert Rev. Vaccines, *2004;3(1): 23–34.)*

production, and induction of transcription factors, such as STAT2 and STAT4, which are associated with T-cell development and activation,[48–50] are also involved.

The immunotherapeutic application of FcR-mediated modulation of the T-cell response includes the use of Fc-conjugated vaccine antigens for immunization to boost protective immunity against microbial pathogens and tumors without the need for additional adjuvants. Beside the use of ICs comprised of specific antibodies and vaccine antigens, Fc-fusion proteins have been used as modified Fc-delivery platforms that prevent possible significant IC-mediated pathologies as secondary complications. Also, DC-based cellular vaccines that involve adoptive transfer of cells pulsed with Fc-targeted antigens as IC or Fc-fusion proteins have been suggested as immunotherapies against microbial pathogens and tumors. Furthermore, an innovative application of the Fc targeting of vaccine antigens that was recently reported is immunization with a vaccine antigen conjugated with a ligand (α-Gal) against which antibodies are already present in the host.[51] Conceptually, the pre-existing antibodies bind to the vaccine conjugate and target the antigen to FcR-bearing antigen-presenting cells, such as DCs, resulting in a rapid immune response against the vaccine antigen. Also, FcR-mediated signaling may be useful for targeting drug delivery to FcR-bearing cells to control inflammatory responses of these cells. Finally, although less dependent on effector cell signaling via FcR engagement, the mucosal vaccine delivery application of the IgG translocation function of FcRn involves targeting vaccine antigens to the FcRn on the mucosal epithelium surface for transepithelial transfer to the underlying antigen-presenting cells. Thus, intranasal immunization of mice with Fc-fused glycoprotein gD of HSV-2 or Fc-fused HIV-Gag, plus the adjuvant CpG in each case, conferred protective immunity against intravaginal challenge by HSV-2 or recombinant vaccinia virus expressing the HIV Gag protein, respectively.[52,53]

Acknowledgments

This work was supported by the Centers for Disease Control and Prevention (CDC) and PHS grants (AI41231, AI65892, AI73139, and 1SC1GM098197) from the National Institutes of Health.

References

1. Okun E, Mattson M, Arumugam T. Involvement of Fc receptors in disorders of the central nervous system. *Neuromolecular Med* 2010;**12**(2):164–78.
2. Nimmerjahn F, Ravetch JV. FcγRs in health and disease. *Curr Top Microbiol Immunol* 2010;**350**:105–25.
3. Ehrhardt G, Cooper M. Immunoregulatory roles for Fc receptor-like molecules. *Curr Top Microbiol Immunol* 2011;**350**:89–104.
4. Davis R. Fc receptor-like molecules. *Annu Rev Immunol* 2007;**25**:525–60.
5. Nimmerjahn F, Ravetch J. Fc-receptors as regulators of immunity. *Adv Immunol* 2007;**96**:179–204.
6. LB I. Cross-regulation of signaling by ITAM-associated receptors. *Nat Immunol* 2009;**10**(4):340–7.
7. Joller N, Weber S, Oxenius A. Antibody–Fc receptor interactions in protection against intracellular pathogens. *Eur J Immunol* 2011;**41**:889–97.
8. Moore T, Ekworomadu C, Eko F, MacMillan L, Ramey K, Ananaba G, et al. Fc receptor-mediated antibody regulation of T cell immunity against intracellular pathogens. *J Infect Dis* 2003;**188**(4):617–24.
9. Arulanandam B, Raeder R, Nedrud JG, Bucher D, Le J, Metzger D. IgA immunodeficiency leads to inadequate Th cell priming and increased susceptibility to influenza virus infection. *J Immunol* 2001;**166**:226–31.
10. Guyre PM, Graziano RF, Goldstein J, Wallace PK, Morganelli PM, Wardwell K, et al. Increased potency of Fc-receptor-targeted antigens. *Cancer Immunol Immunother* 1997;**45**:146–8.
11. Walker D, Olano J, Feng H. Critical role of cytotoxic T lymphocytes in immune clearance of rickettsial infection. *Infect Immun* 2001;**69**(3):1841–6.
12. Feng H, Popov V, Yuoh G, Walker D. Role of T lymphocyte subsets in immunity to spotted fever group *Rickettsiae*. *J Immunol* 1997;**158**(11):5314–20.
13. Efferson CL, Schickli J, Ko BK, Kawano K, Mouzi S, Palese P, et al. Activation of tumor antigen-specific cytotoxic T lymphocytes (CTLs) by human dendritic cells infected with an attenuated influenza A virus expressing a CTL epitope derived from HER-2/neu proto-oncogene. *J Virol* 2003;**77**(13):7411–24.
14. Dorman SE, Holland SM. Interferon-gamma and nterleukin-12 pathway defects and human disease. *Cytokine Growth Factor Rev* 2000;**11**(4):321–33.
15. Rottenberg ME, Gigliotti-Rothfuchs A, Wigzell H. The role of IFN-gamma in the outcome of chlamydial infection. *Curr Opin Immunol* 2002;**14**(4):444–51.
16. Byrne GI, Lehmann LK, Landry GJ. Induction of tryptophan catabolism is the mechanism for gamma interferon-mediated inhibition of intracellular *Chlamydia psittaci* replication in T24 cells. *Infect Immun* 1986;**53**:347–51.
17. Holtmann H, Shemer-Avni Y, Wessel K, Sarov I, Wallach D. Inhibition of growth of *Chlamydia trachomatis* by tumor necrosis factor is accompanied by increased prostaglandin synthesis. *Infect Immun* 1990;**58**:3168–72.
18. Loomis PW, Starnbach MN. T cell responses to *Chlamydia trachomatis*. *Curr Opin Microbiol* 2002;**5**:87–91.
19. Ismail N, Olano JP, Feng HM, Walker DH. Current status of immune mechanisms of killing of intracellular microorganisms. *FEMS Microbiol Lett* 2002;**207**(2):111–20.
20. Kaufmann SHE. Immunity to intracellular bacteria. *Annu Rev Immunol* 1993;**11**:129–63.
21. Casadevall A, Pirofski L. Antibody-mediated regulation of cellular immunity and the inflammatory response. *Trends Immunol* 2003;**24**(9):474–8.
22. Casadevall A. Antibody-mediated immunity against intracellular pathogens: two-dimensional thinking comes full circle. *Infect Immun* 2003;**71**(8):4225–8.
23. Mazanec MB, Nedrud JG, Kaetzel CS, Lamm ME. A three-tiered view of the role of IgA in mucosal defense. *Immunol Today* 1993;**14**:430–5.
24. Corthesy B, Spertini F. Secretory immunoglobulin A: from mucosal protection to vaccine development. *Biol Chem* 1999;**380**(11):1251–62.
25. Brandtzaeg P. Mucosal immunity: integration between mother and the breast-fed infant. *Vaccine* 2003;**21**(24):3382–8.

26. Burton DR, Parren PWHI. Vaccines and the induction of functional antibodies: time to look beyond the molecules of natural infection?. *Nat Med* 2000;**6**(2):123–5.
27. Casadevall A, Pirofski L. A reappraisal of humoral immunity based on mechanisms of antibody-mediated protection against intracellular pathogens. *Adv Immunol* 2006;**91**:1–44.
28. Pleass R, Holder A. Opinion: antibody-based therapies for malaria. *Nat Rev Microbiol* 2005;**3**:893–9.
29. Campodonico V, Llosa N, Grout M, Doring G, Maira-Litran T, Pier G. Evaluation of flagella and flagellin of *Pseudomonas aeruginosa* as vaccines. *Infect Immun* 2010;**78**:746–55.
30. Forthal D, Moog C. Fc receptor-mediated antiviral antibodies. *Curr Opin HIV AIDS* 2009;**4**(5):388–93.
31. Abboud N, Chow S, Saylor C, Janda A, Ravetch J, Scharff M, et al. A requirement for FcγR in antibody-mediated bacterial toxin neutralization. *J Exp Med* 2010;**207**(11):2395–405.
32. Li J, Yager E, Reilly M, Freeman C, Reddy G, Reilly A, et al. Outer membrane protein-specific monoclonal antibodies protect SCID mice from fatal infection by the obligate intracellular bacterial pathogen *Ehrlichia chaffeensis*. *J Immunol* 2001;**166**(3):1855–62.
33. Moore T, Ananaba GA, Bolier J, Bowers S, Belay T, Eko FO, et al. Fc receptor regulation of protective immunity against *Chlamydia trachomatis*. *Immunol* 2002;**105**(2):213–21.
34. Brunham RC, Cohen CR, Kimani J, Bwayo J, Plummer F. Type 1/type 2 immunity and *Chlamydia trachomatis*: insights from the influence of HIV. In: Schachter J, Saikku P, Stephens R, Rank RG, editors. *Chlamydial Infections*. Antalya, Turkey: University Press; 2002. p. 202.
35. Igietseme JU, Eko FO, He Q, Black CM. Antibody regulation of T-cell immunity: implications for vaccine strategies against intracellular pathogens. *Expert Rev Vaccines* 2004;**3**(1):23–34.
36. Swanson J, Hoppe A. The coordination of signaling during Fc receptor-mediated phagocytosis. *J Leukoc Biol* 2004;**76**:1093–103.
37. Igietseme J, He Q, Joseph K, Eko F, Lyn D, Ananaba G, et al. Role of T lymphocytes in the pathogenesis of *Chlamydia* disease. *J Infect Dis* 2009;**200**(6):926–34.
38. Woelbing F, Kostka S, Moelle K, Belkaid Y, Sunderkoetter C, Verbeek S, et al. Uptake of *Leishmania major* by dendritic cells is mediated by Fcgamma receptors and facilitates acquisition of protective immunity. *J Exp Med* 2006;**203**(1):177–88.
39. Maglione P, Xu J, Casadevall A, Chan J. Fc gamma receptors regulate immune activation and susceptibility during *Mycobacterium tuberculosis* infection. *J Immunol* 2008;**180**(5):3329–38.
40. Mara-Koosham G, Hutt J, Lyons C, Wu T. Antibodies contribute to effective vaccination against respiratory infection by type A *Francisella tularensis* strains. *Infect Immun* 2011;**79**(4):1770–8.
41. Yuan R, Clynes R, Oh J, Ravetch J, Scharff M. Antibody-mediated modulation of *Cryptococcus neoformans* infection is dependent on distinct Fc receptor functions and IgG subclasses. *J Exp Med* 1998;**187**(4):641–8.
42. Huber VC, Lynch JM, Bucher DJ, Le J, Metzger DW. Fc receptor-mediated phagocytosis makes a significant contribution to clearance of influenza virus infections. *J Immunol* 2001;**166**:7381–8.
43. Gallo P, Goncalves R, Mosser D. The influence of IgG density and macrophage-Fc(gamma) receptor cross-linking on phagocytosis and IL-10 production. *Immunol Lett* 2010;**133**:70–7.
44. Liu X, Lu L, Yang Z, Palaniyandi S, Zeng R, Gao L, et al. The neonatal FcR-mediated presentation of immune-complexed antigen is associated with endosomal and phagosomal pH and antigen stability in macrophages and dendritic cells. *J Immunol* 2011;**186**(8):4674–86.
45. Baker K, Qiao S, Kuo T, Aveson V, Platzer B, Andersen J, et al. Neonatal Fc receptor for IgG (FcRn) regulates cross-presentation of IgG immune complexes by CD8–CD11b+ dendritic cells. *Proc Natl Acad Sci USA* 2011;**108**(24):9927–32.
46. Heyman B. Feedback regulation by IgG antibodies. *Immunol Lett* 2003;**88**(2):157–61.
47. Kane MM, Mosser DM. The role of IL-10 in promoting disease progression in leishmaniasis. *J Immunol* 2001;**166**(2):1141–7.
48. Rao A, Avni O. Molecular aspects of T-cell differentiation. *Br Med Bull* 2000;**56**(4):969–84.
49. Wurster AL, Tanaka T, Grusby MJ. The biology of Stat4 and Stat6. *Oncogene* 2000;**19**(21):2577–84.
50. Murphy KM, Ouyang J, Farrar D, Yang J, Ranganath S, Asnagli H, et al. Signaling and transcription in T helper development. *Annu Rev Immunol* 2000;**18**:451–94.
51. Abdel-Motal U, Wang S, Awad A, Lu S, Wigglesworth K, Galili U. Increased immunogenicity of HIV-1 p24 and gp120 following immunization with gp120/p24 fusion protein vaccine expressing alpha-Gal epitopes. *Vaccine* 2010;**28**(7):1758–65.
52. Ye L, Zeng R, Bai Y, Roopenian D, Zhu X. Efficient mucosal vaccination mediated by the neonatal Fc receptor. *Nat Biotechnol* 2011;**29**(2):158–63.
53. Lu L, Palaniyandi S, Zeng R, Bai Y, Liu X, Wang Y, et al. A neonatal Fc receptor-targeted mucosal vaccine strategy effectively induces HIV-1 antigen-specific immunity to genital infection. *J Virol* 2011;**85**(20):10542–53.

CHAPTER

16

Fcγ Receptors as Therapeutic Targets

Robert M. Anthony

Center for Immunology and Inflammatory Diseases, Massachusetts General Hospital, Harvard Medical School, Boston, Massachusetts

INTRODUCTION

Therapeutic IgG antibodies and IgG Fc fusions are among the most successful drugs developed in recent decades.[1,2] In fact, over the last 25 years, the U.S. Food and Drug Administration and drug-regulatory agencies of other nations have approved more than 30 IgG-antibody-based therapeutics for various indications. Utilizing the high specificity of their antigen-binding domains, IgG-based therapeutics have been engineered to target specific antigens expressed by cancers, autoreactive lymphocytes, and infectious agents or to neutralize toxins and inflammatory mediators.[3–7]

Research over the last few years has clearly demonstrated that the *in vivo* activity of IgG antibodies is highly dependent the entire IgG molecule.[8–12] The Fab (antigen-binding fragment) portion of IgG antibodies is highly specific and recognizes antigen with high affinity (K_A of $10^9 M^{-1}$). In contrast, the IgG Fc domain is responsible for serum half-life through interactions with the neonatal Fc receptor (FcRn)[13] and proinflammatory and antiinflammatory activities through interactions with Fcγ receptors (FcγRs).[14] Although most Fc interactions with FcγRs are generally quite weak individually (K_A of $10^6 M^{-1}$ across the low-affinity FcγRs[15]), IgG antibodies form immune complexes through Fab–antigen interactions, resulting in multimerization and avidity effects allowing Fc portions to bind and cross-link FcγRs.[8–12] Thus, the relative expression levels and surface densities of activating and inhibitory Fc receptors are important factors contributing to IgG antibody effector functions.

These receptors are classified into two families, activating and inhibitory, where activitating FcγRs signal through an immunoreceptor tyrosine-based activation motif (ITAM) and inhibitory FcγRs contain an immunoreceptor tyrosine-based inhibitory motif (ITIM) in the cytoplasmic domain.[8–10] In the case of FcγRs, ITAM signaling promotes antigen internalization, antigen presentation, leukocyte activation, and target cell killing or antibody-dependent cytotoxicity (ADCC).[16] FcγR-driven ITIM signaling inhibits other signaling pathways and sometimes initiates apoptosis.[17–19] Antibody activity is determined by the types of Fc receptors triggered, which, in turn is affected by the effector leukocyte's repertoire and expression level of FcγRs.[8,10,20] When designing therapeutic antibodies, it is important to empirically determine the FcγR response that promotes the desired IgG effector functions to ensure that appropriate FcγRs are targeted.

Indeed, the importance of FcγR targeting has been supported by studies using murine models that demonstrated that selective targeting of Fc receptors influences the magnitude of the inflammatory response. IgG antibodies of different subclasses, each with Fabs specific for an antigen expressed by the B16–F10 melanoma line, were administered to mice treated with B16–F10 cells. The tumor-specific antibody subclasses that preferential bound activating Fc receptors were most affective at tumor clearance.[20] These results highlight the importance of the Fc and Fc receptor targeting in therapeutic antibody design as discussed below.

TABLE 16.1 A/I Ratios for Mouse and Human IgG Antibody Interactions with FcγRs

IgG	A/I	Bound FcγRs
$mIgG_1$	0.1	FcγRIII/FcγRIIB
$mIgG_{2a}$	69	FcγRIV/FcγRIIB
$mIgG_{2b}$	7	FcγRIV/FcγRIIB
$mIgG_3$	n.b.	
$hIgG_1$	1;13	$FcγRIIIA^{158F}$ $FcγRIIIA^{158V}$/ FcγRIIB
$hIgG_2$	1.5;3.5	$FcγRIIIA^{158F}$ $FcγRIIIA^{158V}$/ FcγRIIB
$hIgG_3$	45;57	$FcγRIIIA^{158F}$ $FcγRIIIA^{158V}$/ FcγRIIB
$hIgG_4$	1	$FcγRIIIA^{158F}$ $FcγRIIIA^{158V}$/ FcγRIIB

Data from Bruhns et al.,[15] Okazaki et al.,[86] Maenaka et al.,[97] and Paetz et al.[98]

Note: n.b. indicates no detectable binding. The ratios are derived by dividing the binding affinity constant of an IgG antibody to activating FcγRs and the inhibitory FcγR. Ratios larger than 1 indicate favored binding to activating FcγRs and enhanced proinflammatory activity; ratios less than 1 represent IgG antibodies that bind the inhibitory FcγR preferentially. The two numbers presented for the human antibodies represent the A/I ratios for the high-affinity ($FcγRIIIA^{158v}$) and low-affinity ($FcγRIIIA^{158F}$) alleles, respectively.

THE A/I RATIO

The proinflammatory activities of IgG antibodies are initiated by activating FcγRs. In addition to the high-affinity receptor, FcγRI, these include FcγRIIA and FcγRIIIA in humans and FcγRIII and FcγRIV in the mouse. Because of its high affinity for IgG, FcγRI is thought to be constantly bound by monomeric IgG and may not be involved in many of the proinflammatory activities ascribed to FcγRs, because the IgG Fc–FcγR interaction occurs independent of the Fab specificity and independent of FcγRI cross-linking. To bind the lower affinity, high-avidity FcγRs, a series of FcγRs must be bound simultaneously by IgG Fcs to form a productive interaction, which is effectively accomplished by immune complexes. This multimerization of IgG antibodies around antigen will productively engage lower affinity FcγRs, inducing signaling and appropriate cellular activation. However, IgG subclasses do not exhibit the same proinflammatory activity, because they bind FcγRs differently. Thus, the inflammatory potential of IgG antibodies *in vivo* is dictated by the relative affinities of the IgG antibodies to the lower affinity FcγRs. In the mouse, the most potent IgG antibody at inducing inflammation is IgG_{2a}, followed closely by IgG_{2b} (Table 16.1). These antibodies have higher affinity for activating FcγRs than the inhibitory FcγR, giving them a high activation-to-inhibitory (A/I) ratio. The A/I ratio compares the relative affinities of Fc receptor types for IgG Fc to predict the *in vivo* activity of IgG antibodies. In short, IgG antibodies with higher ratios display enhanced ADCC.

These observations in murine systems have been supported in the clinic. In humans, alleles of the activating receptors have been described that differ in affinity from those with which IgG antibodies are bound. The FcγRIIIA^{158V} binds IgG_1 with higher affinity than the FcγRIIIA^{158F} allele. Similarly, FcγRIIA^{131H} binds IgG_1 with a higher affinity than FcγRIIA^{131R}. Importantly, breast cancer patients homozygous for the higher affinity receptor, FcγRIIIA^{158V}, have better clinical outcomes following therapy targeting human epidermal growth factor receptor 2 (HER2) than patients with the lower affinity FcγRIIIA^{158F} allele.[21,22] Thus, the HER2 treatment that contains a human IgG_1 Fc portion is more potent *in vivo* with higher A/I ratios, strongly supporting a role for activating FcγRs in anti-HER2-mediated tumor clearance, and indicating that selective targeting of FcγRs enhances clinical outcome.

Fc GLYCAN CONTROL OF FcγR INTERACTIONS

While the peptide backbone of the IgG Fc affects FcγR binding affinity and subsequentally IgG effector function, the IgG glycan also markedly contributes to FcγR binding and is an important consideration for the targeting of IgG Fcs to specific FcγRs by therapeutic antibodies.[23] A highly conserved, complex, biantennary N-linked glycan is attached to the 297 asparagine at the top of the CH2 domain just beneath the hinge on the Fc of IgG antibodies.[24] Briefly, the core heptasacchride is an absolute requirement for IgG binding to mouse and human FcγRs, and thus for initiating the effector functions of wild type IgG antibodies. Furthermore, the Fc glycan is required for interactions of the IgG Fc with the initiator of the classical complement cascade, C1q. However, the core glycan is variably modified by the addition of sugar residues at several positions, and these modifications can significantly affect the biology and effector functions of IgG antibodies.

The addition of fucose to the core *N*-acetlyglucosamine (N-GlcNac), N-GlcNac to the bisecting mannose, or terminal sialic acid to the arms of the glycan all affect IgG effector functions by altering affinity to FcγRs. IgGs with afucosylated Fc glycans have increased affinity to FcγRIIIA, resulting in an A/I ratio shifted 50 to 100 times in favor of activating FcγRs and display enhanced antibody-dependent cell-mediated cytotoxicity (ADCC) *in vitro* and *in vivo*.[25–27] For this reason, the next generation of therapeutic proinflammatory IgG antibodies being developed will lack fucose on the IgG Fc glycan, and a number of approaches are being taken to produce afucosylated IgG antibodies. These include production of recombinant IgG antibodies in cell lines that are deficient in α1,6 fucosyltransferase and thereby unable to add fucose to the glycan.

The presence of the bisecting N-GlcNAc on the IgG Fc glycan enhances affinity to activating FcγRs, also favoring a higher A/I ratio, and IgG antibodies with glycans containing this modification display 10- to 20-fold higher ADCC activity *in vitro*. However, the attachment of the bisecting N-GlcNAc occurs in minor populations of serum IgG antibodies and is not added by CHO, NS0, or Sp2/0 cells, which are widely used to produce recombinant antibodies.[28–30] The enhanced proinflammatory activity obtained by the presence of bisecting N-GlcNAc is both less potent and more difficult to obtain than preventing the addition of fucose.

The addition of sialic acid moieties to the IgG Fc glycan also affects IgG Fc–FcγR interactions. The terminal sialylation of the IgG Fc glycan results in reduced affinity for both activating and inhibitory FcγRs and minimizes interactions of sialylated IgG Fcs with these types of FcγRs *in vivo*.[31] Sialylated IgG antibodies exhibit markedly reduced ADCC.[32] This is independent of sialic acid linkage type, as IgG antibodies

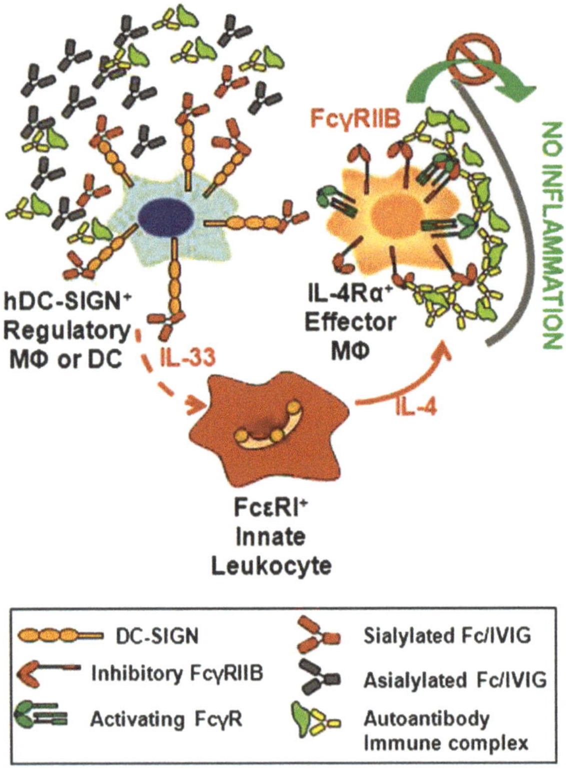

FIGURE 16.1 **Antiinflammatory activity of sFc.** sFcs bind to the antiinflammatory FcγR DC-SIGN, expressed on regulatory macrophages or dendritic cells. This initiates an innate Th2 response, where IL-33 is expressed, and acts on FcγRI+ leukocytes, most likely basophils. The activated basophils increase IL-4 expression, traffic to sites of inflammation, and induce increased surface expression of FcγRIIB in neutrophils and macrophages, thereby preventing autoantibody-induced inflammation

with Fc glycans terminating in either α2,3 or α2,6 sialic acids display reduced FcγR binding affinity and ADCC *in vivo*.[31,32] Sialic acid is generally not added to the IgG Fc glycan by cell lines used to produce recombinant antibodies.

In addition to reducing affinity for FcγRs, the addition of sialic acid to the core glycan converts the effort properties of the Fc to antiinflammatory mediators (Figure 16.1). Interestingly, while IgG Fcs with Fc glycans terminating in α2,6 sialic acids lose affinity to FcγRs, the addition of sialic acid enables binding to the newly defined antiinflammatory FcγR, dendritic cell-specific ICAM-3-grabbing non-integrin (DC-SIGN).[32–34] Importantly, the IgGs with Fc glycans terminating in α2,3 sialic acids do not bind to DC-SIGN, nor do they display antiinflammatory activity.[32,34] The conversion of receptor preference that occurs as a result of the addition of α2,6 sialic acid to the IgG Fc (sFc) is sufficient to initiate a potent antiinflammatory cascade capable of suppressing autoantibody-mediated inflammation.

ACTIVATING AND INHIBITORY FcγR EXPRESSION

As discussed above, the *in vivo* activity of IgG antibodies is dictated by the binding affinity of the IgG Fcs to FcγRs. These interactions are dependent on the IgG antibody subclass and the IgG Fc glycan composition; however, FcγR expression is not static but, like many components of the immune system, is affected by the homeostatic or inflammatory status of an individual. Thus, in addition to the influence that IgG Fc affinity to various FcγRs has over IgG antibody effector functions, the relative expression of FcγRs on effector cell populations also has profound effects on the effector functions triggered by IgG antibodies. Furthermore, not all leukocytes express the same panel of FcγRs. Natural killer (NK) cells express only the activating receptor FcγRIIIA and thus only initiate proinflammatory activities upon immune complex stimulation. Conversely, B cells express only the inhibitory FcγR, and stimulation by immune complexes inhibits other signaling pathways and can instead induce apoptosis.[16,18] In contrast, dendritic cells, monocytes, macrophages, and neutrophils express both activating and inhibitory FcγRs. Interestingly, murine studies have identified a monocyte subset responsible for most of the proinflammatory activities of IgG *in vivo*.[35] In addition to the A/I ratio of IgG binding affinities to FcγRs, the relative expression of these receptors thus plays a role in dictating IgG inflammatory potential. FcγR expression appears to be dynamic and dependent on the inflammatory status among other factors.[10,36,37] In fact, this means of altering FcγR expression has been exploited in a number of studies and is an important consideration during therapeutic antibody administration.

ANTI-INFLAMMATORY IgG MODULATES FcγR EXPRESSION

Intravenous immunoglobulin (IVIG) is a therapeutic preparation of highly purified, polyclonal IgG antibodies from the plasma of tens of thousands of donors. IVIG was developed originally as an IgG antibody replacement therapy for patients unable to produce their own antibodies and was administered at a dose of 400 to 600 mg/kg. However, IVIG displays general antiinflammatory activity when given at high doses of 1 to 2 g/kg.[38,39] For that reason, it is administered to patients suffering from a number of autoimmune and inflammatory diseases, including chronic inflammatory demyelinating neuropathy (CIDP), immune thrombocytopenic purpura (ITP), Kawasaki disease, and multiple sclerosis (MS). The means through which IVIG acts to suppress inflammation is by altering FcγR expression on innate effector cells.[40,41]

The immunomodulatory component of IVIG is sialylated Fcs (sFc, IgG Fcs with glycans terminating in sialic acid).[32,42] This was determined by a series of experiments which first identified the Fc as essential to the immunosuppressive activity of IVIG.[43] Indeed, pediatric immune thrombocytopenic purpura (ITP), in which autoantibodies target platelet antigens leading to platelet destruction and severely low platelet counts, has been successfully treated by infusion with Fcs prepared from IVIG.[44] Next, the glycan on the Fc portion of IgG antibodies was found to be essential for IVIG's antiinflammatory activity.[42] Enzymatic removal of IVIG Fc glycans resulted in loss of antiinflammatory activity. Similarly, enzymatic removal of terminal sialic acid from the Fc glycan abrogated the antiinflammatory activity.[42] Sialylated IgG Fc (sFc) suppresses inflammation by triggering a pathway that culminates in increased surface expression of the inhibitory FcγR on inflammatory cells.[42,45] As shown in Figure 16.1, sFcs bind to DC-SIGN, an antiinflammatory FcγR, resulting in the production of IL-33.[33] IL-33 activates basophils to increase IL-4 expression and traffic to infslammatory sites. IL-4 increases surface expression of the inhibitory FcγR FcγRIIB on inflamsmatory cells including monocytes, macrophages, and neutrophils, which is sufficient to attenuate autoantibody mediated inflammation.

Indeed, increased surface expression of FcγRIIB is associated with a more favorable clinical outcome in IVIG-treated CIDP patients.[46] Interestingly, both circulating memory B cells and monocytes recovered from CIDP patients that responded to IVIG therapy displayed increased FcγRIIB on the cell surface, while cells recovered from nonresponders did not upregulate FcγRIIB surface expression. Indeed, studies using murine models of autoantibody-mediated inflammation have shown that IVIG and sFc administration promotes increased expression of FcγRIIB on the surface of monocytes, macrophages, and neutrophils.[33,43,45] Taken together, these results strongly support a role for FcγRIIB in the antiinflammatory activity of IVIG and sFc and indicate that manipulating the FcγR expression balance has tremendous therapeutic potential.

FcγR REGULATION DURING AUTOIMMUNE DISEASE

FcγR expression has been reported to be perturbed in a number of autoimmune diseases, including ITP, rheumatoid arthritis (RA), SLE, MS, and type I diabetes.[47–51] The high-affinity FcγR, FcγRI, is reported to be upregulated during chronic inflammation, including inflammatory bowel disease and SLE.[52,53] FcγR expression on macrophages recovered from synovia of RA-afflicted and healthy individuals was analyzed. Higher surface expression of activating receptors FcγRIIA and FcγRIIIA were detected on cells recovered from the inflammatory autoimmune environment. Further, the macrophages recovered from RA patients produced higher levels of the inflammatory cytokine TNFα following immune complex stimulation, compared to macrophages recovered from healthy donors.[54] Consistent with this observation, neutrophils stimulated *in vitro* with TNFα demonstrate upregulation of the activating FcγR FcγRIIA. RA patients treated with infliximab, a therapeutic used to neutralize TNFα, displayed decreased surface expression of FcγRIIA compared to untreated RA patients.[54] These results support a positive feedback loop of FcγR and immune-complex-driven inflammation and inflammatory cytokine production. Conversely, surface expression of the inhibitory FcγR FcγRIIB was observed to be reduced on memory B cells from CIDP patients compared to healthy controls. Similarly, patients suffering from systemic lupus erythematosus (SLE) exhibited decreased surface expression of FcγRIIB on memory B cells and plasma cells compared to healthy donors. These observations support the notion of a shift toward activating and away from inhibitory FcγR expression profiles during pro-inflammatory settings.

FcγR REGULATION DURING INFECTION

As mentioned above, the inflammatory milieu also contributes to FcγR expression levels. Administration of the Gram-negative bacterial cell wall component lipopolysaccharide (LPS) to mice resulted in increased expression of activating receptors FcγRIII and FcγRIV (Lunnon et al.[37] and R.M. Anthony and J.V. Ravetch, unpublished). Viral infections, including HIV, have been reported to alter FcγR expression. Increased FcγRI expression on inflammatory leukocytes, including neutrophils and monocytes, has been observed during acute HIV infection, which is attributed to increased levels of IFN-γ.[36,55,56] However, chronic HIV patients are reported to have lower expression levels of FcγRII and FcγRIIIA.[36] Further, monocytes recovered from AIDS patients displayed increased levels of FcγRIIIA compared to healthy controls.[55] Indeed, FcγR expression is an important consideration for treatment of HIV patients with passively administered antibodies.

Approximately half of ITP patients with *Helicobacter pylori* infections exhibit marked recovery of platelet numbers followed clearance of *H. pylori* infection.[57–61] It has been proposed that antibodies cross-react with *H. pylori* and platelet antigens, and that infection promotes development of autoreactive B cells.[62–64] However, FcγR expression is also affected by the inflammatory status of patients afflicted both by ITP and *H. pylori* infections. In fact, the rebound of platelet numbers associated with eradication of the *H. pylori* infection also correlates with increased expression of FcγRIIB on monocytes.[65] This observation is consistent with the proposed anti-inflammatory mechanism of IVIG and sFc (Figure 16.1) proposed by Ravetch and colleagues, and with published results suggesting increased expression of FcγRIIB is important for the resolution of ITP symptoms.[33,40,41,45,66]

FcγR REGULATION DURING CANCER

As discussed above, much attention has been given to activating FcγR alleles and responsiveness to various cancer monoclonal antibody therapies. For example, follicular lymphoma patients with high affinity binding alleles FcγRIIIA$^{v/v158}$ and FcγRIIA$^{h/h131}$ respond better to rituximab.[67] Similarly, the FcγRIIA$^{h/h131}$ genotype was significantly correlated with complete response to rituximab compared to patients with the FcγRIIA$^{r/r131}$ allele in non-Hodgkin lymphoma patients.[68–70] These observations strongly support the notion of specific targeting of activating FcγRs to promote enhanced anti-tumor monoclonal antibody therapy.

Higher expression levels of FcγRs have been reported in patients with lung small cell carcinoma, as indicated by increased rosette formation by heat-aggregated IgG. Unfortunately, this assay cannot distinguish between inhibitory and activating FcγRs. However, these patients exhibited even higher rosette formation following treatment with IFN-?. Thus, treatment with IFN-? increased FcγR expression, which would be expected to affect a patient's subsequent response to therapeutic IgG antibodies. In the setting of combination therapies, the effect of various chemotherapies on FcγR expression is an important consideration.[71,72] Anti-Her2 therapy in combination with chemotherapy did improve survival in patients suffering from gastric cancer, compared to patients receiving only chemotherapy.[73] However, there have been reports linking anti-CD20 (Rituximab) treatment with late onset neutropenia, in which neutrophil depletion is further associated with the high affinity FcγRIIA$^{v/v158}$allele.[74,75] How this loss of neutrophils might affect subsequent monoclonal antibody therapy needs further experimentation.

Interestingly, malignant melanoma tumors have been reported to express the inhibitory FcγR.[76,77] Similarly, FcγRIIB is highly expressed on B cell malignancies.[78–81] This expression of FcγRIIB has been suggested to be an effective means to evade the host-anti-tumor response, as the cancer expressed FcγRs compete with leukocyte FcγRs for anti-tumor IgG antibodies. However, therapeutic IgG Fcs engineered to selectively bind activating FcγRs would be an effective means circumvent this. Also, it has been proposed that targeting FcγRIIB with therapeutic monoclonal antibodies might be a means to address tumors expressing this receptor.[82] However, as discussed, the wide cellular distribution of FcγRIIB would most likely make this an ineffective cancer target antigen. An interesting approach to target immune responses to tumors forced surface expression of IgG Fcs on the surface of solid tumors in mice.[83] Adenoviral vectors expressing membrane bound murine IgG_{2a} Fcs, which have an A/I ratio favoring the activating murine FcγRIV (Table 16.1), were used to infect the murine B16-F10 melanoma line. Indeed, this approach was effective at targeting the tumor cells to effector leukocytes, but it remains to be determined if this approach is clinically valid.

ENGINEERING IgG IMMUNE RESPONSES

Manipulating FcγR accessibility has also been employed to promote IgG-mediated responses. Human monocyte-derived dendritic cells were cultured in sera, in the presence of an antibody that blocking binding to the inhibitory FcγR, FcγRIIB. Under these conditions, the presence of normal sera was sufficient to trigger dendritic cell activation, which included increased surface expression of MHC II molecules, upregulation of costimulatory molecules CD80 and CD86, and production of IL-12p70.[84] This activated phenotype of dendritic cells was driven by Stat1 and resulted in a characteristic type-1 interferon program of gene expression, indicating the magnitude of influence the ITIM signaling motif on the cytoplasmic tail of FcγRIIB has over leukocyte.[85] This strategy of blocking or inhibiting FcγRIIB to enhance DC activation is an appealing strategy to enhance a pro-inflammatory immune response. However, the wide cellular expression and tissue distribution of FcγRIIB is such that blockade of this receptor *in vivo* would not selectively target dendritic cells. FcγRIIB expressed by B cells, as well as macrophages and neutrophils, would also be targeted by FcγRIIB blocking antibodies, and thereby dilute the effects on dendritic cells. Perhaps, antibodies that recognized activating FcγRs that are expressed more selectively by antigen presenting cells, including FcγRIIA, might be an effective means to activate dendritic cells and macrophages.

TARGETING Fcs TO FcγRs

As discussed above, there is substantial evidence that selective binding of FcγRs by therapeutic IgG can improve the effector functions of antibodies. In order to control the effector mechanisms employed, a number of strategies have been employed to selectively target the Fc portion to defined FcγRs. These approaches attempt to skew the A/I ratio toward the desired effector function, and frequently focus on preferential binding to activating FcγRs. However, a thorough characterization of the therapeutic antibody of interest is required to accurately identify the appropriate FcγR to target.

A well-documented approach to enhancing pro-inflammatory IgG effector functions is to ensure the Fc glycan has the appropriate modifications. To preferentially bind activating FcγRs, the Fc glycan should lack fucose and sialic acid, but possess the bisecting N-GlcNAc.[25–27,31,32,86] However, the regulation of the variable sugar additions to the glycan is poorly understood.[87] It has been reported that during some inflammatory conditions, including chronic inflammation, they promote secretion of IgGs with reduced sialic acid and fucose, which is consistent with pro-inflammatory environments promoting IgG production with enhanced A/I ratios.[88–92] Aglycosylated IgG Fc mutants that productively engage FcγRs have been identified through yeast cell surface display screens.[93] While the affinities for these IgG antibodies for FcγRs was not as strong as afucosylated IgG, this might be a productive benchmark for the development of a generation of aglycosylated therapeutic IgG antibodies.

ENGINEERING THE Fc PEPTIDE BACKBONE

Other strategies undertaken to target specific FcγRs have involved mutations near the FcγR contract points, to engineer Fc peptide backbones that bind specific FcγRs. A series of Fc mutants have been identified that have selective affinity for FcγRs.[94,95] Development of mutants has focused on IgG_1, with the attempts to skew its binding towards activating or inhibitory FcγRs, depending on the intended application. As predicted by A/I ratio, mutants with affinity constants favoring activating FcγRs display increased ADCC in a number of *in vivo* assays.

However, while the A/I ratio will accurately predict the inflammatory potential of an IgG antibody, this is not necessary akin to the desired effector function. For example, the adjuvant activity of anti-CD40 antibodies is well documented, as this treatment promotes dendritic cell activation and enhances antigen-specific $CD8^+$ T cell responses in a number of immunization models. Surprisingly, this pro-inflammatory activity of the anti-CD40 antibody required the inhibitory FcγR.[96] Mice deficient in FcγRIIB were unresponsive to the effects of this treatment. Further, IgG Fc mutants with A/I ratio favoring binding to FcγRIIB displayed enhanced adjuvant activity, but mutants favoring activating FcγRs had reduced activity. It is not clear how binding of FcγRIIB by anti-CD40 antibodies triggers a pro-inflammatory response, nor whether signaling through the FcγRIIB ITIM is initiated by anti-CD40 antibodies. Regardless, these observations underscore the importance of testing the appropriate FcγR to target.

OUTLOOK AND PERSPECTIVES

There is tremendous therapeutic potential in targeting FcγRs, and this approach can be applied to a number of diseases. The selective targeting of FcγRs provides a powerful means to engineer the magnitude of IgG antibody effector functions. Indeed, IgG antibodies and recombinant proteins with IgG Fc portions have proven to be highly effective therapeutically. Further, the dogma that IgG antibodies are merely neutralizing agents is obsolete, as the importance of FcγRs in the effector function of antibodies has been highlighted in recent years. Thus, it is expected that the coming generations of IgG antibody-based drugs will be more effective, more specific, and will appropriately target FcγR to initiate enhanced immune responses.

FcγRs can promote or inhibit inflammation, dictated by the type of signaling motif that is triggered by the receptor (Figure 16.2). Activating FcγRs in humans include FcγRI, FcγRIIA, and FcγRIIIA, while in mouse the activating FcγRs are FcγRI, FcγRIII, and FcγRIV. The inhibitory FcγRIIB is conserved in both species. The expression of these receptors differs by leukocyte population, and also can be dynamic. NK cells only express activating FcγRIIIA, B cells on express inhibitory FcγRIIB, and macrophages, neutrophils, and dendritic cells express both activating and inhibitory FcγRs.

A number of strategies have been employed to target IgG antibodies to specific FcγRs. These include manipulating the IgG Fc glycan to favor interactions with particular FcγRs. Specifically, removal of fucose or the presence of bisecting N-GlcNAc both result in preferential binding to inhibitory FcγRs. The additional of terminal sialic acid to the Fc glycan reduces binding capacity to activating and inhibitory FcγRs, but instead allows binding to the anti-inflammatory FcγR, DC-SIGN. Alternatively, mutations in the IgG Fc peptide backbone have been reported that bestow selective FcγR binding affinity. Importantly, FcγR binding affinity predicts IgG Fc activity *in vivo*, as IgG antibodies with enhanced binding to activating FcγRs exhibit increased ADCC activity. This has been supported in the clinic as patients with FcγR alleles that bind IgG antibodies with higher affinity often have better outcomes following therapeutic antibody treatment.

An important consideration for targeting FcγRs is the dynamics of FcγR expression. In general, inflammatory conditions favor upregulation of activating FcγRs. This appears to be consistent in a number of autoimmune diseases, and also following treatment with inflammatory stimulants. Conversely, some diseases that promote an immunocompromised state skew FcγR expression towards an inhibitory FcγR binding. For example, HIV infection is associated with decreased expression of activating FcγRs. Further, some cancers have been shown to upregulate the inhibitory FcγRIIB, which can interfere with ADCC. The expression pattern of FcγRs is an important consideration when therapeutically targeting FcγRs.

In fact, altering the expression pattern of FcγRs is an effective means to suppress autoantibody driven inflammation. Studies examining the anti-inflammatory therapeutic high dose IVIG have demonstrated that leukocytes display increased expression of FcγRIIB following treatment. Mice lacking FcγRIIB are unresponsive to high dose IVIG in a number of autoimmune models. Further, increased surface expression following IVIG treatment was found to be associated with better clinical outcomes in CIDP patients. Conversely, an additional means to skew the A/I ratio to favor activating FcγRs might be an intervention that reduces expression of the inhibitory FcγRIIB or increases expression of activating FcγRs.

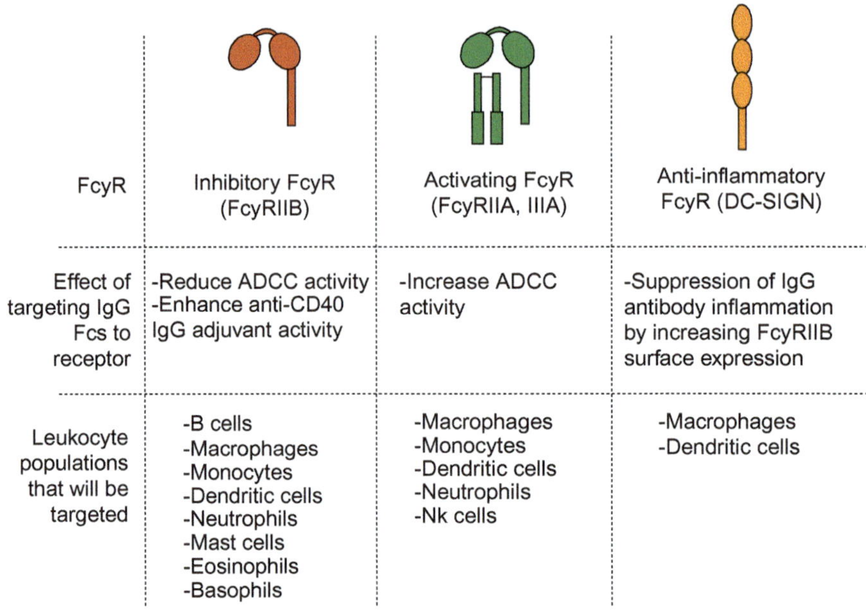

FIGURE 16.2 **The outcomes of targeting IgG Fcs to specific FcγRs.** Targeting IgG antibodies to bind inhibitory FcγRIIB (red) can result in dampened and attenuated IgG effector functions, including ADCC. Also, targeting this FcγR enhances the adjuvant activity of anti-CD40 IgG antibodies. IgG antibodies engineered to target activating FcγRs (green) exhibit enhanced proinflammatory activities, including ADCC. Fc portions that selectively bind the inhibitory FcγR DC-SIGN (yellow), including sialylated IgG Fcs, promote an antiinflammatory response that culminates in the increased expression of the inhibitory FcγRIIB on inflammatory leukocytes, which is effective at suppressing IgG antibody-induced inflammation.

Harnessing FcγRs by targeting IgG Fc or by manipulating their expression and accessibility is a powerful means to enhancing IgG effector functions. Targeting IgG Fcs to specific FcγRs can be achieved by manipulating the IgG Fc glycan, or mutating the Fc peptide backbone. The inflammatory milieu of an individual appears to affect FcγR expression patterns, such that ongoing inflammation results in upregulation of activating FcγRs, while anti-inflammatory and immunosuppressive responses increase expression of the inhibitory FcγRIIB. Understanding which FcγR is most appropriate to target is of paramount importance. As demonstrated in experiments examining anti-CD40 adjuvant antibody, pro-inflammatory responses might require inhibitory FcγRs. These considerations will improve the design and use of therapeutic antibodies.

References

1. Beck A, Wurch T, Bailly C, Corvaia N. Strategies and challenges for the next generation of therapeutic antibodies. *Nat Rev Immunol* 2010;**10**(5):345–52.
2. Chan AC, Carter PJ. Therapeutic antibodies for autoimmunity and inflammation. *Nat Rev Immunol* 2010;**10**(5):301–16.
3. Becker YT, Samaniego-Picota M, Sollinger HW. The emerging role of rituximab in organ transplantation. *Transpl Int* 2006;**19**(8):621–8.
4. Maloney DG, Grillo-Lopez AJ, White CA, Bodkin D, Schilder RJ, Neidhart JA, et al. IDEC-C2B8 (rituximab) anti-CD20 monoclonal antibody therapy in patients with relapsed low-grade non-Hodgkin's lymphoma. *Blood* 1997;**90**(6):2188–95.

5. Sonnenday CJ, Warren DS, Cooper M, Samaniego M, Haas M, King KE, et al. Plasmapheresis, CMV hyperimmune globulin, and anti-CD20 allow ABO-incompatible renal transplantation without splenectomy. *Am J Transplant* 2004;**4**(8):1315–22.
6. Hudziak RM, Lewis GD, Winget M, Fendly BM, Shepard HM, Ullrich A. p185HER2 monoclonal antibody has antiproliferative effects *in vitro* and sensitizes human breast tumor cells to tumor necrosis factor. *Mol Cell Biol* 1989;**9**(3):1165–72.
7. Wong WM. Drug update: trastuzumab: anti-HER2 antibody for treatment of metastatic breast cancer. *Cancer Pract* 1999;**7**(1):48–50.
8. Nimmerjahn F, Ravetch JV. Fcγ receptors: old friends and new family members. *Immunity* 2006;**24**(1):19–28.
9. Nimmerjahn F, Ravetch JV. Antibodies, Fc receptors and cancer. *Curr Opin Immunol* 2007;**19**(2):239–45.
10. Nimmerjahn F, Ravetch JV. Fcγ receptors as regulators of immune responses. *Nat Rev Immunol* 2008;**8**(1):34–47.
11. Ravetch JV, Bolland S. IgG Fc receptors. *Annu Rev Immunol* 2001;**19**:275–90.
12. Ravetch JV, Nimmerjahn F. Fc receptors and their role in immune regulation and inflammation. In: Paul WE, editor. *Fundamental immunology* 6th ed.. Philadelphia PA: Lippincott Williams & Wilkins; 2008. p. 684–705.
13. Junghans RP, Anderson CL. The protection receptor for IgG catabolism is the beta2-microglobulin-containing neonatal intestinal transport receptor. *Proc Natl Acad Sci USA* 1996;**93**(11):5512–6.
14. Boruchov AM, Heller G, Veri MC, Bonvini E, Ravetch JV, Young JW. Activating and inhibitory IgG Fc receptors on human DCs mediate opposing functions. *J Clin Invest* 2005;**115**(10):2914–23.
15. Bruhns P, Iannascoli B, England P, Mancardi DA, Fernandez N, Jorieux S, et al. Specificity and affinity of human Fcgamma receptors and their polymorphic variants for human IgG subclasses. *Blood* 2009;**113**(16):3716–25.
16. Isakov N. ITIMs and ITAMs. The Yin and Yang of antigen and Fc receptor-linked signaling machinery. *Immunol Res* 1997;**16**(1):85–100.
17. Muta T, Kurosaki T, Misulovin Z, Sanchez M, Nussenzweig MC, Ravetch JV. A 13-amino-acid motif in the cytoplasmic domain of Fc gamma RIIB modulates B-cell receptor signalling. *Nature* 1994;**368**(6466):70–3.
18. Ono M, Okada H, Bolland S, Yanagi S, Kurosaki T, Ravetch JV. Deletion of SHIP or SHP-1 reveals two distinct pathways for inhibitory signaling. *Cell* 1997;**90**(2):293–301.
19. McGaha TL, Karlsson MC, Ravetch JV. FcγRIIB deficiency leads to autoimmunity and a defective response to apoptosis in Mrl–MpJ mice. *J Immunol* 2008;**180**(8):5670–9.
20. Nimmerjahn F, Ravetch JV. Divergent immunoglobulin g subclass activity through selective Fc receptor binding. *Science* 2005;**310**(5753):1510–2.
21. Tamura K, Shimizu C, Hojo T, Akashi-Tanaka S, Kinoshita T, Yonemori K, et al. FcγR2A and 3A polymorphisms predict clinical outcome of trastuzumab in both neoadjuvant and metastatic settings in patients with HER2-positive breast cancer. *Ann Oncol* 2011;**22**(6):1302–7.
22. Zhang W, Gordon M, Schultheis AM, Yang DY, Nagashima F, Azuma M, et al. FCGR2A and FCGR3A polymorphisms associated with clinical outcome of epidermal growth factor receptor expressing metastatic colorectal cancer patients treated with single-agent cetuximab. *J Clin Oncol* 2007;**25**(24):3712–8.
23. Mimura Y, Jefferis R, Mimura-Kimura Y, Abrahams J, Rudd PM. Glycosylation of therapeutic IgGs. In: An Z, editor. *Therapeutic monoclonal antibodies: from bench to clinic*. New York: John Wiley & Sons; 2009. p. 67–90.
24. Arnold JN, Wormald MR, Sim RB, Rudd PM, Dwek RA. The impact of glycosylation on the biological function and structure of human immunoglobulins. *Annu Rev Immunol* 2007;**25**:21–50.
25. Shields RL, Lai J, Keck R, O'Connell LY, Hong K, Meng YG, et al. Lack of fucose on human IgG1 N-linked oligosaccharide improves binding to human Fcgamma RIII and antibody-dependent cellular toxicity. *J Biol Chem* 2002;**277**(30):26733–40.
26. Natsume A, Wakitani M, Yamane-Ohnuki N, Shoji-Hosaka E, Niwa R, Uchida K, et al. Fucose removal from complex-type oligosaccharide enhances the antibody-dependent cellular cytotoxicity of single-gene-encoded antibody comprising a single-chain antibody linked the antibody constant region. *J Immunol Meth* 2005;**306**(1–2):93–103.
27. Shoji-Hosaka E, Kobayashi Y, Wakitani M, Uchida K, Niwa R, Nakamura K, et al. Enhanced Fc-dependent cellular cytotoxicity of Fc fusion proteins derived from TNF receptor II and LFA-3 by fucose removal from Asn-linked oligosaccharides. *J Biochem* 2006;**140**(6):777–83.
28. Jefferis R. Glycosylation of recombinant antibody therapeutics. *Biotechnol Prog* 2005;**21**(1):11–16.
29. Jefferis R. Glycosylation as a strategy to improve antibody-based therapeutics. *Nat Rev Drug Discov* 2009;**8**(3):226–34.
30. Jefferis R. Glycosylation of antibody therapeutics: optimisation for purpose. *Meth Mol Biol* 2009;**483**:223–38.
31. Scallon BJ, Tam SH, McCarthy SG, Cai AN, Raju TS. Higher levels of sialylated Fc glycans in immunoglobulin G molecules can adversely impact functionality. *Mol Immunol* 2007;**44**(7):1524–34.
32. Anthony RM, Nimmerjahn F, Ashline DJ, Reinhold VN, Paulson JC, Ravetch JV. Recapitulation of IVIG anti-inflammatory activity with a recombinant IgG Fc. *Science* 2008;**320**(5874):373–6.
33. Anthony RM, Kobayashi T, Wermeling F, Ravetch JV. Intravenous gammaglobulin suppresses inflammation

through a novel T(H)2 pathway. *Nature* 2011;**475**(7354):110–3.

34. Anthony RM, Wermeling F, Karlsson MC, Ravetch JV. Identification of a receptor required for the anti-inflammatory activity of IVIG. *Proc Natl Acad Sci USA* 2008;**105**(50):19571–8.
35. Biburger M, Aschermann S, Schwab I, Lux A, Albert H, Danzer H, et al. Monocyte subsets responsible for immunoglobulin g-dependent effector functions *in vivo*. *Immunity* 2011;**35**(6):932–44.
36. Dugast AS, Tonelli A, Berger CT, Ackerman ME, Sciaranghella G, Liu Q, et al. Decreased Fc receptor expression on innate immune cells is associated with impaired antibody-mediated cellular phagocytic activity in chronically HIV-1 infected individuals. *Virology* 2011;**415**(2):160–7.
37. Lunnon K, Teeling JL, Tutt AL, Cragg MS, Glennie MJ, Perry VH. Systemic inflammation modulates Fc receptor expression on microglia during chronic neurodegeneration. *J Immunol* 2011;**186**(12):7215–24.
38. Imbach P, Barandun S, Baumgartner C, Hirt A, Hofer F, Wagner HP. High-dose intravenous gammaglobulin therapy of refractory, in particular idiopathic thrombocytopenia in childhood. *Helv Paediatr Acta* 1981;**36**(1):81–6.
39. Imbach P, Barandun S, d'Apuzzo V, Baumgartner C, Hirt A, Morell A, et al. High-dose intravenous gammaglobulin for idiopathic thrombocytopenic purpura in childhood. *Lancet* 1981;**1**(8232):1228–31.
40. Nimmerjahn F, Ravetch JV. The antiinflammatory activity of IgG: the intravenous IgG paradox. *J Exp Med* 2007;**204**(1):11–15.
41. Nimmerjahn F, Ravetch JV. Anti-inflammatory actions of intravenous immunoglobulin. *Annu Rev Immunol* 2008;**26**:513–33.
42. Kaneko Y, Nimmerjahn F, Ravetch JV. Anti-inflammatory activity of immunoglobulin G resulting from Fc sialylation. *Science* 2006;**313**(5787):670–3.
43. Bruhns P, Samuelsson A, Pollard JW, Ravetch JV. Colony-stimulating factor-1-dependent macrophages are responsible for IVIG protection in antibody-induced autoimmune disease. *Immunity* 2003;**18**(4):573–81.
44. Debre M, Bonnet MC, Fridman WH, Carosella E, Philippe N, Reinert P, et al. Infusion of Fc gamma fragments for treatment of children with acute immune thrombocytopenic purpura. *Lancet* 1993;**342**(8877):945–9.
45. Samuelsson A, Towers TL, Ravetch JV. Anti-inflammatory activity of IVIG mediated through the inhibitory Fc receptor. *Science* 2001;**291**(5503):484–6.
46. Tackenberg B, Jelcic I, Baerenwaldt A, Oertel WH, Sommer N, Nimmerjahn F, et al. Impaired inhibitory Fcgamma receptor IIB expression on B cells in chronic inflammatory demyelinating polyneuropathy. *Proc Natl Acad Sci USA* 2009;**106**(12):4788–92.
47. Prins JB, Todd JA, Rodrigues NR, Ghosh S, Hogarth PM, Wicker LS, et al. Linkage on chromosome 3 of autoimmune diabetes and defective Fc receptor for IgG in NOD mice. *Science* 1993;**260**(5108):695–8.
48. Frank MM, Hamburger MI, Lawley TJ, Kimberly RP, Plotz PH. Defective reticuloendothelial system Fc-receptor function in systemic lupus erythematosus. *N Engl J Med* 1979;**300**(10):518–23.
49. Zuniga R, Ng S, Peterson MG, Reveille JD, Baethge BA, Alarcon GS, et al. Low-binding alleles of Fcgamma receptor types IIA and IIIA are inherited independently and are associated with systemic lupus erythematosus in Hispanic patients. *Arthritis Rheum* 2001;**44**(2):361–7.
50. Van Weyenbergh J, Lipinski P, Abadie A, Chabas D, Blank U, Liblau R, et al. Antagonistic action of IFN-beta and IFN-gamma on high affinity Fc gamma receptor expression in healthy controls and multiple sclerosis patients. *J Immunol* 1998;**161**(3):1568–74.
51. Salmon JE, Pricop L. Human receptors for immunoglobulin G: key elements in the pathogenesis of rheumatic disease. *Arthritis Rheum* 2001;**44**(4):739–50.
52. Li Y, Lee PY, Sobel ES, Narain S, Satoh M, Segal MS, et al. Increased expression of FcγRI/CD64 on circulating monocytes parallels ongoing inflammation and nephritis in lupus. *Arthritis Res Ther* 2009;**11**(1):R6.
53. Tillinger W, Jilch R, Jilma B, Brunner H, Koeller U, Lichtenberger C, et al. Expression of the high-affinity IgG receptor FcRI (CD64) in patients with inflammatory bowel disease: a new biomarker for gastroenterologic diagnostics. *Am J Gastroenterol* 2009;**104**(1):102–9.
54. Belostocki K, Park MS, Redecha PB, Masuda E, Salmon JE, Pricop L. FcgammaRIIa is a target for modulation by TNFalpha in human neutrophils. *Clin Immunol* 2005;**117**(1):78–86.
55. Capsoni F, Minonzio F, Ongari AM, Bonara P, Pinto G, Carbonelli V, et al. Fc receptors expression and function in mononuclear phagocytes from AIDS patients: modulation by IFN-gamma. *Scand J Immunol* 1994;**39**(1):45–50.
56. Bender BS, Davidson BL, Kline R, Brown C, Quinn TC. Role of the mononuclear phagocyte system in the immunopathogenesis of human immunodeficiency virus infection and the acquired immunodeficiency syndrome. *Rev Infect Dis* 1988;**10**(6):1142–54.
57. Fujimura K. *Helicobacter pylori* infection and idiopathic thrombocytopenic purpura. *Int J Hematol* 2005;**81**(2):113–8.
58. Candelli M, Nista EC, Pignataro G, Gasbarrini G, Gasbarrini A. Idiopathic thrombocytopenic purpura and *Helicobacter pylori* infection. *Scand J Gastroenterol* 2003;**38**(5):569–70.

59. Gasbarrini A, Franceschi F, Tartaglione R, Landolfi R, Pola P, Gasbarrini G. Regression of autoimmune thrombocytopenia after eradication of *Helicobacter pylori*. *Lancet* 1998;**352**(9131):878.
60. Fujimura K, Kuwana M, Kurata Y, Imamura M, Harada H, Sakamaki H, et al. Is eradication therapy useful as the first line of treatment in *Helicobacter pylori*-positive idiopathic thrombocytopenic purpura? Analysis of 207 eradicated chronic ITP cases in Japan. *Int J Hematol* 2005;**81**(2):162–8.
61. Franchini M, Veneri D. *Helicobacter pylori*-associated immune thrombocytopenia. *Platelets* 2006;**17**(2):71–7.
62. Takahashi T, Yujiri T, Shinohara K, Inoue Y, Sato Y, Fujii Y, et al. Molecular mimicry by *Helicobacter pylori* CagA protein may be involved in the pathogenesis of *H. pylori*-associated chronic idiopathic thrombocytopenic purpura. *Br J Haematol* 2004;**124**(1):91–6.
63. Michel M, Khellaf M, Desforges L, Lee K, Schaeffer A, Godeau B, et al. Autoimmune thrombocytopenic *Purpura* and *Helicobacter pylori* infection. *Arch Intern Med* 2002;**162**(9):1033–6.
64. Yamanishi S, Iizumi T, Watanabe E, Shimizu M, Kamiya S, Nagata K, et al. Implications for induction of autoimmunity via activation of B-1 cells by *Helicobacter pylori* urease. *Infect Immun* 2006;**74**(1):248–56.
65. Asahi A, Nishimoto T, Okazaki Y, Suzuki H, Masaoka T, Kawakami Y, et al. *Helicobacter pylori* eradication shifts monocyte Fcgamma receptor balance toward inhibitory FcgammaRIIB in immune thrombocytopenic purpura patients. *J Clin Invest* 2008;**118**(8):2939–49.
66. Anthony RM, Ravetch JV. A novel role for the IgG Fc glycan: the anti-inflammatory activity of sialylated IgG Fcs. *J Clin Immunol* 2010;**30**(Suppl. 1):S9–S14.
67. Weng WK, Levy R. Two immunoglobulin G fragment C receptor polymorphisms independently predict response to rituximab in patients with follicular lymphoma. *J Clin Oncol* 2003;**21**(21):3940–7.
68. Paiva M, Marques H, Martins A, Ferreira P, Catarino R, Medeiros R. FcgammaRIIa polymorphism and clinical response to rituximab in non-Hodgkin lymphoma patients. *Cancer Genet Cytogenet* 2008;**183**(1):35–40.
69. Khan KD, Emmanouilides C, Benson Jr DM, Hurst D, Garcia P, Michelson G, et al. A Phase 2 study of rituximab in combination with recombinant interleukin-2 for rituximab-refractory indolent non-Hodgkin's lymphoma. *Clin Cancer Res* 2006;**12**(23):7046–53.
70. Cartron G, Dacheux L, Salles G, Solal-Celigny P, Bardos P, Colombat P, et al. Therapeutic activity of humanized anti-CD20 monoclonal antibody and polymorphism in IgG Fc receptor FcgammaRIIIa gene. *Blood* 2002;**99**(3):754–8.
71. Pujol JL, Gibney DJ, Su JQ, Maksymiuk AW, Jett JR. Immune response induced in small-cell lung cancer by maintenance therapy with interferon gamma. *J Natl Cancer Inst* 1993;**85**(22):1844–50.
72. Rhodes J, Jones DH, Bleehen NM. Increased expression of human monocyte HLA-DR antigens and Fc gamma receptors in response to human interferon *in vivo*. *Clin Exp Immunol* 1983;**53**(3):739–43.
73. Bang YJ, Van Cutsem E, Feyereislova A, Chung HC, Shen L, Sawaki A, et al. Trastuzumab in combination with chemotherapy versus chemotherapy alone for treatment of HER2-positive advanced gastric or gastro-oesophageal junction cancer (ToGA): a Phase 3, open-label, randomised controlled trial. *Lancet* 2010;**376**(9742):687–97.
74. Keane C, Nourse JP, Crooks P, Nguyen-Van D, Mutsando H, Mollee P, et al. Homozygous FCGR3A-158V alleles predispose to late onset neutropenia after CHOP-R for diffuse large B-cell lymphoma. *Intern Med J* 2011;**42**(10):1113–9.
75. Wolach O, Shpilberg O, Lahav M. Neutropenia after rituximab treatment: new insights on a late complication. *Curr Opin Hematol* 2012;**19**(1):32–8.
76. Cassard L, Cohen-Solal JF, Fournier EM, Camilleri-Broet S, Spatz A, Chouaib S, et al. Selective expression of inhibitory Fcgamma receptor by metastatic melanoma impairs tumor susceptibility to IgG-dependent cellular response. *Int J Cancer* 2008;**123**(12):2832–9.
77. Cassard L, Cohen-Solal JF, Galinha A, Sastre-Garau X, Mathiot C, Galon J, et al. Modulation of tumor growth by inhibitory Fc(gamma) receptor expressed by human melanoma cells. *J Clin Invest* 2002;**110**(10):1549–57.
78. Callanan MB, Le Baccon P, Mossuz P, Duley S, Bastard C, Hamoudi R, et al. The IgG Fc receptor, FcγRIIB, is a target for deregulation by chromosomal translocation in malignant lymphoma. *Proc Natl Acad Sci USA* 2000;**97**(1):309–14.
79. Chen W, Palanisamy N, Schmidt H, Teruya-Feldstein J, Jhanwar SC, Zelenetz AD, et al. Deregulation of FCGR2B expression by 1q21 rearrangements in follicular lymphomas. *Oncogene* 2001;**20**(52):7686–93.
80. Zusman T, Gohar O, Eliassi H, Avivi Y, Lisansky E, Sautes C, et al. The murine Fc-gamma (Fc gamma) receptor type II B1 is a tumorigenicity-enhancing factor in polyoma-virus-transformed 3T3 cells. *Int J Cancer* 1996;**65**(2):221–9.
81. Camilleri-Broet S, Cassard L, Broet P, Delmer A, Le Touneau A, Diebold J, et al. FcgammaRIIB is differentially expressed during B cell maturation and in B-cell lymphomas. *Br J Haematol* 2004;**124**(1):55–62.
82. Rankin CT, Veri MC, Gorlatov S, Tuaillon N, Burke S, Huang L, et al. CD32B, the human inhibitory Fc-gamma receptor IIB, as a target for monoclonal antibody therapy of B-cell lymphoma. *Blood* 2006;**108**(7):2384–91.

83. Riddle DS, Sanz L, Chong H, Thompson J, Vile RG. Tumor cell surface display of immunoglobulin heavy chain Fc by gene transfer as a means to mimic antibody therapy. *Hum Gene Ther* 2005;**16**(7):830–44.
84. Dhodapkar KM, Kaufman JL, Ehlers M, Banerjee DK, Bonvini E, Koenig S, et al. Selective blockade of inhibitory Fcgamma receptor enables human dendritic cell maturation with IL-12p70 production and immunity to antibody-coated tumor cells. *Proc Natl Acad Sci USA* 2005;**102**(8):2910–5.
85. Dhodapkar KM, Banerjee D, Connolly J, Kukreja A, Matayeva E, Veri MC, et al. Selective blockade of the inhibitory Fcγ receptor (FcγRIIB) in human dendritic cells and monocytes induces a type I interferon response program. *J Exp Med* 2007;**204**(6):1359–69.
86. Okazaki A, Shoji-Hosaka E, Nakamura K, Wakitani M, Uchida K, Kakita S, et al. Fucose depletion from human IgG1 oligosaccharide enhances binding enthalpy and association rate between IgG1 and FcγRIIIa. *J Mol Biol* 2004;**336**(5):1239–49.
87. Wang J, Balog CI, Stavenhagen K, Koeleman CA, Scherer HU, Selman MH, et al. Fc-glycosylation of IgG1 is modulated by B-cell stimuli. *Mol Cell Proteomics* 2011;**10**(5) M110.004655.
88. Guo N, Liu Y, Masuda Y, Kawagoe M, Ueno Y, Kameda T, et al. Repeated immunization induces the increase in fucose content on antigen-specific IgG N-linked oligosaccharides. *Clin Biochem* 2005;**38**(2):149–53.
89. Nakagawa H, Hato M, Takegawa Y, Deguchi K, Ito H, Takahata M, et al. Detection of altered N-glycan profiles in whole serum from rheumatoid arthritis patients. *J Chromatogr B Analyt Technol Biomed Life Sci* 2007;**853**(1–2):133–7.
90. Espy C, Morelle W, Kavian N, Grange P, Goulvestre C, Viallon V, et al. Sialylation levels of anti-proteinase 3 antibodies are associated with the activity of granulomatosis with polyangiitis (Wegener's). *Arthritis Rheum* 2011;**63**(7):2105–15.
91. Selman MH, Niks EH, Titulaer MJ, Verschuuren JJ, Wuhrer M, Deelder AM. IgG Fc N-glycosylation changes in Lambert–Eaton myasthenic syndrome and myasthenia gravis. *J Proteome Res* 2011;**10**(1):143–52.
92. van de Geijn FE, Wuhrer M, Selman MH, Willemsen SP, de Man YA, Deelder AM, et al. Immunoglobulin G galactosylation and sialylation are associated with pregnancy-induced improvement of rheumatoid arthritis and the postpartum flare: results from a large prospective cohort study. *Arthritis Res Ther* 2009;**11**(6):R193.
93. Sazinsky SL, Ott RG, Silver NW, Tidor B, Ravetch JV, Wittrup KD. Aglycosylated immunoglobulin G1 variants productively engage activating Fc receptors. *Proc Natl Acad Sci USA* 2008;**105**(51):20167–72.
94. Lazar GA, Dang W, Karki S, Vafa O, Peng JS, Hyun L, et al. Engineered antibody Fc variants with enhanced effector function. *Proc Natl Acad Sci USA* 2006;**103**(11):4005–10.
95. Chu SY, Vostiar I, Karki S, Moore GL, Lazar GA, Pong E, et al. Inhibition of B cell receptor-mediated activation of primary human B cells by coengagement of CD19 and FcgammaRIIb with Fc-engineered antibodies. *Mol Immunol* 2008;**45**(15):3926–33.
96. Li F, Ravetch JV. Inhibitory Fcγ receptor engagement drives adjuvant and anti-tumor activities of agonistic CD40 antibodies. *Science* 2011;**333**(6045):1030–4.
97. Maenaka K, van der Merwe PA, Stuart DI, Jones EY, Sondermann P. The human low affinity Fcγ receptors IIa, IIb, and III bind IgG with fast kinetics and distinct thermodynamic properties. *J Biol Chem* 2001;**276**(48):44898–904.
98. Paetz A, Sack M, Thepen T, Tur MK, Bruell D, Finnern R, et al. Recombinant soluble human Fcgamma receptor I with picomolar affinity for immunoglobulin G. *Biochem Biophys Res Commun* 2005;**338**(4):1811–7.

CHAPTER

17

Fc Protein Engineering

Roy Jefferis

University of Birmingham, Birmingham, West Midlands, United Kingdom

INTRODUCTION

We live in a hostile environment and are constantly exposed to potential pathogens but are mostly unaware of these insults due to protective innate and adaptive immune responses (AIRs).[1,2] The innate immune response provides immediate protection, while the AIR requires time to develop; when established, it provides a rapid and heightened response with immunological memory. A defining feature of the AIR is the ability to generate a virtually infinite repertoire of antigen-binding sites through somatic hypermutation of genes encoding the variable regions of antibody molecules. Consequently, each specific antibody molecule has a unique sequence at its antigen binding site (paratope). A recombinant antibody therapeutic will most likely present a unique (non-self) sequence to each patient and has the potential to be immunogenic with production of anti-drug antibody (ADA; anti-idiotypic). Although the binding of an antibody to its antigen may neutralize toxicity and/or limit diffusion of a pathogen from the site of entry, the immune complexes formed must still be removed and destroyed. The biologic effector mechanisms activated by such immune complexes differ according to the class, or mixture of classes, of antibody forming the complex. Humans have the potential to produce five classes of antibody (IgM, IgD, IgG, IgA, IgE), and there are four subclasses of IgG and two of IgA. Because each class and subclass is expressed in all normal individuals the protein products (antibodies) are referred to as *isotypes*. The genes encoding the nine isotypes are closely linked on chromosome 14;[3–5] however, there are polymorphisms (allotypes) within the classes and subclasses of IgG and IgA that are inherited as a haplotype. The separation of populations over the course of human evolution has resulted in a characteristic distribution of haplotypes among racial groups. Each antibody isotype has unique structural properties and a unique profile of biologic effector activities that may be triggered upon the formation of antibody–antigen immune complexes. The unique properties of each isotype can be exploited in the development and clinical application of monoclonal antibody therapeutics. To date the IgG class of antibody has been the predominant format developed.

In spite of the diversity of the antibody response, humans remain susceptible to infections by microorganisms, particularly in early

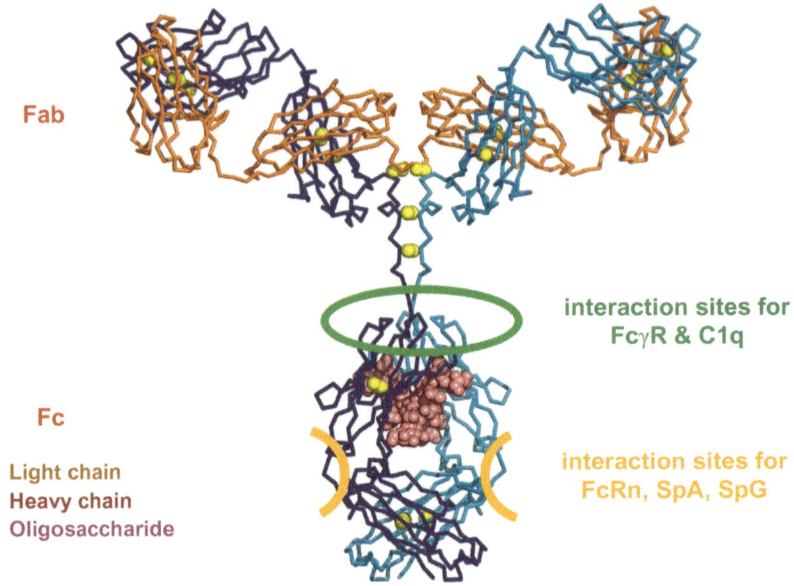

FIGURE 17.1 **The α-chain backbone structures the IgG molecule.** The location of interaction sites for IgG-Fc ligands is indicated. (Structure generated by Peter Artymiuk, University of Sheffield, using PyMOL: http://pymol.sourceforge.net.)

life before the immune system is fully developed and in later life when it is on the wane. Research increasingly reveals mechanisms by which pathogens frustrate and/or negate immune responses, in some cases subverting the immune response to enhance survival and proliferation of the pathogen. The most widely recognized escape mechanism is antigenic variation, resulting in ineffective binding/neutralization of the pathogen by previously protective antibody specificities. These are properties of the Fab region of IgG molecules (IgG-Fab); however, while modulation of the IgG-Fc (Figure 17.1) domain's effector activities can be mediated by "natural" IgG-Fc sequences as has been discussed, there has been a great deal of interest in approaches aimed at enhancing, diminishing, or abrogating IgG-Fc biologic function by protein engineering (i.e., creating mutant antibody molecules). This review will attempt to summarize the objectives, successes, and limitations resulting from protein engineering of the IgG-Fc. Considerable success has been reported but it must be born in mind that protein engineering results in the generation of non-self molecules that may potentiate immunogenicity. Although the mutant IgG-Fc antibodies generated have been evaluated for binding/activation to self IgG-Fc ligands, they have not been similarly evaluated for interactions with pathogen elaborated ligands.

THE IgG SUBCLASSES

The four human IgG subclasses are enumerated according to their relative concentrations in normal serum; thus, IgG_1, IgG_2, IgG_3, and IgG_4 account for approximately 60%, 25%, 10%, and 5% of plasma IgG, respectively. The genes encoding the immunoglobulin heavy chains are inherited within a closely linked complex; however, mutations and cross-overs have occurred over evolutionary time such that characteristic haplotype differences exist among population groups.[6] The IgG antibody class predominates in human blood, equilibrates with the extravascular space, and activates a wide range of effector functions that can result in the killing, removal, and destruction of specifically targeted pathogens. Evaluation of biologic activities *in vitro* demonstrates that each IgG subclass exhibits a unique profile of effector functions.[3–7] Multiple parameters influence the antibody isotype profile of a natural protective immune response to a given pathogen, and it is presumed to be "orchestrated" to maximize the benefit to the host.[3–8] Within the IgG class the broad generalization can be made that protein antigens provoke predominantly IgG_1 and IgG_3 responses; carbohydrate antigens provoke an IgG_2 response; and IgG_4 responses may predominate as a consequence of chronic antigen stimulation.[7,8] When developing a rMAb therapeutic, the choice of IgG subclass is predicated on the presumption that one can extrapolate from activities demonstrated *in vitro* to *in vivo* mechanisms; importantly, this presumption may be naïve. Early therapeutic success was reported for the treatment of non-Hodgkin lymphoma with the chimeric mouse-human IgG_1 anti-CD20 antibody rituximab and the treatment of rheumatoid arthritis with the chimeric mouse-human IgG_1 TNFα neutralizing antibody infliximab. It has now become evident that antibodies specific for the same target (e.g., CD20) but with different epitopes may activate differing downstream biologic mechanisms and variable efficacy.

IgG-Fc BINDING LIGAND: AN OVERVIEW

Three classes or subtypes, six isotypes, of cell membrane-bound IgG-Fc receptors (FcγRs) are defined that are co-expressed or differentially expressed on multiple leukocyte cell types.[9–12] The FcγRs are structurally homologous, and their engagement by immune complexes results in one or more of multiple possible outcomes, including antibody-dependent cellular cytotoxicity (ADCC), antibody-dependent cell-mediated phagocytosis (ADCP), release of inflammatory mediators, induction of cellular apoptosis, and regulation of immune system cell activation.[9–12] Early studies demonstrating the binding of monomeric IgG or IgG-Fc to the cell surface of leukocytes (monocytes) led to the identification of a receptor referred to, subsequently, as the high-affinity Fc gamma receptor (FcγRI).[12] Studies of eluted membrane proteins binding to aggregated or immobilized IgG led to the identification of low-affinity FcγRs (FcγRII, FcγRIII). Subsequently, further subtypes of FcγR were identified (FcγRIIa, FcγRIIb, FcγRIIc, FcγRIIIa, and FcγRIIIb) and consolidated with sequencing of the FcγR gene locus at chromosome 1q23.[13] Polymorphisms within and between population groups for the FcγR genes is also observed. Engagement of the FcγR results in cellular activation, mediated through the immunoreceptor tyrosine-based activation motif (ITAM), except for FcγRIIb, which is an inhibitory receptor mediating activity through the immunoreceptor tyrosine-based inhibition motif (ITIM).[8–13]

Early studies directed toward mapping structural features of IgG-Fc that facilitate FcγR binding and activation established that glycosylation at asparagine 297 is essential; subsequently, it was shown that some residual activity may be evident when the target is sensitized with high levels of antibody.[14–16] The profile of human IgG subclass proteins and IgGs of other species binding or not binding to FcγRI suggested that the unique sequence $-L_{234}-L-G-G_{237}-$ is associated with binding.[17] This sequence is proximal to the hinge region of the CH2 domain and present in FcγRI binding human IgG_1-Fc and IgG_3-Fc and mouse IgG_{2a}-Fc subclasses but not mouse IgG_{2b}-Fc, the latter having the sequence $-L_{234}-E-G-G_{237}-$. The mouse IgG_{2b} sequence was engineered to replace the glutamic acid with leucine and this mutant protein bound FcγRI with an affinity equal to that of mouse IgG_{2a}.[18] Human IgG_2, which does not bind FcγRI, has the sequence $–V_{234}–A–G–$ with a deletion at 237; IgG_4, which binds FcγRI with lower affinity, has the sequence $–F_{234}–L–G–G_{237}–$.[7,8] Subsequently, extensive protein engineering has been applied in attempts to generate panels of IgG_1 proteins exhibiting increased, decreased, and/or selective FcγR binding (see below). Four antibody-based therapeutics bearing modified IgG-Fc regions are U.S. Food and Drug Administration (FDA) approved: abatacept, ecilizumab, catumaxomab, and belatacept. Seven others are in clinical trials: teplizumab, tanezumab, ertumaxomab, LY2469298, ponezumab, PRO-131921, and TRU-015.

Immune complexes of IgG_1 and IgG_3 subclass antibodies bind and activate the C1q component of the classical complement system.[4,5,19] This triggers a cascade of enzyme proteolytic events, from C1 to C9, that results in the addition of complement breakdown components to the immune complex. The immune complex-bound complement proteins may be recognized by cell membrane-bound complement receptors, expressed on leukocytes, to enhance opsonization and uptake by phagocytosis. Other complement breakdown products, in the fluid phase, form the "membrane attack complex," a hydrophobic complex that inserts into cellular membranes and forms a pore that allows ingress and egress of water and molecules resulting in loss of cellular integrity and osmotic control.

A significant factor that contributes to the success of antibody therapeutics is their long half-lives: approximately 21 days for IgG_1, IgG_2, and IgG_4 and 7 days for IgG_3.[7,8,19] This means that each infusion of antibody can provide protection over an extended period of time, reducing the frequency of attendance at clinics and contributing positively to the cost of treatment (CoT). Catabolism of IgG is delayed due to recycling mechanisms mediated by the neonatal (FcRn) receptor expressed within the cellular membrane of many cell types that take up IgG, from the external medium, within pinocytotic vesicles that form vacuoles. Subsequent lowering of pH promotes IgG binding to FcRn and protection from cleavage by enzymes present in the vacuole; unbound IgG is not protected and is degraded.[20] When the membrane of the vacuole is recycled to the cellular membrane the IgG–FcRn complex is exposed to extravascular fluid, at pH 7.2, and released. Protein engineering to increase the affinity of a monoclonal antibody (mAb) for FcRn will offer preferential protection from degradation relative to natural polyclonal IgG. The resulting half-life extension further enhances therapeutic efficacy and reduces the CoT, particularly for treatment with mAbs formulated at high concentrations for self-administration.

A continuing problem associated with antibody therapy is immunogenicity and the development of antibodies that may neutralize the therapeutic antibody or give rise to adverse reactions on re-exposure. While these responses are mostly limited to unique variable region sequences (idiotypes) it should be appreciated that protein engineering of the IgG-Fc creates unique non-self structures. In addition, the relationship between co-evolved human pathogens and protective innate and adaptive immune responses may be compromised. Numerous pathogen-produced ligands that target the IgG-Fc have been identified: staphylococcal protein A (SpA),[21,22] streptococcal protein G (SpG),[23] and virus-encoded IgG-Fc receptors.[24–28] The impact of IgG-Fc engineering on interactions with these ligands has not been investigated.

EVALUATION OF IgG-Fc ENGINEERED PROTEINS

Before reviewing the consequences of IgG-Fc engineering, I would emphasize that the claimed outcomes need to be evaluated in context with the protocols employed (e.g., glycoform of IgG-Fc, target cell line, effector cell). The most widely investigated activity has been increased or decreased FcγR binding and cellular activation. Early studies employed recombinant extracellular domains of FcγR, produced in *Escherichia coli* or a variety of non-human cell types, with binding assessed by surface plasmon resonance (SPR) or cell ELISA protocols. In each case, the immobilization protocol may alter the conformation of bound ligand and impact binding. Until relatively recently the impact of IgG-Fc engineering on the glycoform profile had not been appreciated and consequently its impact on FcγR and C1q binding was not taken account of in early studies. Similarly, it has been shown that the FcγR glycoform may also have a profound impact on FcγR binding and activation *in vitro* and when expressed as membrane integrated proteins.[29,30] Therefore, when binding or activation of cellular expressed FcγR is investigated in *in vitro* studies, outcomes may vary significantly depending on the cell line evaluated; likewise, *in vivo* studies of FcγR activity in transgenic mice may possess similar confounding factors. It is not within the scope of this review to critically evaluate the impact of these many parameters on outcomes and conclusions drawn for IgG-Fc mutants; however, the reader should be aware of these possible limitations.

IgG_1 AND IgG_3 BINDING AND ACTIVATION OF FcγR

Because IgG_1 predominates in human serum and has been readily available as a monoclonal protein isolated from the serum of patients with plasma cell cancers (multiple myeloma), early structural and functional studies were focused on this IgG subclass. It transpired that IgG_1 defined all of the IgG-Fc-mediated ligand binding and effector activation functions. Comparative studies demonstrated that IgG_3 mediates comparable functional activity, while IgG_2 and IgG_4 exhibit restrictions in one or more activity. The IgG constant region genes are polymorphic, and this is reflected in inheritance of IgG gene haplotypes and consequent differences in IgG-Fc protein sequences.[29] Few studies have addressed the impact of IgG-Fc polymorphisms on structure and function; however, IgG_3 exhibits a very extensive polymorphism with allotypic forms that differ in their ability to bind SpA.[32] By contrast, some studies have focused on possible influences of IgG polymorphisms on clinical responses to infective agents.[33,34]

Following the initial scan of mutant IgG_1-Fc for binding and activation of FcγRI,[17,18] Shields et al.[35] published a comprehensive study that employed full-length chimeric IgG_1, IgG_2, IgG_3, and IgG_4 variants of an anti-IgE antibody. All solvent-exposed residues of the IgG_1 isotype were sequentially substituted by alanine. The IgG proteins and His-tagged extracellular domains of FcγR and FcRn were expressed in HEK293 cells, now shown to generate atypical FcγRIIIa glycoforms. The IgG protein products were classified according to their binding to the subtypes of FcγR and FcRn in an ELISA assay: Class 1 exhibited reduced binding to all FcγRs; Class 2, reduced binding to FcγRII and FcγRIIIa; Class 3, improved binding to FcγRII and FcγRIIIa; etc. Significantly, residues in the lower hinge region, embracing the $–L_{234}–L–G–G_{237}–$ sequence, were shown to influence binding to all FcγR subtypes tested but not FcRn. These data were counterintuitive at the time, as the $–L_{234}–L–G–G_{237}–$ sequence did not yield defined conformation in the Deisenhofer IgG-Fc structure[18] and was assumed to be mobile; this conundrum was resolved with publication of an x-ray crystal structure for IgG_1-Fc in complex with an aglycosylated form of FcγRIIIb that showed binding to be in the lower hinge region and embracing the $–L_{234}–L–G–G_{237}–$ sequence that assumed defined structure within the complex.[37,38] Flexibility within the hinge region of the intact IgG molecule allows each Fab region to engage its specific antigen with the generation of an equilibrium of IgG-Fc conformers that may, separately, accommodate binding to an individual FcγR. The subtlety of IgG-Fc conformation and FcγR recognition is underlined by the finding that substitution of certain residues within the CH3 domain also influenced FcγR binding affinity. In a subsequent publication, Shields et al.[38] demonstrated a 50-fold increase in the binding affinity of a non-fucosylated glycoform of IgG-Fc for FcγRIIIa and a consequent increase in NK-cell-mediated ADCC. In the decade following these landmark publications, research has been directed towards differentially maximizing or minimizing binding to and activation of selected FcγR and FcRn, with the aim of generating antibody therapeutics with an effector function profile that might be optimal for a given disease indication *in vivo*. A particular goal has been to differentially up- or downregulate interaction with activating and inhibitory FcγR.

Initial evaluation of the mechanism of action of rituximab indicated ADCC, mediated through engagement of FcγRIIIa expressed on NK cells. This conclusion was supported by the finding that disease remission in non-Hodgkin lymphoma was linked to polymorphic variants of the FcγRIIIa receptor that differ in their affinity for IgG_1-Fc.[39,40] The allelic products differ in the presence of valine (V) or phenylalanine (F) at position 158 (FcγRIIIa-V158 and FcγRIIIa-F158) in the extracellular domain. These residues were later shown to be located within the IgG-Fc/FcγRIII interaction site.[36,37] Consequently, research has been directed toward generating antibodies with IgG-Fc mutations that result in increased binding affinity for products of each FcγRIIIa allele, with the expectation of a consequent increase in ADCC irrespective of a patient's FcγRIIIa haplotype. The earlier demonstration of increased affinity for afucosylated IgG_1-Fc was consolidated with the development of stable production cell lines generating non-fucosylated antibodies.[38,41,42] The improved efficacy for killing cancer cells demonstrated *in vitro* for these antibodies encouraged other research groups and companies to attempt to improve FcγRIIIa-mediated ADCC through protein engineering. In addition to the intellectual challenge, success could generate significant intellectual property (IP) and opportunities for patent acquisition that might be exploited for the generation of biobetter therapeutics.

Using computational design algorithms and high-throughput screening, Xencor has generated an extensive panel of IgG-Fc mutants exhibiting altered profiles of FcγR binding and biologic activities.[43–46] A "core" mutation appeared to be the exchange of residues S239D/I332E to yield an IgG-Fc that exhibited ~40-fold increased affinity for both polymorphic forms of FcγRIIIa and an ~10-fold increase for FcγRIIa and FcγRIIb.[44] An anti-CD40 antibody bearing the S239D/I332E mutation exhibited an ~150-fold increase in ADCC for leukemic cells, compared to the wild-type IgG_1 protein; in contrast, FcγR binding was abrogated for the double mutant G236R/L328R.[44] It was further shown that generation of an aglycosylated form of IgG-Fc having the sequence N297D/A330Y/I332E restored ~43% binding affinity for FcγRIIIa.[45,46] A challenge remained to generate increased affinity for the activating FcγRIIa receptor but lower affinity for the inhibitory FcγRIIb receptor. The S239D/I332E/G236 mutant exhibited this property;[46] the G236A mutation alone delivered ~70-fold greater FcγRIIa affinity and mediated enhanced ADCP by macrophages.[47] Interestingly, this mutant was shown to have minimal affect on FcγRI binding, in contrast to previous reports of diminished or lost FcγRI binding and activation.[48,49] Sazinsky et al.[50] focused attention on residues 296 to 300 and showed that a N297/S298G/T299A mutant IgG was aglycosylated when produced in HEK293 cells, yet exhibited affinities for FcγRIIa and FcγRIIb comparable to wild-type IgG-Fc. Mutants with increased affinity for FcγRIIIa were generated by Macrogenics employing a functional genetic screen via yeast display technology. A series of IgG proteins were isolated with substitutions in both the CH2 and CH3 domains that exhibited individual profiles of FcγR recognition. An anti-HER2 antibody was developed bearing an Fc with five substitutions (L235V, F243L, R292P, Y300L P396L) that exhibited enhanced binding to FcγRIIIa but reduced binding to the inhibitory FcγRIIb receptor. This construct exhibited enhanced killing of HER2-expressing cancer cells, showing an ~100-fold increased rate of lysis compared to wild-type protein.[51,52]

A comprehensive panel of aglycosylated IgG-Fc was generated by substitution of asparagine 297 by each of the alternative amino acids. The N297Y mutant was selected for Gene Site Saturation Mutagenesis™ (GSSM™), with the generation of 222 further mutants that were screened for binding to FcγR, FcRn, and C1q and for their ability to promote phagocytosis.[53] As expected, a majority of mutants exhibited lower or no binding activity; however, mutants with 32-, 15-, and 11-fold increases in binding to FcγRIIIa were reported for variants N297Y/Ser254W, N297YQ418W, and N297Y/V259Y, respectively. Many mutants had binding activity for FcγRI similar to or increased relative to wild-type and/or increased binding to FcRn; by contrast, binding to FcγRIIa was virtually abolished for each of the mutants. Surprisingly, the N297A mutant was reported to have near wild-type activity, in contrast to previous reports of loss of binding for FcγRI.[54]

Jung et al.[55] took advantage of the inability of *Escherichia coli* to effect glycosylation using expression to screen a combinatorial library of IgG-Fc mutants binding to FcγR. They characterized the double mutant, E382V/M428I, within the CH3 region, which conferred binding to FcγRI with an affinity nearly identical to that of glycosylated IgG_1 antibodies.[55,56] Binding to all other FcγRs was ablated; interestingly, binding to all FcγRs was observed for the glycosylated form of this antibody mutant when produced in HEK293 cells. When introduced into the anti-HER2 antibody trastuzumab and produced in *E. coli*, the product effected dendritic cell-mediated ADCC, in contrast to wild-type glycosylated trastuzumab.[55,56] It is remarkable that these substitutions within the CH3 domain should have such a profound influence on FcγR binding at the lower hinge site; however, the E382V/M428I residues are contact residues at the CH2–CH3 interface, and, presumably, perturbation of this interaction can influence conformation at a distance.

Error-prone ribosome display has been employed to generate panels of IgG-Fc mutants that were screened for enhanced binding to FcγRIIIa.[57] The F243L/T393A/H433P mutant had increased binding affinity for FcγRIIIa and was shown to mediate ~fourfold enhanced ADCC. Evidence was presented to suggest that the F243L mutation was mostly responsible for the enhanced activity; however, improved function may correlate more closely with the observed increase in the levels of glycoforms lacking fucose but expressing bisecting N-acetylglucosamine. Earlier studies reported that a F243A mutant, produced in CHO cells, was fucosylated and exhibited high levels of galactosylated and sialylation with significant reduction in FcγRI binding.[58]

IgG_2 BINDING AND ACTIVATION OF FcγR

When the objective is to kill cancer cells, antibodies exhibiting maximal effector activities are presumed to be most beneficial; however, care has to be exercised to anticipate or avoid collateral damage (i.e., the killing of normal cells expressing the target antigen). For other disease indications (e.g., chronic diseases such as rheumatoid arthritis), the activation of inflammatory cascades may be contraindicated.

The limited FcγR binding profile and inability to activate the complement cascade suggest that IgG_2 could be the isotype of choice. It is widely reported that IgG_2 exhibits higher functional activity for the polymorphic form of FcγRIIa bearing histidine at residue 134 (FcγRIIa-H134) compared with the arginine 134 form present (FcγRIIa-R134);[59,60] however, functional activity for both polymorphic forms of FcγRIIIa has been demonstrated for non-fucosylated IgG_2.[61] Analysis of the crystal structure of an IgG_1-Fc–FcγRIIa complex provides evidence for the IgG subclass binding specificity and the preferential binding of IgG_2-Fc to the FcγRIIa-H134 variant. It was noted that the inhibitory FcγRIIb receptor has arginine at residue 134; therefore, it might be anticipated that the IgG_2-Fc will bind with low affinity to FcγRIIb, as for FcγRIIa-R134.[61] The interaction site of IgG_1-Fc for FcγRIIa embraces the –L_{234}–L–G–G_{237}– sequence and residues S_{239}, D_{265}, S267, V_{266}, N_{297}; the latter residues are present in the IgG_2-Fc and may account for its binding to FcγRIIb, as the lower hinge sequence of IgG_2-Fc is –V_{234}–A–gap–G_{237}–. These differences may account for the fact that IgG_2-Fc does not bind FcγRI and exhibits differential binding to the polymorphic variants of FcγRIIa.[62]

The first approved antibody therapeutic was a mouse anti-CD3 that had efficacy in treatment of transplant patients undergoing acute graft rejection. It was converted to a chimeric mouse–human IgG_1 antibody that depleted CD3-positive T cells with subsequent profound immune suppression. A less active isotype was sought, and IgG_2 was selected for the development of a format exhibiting minimal binding and activation of FcγR. This aim was achieved when the lower hinge region sequence –V_{234}–A–gap–G_{237}– was mutated to –A_{234}–A–gap–A_{237}– to give a protein product that bound CD3 on T cells to induce transitory anergy.[63,64] Loss of both FcγR and C1q binding was achieved for an anti-porcine VCAM IgG_2/4 chimeric antibody comprised of the CH1 domain and hinge sequence of IgG_2 combined with the CH2 and CH3 sequence of IgG_4.[65] This format was subsequently used to develop the approved antibody therapeutic eculizumab, which has specificity for the C5 component of complement and inhibits haemolysis.[66] A similar outcome was achieved for another IgG_2/IgG_4 hybrid (IgG_2m4) based, principally, on the IgG_2 isotype with four key amino acid residue changes derived from IgG_4 (H268Q, V309L, A330S, and P331S).[67]

There is continuing interest in the development of IgG_2 antibodies; however, it has recently been demonstrated that both natural and recombinant IgG_2 displays heterogeneity in inter- and intrachain disulfide bridge formation. Three or more distinct structural isomers have been identified and result from disulfide shuffling within the upper hinge region. The possible impact of these structural isomers on effector functions was examined for a series of cysteine to serine mutations made on a human IgG_2 backbone. Disulfide hetergeneity was observed among these mutants; however, no difference in binding to FcγR or C1q and the wild-type IgG_2 was observed.[68,69] A further heterogeneity may arise from the formation of trisulfides in the light-/heavy-chain disulfide bond, in both recombinant and natural antibodies. For recombinant antibodies, this heterogeneity could be controlled by the presence of reducing agent (2 mM cysteine) present in culture media.[70]

IgG_4 BINDING AND ACTIVATION OF FcγR

The IgG_4 subclass has enjoyed a checkered history, being in favor, neglected, and in favor again. Within my memory, IgG_4 was particularly associated with research in allergy and the development of IgG anti-allergen antibody responses, particularly following desensitization protocols. These early practices were discontinued due to adverse reactions occasioned through the use of impure allergen preparations. In the modern era, the availability of recombinant allergens has given rise to the reintroduction of desensitization therapies. Early studies of polyclonal IgG_4 anti-allergen responses led to reports that IgG_4 antibodies are of lower affinity than antibodies of the other IgG isotypes and/or are bispecific; that is, each Fab region is specific for a different antigen. At the time, the evidence was not convincing; however, recent studies have confirmed earlier conclusions. The current view may be summarized as: (1) Chronic antigen stimulation, as by allergen, can result in a switch from a predominant IgG_1/IgG_3 isotype response to an IgG_4 response; (2) IgG_4 present in human serum can exhibit dual specificity due to its propensity to dissociate into half-molecules (HLs) and reform the H2L2 format by random reassociation; (3) the production of IgG_4 antibodies is associated with allergen desensitization therapy; and (4) raised levels of IgG_4 are associated with a number of inflammatory disease entities.[71–75]

When the biopharmaceutical industry first considered generating antibody therapeutics with reduced effector activities, relative to IgG_1, for reasons not apparent to me, they chose the IgG_4 isotype. Choice of the IgG_4 format may have been influenced by a report that an IgG_1 anti-TNFα antibody, but not an IgG_4 version, resulted in efficient killing of the TNFα-expressing cells by both ADCC and CDC.[76] The choice of the IgG_4 format for an anti-CD28 antibody may, in part at least, have contributed to the disaster that ensued at "first in man" clinical trials of TGN 1412.[77] From the earliest studies, IgG_4 was reported to bind and activate FcγRI, although with lower affinity than IgG_1, due in part to replacement of the IgG_1 L234 residue by F234. The FcγRI receptor binding activity of an IgG_4 anti-CD4 antibody was downregulated in a S228P,L235E mutant,[78] and the non-fucosylated form of IgG_4 has been shown to bind and activate FcγRIIIa.[60]

A common observation for recombinant and serum-derived IgG_4 molecules is, in addition to the H2L2 form, the presence of HL species on sodium dodecyl sulfate polyacrylamide gel electrophoresis (SDS-PAGE) under non-reducing conditions. This composition was shown to be due to the presence of H2L2 molecules that lacked inter-heavy-chain disulfide bridges normally present in the hinge region.[72] Under physiologic conditions, the H2L2 format is achieved due to the non-covalent interactions between the CH3 domains; however, these interactions are relatively weak compared to those for the other IgG subclasses, with the result that dissociation and reassociation can occur *in vivo*.[71] The inter-heavy-chain disulfide bridges in IgG_1 are formed by the sequence $-T_{223}$–H–T–C–P–P–C–P–A–P_{232}–; the proline residues generate a "twist" in the conformation that prevents the formation of a C_{226}–C_{229} disulfide bond. The sequence in IgG_4 is –G_{223}–P–P–C–P–S–C–P–A–P_{332}–, which does allow for formation of an intra-disulfide bond. Mutant recombinant IgG_4 molecules have been generated in which S_{228} is replaced with P_{228} with suppression of HF formation.[79] Nine residues within the CH3 domain of IgG_1 have been identified as contributing to the non-covalent CH3–CH3 interaction: T366, L368, F405, Y407, K409, K370, D399, E357, and S364. These residues point directly into the CH3–CH3 interface. In the IgG_4 molecule, K409 is replaced by R409. Replacement of the IgG_4-Fc R409 residue with K409 was shown to increase the affinity of the CH3–CH3 interaction and to limit the formation of half-molecules; interestingly, exchange of F405 with Q405 resulted in virtually quantitative half-molecule formation.[80]

THE NEONATAL RECEPTOR FcγRn: TRANSCYTOSIS AND CATABOLISM

The FcγRn receptor was first identified from studies of the transport of IgG across the gut of newborn rats and designated the neonatal Fc receptor—hence, FcRn. Subsequently, the human homolog was identified in human placenta and was presumed to effect transport IgG from mother to foetus.[81–84] The catabolism of human IgG antibodies is also impacted by FcRn that is expressed in the cellular membrane of many tissues.[4,81–85] The interaction site on IgG-Fc is at the CH2–CH3 interface, and the CH3 sequence $-H_{433}$–N–H–Y–H_{437}–[85,86] is of functional significance, because titration of these histidine residues accounts for the observed binding of IgG to FcRn at pH 6.0 to 6.5 and its release at pH 7.0 to 7.5.[81–87] The interaction of IgG-Fc with FcRn appears not to be influenced by the natural IgG-Fc glycoform profile, or indeed the presence or absence of oligosaccharides. On the contrary, the N-glycans in FcRn contribute to the steady-state membrane distribution and direction of IgG transport.[84] An additional role for FcRn is emerging with the demonstration that in monocyte-derived dendritic cells FcRn-bound immune complexes determine the pathway of degradation that can result in antigen cross-presentation.[88,89] It has been reported that cross-presentation is enhanced for mice overexpressing (bovine) FcRn. The rationale is that overexpression of FcRn results in increased salvage of IgG, resulting in increased total IgG levels; consequently, IgG–immune complexes are not salvaged but directed to the degradation pathway that leads to presentation.[90]

Transcytosis

Each of the four human IgG subclasses is transferred across the placenta but with differing facility. Cord blood levels of IgG_1 may be higher than in matched maternal blood, while IgG_3 and IgG_4 levels are equivalent. The level of IgG_2 is ~80 % of the concentration in maternal blood.[91] It is of interest to note that IgG_3 is transferred with equal efficacy to IgG_1 although it has a shorter half-life, suggesting that its interaction with FcRn in the environment of the placenta may be different from that in endosomes in the catabolic pathway. During pregnancy, the level of galactosylation of maternal IgG increases and there is evidence for preferential transport of galactosylated IgG across the placenta.[92–94] This observation provides circumstantial evidence to suggest that the affinity of IgG for FcRn may differ between glycoforms, under conditions operative at the interface between the mother and the placenta. A further development opens a new route for administration, as it has been shown that FcRn is expressed in the central and upper airways of the lung and that drug–IgG-Fc fusion proteins delivered to these sites can be transported, by transcytosis, to the systemic circulation. Potential protein therapeutics that have a short half-life, such as cytokines, are being generated as fusion proteins with IgG-Fc to extend plasma circulation; it may be that they may be self-administered by inhalation, an exciting development with considerable promise and significance.[95,96]

Catabolism

Catabolism of IgG is mediated through FcRn-expressing cells that take up extracellular fluid within pinocytotic vesicles with the formation of vacuoles; subsequent lowering of pH results in the binding of IgG to membrane-bound FcRn and protection from degradation by enzymes present in the vacuole, and unbound IgG is degraded.[4,81] When the membrane of the vacuole is recycled to the cellular membrane, the IgG–FcRn complex is exposed to pH 7.2 and released into the extravascular fluid. The catabolic half-life of human IgG_1, IgG_2, and IgG_4 is ~21 days; for IgG_3, it is ~7 days. IgG_3 data have been obtained for IgG_3 molecules of G3m(b) and G3m(g) allotypes in which the histidine 435 residue, present in IgG_1, IgG_2, and IgG_4, is replaced with arginine.[7] It has been reported (U.S. Patent Application 20110003336) that replacement of this arginine residue by histidine increases the affinity for

FcRn. The IgG allotype G3m(s,t), present within Mongoloid populations, has a histidine residue at position 435 and presumed higher binding affinity for FcRn.[7,31] The catabolic half-life of IgG mediated through FcRn does not appear to be influenced by the IgG-Fc glycoform;[81–87] however, it should be emphasized that only glycoforms of IgG bearing neutral oligosaccharides have been evaluated. It might be anticipated that sialylation could influence IgG–FcRn interactions as it introduces a negative charge in the vicinity of the histidine residues involved in FcRn binding. There is evidence that glycoproteins expressing terminal *N*-acetylglucosamine residues may be cleared through the mannose receptor which accounts for the enhanced clearance of the IgG-Fc–TNF receptor fusion protein therapeutic (lenercept) having exposed terminal *N*-acetylglucosamine residues.[97,98]

Protein engineering of IgG-Fc has been directed towards increased binding affinity for FcRn at ~pH 6.0, in anticipation of increasing catabolic half-life. Early studies reported engineered IgG-Fc with increased affinity for FcRn at ~pH 6.0 that did not allow for release at pH 7.0. If successful and combined with an ability to formulate antibody therapeutic at high concentration for subcutaneous self-administration, the resulting benefits of convenience, shorter administration time, and lower administration costs (CoT) are anticipated. These objectives have been achieved for the anti-TNFα drugs Humira® (adalimumab) and Enbrel® (etanercept). Genentech is developing formulations for recombinant protein therapeutics that include recombinant human hyaluronidase (rHuPH20), which temporarily degrades hyaluronan in the skin and facilitates the dispersion and absorption of drugs and fluids. Such formulations for Herceptin® and MabThera® are understood to be at an advanced stage of development. Mutational analysis of wild-type and mutated Fc fragments derived from human IgG_1 indicates that I253, H310, and H435 play a central role in regulating serum half-life in mice. Reduced serum half-life for mutated Fc fragments correlates with decreased binding to FcRn. Analysis of an Fc fragment with H435A mutation demonstrates that the sequence difference at this position between human IgG_1 (H435) and IgG_3 (R435) most likely accounts for the shorter serum half-life of IgG_3 relative to IgG_1.[35,97,99] Hinton et al.[100] adopted an indirect approach to circumvent residues protected by patent and employed molecular modeling to identify IgG-Fc residues proximal to the FcRn binding site that, when mutated, might alter the architecture of the IgG_1-Fc binding site for FcRn. Following mutagenesis, several IgG_2 mutants with increased binding affinity to human FcRn at pH 6.0 were identified, at IgG-Fc residues 250 and 428, that did not bind human FcRn at pH 7.5. A pharmacokinetic study of two mutants of the IgG_{2M3} antibody[63] with increased FcRn binding affinity indicated that they had serum half-lives, in rhesus monkeys, ~twofold longer than the wild-type antibody.[100] It was suggested that increased affinity of a mutant IgG-Fc molecule for FcRn would compete with natural IgG for binding the FcRn, resulting in enhanced catabolism for the latter. Such activity could be beneficial in enhancing the catabolism (degradation) of autoantibodies present in a patient's serum; such antibodies have been designated as "Abdegs" (antibodies that enhance IgG degradation).[101] This objective was achieved, in a mouse model, for the human IgG-Fc M252Y/S254T/T256E mutant, which exhibits an ~tenfold increase in binding to FcRn at pH 6.0 with efficient release at pH 7.2; when this mutation was combined with the S239DA330L/I332E mutation,[63] enhanced binding for both FcRn and FcγRIIIa was achieved.[102]

The relationship between the binding affinity of IgG_1-Fc for FcRn and pharmacokinetics has been shown to be complex and may be dependent on the species in which mutant proteins are evaluated. The IgG-Fc mutant T250Q/M428L was shown to exhibit enhanced binding affinity for human, rhesus, and mouse FcRn that translated to increased half-life *in vivo* in rhesus primates and the mouse; however, the pharmacokinetics in cynomolgous primates was the same as for the wild-type IgG-Fc.[103] The relationship between IgG_1-Fc–FcRn affinity (off rates) and *in vivo* half-lives was explored for IgG_1 mutants generated by proximity-guided mutagenesis and selection.[104] Seven mutants of N434 (N434W, -F, -Y, -A, -S, -H, and -Q) delivered enhanced binding at pH 6.0. The N434A and N434W IgG_1-Fc mutants exhibited ~4- and 80-fold improvements in pH 6 binding affinity to both human and non-human primate FcRn; however, the N434W mutant was shown to exhibit significant binding at pH 7.4 and (consequently?) no decrease in clearance in cynomolgous monkeys, whereas the N434A mutant exhibited an ~twofold decrease in clearance. Thus, a modest increase in affinity can result in improved pharmacokinetics in primates.[102] Application of computational electrostatic optimization identified the additional N434K mutant as an affinity-enhancing residue in human IgG_1.[105,106] Increased half-life has been demonstrated for M428L/N434S mutants of the approved antibody therapeutics Avastin® and cetuximab.[107]

CLASSICAL PATHWAY OF COMPLEMENT ACTIVATION

Complement-dependent cytotoxicity (CDC) may be activated by mechanisms within both the innate and adaptive immune protection, particularly through lysis of antibody-sensitized bacteria. Antibody-sensitized cancer cells may be lysed by CDC similarly. Activation of complement through the classical route is initiated by binding and activation of the C1 component by immune complexes comprised of IgM, IgG_1, or IgG_3 antibody.[108–110] This leads to a cascade of enzymatic amplification reactions, resulting in formation of the "membrane attack complex" that inserts into the cellular membrane to form a pore and a loss of cellular integrity. The reaction cascade generates chemotactic agents that attract inflammatory cells into the site of infection and opsonic molecules that bind to the surface of the target to further sensitize for phagocytosis through complement receptor-bearing leukocytes. A low level of complement activation occurs naturally; however, normal cells are protected from any deleterious consequences through their expression of proteins (complement decay factors) that can degrade complement components generated at their surface.

Numerous studies have attempted to define the interaction site on IgG, of differing species, for the C1q component. An early alanine replacement study revealed that N297, E318, K320, and K322 in murine IgG_{2b} are important for guinea pig C1q binding, and the study suggested that E318, K320, and K322 are the core of the C1q binding site.[111] This publication has often been cited as evidence that the same residues also influence C1q binding for human IgG; however, the study of Morgan et al.[111] showed that the K320A mutation in human IgG_1 had no effect on C1q binding or CDC, while alanine replacement of residues 231 to 238 variously affected activity. A further study confirmed that alanine replacements of E318 and K320 did not influence C1q binding of human IgG_1 when challenged with human, rabbit, or guinea pig complement, whereas alanine substitution at positions D270, K322, P329, and P331 significantly reduced the ability of rituximab to bind C1q and activate complement; these residues were claimed to define the epicenter of the interaction site.[112] Replacement of the IgG_4 S331 residue with proline (P331) conferred complement-activating properties to this isotype.[110–112] The further mutations K326W and E333S were shown to enhance CDC, and transfer of these residues to IgG_2 conferred CDC activity.[113]

Domain "swapping" has been a favored approach to the generation of IgG molecules with altered effector activity profiles. Although IgG_3 has been reported to express enhanced complement activation relative to IgG_1, this isotype has not been favored due to its extended hinge region that is very susceptible to enzymatic cleavage; however, a chimeric IgG_1/IgG_3 molecule was shown to have significantly enhanced complement activity while retaining FcγR activity of the wild type, as both fucosylated and non-fucosylated glycoforms.[114] The chimeric molecule comprised of the CH1 and hinge of IgG_1 and the CH2 and CH3 domains of IgG_3 (designated 1133) was shown to exhibit maximal activity. This molecule did not bind Protein A; therefore, the further mutation of arginine 435 to histidine was introduced (designated 1133F) and SpA binding was restored.[114–116] This antibody format is patented and available as the Complegent® platform (http://www.biowa.com/technologies/complegent).

Having generated antibody mutants that individually enhanced CDC, ADCC, and ADCP, a comprehensive study was performed to evaluate the effector function profile of molecules comprised of combinations of the amino acid replacements.[117] The mutant S267E/H268F/S324T had the tightest C1q binding affinity and a 47-fold increase in CDC compared to wild-type IgG_1 and 6.9-fold compared to the 1133F molecule. The mutant comprised of S267E/H268F/S324T + G236A/I332E had similarly increased CDC and retained native FcγR-mediated activities, while H268F/S324T + G236A/I332E and H268F/S324T + S239D/I332E mutants simultaneously enhanced CDC, ADCC, and ADCP.[117]

IMMUNOGENICITY AND ADVERSE EVENTS

The development of an immune response to a protein therapeutic may nullify its beneficial activity or result in adverse events. Immunogenicity is, therefore, a major concern for clinicians, regulatory authorities, and the biopharmaceutical industry.[118–120] These concerns are particularly acute for the treatment of chronic diseases, as opposed to cancer, that may require repeated exposure to therapeutic over extended cycles of remission and relapse. There are many parameters that may be contributory to immunogenicity; however, the *bête noir* for the past decade has been aggregation.[118–122] I have argued that antibody therapeutics are intrinsically immunogenic since even "fully human" antibodies, whether generated from phage display libraries or transgenic "humanized" mice, are formed from combinations of heavy and light chains that would be recognized as anti-self during development of the endogenous immune repertoire and be eliminated to maintain self tolerance.[122] Antibody therapy thus represents the administration of anti-self antibody (autoantibody!) and as such violates a fundamental protective feature of the immune system, namely tolerance to self. Autoimmunity can result from or precipitate disregulation of multiple immune or non-immune pathways. The reported incidence of anti-drug antibody (ADA) responses has increased as progressively more sensitive assays have been developed. The presence of ADAs may impact patient management and, in some cases, may be modulated by the administration of mild immunosuppressive agents.[123,124] Review of the prescribing instructions for approved antibody therapeutics, over time, reveals a consistent increase in the warning of hypersensitivity reactions.[125]

It may not be surprising that the unique structure of a recombinant antibody molecule is recognized as non-self and (idiotype) immunogenicity is encountered for virtually all recombinant protein therapeutics, but in a proportion of patients manipulation of antibody effector mechanisms through protein engineering introduces further non-self sequences and may, therefore, further potentiate immunogenicity, either directly or because of altered intrinsic stability and consequent loss of structural integrity. Differential scanning microcalorimetry employed to determine the intrinsic stability of the IgG-Fc generated from serum-derived IgG has shown the melting temperature of the CH2 domain to be ~71°C, which reduced to ~68°C for deglycosylated IgG-Fc;[126,127] however, the melting temperature for the CH2 domain of the S239D/A330L/I332E mutant, shown to exhibit enhanced FcγR binding,[43] was reported as 48°C.[128] This decrease represents a radical destabilization of the molecular structure.

HUMAN IgG-Fc BINDING LIGANDS IN NATURE

Purification of antibody therapeutics of the IgG_1, IgG_2, and IgG_4 isotypes has depended on their binding to staphylococcal protein A (SpA), expressed by *Staphylococcus aureus*. We might pause to consider the possible significance of this property for the host/parasite relationship. It is most likely an evolved strategy that allows *S. aureus* to evade immune recognition by absorbing to its surface host protein (i.e., IgG); interestingly SpA is also a polyclonal activator ("super-antigen") that stimulates a subset of human B cells.[129] In fact, the elaboration of IgG binding proteins by bacteria is a common feature.[130–132] Virus seeks to subvert the immune system to enhance infectivity through the expression of virus-encoded "Fc-like receptors." Presumably, antibody–virus immune complexes may be taken up by infected cells, resulting in increased virus load. Virus shown to encode "Fc-like receptors" include herpes simplex virus-1 and herpes simplex virus-2,[133] cytomegalovirus,[134] varicella-zoster,[135] and hepatitis C virus[136] (Figure 17.2). An intriguing feature of these ligands is their common binding specificity at the CH2–CH3 domain interface. It is to be expected that the multiple mutations reviewed will impact on one or more of the pathogen-encoded IgG-Fc binding ligands; however, to my knowledge no study has investigated the consequences.

CONCLUDING REMARKS

The total global sales for biologics in 2011 was estimated at $115 billion; the market for mAbs is estimated at $57 billion and projected to grow by 9 to 15% by 2015. These projections explain the interest the biopharmaceutical industry has in the further development of mAbs, particularly mAbs exhibiting unique profiles of biologic activities that may be selected as optimal for individual disease indications. As I conclude this review, the first glycol-engineered mAb (mogamulizumab) has been approved for the treatment of relapsed or refractory CCR4-positive adult T-cell leukemia–lymphoma.[137,138] In addition to biosimilar rituximab five potentially biobetter anti-CD20 antibodies are in clinical trials.[46] Much of the basic research has been initiated by small biopharmaceutical companies with the aim of securing patents for next-generation antibody therapeutics. Although the development of biobetters is potentially of benefit to patients, bringing new drugs to the market is very expensive, as reflected in high costs of treatment. A high CoT can result in limited patient access due to decisions made on a cost/benefit basis. Where the decision is in favor of access it may not be affordable to a majority of patients worldwide. The present and near future may be dominated by access to biosimilar mAbs generated and produced in the BRIC countries (i.e., Brazil, Russia, India, and China) and identified as providing substantial emerging markets. Pressure on pricing is increasing in both developed and emerging markets and presents both social and political challenges.

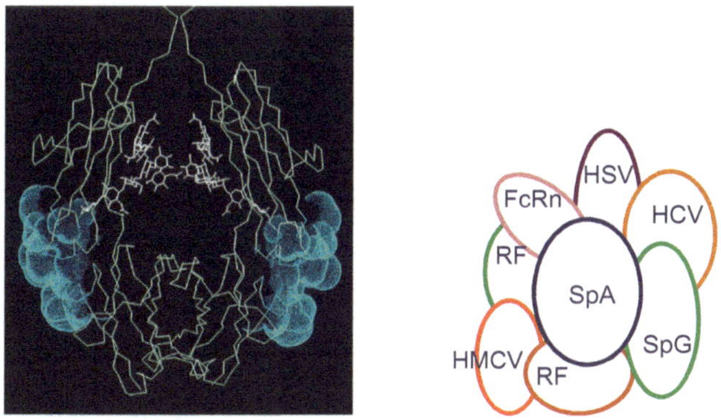

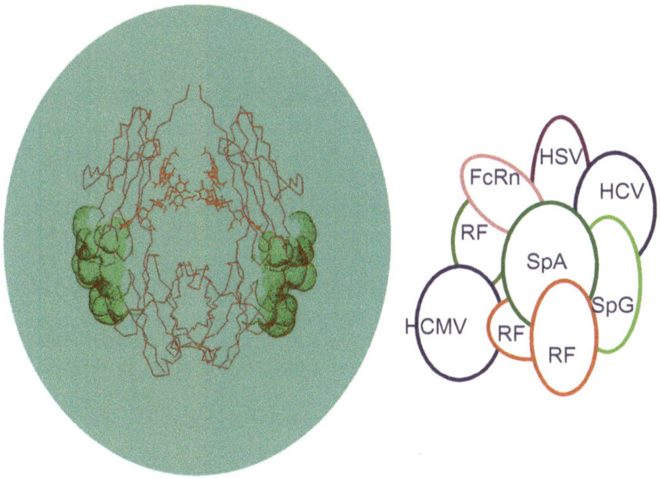

FIGURE 17.2 van der Waals binding surface of IgG_1-Fc for SpG[21] and Venn diagram of overlapping ligand interaction sites at the CH2–CH3 interface region.

References

1. Iwasaki A, Medzhitov R. Regulation of adaptive immunity by the innate immune system. *Science* 2010;**327**:291–5.
2. Gardy JL, Lynn DJ, Brinkman FS, et al. Enabling a systems biology approach to immunology: focus on innate immunity. *Trends Immunol* 2009;**30**:249–62.
3. Nezlin R. *The immunoglobulins: structure and function*. Amsterdam: Elsevier; 1998.
4. Nezlin R, Ghetie V. Interactions of immunoglobulins outside the antigen-combining site. *Adv Immunol* 2004;**82**:155–215.
5. Schroeder Jr HW, Cavacini L. Structure and function of immunoglobulins. *Allergy Clin Immunol* 2010;**125**(Suppl. 2):S41–52.
6. Woof JM, Burton DR. Human antibody–Fc receptor interactions illuminated by crystal structures. *Nat Rev Immunol* 2004;**4**:89–99.
7. Jefferis R. Isotype and glycoform selection for antibody therapeutics. *Arch Biochem Biophys* 2012;**526**(2): 159–66.
8. http://ednieuw.home.xs4all.nl/IgGsubclasses/subkl.htm
9. Nimmerjahn F, Ravetch JV. FcγRs in health and disease. *Curr Top Microbiol Immunol* 2011;**350**:105–25.

10. Concetti F, Napolioni V. Insights into the role of Fc gamma receptors (FcgammaRs) genetic variations in monoclonal antibody-based anticancer therapy. *Recent Pat Anticancer Drug Discov* 2010;**5**:197–204.
11. van de Winkel JG. Fc receptors: role in biology and antibody therapy. *Immunol Lett* 2010;**128**:4–5.
12. van der Poel CE, Spaapen RM, van de Winkel JG, et al. Functional characteristics of the high affinity IgG receptor, FcγRI. *J Immunol* 2011;**186**:2699–704.
13. Breunis WB, van Mirre E, Geissler J, et al. Copy number variation at the FCGR locus includes FCGR3A, FCGR2C and FCGR3B but not FCGR2A and FCGR2B. *Hum Mutat* 2009;**30**:E640–50.
14. Nose M, Wigzell H. Biologic significance of carbohydrate chains on monoclonal antibodies. *Proc Natl Acad Sci USA* 1983;**80**:6632–6.
15. Leatherbarrow RJ, Rademacher TW, Dwek RA, et al. Effector functions of a monoclonal aglycosylated mouse IgG2a: binding and activation of complement component C1 and interaction with human monocyte Fc receptor. *Mol Immunol* 1985;**22**:407–15.
16. Pound JD, Lund J, Jefferis R. Aglycosylated chimaeric human IgG3 can trigger the human phagocyte respiratory burst. *Mol Immunol* 1993;**30**:233–41.
17. Woof JM, Partridge LJ, Jefferis R, et al. Localisation of the monocytebinding region on human immunoglobulin G. *Mol Immunol* 1986;**23**:319–30.
18. Duncan AR, Woof JM, Partridge LJ, et al. Localization of the binding site for the human high-affinity Fc receptor on IgG. *Nature* 1988;**332**:563–4.
19. Brekke OH, Michaelsen TE, Sandlie I. The structural requirements for complement activation by IgG: does it hinge on the hinge?. *Immunol Today* 1995;**16**:85–90.
20. Kuo TT, Aveson VG. Neonatal Fc receptor and IgG-based therapeutics. *MAbs* 2011;**3**:422–30.
21. Deisenhofer J. Crystallographic refinement and atomic models of a human Fc fragment and its complex with fragment B of Protein A from *Staphyloccus aureus* at 2.9- and 2.8-Angstrom resolution. *Biochemistry* 1981;**20**:2361–70.
22. Potter KN, Yucheng L, Mageed RA, et al. Anti-idiotypic antibody D12 and superantigen SpA both interact with human VH3 encoded antibodies on the external face of the heavy chain involving FR1, CDR2 and FR3. *Molec Immunol* 1993;**35**:1170–87.
23. Sauer-Eriksson AE, Kleywegt GJ, Uhlén M, et al. Crystal structure of the C2 fragment of streptococcal protein G in complex with the Fc domain of human IgG. *Structure* 1995;**3**:265–78.
24. Atherton A, Armour KL, Bell S, Minson AC, Clark MR. The herpes simplex virus type 1 Fc receptor discriminates between IgG1 allotypes. *Eur J Immunol* 2000;**30**(9):2540–7.
25. Sprague ER, Wang C, Baker D, Bjorkman PJ. Crystal structure of the HSV-1 Fc receptor bound to Fc reveals a mechanism for antibody bipolar bridging. *PLoS Biol* 2006;**4**(6):e148.
26. Antonsson A, Johansson PJ. Binding of human and animal immunoglobulins to the IgG Fc receptor induced by human cytomegalovirus. *J Gen Virol* 2001;**82**(Pt. 5):1137–45.
27. Sprague ER, Reinhard H, Cheung EJ, Farley AH, Trujillo RD, Hengel H, et al. The human cytomegalovirus Fc receptor gp68 binds the Fc CH2–CH3 interface of immunoglobulin G. *J Virol* 2008;**82**(7):3490–9.
28. Lubinski JM, Lazear HM, Awasthi S, Wang F, Friedman HM. The herpes simplex virus 1 IgG fc receptor blocks antibody-mediated complement activation and antibody-dependent cellular cytotoxicity *in vivo*. *J Virol* 2011;**85**(7):3239–49.
29. Ferrara C, Grau S, Jäger C, Sondermann P, Brünker P, Waldhauer I, et al. Unique carbohydrate–carbohydrate interactions are required for high affinity binding between FcgammaRIII and antibodies lacking core fucose. *Proc Natl Acad Sci USA* 2011;**108**(31):12669–74.
30. Zeck A, Pohlentz G, Schlothauer T, Peter-Katalinic J, Regula JT. Cell type-specific and site directed N-glycosylation pattern of FcγRIIIa. *J Proteome Res* 2011;**10**(7):3031–9.
31. Jefferis R, Lefranc M-P. Human immunoglobulin allotypes: possible implications for immunogenicity. *MAbs* 2009;**1**(4):332–8.
32. Stapleton NM, Andersen JT, Stemerding AM, Bjarnarson SP, Verheul RC, et al. Competition for FcRn-mediated transport gives rise to short half-life of human IgG3 and offers therapeutic potential. *Nat Commun* 2011;**2**:599.
33. Pandey JP. Genetic polymorphism of Fc. *Science* 2006;**311**:1376–7.
34. Pandey JP, Namboodiri AM, Luo Y, Wu Y, Elston RC, Thomas DL, et al. Genetic markers of IgG influence the outcome of infection with hepatitis C virus. *J Infect Dis* 2008;**198**(9):1334–6.
35. Shields RL, Namenuk AK, Hong K, et al. High resolution mapping of the binding site on human IgG1 for FcγRI, FcγRII, FcγRIII, and FcRn and design of IgG1 variants with improved binding to the FcγR. *J Biol Chem* 2000;**276**:6591–604.
36. Sondermann P, Huber R, Oosthuizen V, et al. The 3.2-A crystal structure of the human IgG1 Fc–FcRγIIIb complex. *Nature* 2000;**406**:267–73.
37. Radaev S, Motyka S, Fridman WH, et al. The structure of human type FcIII receptor in complex with Fc. *J Biol Chem* 2001;**276**:16469–77.
38. Shields RL, Lai J, Keck R, et al. Lack of fucose on human IgG1 Nlinked oligosaccharide improves

binding to human FcRγIII and antibody-dependent cellular toxicity. *J Biol Chem* 2002;**277**:26733–40.
39. Koene HR, Kleijer M, Algra J, et al. FcRγIIIa-158V/F polymorphism influences the binding of IgG by natural killer cell FcRγIIIa, independently of the Fc RIIIa-48L/R/H phenotype. *Blood* 1997;**90**:1109–14.
40. Cartron G, Dacheux L, Salles G, et al. Therapeutic activity of humanized anti-CD20 monoclonal antibody and polymorphism in IgG Fc receptor FcRγIIIa gene. *Blood* 2002;**99**:754–8.
41. Yamane-Ohnuki N, Satoh M. Production of therapeutic antibodies with controlled fucosylation. *MAbs* 2009;**1**(3):230–6.
42. Mössner E, Brünker P, Moser S, Püntener U, Schmidt C, et al. Increasing the efficacy of CD20 antibody therapy through the engineering of a new type II anti-CD20 antibody with enhanced direct and immune effector cell-mediated B-cell cytotoxicity. *Blood* 2010;**115**(22):4393–402.
43. Lazar GA, Dang W, Karki S, Vafa O, Peng JS, Hyun L. Engineered antibody Fc variants with enhanced effector function. *Proc Natl Acad Sci USA* 2006;**103**(11):4005–10.
44. Lazar GA, Chirino AJ, Dang W, Desjarlais JR, Doberstein SK, Hayes RJ, et al. Optimized Fc variants and methods for their generation. U.S. Patent No. 20090092599.
45. Horton HM, Bernett MJ, Peipp M, Pong E, Karki S, Chu SY, et al. Fc-engineered anti-CD40 antibody enhances multiple effector functions and exhibits potent *in vitro* and *in vivo* antitumor activity against hematologic malignancies. *Blood* 2010;**116**(16):3004–12.
46. Desjarlais JR, Lazar GA. Modulation of antibody effector functions. *Exp Cell Res* 2011;**317**(9):1278–85.
47. Richards JO, Karki S, Lazar GA, Chen H, Dang W, Desjarlais JR. Optimization of antibody binding to FcgammaRIIa enhances macrophage phagocytosis of tumor cells. *Mol Cancer Ther* 2008;**7**(8):2517–27.
48. Lund J, Winter G, Jones PT, Pound JD, Tanaka T, Walker MR, et al. Human Fc gamma RI and Fc gamma RII interact with distinct but overlapping sites on human IgG. *J Immunol* 1991;**147**(8):2657–62.
49. Moldt B, Schultz N, Dunlop DC, Alpert MD, Harvey JD, Evans DT, et al. A panel of IgG1 b12 variants with selectively diminished or enhanced affinity for Fcγ receptors to define the role of effector functions in protection against HIV. *J Virol* 2011;**85**(20):10572–81.
50. Sazinsky SL, Ott RG, Silver NW, Tidor B, Ravetch JV, Wittrup KD. Aglycosylated immunoglobulin G1 variants productively engage activating Fc receptors. *Proc Natl Acad Sci USA* 2008;**105**(51):20167–72.
51. Nordstrom JL, Gorlatov S, Zhang W, Yang Y, Huang L, Burke S. Anti-tumor activity and toxicokinetics analysis of MGAH22, an anti-HER2 monoclonal antibody with enhanced Fcγ receptor binding properties. *Breast Cancer Res* 2011;**13**(6):R123.
52. Stavenhagen JB, Gorlatov S, Tuaillon N, Rankin CT, et al. Enhancing the potency of therapeutic monoclonal antibodies via Fc optimization. *Adv Enzyme Regul* 2008;**48**:152–64.
53. Verenium Corp, et al. Aglycosylated antibodies and methods of making and using those antibodies, Patent No. WO/2008/030564.
54. Jefferis R. Aglycosylated antibodies and methods of making and using them: WO2008030564. *Expert Opin Ther Pat* 2009;**19**(1):101–5.
55. Jung ST, Reddy ST, Kang TH, Borrok MJ, Sandlie I, Tucker PW, et al. Aglycosylated IgG variants expressed in bacteria that selectively bind FcgammaRI potentiate tumor cell killing by monocyte-dendritic cells. *Proc Natl Acad Sci USA* 2010;**107**(2):604–9.
56. Jung ST, Kang TH, Kelton W, Georgiou G. Bypassing glycosylation: engineering aglycosylated full-length IgG antibodies for human therapy. *Curr Opin Biotechnol* 2011;**22**(6):858–67.
57. Stewart R, Thom G, Levens M, Güler-Gane G, Holgate R, Rudd PM, et al. A variant human IgG1-Fc mediates improved ADCC. *Protein Eng Des Sel* 2011;**24**(9):671–8.
58. Lund J, Takahashi N, Pound J, Goodall M, Jefferis R. Multiple interactions of IgG with its core oligosaccharide can modulate recognition by complement and human FcRγI and influence the synthesis of its oligosaccharide chains. *J Immunol* 1996;**157**:4963–9.
59. Parren PW, Warmerdam PA, Boeije LC, Arts J, Westerdaal NA, Vlug A, et al. On the interaction of IgG subclasses with the low affinity Fc gamma RIIa (CD32) on human monocytes, neutrophils, and platelets. Analysis of a functional polymorphism to human IgG2. *J Clin Invest* 1992;**90**:1537–46.
60. Niwa R, Natsume A, Uehara A, Wakitani M, Iida S, Uchida K, et al. IgG subclass-independent improvement of antibodydependent cellular cytotoxicity by fucose removal from Asn297-linked oligosaccharides. *J Immunol Meth* 2005;**306**(1–2):151–60.
61. Ramsland PA, Farrugia W, Bradford TM, Sardjono CT, Esparon S, et al. Structural basis for FcγRIIa recognition of human IgG and formation of inflammatory signaling complexes. *J Immunol* 2011;**187**(6):3208–17.
62. Schneider-Merck T, Lammerts van Bueren JJ, Berger S, Rossen K, van Berkel PH, et al. Human IgG2 antibodies against epidermal growth factor receptor effectively trigger antibody-dependent cellular cytotoxicity but, in contrast to IgG1, only by cells of myeloid lineage. *Immunology* 2010;**184**(1):512–20.
63. Cole MS, Anasetti C, Tso JY. Human IgG2 variants of chimeric anti-CD3 are nonmitogenic to T cells. *J Immunol* 1997;**159**(7):3613–21.

64. Chau LA, Tso JY, Melrose J, Madrenas J. HuM291(Nuvion), a humanized Fc receptor-nonbinding antibody against CD3, anergizes peripheral blood T cells as partial agonist of the T cell receptor. transplantation. *Transplantation* 2001;**71**(7):941–50.
65. Mueller JP, Giannoni MA, Hartman SL, Elliott EA, Squinto SP, et al. Humanized porcine VCAM-specific monoclonal antibodies with chimeric IgG2/G4 constant regions block human leukocyte binding to porcine endothelial cells. *Mol Immunol* 1997;**34**(6):441–52.
66. Hillmen P, Elebute M, Kelly R, Urbano-Ispizua A, Hill A, Rother RP, et al. Long-term effect of the complement inhibitor eculizumab on kidney function in patients with paroxysmal nocturnal hemoglobinuria. *Am J Hematol* 2010;**85**(8):553–9.
67. An Z, Forrest G, Moore R, Cukan M, Haytko P, Huang L, et al. IgG2m4, an engineered antibody isotype with reduced Fc function. *MAbs* 2009;**1**(6):572–9.
68. Lightle S, Aykent S, Lacher N, Mitaksov V, Wells K, Zobel J, et al. Mutations within a human IgG2 antibody form distinct and homogeneous disulfide isomers but do not affect Fc gamma receptor or C1q binding. *Protein Sci* 2010;**19**(4):753–62.
69. Liu H, May K. Disulfide bond structures of IgG molecules: structural variations, chemical modifications and possible impacts to stability and biological function. *MAbs* 2012;**4**(1):17–23.
70. Gu S, Wen D, Weinreb PH, Sun Y, Zhang L, Foley SF, et al. Characterization of trisulfide modification in antibodies. *Anal Biochem* 2010;**400**(1):89–98.
71. van der Neut Kolfschoten M, Schuurman J, Losen M, Bleeker WK, Martínez-Martínez P, et al. Anti-inflammatory activity of human IgG4 antibodies by dynamic Fab arm exchange. *Science* 2007;**317**(5844):1554–7.
72. Aalberse RC, Stapel SO, Schuurman J, Rispens T. Immunoglobulin G4: an odd antibody. *Clin Exp Allergy* 2009;**39**(4):469–77.
73. Rose RJ, Labrijn AF. Quantitative analysis of the interaction strength and dynamics of human IgG4 half molecules by native mass spectrometry. *Structure* 2011;**19**(9):1274–82.
74. Fujita H, Soyka MB, Akdis M, Adkis CA. Mechanisms of allergenspecific immunotherapy. *Clin Transl Allergy* 2012;**2**(1):2.
75. Stone JH, Zen Y, Deshpande V. IgG4 related disease. *N Engl J Med* 2012;**366**(6):539–51.
76. Scallon BJ, Moore MA. Chimeric anti-TNF-alpha monoclonal antibodycA2 binds recombinant transmembrane TNF-alpha and activates immune effector functions. *Cytokine* 1995;**7**(3):251–9.
77. Eastwood D, Findlay L, Poole S, Bird C, Wadhwa M, Moore M, et al. Monoclonal antibody TGN1412 trial failure explained by species differences in CD28 expression on CD4+ effector memory T-cells. *Br J Pharmacol* 2010;**161**(3):512–26.
78. Newman R, Hariharan K, Reff M, Anderson DR, Braslawsky G, Santoro D, et al. Modification of the Fc region of a primatized IgG antibody to human CD4 retains its ability to modulate CD4 receptors but does not deplete CD4(+) T cells in chimpanzees. *Clin Immunol* 2001;**98**(2):164–74.
79. Stubenrauch K, Wessels U, Regula JT, Kettenberger H, Schleypen J, Kohnert U. Impact of molecular processing in the hinge region of therapeutic IgG4 antibodies on disposition profiles in cynomolgus monkeys. *Drug Metab Dispos* 2010;**3**(1):84–91.
80. Rose RJ, Labrijn AF, van den Bremer ETJ, Loverix S, Lasters I, et al. Quantitative analysis of the interaction strength and dynamics of human IgG4 half molecules by native mass spectrometry. *Structure* 2011;**19**(9):1274–82.
81. Roopenian DC, Akilesh S. FcRn: the neonatal Fc receptor comes of age. *Nat Rev Immunol* 2007;**7**:715–25.
82. Ward ES, Ober RJ. Multitasking by exploitation of intracellular transport functions the many faces of FcRn. *Adv Immunol* 2009;**103**:77–115.
83. Tesar DB, Björkman PJ. An intracellular traffic jam: Fc receptormediated transport of immunoglobulin G. *Curr Opin Struct Biol* 2010;**20**:226–33.
84. Kuo TT, de Muinck EJ, Claypool SM, et al. N-glycan moieties in neonatal Fc receptor determine steady-state membrane distribution and directional transport of IgG. *J Biol Chem* 2009;**284**:8292–300.
85. Kuo TT, Aveson VG. Neonatal Fc receptor and IgG therapeutics. *MAbs* 2011;**3**(5):422–30.
86. Martin WL, West Jr AP, Gan L, Bjorkman PJ. Crystal structure at 2.8 Å of an FcRn/heterodimeric Fc complex: mechanism of pH-dependent binding. *Mol Cell* ;**7**(4):867–877.
87. Mezo AR, Sridhar V, Badger J, Sakorafas P, Nienaber V. X-ray crystal structures of monomeric and dimeric peptide inhibitors in complex with the human neonatal Fc receptor. *J Biol Chem* 2010;**285**(36):27694–701.
88. Liu X, Lu L, Yang Z, Palaniyandi S, Zeng R, Gao LY, et al. The neonatal FcR-mediated presentation of immune-complexed antigen is associated with endosomal and phagosomal pH and antigen stability in macrophages and dendritic cells. *J Immunol* 2011;**186**(8):4674–86.
89. Baker K, Qiao SW, Kuo TT, Aveson VG, Platzer B, Andersen JT, et al. Neonatal Fc receptor for IgG (FcRn) regulates cross-presentation of IgG immune complexes by CD8–CD11B+ dendritic cells. *Proc Natl Acad Sci USA* 2011;**108**(24):9927–32.
90. Kacskovics I, Cervenak J, Erdei A, Goldsby RA, Butler JE. Recent advances using FcRn overexpression in transgenic animals to overcome impediments of

standard antibody technologies to improve the generation of specific antibodies. *MAbs* 2011;**3**(5):431–9.
91. Pentsuk N, van der Laan JW. An interspecies comparison of placental antibody transfer: new insights into developmental toxicity testing of monoclonal antibodies. *Birth Defects Res B* 2009;**86**:328–44.
92. Kibe T, Fujimoto S, Ishida C, et al. Glycosylation and placental transport of immunoglobulin G. *J Clin Biochem Nutr* 1996;**21**:57–63.
93. Alavi A, Arden N, Spector TD, et al. Immunoglobulin G glycosylation and clinical outcome in rheumatoid arthritis during pregnancy. *J Rheumatol* 2000;**27**:1379–85.
94. van de Geijn FE, Wuhrer M, Selman MH, et al. Immunoglobulin G galactosylation and sialylation are associated with pregnancy-induced improvement of rheumatoid arthritis and the postpartum flare: results from a large prospective cohort study. *Arthritis Res Ther* 2009;**11**:R193.
95. Dumont JA, Low SC, Peters RT, Bitonti AJ. Monomeric Fc fusions: impact on pharmacokinetic and biological activity of protein therapeutics. *BioDrugs* 2006;**20**(3):151–60.
96. Lee CH, Woo JH, Cho KK, Kang SH, Kang SK, Choi YJ. Expression and characterisation of human growth hormone-Fc fusion proteins for transcytosis induction. *Biotechnol Appl Biochem* 2007;**46**(Pt. 4):211–7.
97. Jones AJ, Papac DI, Chin EH, et al. Selective clearance of glycoforms of a complex glycoprotein pharmaceutical caused by terminal Nacetylglucosamine is similar in humans and cynomolgus monkeys. *Glycobiology* 2007;**17**:529–40.
98. Keck R, Nayak N, Lerner L, et al. Characterization of a complex glycoprotein whose variable metabolic clearance in humans is dependent on terminal N-acetylglucosamine content. *Biologicals* 2008;**36**:49–60.
99. Kim JK, Firan M, Radu CG, Kim CH, Ghetie V, Ward ES. Mapping the site on human IgG for binding of the MHC class I-related receptor, FcRn. *Eur J Immunol* 1999;**29**:2819–25.
100. Hinton PR, Johlfs MG, Xiong JM, Hanestad K, Ong KC, Bullock C, et al. Engineered human IgG antibodies with longer serum half-lives in primates. *J Biol Chem* 2004;**279**(8):6213–6.
101. Vaccaro C, et al. Engineering the Fc region of immunoglobulin G to modulate *in vivo* antibody levels. *Nat Biotechnol* 2005;**23**(10):1283–8.
102. Dall'Acqua WF, Kiener PA, Wu H. Properties of human IgG1s engineered for enhanced binding to the neonatal Fc receptor (FcRn). *J Biol Chem* 2006;**281**(33):23514–24.
103. Datta-Mannan A, Witcher DR, Tang Y, Watkins J, Jiang W, Wroblewski VJ. Humanized IgG1 variants with differential binding properties to the neonatal Fc receptor: relationship to pharmacokinetics in mice and primates. *Drug Metab Dispos* 2007;**35**(1):86–94.
104. Yeung YA, Leabman MK, Marvin JS, Qiu J, Adams CW, Lien S, et al. Engineering human IgG1 affinity to human neonatal Fc receptor: impact of affinity improvement on pharmacokinetics in primates. *J Immunol* 2009;**182**(12):7663–71.
105. Fitzgerald J, Lugovskoy A. Rational engineering of antibody therapeutics targeting multiple oncogene pathways. *MAbs* 2011;**3**:299–309.
106. Lugovskoy AA, Rechert JM, Beck A. 7th Annual European Antibody Congress 2011: November 29–December 1, 2011, Geneva, Switzerland. *MAbs* 2012;**4**(2) [Epub ahead of print]..
107. Zalevsky AK, Chamberlain HM, Horton S, Karki IW, Leung TJ, et al. Enhanced antibody half-life improves *in vivo* activity. *Nat Biotechnol* 2010;**28**(2):157–9.
108. Ricklin D, Hajishengallis G, Yang K, Lambris JD. Complement: a key system for immune surveillance and homeostasis. *Nat Immunol* 2010;**11**(9):785–97.
109. Schneider S, Zacharias M. Atomic resolution model of the antibody Fc interaction with the complement C1q component. *Mol Immunol* 2012;**51**(1):66–72.
110. Daha NA, Banda NK, Roos A, Beurskens FJ, Bakker JM, Daha MR, et al. Complement activation by (auto-) antibodies. *Mol Immunol* 2011;**48**(14):1656–65.
111. Morgan A, Jones ND, Nesbitt AM, Chaplin L, Bodmer MW, Emtage JS. The N-terminal end of the CH2 domain of chimeric human IgG1 anti-HLA-DR is necessary for C1q, FcgRI and FcgRIII binding. *Immunology* 1995;**86**(2):319–24.
112. dusogie EE, Presta LG, Gazzano-Santoro H, Totpal K, Wong PY, Ultsch M, et al. Mapping of the C1q binding site on rituxan, a chimeric antibody with a human IgG1 Fc. *J Immunol* 2000;**164**(8):4178–84.
113. Idusogie EE, Wong PY, Presta LG, Gazzano-Santoro H, Totpal K, Ultsch M, et al. Engineered antibodies with increased activity to recruit complement. *J Immunol* 2001;**166**(4):2571–5.
114. Natsume A, In M, Takamura H, Nakagawa T, Shimizu Y, et al. Engineered antibodies of IgG1/IgG3 mixed isotype with enhanced cytotoxic activities. *Cancer Res* 2008;**68**(10):3863–72.
115. Natsume A, Shimizu-Yokoyama Y, Satoh M, et al. Engineered anti- CD20 antibodies with enhanced complement-activating capacity mediate potent antilymphoma activity. *Cancer Sci* 2009;**100**:2411–8.
116. Kaneko E, Niwa R. Optimizing therapeutic antibody function: progress with Fc domain engineering. *BioDrugs* 2011;**25**(1):1–11.
117. Moore GL, Chen H, Karki S, Lazar GA. Engineered Fc variant antibodies with enhanced ability to recruit complement and mediate effector functions. *MAbs* 2010;**2**(2):181–9.

118. Rosenberg AS. Effects of protein aggregation: an immunologic perspective. *AAPS J* 2006;**8**:E501–7.
119. Brinks V, Jiskoot W, Schellekens H. Immunogenicity of therapeutic proteins: the use of animal models. *Pharm Res* 2011;**28**(10):2379–85.
120. Büttel IC, Chamberlain P, Chowers Y, Ehmann F, Greinacher A, Jefferis R, et al. Taking immunogenicity assessment of therapeutic proteins to the next level. *Biologicals* 2011;**3**:100–9.
121. van Beers MM, Jiskoot W, Schellekens H. On the role of aggregates in the immunogenicity of recombinant interferon beta in patients with multiple sclerosis. *J Interferon Cytokine Res* 2010;**30**:767–75.
122. Jefferis R. Aggregation, immune complexes and immunogenicity. *MAbs* 2011;**3**:503–4.
123. Hale G, Rebello P, Al Bakir I, Bolam E, Wiczling P, Jusko WJ. Pharmacokinetics and antibody responses to the CD3 antibody otelixizumab used in the treatment of type 1 diabetes. *J Clin Pharmacol* 2010;**50**(11):1238–48.
124. Pan J, Small T, Qin D, Li S, Wang L, Chen D, et al. Comparison of the NIDS rapid assay with ELISA methods in immunogenicity of two biotherapeutics. *J Pharmacol Toxicol Meth* 2011;**63**:150–9.
125. Kleyman K, Weintraub D. Monoclonal antibodies: longitudinal prescribing information analysis of hypersensitivity reactions. *MAbs* 2012;**4**:392–7.
126. Mimura Y, Church S, Ghirlando R, Dong S, Goodall M, Lund J, et al. The influence of glycosylation on the thermal stability and effector function expression of human IgG1-Fc: properties of a series of truncated glycoforms. *Mol Immunol* 2000;**37**:697–706.
127. Krapp S, Mimura Y, Jefferis R, Huber R, Sondermann P. Structural analysis of human IgG glycoforms reveals a correlation between oligosaccharide content, structural integrity and Fc-receptor affinity. *J Mol Biol* 2003;**325**(5):979–89.
128. Oganesyan V, Damschroder MM, Leach W, Wu H, Dall'Acqua WF. Structural characterization of a mutated, ADCC-enhanced human Fc fragment. *Mol Immunol* 2008;**45**(7):1872–82.
129. Bekeredjian-Ding I, Inamura S, Giese T, Moll H, Endres S, Sing A, et al. *Staphylococcus aureus* protein A triggers T cell-independent B cell proliferation by sensitizing B cells for TLR2 ligands. *J Immunol* 2007;**178**(5):2803–12.
130. Sidorin EV, Solov'eva TF. IgG_binding proteins of bacteria. *Biochemistry (Mosc)* 2011;**76**(3):295–308.
131. Wines BD, Trist HM, Farrugia W, Ngo C, Trowsdale J, Areschoug T, et al. A conserved host and pathogen recognition site on immunoglobulins: structural and functional aspects. *Adv Exp Med Biol* 2012;**946**:87–112.
132. Laboratory of Bacterial Pathogenesis and Immunology *Surface proteins on gram-positive bacteria*. New York: The Rockefeller University; 2013. <http://www.rockefeller.edu/vaf/surfdata.php>.
133. Lubinski JM, Lazear HM, Awasthi S, Wang F, Friedman HM. The herpes simplex virus 1 IgG fc receptor blocks antibody-mediated complement activation and antibody-dependent cellular cytotoxicity *in vivo*. *J Virol* 2011;**85**(7):3239–49.
134. Lilley BN, Ploegh HL, Tirabassi RS. Human cytomegalovirus open reading frame TRL11/IRL11 encodes an immunoglobulin G Fcbinding protein. *J Virol* 2001;**75**:11218–21.
135. Litwin V, Jackson W, Grose C. Receptor properties of two varicellazostervirus glycoproteins, gpI and gpIV, homologous to herpes simplex virus gE and gI. *J Virol* 1992;**66**:3643–51.
136. Maillard P, et al. Fcγ receptor-like activity of hepatitis C virus core protein. *J Biol Chem* 2004;**279**:2430–7.
137. Beck A, Reichert J. Marketing approval of mogamulizumab: a triumph for glyco-engineering. *MAbs* 2012;**4**:419–25.
138. http://www.kyowa-kirin.co.jp/english/news/2012/e20120529_02.html

CHAPTER

18

Bacterial Modulation of Fc Effector Functions

Mattias Collin[a,*] *and Mogens Kilian*[b,*]

[a]Division of Infection Medicine, Department of Clinical Sciences, Lund University, Lund, Sweden, [b]Medical Microbiology and Immunology, Department of Biomedicine, Aarhus University, Aarhus, Denmark

INTRODUCTION

This entire volume clearly stresses that Fc-mediated effector functions are fundamental to our adaptive responses against invading microorganisms and also serve as a bridge between adaptive and innate immunity. Therefore, it is not at all surprising that microorganisms through co-evolution with their mammalian hosts have developed a molecular arsenal to circumvent or control this central immunological pathway. In this chapter, we will try to give an overview of the vast amount of accumulated knowledge about bacterial subversion of Fc-mediated responses. It is virtually impossible to cite all of the original studies describing such activities; therefore, we will sometimes refer to particularly helpful review articles. We encourage the reader, however, to dig deeper and critically evaluate the underlying original research, as this chapter represents the tip of the iceberg of a field that has developed during the last 50 or more years.

* Corresponding Author

IMMUNOGLOBULIN-BINDING PROTEINS

Surface-Associated Immunoglobulin-Binding Proteins

Immunoglobulin-binding proteins (proteins A, G, and L) have become essential laboratory tools that many of us take for granted with little thought about where they came from and why they exist. There are a few things one needs to know about the bacteria that express these proteins in order to appreciate their biological function. Gram-positive (G+) bacteria have one bilayered cytoplasmic membrane. This membrane is not entirely "naked" but serves as the anchoring point for lipoproteins, many of which serve as transporters for small molecules such as oligopeptides, amino acids, and metal ions. However, in G+ species, this vulnerable membrane is protected by a relatively rigid peptidoglycan layer that also serves as an exoskeleton ensuring cellular shape and integrity. Most G+ proteins intended to interact with the environment are covalently attached to the peptidoglycan via a transpeptidase activity of the so-called sortases. The discovery of the LPXTG motif signaling cell-wall anchoring of proteins has been instrumental in deciphering their involvement in bacterial pathogenesis and immune evasion.[1]

Protein A from *Staphylococcus aureus* (SpA) is the prototypic immunoglobulin-binding, cell-wall-anchored protein that for a very long time has been the laboratory and industry standard for purification and detection of IgG. A PubMed search using the terms "protein A" and "Staphylococcus" results in more than 2000 papers, so all of the proposed roles for SpA alone or during *S. aureus* infections are virtually impossible to cover here. In 1958, Jensen suggested that *S. aureus* could precipitate immunoglobulins,[2] and SpA was subsequently identified by Forsgren et al.[3] Numerous subsequent studies by several groups have defined the immunoglobulin-binding properties. SpA binds IgG from many mammalian species, and binding predominantly takes place in the Cγ2–Cγ3 interface in the Fc portion, although SpA also binds Fab weakly (for a recent review on staphylococcal immune evasion strategies, including Ig binding, see Kim et al.[4]). It has been known for quite some time that additional G+ bacteria, such as *Streptococcus pyogenes* (group A streptococci), and *Streptococcus dysgalactiae* subsp. *equisimilis* (group C and G streptococci) have the capability of binding human immunoglobulin G through the Fc portion,[5] of which protein G from group G streptococci has been extensively characterized and turned into a standard IgG purification tool.[6] Among the streptococcal IgG-binding proteins, protein H from *S. pyogenes* stands out, as it is highly specific for human IgG.[7] Protein H is a member of the M protein family in *S. pyogenes* that also comprises additional Ig binding proteins.[8–10] One member of the M protein family, Arp, does not bind IgG but instead specifically binds human IgA,[11,12] while another, Sir, binds both IgG and IgA.[13] Peptides derived from these proteins can be used for specific detection and purification of human IgA.[14,15] Also, *S. agalactiae* (group B streptococci) have the capacity to bind IgA through the β protein (Jerlström et al.).[16]

The commensal and opportunistic pathogen *Finegoldia magna* (formerly *Peptostreptococcus magnus*) is an anaerobic G+ bacterium that also has the ability to bind immunoglobulins, but instead of interacting with the Fc portion this bacterium binds Ig light chains.[18] This binding is attributed to the LPXTG-anchored protein L that binds κ light chains through repeated binding units.[19–22] Protein L and hybrids of protein L and protein A or G have been developed as immunoglobulin detection and purification tools.[23–25] Even though most of the known Ig-binding proteins are from G+ bacteria, it has been known for a long time that some Gram-negative (G–) bacteria also bind Ig, particularly IgD.[26] In G– bacteria, surface proteins interacting with the environment are often lipoproteins anchored in the outer of the two lipid membranes (outer membrane proteins). Subsequent studies have identified specific IgD-binding surface proteins in the G– pathogens *Haemophilus influenzae* (protein D) and *Moraxella catarrhalis* (MID).[27,28] The protein MID from *M. catarrhalis* can be used to purify human IgD from serum.[29] Key properties and biological activities of surface-associated Ig-binding proteins are summarized in Table 18.1 and a visual summary of interactions can be seen in Figure 18.1.

TABLE 18.1 Bacterial Proteins Interfering with Fc Function

Protein	Species	Mode of Action	Biological Effects/ Additional Features	Refs.
Cell Wall Ig-binding Proteins				
Protein A	*S. aureus*	IgG Fc binding	Inhibition of opsonophagocytic clearance, superantigen, B-cell depletion	Jensen,[2] Forsgren and Sjöquist,[3] Kim et al.[4]
Protein G	Group G *Streptococcus*	IgG Fc binding	Also binds IgG Fab	Kronvall,[5] Björck and Kronvall[6]
Protein L	*F. magna*	κ light-chain binding	Superantigen, mast cell activation	Björck,[21] Genovese et al.[111]
Protein H	*S. pyogenes*	IgG Fc binding	Inhibition of opsonophagocytic killing, complement inhibition	Åkesson,[7] Berge et al.[112]
M proteins	*S. pyogenes*	IgG Fc binding	Inhibition of opsonophagocytic killing	Navarre and Schneewind,[1] Fischetti[113]
Protein ARP	*S. pyogenes*	IgA binding	Also binds the complement regulator C4BP and thereby inhibits complement at the bacterial surface	Lindahl et al.[12]
Protein Sir	*S. pyogenes*	IgG, IgA binding	Also binds the complement regulator C4BP and thereby inhibits complement at the bacterial surface	Stenberg et al.,[13] Thern et al.[114]
β protein	*S. agalactiae*	IgA binding	Protection against IgA-mediated bacterial killing	Lindahl et al.,[11] Jerlström et al.,[16] Hedén et al.,[17] Russell-Jones et al.[115]
MID	*M. catharralis*	IgD binding	Activates B cells	Forsgren et al.,[28] Gjörloff et al.[116]
Protein D	*H. influenzae*	IgD binding	Histamine release, degranulation of mast cells	Akkoyunlu et al.,[27] Ruan et al.[117]
Secreted Ig-binding Proteins				
Sbi	*S. aureus*	IgG binding	Inhibition of opsonization, complement inhibition	Zhang et al.,[30] Smith et al.[31]
SibA	*S. pyogenes*	IgG, IgA, and IgM binding	—	Fagan et al.[33]
Lzp	*S. pyogenes*	IgG, IgA, and IgM binding	—	Okamoto et al.[34]
Ig Proteases				
IgA1 protease	*N. meningitidis*, *N. gonorrhoeae*	Cleavage in the hinge region	Serine-type proteases; cleavage eliminates agglutination and all Fc-mediated effector functions	Plaut et al.,[118] Mulks and Plaut[119]

(Continued)

TABLE 18.1 (Continued)

Protein	Species	Mode of Action	Biological Effects/ Additional Features	Refs.
IgA1 protease	*S. pneumoniae*, *S. mitis*, *S. oralis*, *Gemella haemolysans*	Cleavage in the hinge region	Zinc metalloproteases; cleavage eliminates agglutination and all Fc-mediated effector functions	Kilian et al.[120]
IgA1 protease	*H. influenzae*, *H. aegypticus*	Cleavage in the hinge region	Serine-type proteases; cleavage eliminates agglutination and all Fc-mediated effector functions	Kilian et al.[120]
IgA1 protease	*Prevotella* species	Cleavage in the hinge region	Cysteine protease; cleavage eliminates agglutination and all Fc-mediated effector functions	Kilian[76]
IgA1 protease	*Capnocytophaga* species	Cleavage in the hinge region	Metallo protease; only in human-associated species	Kilian[76]
IgG protease	*P. mirabilis*	Cleavage in the hinge region		Loomes et al.[80]
SpeB	*S. pyogenes*	Cleavage of IgG, IgA, IgM in the hinge region; degradation of IgD and IgE	Cysteine protease; cleavage of M-protein-specific IgG inhibits opsonophagocytic killing	Collin et al.[83,84]
IgG Glycan Hydrolysis				
EndoS	*S. pyogenes*	Complete hydrolysis of IgG Fc-glycans in the chitobiose core	Endo-β-*N*-acetylglucosamnidase with no major effect on bacterial virulence in invasive disease; shows potential as therapy against antibody-mediated autoimmunity and as a biotechnological tool	Collin et al.[84,90]
EndoE	*E. faecalis*	Hydrolysis of mono-antennary glycans on native human IgG	Dual-domain (family 18 and family 20) glycan hydrolase with additional activity on high-mannose glycans on RNase B and lactoferrin	Collin et al.,[104] Garbe et al.[105]
EndoC/ EndoSE	Human group C streptococci *S. equi* subspecies *equi* and *zooepidemicus*	Complete hydrolysis of IgG Fc-glycans in the chitobiose core	True homolog to EndoS, both genetically and functionally	Collin and Olsén,[106] Flock et al.,[107] Garbe and Collin,[110] unpublished observations in the Collin laboratory
$EndoS_2$	*S. pyogenes* serotype M49	Complete hydrolysis of IgG Fc-glycans in the chitobiose core	Endo-β-*N*-acetylglucosaminidase with additional activity on the acute-phase protein orosomucoid (α-acid glycoprotein)	Sjögren et al., manuscript in preparation

(Continued)

TABLE 18.1 (Continued)

Protein	Species	Mode of Action	Biological Effects/ Additional Features	Refs.
EndoD	*S. pneumoniae*	Hydrolysis of complex *N*-linked glycans	Endoglycosidase with activity on several glycoproteins, including IgG	Muramatsu et al.[121,122]
StrH	*S. pneumoniae*	Hydrolysis of *N*-acetylglucosamine β1 linked to mannose	Exoglycosidase activity on several glycoproteins, including IgA_1	King et al.[123]
NanA	*S. pneumoniae*	Hydrolysis of sialic acid α2–3 or α2–3 linked to galactose	Exoglycosidase activity on several glycoproteins, including IgA_1	King et al.,[123] Burnaugh et al.[124]
BgaA	*S. pneumoniae*	Hydrolysis of galactose β1–4 linked to *N*-acetylglucosamine	Exoglycosidase activity on several glycoproteins, including IgA_1	King et al.[123]
SiaC	*C. carnimorsus*	unknown	Exoglycosidase activity on IgG	Renzi et al.[125]
GpdC	*C. carnimorsus*	Hydrolysis of complex *N*-linked glycans	Exoglycosidase activity on IgG	Renzi et al.[125]

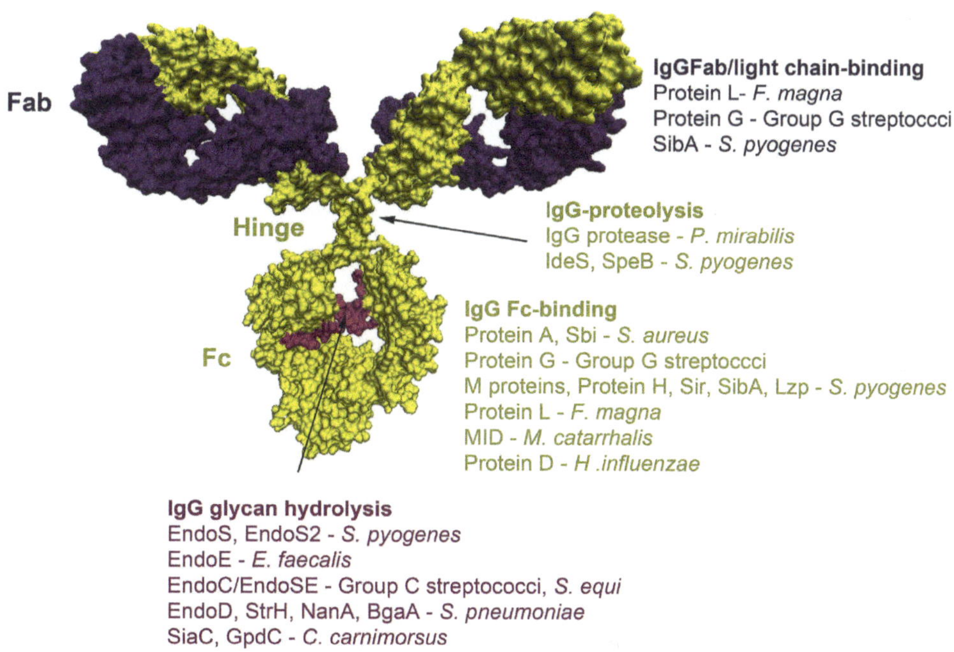

FIGURE 18.1 **Visual summary of interactions between bacterial proteins and human IgG.** Structural representation of glycosylated IgG_1 visualized using VMD 1.9.1 and Tachyon ray tracer based on a model deposited in PDB by M. Clark. IgG heavy chains are represented in yellow, the light chains in blue, and the conserved *N*-linked glycan on Asn297 of the heavy chain in purple. Bacterial proteins binding to Fab and/or light chains are written in blue text; proteins binding to and hydrolyzing the IgG heavy chain are written in green text; and enzymes hydrolyzing the IgG-Fc glycan are written in purple text.

Secreted Immunoglobulin Binding Proteins

In addition to the vast number of described cell-surface-associated Ig-binding proteins, there are also a few examples of secreted Ig binders (see Table 18.1 and Figure 18.1). Interestingly, these are found in bacteria that also express cell-wall-anchored Ig-binding proteins. In *Staphylococcus aureus* the protein Sbi is secreted but is also associated with the bacterial surface.[30,31] When associated with the surface the protein predominantly binds IgG, but in solution Sbi interacts with complement factor C3 and inhibits the complement cascade.[32] In *Streptococcus pyogenes*, two secreted Ig-binding proteins have recently been identified. SibA binds to both Fab and Fc of IgG and also binds IgA and IgM,[33] and the secreted leucine zipper protein Lzp binds to IgG, IgA, and IgM.[34] In addition to truly secreted Ig-binding proteins, it has been shown that several cell-wall-anchored Ig-binding proteins are released more or less specifically by endogenous bacterial proteases. For example, the secreted cysteine proteinase SpeB from *S. pyogenes* releases biologically active fragments of IgG-binding M- and M-like proteins that can activate complement at a distance from the bacteria.[35,36]

IMMUNOGLOBULIN PROTEASES

IgA Proteases

IgA Protease-Producing Bacteria

Several bacterial species with a primary habitat on human mucosal surfaces, particularly in the upper respiratory tract, produce endoproteases that are capable of cleaving a single peptide bond in the extended and abundantly glycosylated hinge region of human IgA_1 and its normally protease-resistant secreted form, S-IgA_1. IgA_1 is vastly predominant in secretions of the upper respiratory tract and in serum and is exclusively present in humans and hominoid primates (chimpanzees, gorillas, and orangutans). The genetic diversity and the fact that IgA_1 protease is present exclusively in bacteria associated with these hosts suggest that these enzymes arose independently in several bacterial species as a response to the emergence of the IgA_1 subclass approximately 7 million years ago. Sequence comparisons show that IgA_1 protease genes are members of families of paralogous genes and arose by gene duplication and subsequent specialization of already existing genes encoding proteases with other functions.

IgA_1 proteases are produced by all members of the species *Neisseria meningitidis, Streptococcus pneumoniae*, and *Haemophilus influenzae*, which are the principal causes of bacterial meningitis (for a review, see Kilian et al.[37]). In addition, several bacteria genetically related to these important pathogens produce IgA_1 proteases, reflecting either shared ancestry or, in some cases, horizontal gene transfer.[37,38] The biological significance of IgA_1 proteases is indirectly supported by the fact that they are a striking result of convergent evolution along at least five independent lineages. In spite of virtually identical enzymatic function, IgA_1 proteases of different bacteria belong to all major protease families (i.e., serine proteases, metalloproteases, and thiol proteases). Whereas the IgA_1 proteases of *Neisseria* and *Haemophilus* species and *Ureaplasma urealyticum* are serine proteases, those produced by some species belonging to the genera *Streptococcus, Gemella*, and the Gram-negative *Capnocytophaga* are zinc metalloproteases. The thiol protease version of IgA_1 proteases is present in all human-associated species of the genus *Prevotella* (Figure 18.2). For references to the individual findings, see Kilian et al.,[37] Bek-Thomsen et al.,[39] and Table 18.1.

A striking example of adaptation to its preferred habitat is the IgA protease produced by the gut bacterium *Clostridium ramosum*, which cleaves both IgA_1 and the A2m(1) allotype of IgA_2, which are represented in approximately

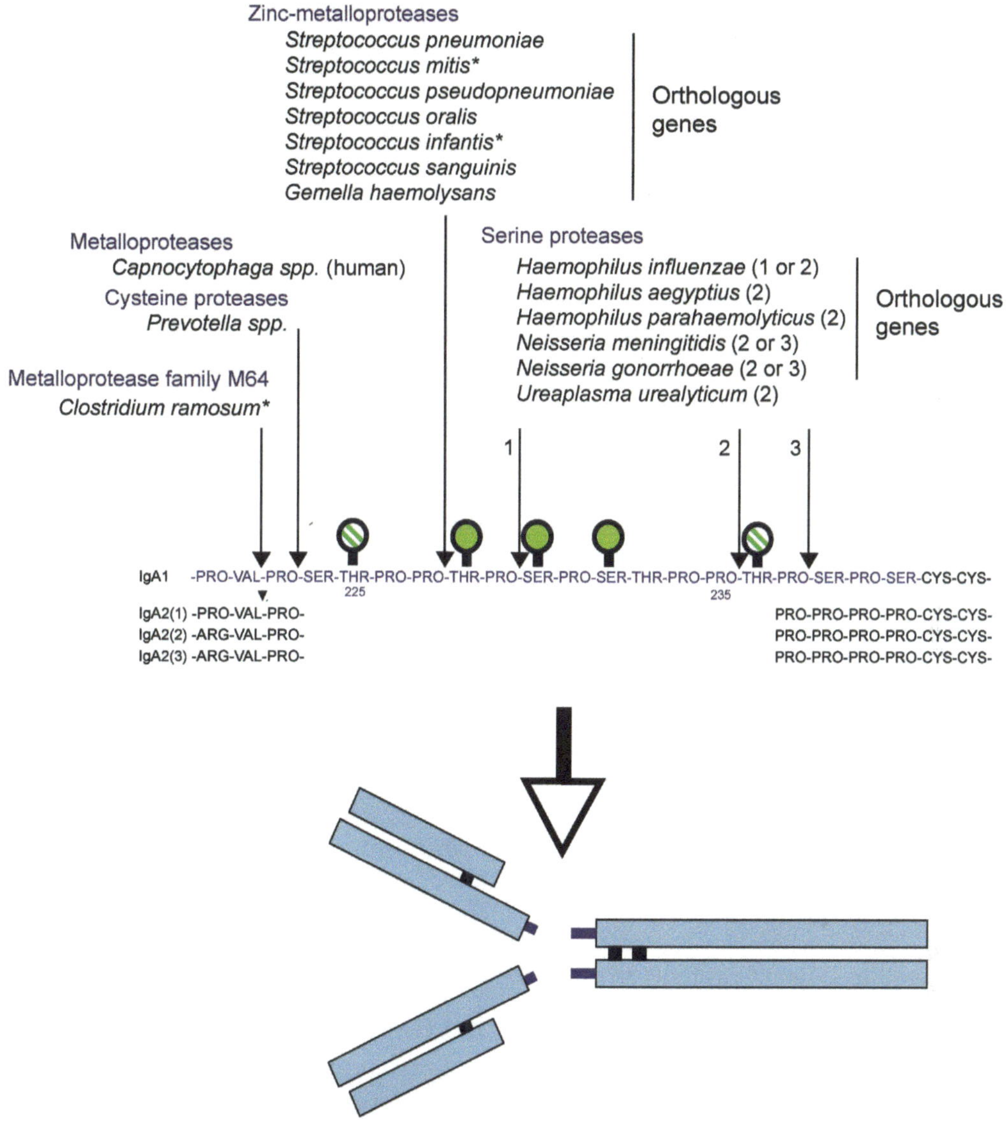

FIGURE 18.2 **Sites of IgA_1 protease-induced cleavage within the hinge region of human IgA.** Note that strains of *Haemophilus influenzae, Neisseria meningitidis,* and *Neisseria gonorrhoeae* may cleave either a Pro–Ser peptide bond (type 1 protease) or a Pro–Thr peptide bond (type 2 protease). The *Clostridium ramosum* IgA protease cleaves both IgA_1 and the IgA_2 allotype A2m(1), as indicated by the arrow. The green circles indicate carbohydrate side-chains in the IgA_1 hinge region, those that are hatched being variably present in IgA_1 molecules. An asterisk next to a species name indicates that not all strains of the species produce IgA_1 protease.

even proportions in intestinal secretions.[40,41] The increased conformational freedom of the two antigen-binding domains of IgA_1 antibodies attained by the extended hinge region was achieved at the expense of introducing an open stretch that potentially is more susceptible to attack by proteolytic enzymes. This potential weakness has been counteracted by an unusual proline-rich amino acid sequence combined with extensive *O*-glycosylation of several serine and threonine residues (Figure 18.2), which render the IgA_1 hinge resistant to traditional proteolytic enzymes. All IgA_1 proteases are strikingly specialized endopeptidases that cleave one of the several prolyl–seryl or prolyl–threonyl peptide bonds present in the IgA_1 hinge and adjacent to a carbohydrate side chain. The *C. ramosum* protease cleaves IgA_1 and the A2m(1) allotype of IgA_2 at the prolyl–valyl bond shared by these two human α-chains just before the hinge (Figure 18.2).

The serine IgA_1 proteases in *Neisseria meningitidis*, *N. gonorrhoeae*, *Haemophilus influenzae*, *H. aegyptius*, and *H. parahaemolyticus* are actively secreted to the extracellular environment by a type V auto-secretion system.[42,43] In contrast, the IgA_1 protease of *Streptococcus pneumoniae* and several commensal streptococci remain linked to the cell surface by a cell-wall-anchor LPXTG motif, which, in contrast to all other known wall-associated proteins in Gram-positive bacteria, is located in the N-terminal part of the molecule.[44,45]

Although the pneumococcal IgA_1 protease is clearly associated with virulence,[46,47] homologous proteins are also expressed by several commensal *Streptococcus* species. In most of the commensal species, the *iga* gene and IgA_1 protease activity are variably present. Phylogenetic analyses suggest that the *iga* gene evolved in the common ancestor of these phylogenetically related streptococci and was subsequently lost within multiple lineages of commensal streptococci due to a more subtle relationship with the adaptive mucosal immune system than that of pneumococci.[39,48] This is supported by evidence of a significantly higher selective pressure for sequence divergence in *iga* genes of the pathogenic *S. pneumoniae* than in the commensal streptococci.[39]

The primary function of the IgA_1 protease in *Streptococcus pneumoniae*, *Haemophilus influenzae*, and *Neisseria meningitidis* is assumed to be the evasion of IgA_1 antibodies. However, the observation that the pneumococcal IgA_1 protease is crucial for experimental infections in mice, in spite of the fact that the protease does not cleave murine IgA,[46,47,49] indicates that it has additional, but yet unidentified virulence-associated properties.

IgA Protease Strain Variations

Comparative studies of the IgA_1 protease activity released from cultures of numerous bacterial strains reveal significant inter- and intraspecies differences.[50] Although there is no overall relationship between pathogenicity of species and IgA_1 protease activity, it is notable that meningococci generally show activities that may be several hundred times higher than those of some of the commensal streptococci. Significant variations are also seen within species,[50] and isolates of *Neisseria meningitidis* and *Haemophilus influenzae* from invasive infections are reported to produce more IgA_1 protease than isolates from healthy carriers.[51,52]

In Vivo *Activity of IgA_1 Proteases*

IgA_1 proteases are not inhibited by physiological protease inhibitors (e.g., 2-macroglobulin and 1-protease inhibitor), in contrast to many other microbial proteinases;[53] however, human milk lactoferrin is reported to inactivate IgA_1 protease from *Haemophilus influenzae* by releasing the autotransporter protein from the bacterial cell membrane.[54] Under conditions that allow prolonged exposure of S-IgA_1 in mucosal secretions to IgA_1 protease-producing bacteria it is possible to demonstrate characteristic fragments of S-IgA_1.[55,56] However, the failure to demonstrate characteristic cleavage fragments of IgA in vaginal secretions of women with gonococcal infection[57] and in nasal rinses from healthy human adults colonized with IgA_1 protease-producing bacteria[58] suggests that cleavage, in most cases, is restricted to the microenvironment of the individual bacterial cells.

Functional Significance of IgA_1 Proteases

Due to the specificity for human IgA_1, animal models that allow evaluation of the contribution of IgA_1 proteases to pathogenicity are not available. Two studies used human organ culture models. Isogenic strains of *Neisseria gonorrhoeae* and *Haemophilus influenzae* with or without IgA_1 protease activity were used to infect human fallopian tube and nasopharyngeal organ cultures, with no observed differences in the ability to attach to or penetrate the mucosal tissues.[59,60] As these models lacked specific IgA_1 antibodies, they do not elucidate potential effects related to IgA_1 cleavage. The same limitation probably applies to studies using a human infection model of initial gonococcal infection that, likewise, failed to reveal signs of reduced infectivity of IgA_1-protease-negative mutants.[61]

It is conceivable that IgA_1-protease-induced cleavage of IgA_1 efficiently eliminates secondary Fc_α-mediated effector functions of IgA_1 antibodies. These include IgA_1-mediated agglutination, mucus trapping, inhibition of adherence, and opsonization for interaction with various white blood cells, including phagocytes (for a review, see Kilian and Russell[62]). However, two points are crucial to understanding the complexity of these interactions. First, the mentioned consequences of IgA_1 cleavage are relevant to the protease-producing bacterium only in the presence of IgA_1 antibodies specific to the producer. Second, the monomeric Fab fragments released from the cleaved IgA_1 molecules retain their antigen-binding activity.[63] Again, providing specificity of the IgA_1 antibodies, the protease-producing bacterial cell will become coated with these Fab fragments.[56] These Fabα fragments conceivably block access of intact antibodies of other isotypes and interfere with complement activation and complement-mediated lysis in the presence of IgM and IgG antibodies.[64] Studies using pneumococci with and without IgA_1 protease activity further suggest that coating with hydrophobic Fab fragments of IgA_1 antibodies to capsular polysaccharides even may be a prerequisite for the ability of encapsulated bacteria to adhere to epithelial cells.[65] In this way, IgA_1 proteases allow the bacteria to take advantage of IgA_1 antibodies to their surface components. Based on these observations, it has been hypothesized that one factor in the pathogenesis of invasive disease due to *Haemophilus influenzae*, *Neisseria meningitidis*, and *Streptococcus pneumoniae* is the presence of preexisting IgA_1 antibodies to the capsular polysaccharide as a result of prior colonization with cross-reactive enterobacteria (e.g., *Escherichia coli* K100 in the case of *H. influenzae* type b, *E. coli* K1 in the case of *N. meningitidis* group B). In this situation, the pathogen encounters preexisting IgA_1 antibodies to its surface epitopes but no antibodies that will neutralize its IgA_1 protease.[66]

IgG Proteases

IdeS from **Streptococcus pyogenes**

Until quite recently, no bacterial IgG proteases with the kind of strict specificity as can be seen for IgA proteases had been described, though there were numerous reports on proteases that among other substrates also hydrolyze IgG (see next section). The strictly human pathogen *Streptococcus pyogenes* has proven to be a real treasure trove for finding novel immunomodulating molecules (for a review, see Nizet[67]); therefore, it might not be surprising that it was in this bacterium that the first IgG-specific protease, IdeS, was discovered. IdeS is a secreted cysteine proteinase that specifically hydrolyzes all subclasses of human IgG in the hinge region just below the disulfide bridge, thus generating $F(ab')_2$ and monomeric Fc fragments (1/2 Fc).[68] The biological significance of this activity is quite obvious: Bacteria are protected from IgG-mediated phagocytic killing,[69] but it also turns out that the IdeS generated soluble 1/2 Fc that unspecifically can prime neutrophils and thus reduce phagocytic killing of bacteria.[70] IdeS has been extensively characterized functionally and structurally (for reviews, see Pawel-Rammingen[71,72]). One of the intriguing avenues taken with this enzyme is the development of IdeS as a novel pharmaceutical against autoimmunity spurred by the strict selectivity for IgG also *in vivo*.[73–75] Furthermore, the $F(ab')_2$-generating capacity has proven to be an excellent tool, especially in combination with protein G, for efficient purification of Fc free antibodies for research purposes.

Broad-Spectrum Proteases with Activity on Immunoglobulins

Several microorganisms produce broad-spectrum proteases that degrade human immunoglobulins. This is the case with the putative periodontal pathogen *Porphyromonas gingivalis*, which degrades IgG, IgM, IgA_1, and IgA_2 and many other host proteins into small fragments.[76] Likewise, *Pseudomonas aeruginosa*, a notable opportunistic pathogen, cleaves IgA, S-IgA, SC, and IgG into multiple fragments.[77,78] A protease from *Proteus mirabilis* cleaves IgA between the CH2 and CH3 domains and IgG at either side of the hinge region.[79,80] One of the most studied proteases from any pathogen is the secreted cysteine proteinase, SpeB, from *Streptococcus pyogenes*. It is one of the most abundant secreted proteins from this bacterium, and in most infection models and clinical studies it is viewed as an important virulence factor (for two recent reviews on SpeB, see Carroll and Musser[81] and Nelson et al.[82]). Even though all of the described substrates for SpeB might not be physiologically relevant, one activity of particular interest in this context is the ability of SpeB to hydrolyze human immunoglobulins. SpeB cleaves IgG, IgA, and IgM in the hinge regions and completely degrades IgD and IgE.[83] Even though the contribution of this particular activity among all the other activities attributed to SpeB in colonization and virulence *in vivo* is unclear, it has been shown *in vitro* that SpeB hydrolysis of human IgG directed toward the cell-wall-anchored M protein protects bacteria from opsonophagocytic killing in human blood.[84]

IMMUNOGLOBULIN GLYCAN HYDROLASES

Immunoglobulin Glycosylation

Among the latest additions to the family of microbial products with activity on immunoglobulins are the immunoglobulin glycan hydrolases. The discovery of these enzymes has been spurred by the increasing worldwide interest in glycoimmunology. Not very surprising, at least not to glycobiologists, many if not all immunological pathways are influenced by the glycosylation status of key proteins.[85] Immunoglobulins certainly belong to this group of key glycoproteins as outlined in previous chapters. All mammalian antibodies of all subclasses are glycosylated to varying extents. IgG represents the simplest glycoprotein with one complex *N*-linked glycan on Asn297 in the constant region of the heavy chain (see Figure 18.1). Depending on the composition of the variable part, all antibodies can harbor additional *N*- or *O*-linked glycan in the Fab portion. As described in previous chapters, minor changes in this complex biantennary glycan have profound effects on the function of IgG Fc.[86] IgA, and in particular S-IgA, are heavily glycosylated with both *N*-linked and *O*-linked glycan chains that are important for their conformation, net charge, hydrophilicity, and for resistance to proteolytic enzymes.[87–89] Thus, it is conceivable that bacteria-induced alterations of the glycosylation of IgA molecules can interfere with their antibody function; however, the *in vivo* significance of this hypothesis has not been examined.

Glycosidases with Activity on Immunoglobulins

Specific Immunoglobulin Glycan Hydrolases

EndoS, a recently discovered secreted endoglycosidase *Streptococcus pyogenes*, represents a novel mode of targeting the adaptive branch of the immune system. EndoS specifically hydrolyzes the *N*-linked glycan at Asn297 in IgG.[90] In contrast to many related endoglycosidases, EndoS only hydrolyzes native IgG, suggesting that protein–protein interactions, in addition to protein–glycan interactions, between the enzyme and IgG provide this unique specificity.[83] Treatment of human IgG directed toward the bacteria with EndoS almost completely abolishes binding to white blood cells, decreases complement activation through the classical pathway, and increases bacterial survival in blood.[84] From the bacterial point of view, this strategy makes perfect sense with evasion of adaptive immunity, but EndoS does not seem to be a major virulence factor, at least not during systemic infections.[91] The unique specificity of EndoS could also be exploited for other purposes, especially considering that immunoglobulin glycans are instrumental in fine-tuning IgG effector functions.[92] Autoimmune disorders constitute a large group of diseases with various manifestations from mild to severe, but they all have in common that the immune system attacks and damages endogenous tissues and organs. Accumulating evidence suggests that autoantibodies are more important than previously appreciated for the development of disease.[93] This is also true for acute and chronic rejection of transplanted organs, where recent studies have shown that antibodies account for a substantial portion of graft rejection episodes.[94] There is a great need for novel pharmaceuticals for treating these diseases, and *in vivo* or *ex vivo* glycan modification could possibly meet this need. Indeed, EndoS has proven efficient as an experimental treatment in a number of passive, active, and spontaneous animal models of antibody-mediated autoimmunity. These include arthritis, systemic lupus erythematosus (SLE), autoimmune thrombocytopenia, autoimmune hemolysis, bullous skin disease, autoimmunity of the kidney, and multiple sclerosis.[95–102] Furthermore, it has recently been demonstrated that pathogenic antibodies from neuromyelitis optica can be transformed into potentially therapeutic antibodies by *ex vivo* treatment with EndoS.[103]

Since the discovery of EndoS, several structurally or functionally related enzymes have been identified in other bacterial pathogens. EndoE from *Enterococcus faecalis* has dual functions, with activity on IgG glycans and broader activity on additional human glycoproteins.[104,105] Furthermore, true EndoS homologs both functionally and structurally have been found in the predominantly animal pathogens *Streptococcus equi* subspecies *equi* and zooepidemicus, as well as in human isolates of group C streptococci (it is at present not clear what streptococcal species these isolates are). (Table 18.1 and Figure 18.1).[106,107]

Broad-Spectrum Glycan Hydrolases with Activity on Immunoglobulins

In addition to enzymes that are quite specific for immunoglobulins, several other bacterial pathogens have developed enzymes or enzyme complexes that can modify both *N*- and *O*-linked glycans on many glycoproteins, including immunoglobulins. As an example, *Streptococcus pneumoniae* and the oral streptococcal species *S. oralis* and *S. mitis* are capable of stripping IgA_1 molecules of all their carbohydrate side chains.[89,108] Other microorganisms selectively remove part of the oligosaccharide chains, such as the terminal sialic acid residues.[89,109] Some of these activities are summarized in Table 18.1 and Figure 18.1 and have been reviewed in Garbe and Collin.[110]

CONCLUDING REMARKS

We sincerely hope that this chapter has made it evident that bacterial co-evolution with our immune system has generated an amazing array of mechanisms to avoid IgFc-mediated effector functions. We have clearly not been able to cover every aspect of bacterial avoidance of Fc-functions. Nevertheless, we hope to have stimulated further reading, and we anticipate many exciting future discoveries emanating from studies of the interface between pathogens and the human immune system. After all, pathogens are the true experts of our immune system!

Acknowledgments

Mattias Collin is supported by grants from the Swedish Research Council (2010-57X-20240), the Foundations of Wiberg, Österlund, Hedlund, Söderberg, the Royal Physiografic Society, King Gustaf V's Memorial Fund, the Medical Faculty at Lund University, and Hansa Medical AB. Mogens Kilian is supported by a grant from the Danish Medical Research Council. The funders had no role in preparation of the manuscript or decision to publish.

References

1. Navarre WW, Schneewind O. Surface proteins of Gram-positive bacteria and mechanisms of their targeting to the cell wall envelope. *Microbiol Mol Biol Rev* 1999;**63**:174–229.
2. Jensen K. A normally occurring *Staphylococcus* antibody in human serum. *Acta Path Microbiol Scand* 1958;**44**:421–8.
3. Forsgren A, Sjöquist J. "Protein A" from *S. aureus*. I. Pseudo-immune reaction with human γ-globulin. *J Immunol* 1966;**97**:822–7.
4. Kim HK, Thammavongsa V, Schneewind O, Missiakas D. Recurrent infections and immune evasion strategies of *Staphylococcus aureus*. *Curr Opin Microbiol* 2012;**15**:92–9.
5. Kronvall G. A surface component in group A, C, and G streptococci with non-immune reactivity for immunoglobulin G. *J Immunol* 1973;**111**:1401–6.
6. Björck L, Kronvall G. Purification and some properties of streptococcal protein G, a novel IgG-binding reagent. *J Immunol* 1984;**133**:969–74.
7. Åkesson P, Cooney J, Kishimoto F, Björck L. Protein H—a novel IgG binding bacterial protein. *Mol Immunol* 1990;**27**:523–31.
8. Åkesson P, Schmidt KH, Cooney J, Björck L. M1 protein and protein H: IgGFc- and albumin-binding streptococcal surface proteins encoded by adjacent genes. *Biochem J* 1994;**300**(Pt. 3):877–86.
9. O'Toole PW, O'Toole P, Stenberg L, Rissler M, Lindahl G. Two major classes in the M protein family in group A streptococci. *Proc Natl Acad Sci USA* 1992;**89**:8661–5.
10. Stenberg L, O'Toole P, Lindahl G. Many group A streptococcal strains express two different immunoglobulin-binding proteins, encoded by closely linked genes: characterization of the proteins expressed by four strains of different M-type. *Mol Microbiol* 1992;**6**:1185–94.
11. Lindahl G, Åkerström B, Vaerman JP, Stenberg L. Characterization of an IgA receptor from group B streptococci: specificity for serum IgA. *Eur J Immunol* 1990;**20**:2241–7.
12. Lindahl G, Åkerström B. Receptor for IgA in group A streptococci: cloning of the gene and characterization of the protein expressed in *Escherichia coli*. *Mol Microbiol* 1989;**3**:239–47.
13. Stenberg L, O'Toole PW, Mestecky J, Lindahl G. Molecular characterization of protein Sir, a streptococcal cell surface protein that binds both immunoglobulin A and immunoglobulin G. *J Biol Chem* 1994;**269**:13458–64.
14. Johnsson E, Areschoug T, Mestecky J, Lindahl G. An IgA-binding peptide derived from a streptococcal surface protein. *J Biol Chem* 1999;**274**:14521–4.
15. Sandin C, Linse S, Areschoug T, Woof JM, Reinholdt J, Lindahl G. Isolation and detection of human IgA using a streptococcal IgA-binding peptide. *J Immunol* 2002;**169**:1357–64.
16. Jerlström PG, Talay SR, Valentin-Weigand P, Timmis KN, Chhatwal GS. Identification of an immunoglobulin A binding motif located in the beta-antigen of the C protein complex of group B streptococci. *Infect Immun* 1996;**64**:2787–93.
17. Hedén L-O, Frithz E, Lindahl G. Molecular characterization of an IgA receptor from group B streptococci: sequence of the gene, identification of a proline-rich region with unique structure and isolation of N-terminal fragments with IgA-binding capacity. *Eur J Immunol* 1991;**21**:1481–90.
18. Myhre EB, Erntell M. A non-immune interaction between the light chain of human immunoglobulin

and a surface component of a *Peptococcus magnus* strain. *Mol Immunol* 1985;**22**:879–85.
19. Kastern W, Sjöbring U, Björck L. Structure of peptostreptococcal protein L and identification of a repeated immunoglobulin light chain-binding domain. *J Biol Chem* 1992;**267**:12820–5.
20. Nilson BH, Solomon A, Björck L, Åkerström B. Protein L from *Peptostreptococcus magnus* binds to the kappa light chain variable domain. *J Biol Chem* 1992;**267**:2234–9.
21. Björck L. Protein L. A novel bacterial cell wall protein with affinity for Ig L chains. *J Immunol* 1988;**140**:1194–7.
22. de Château M, Nilson B, Erntell M, et al. On the interaction between protein L and immunoglobulins of various mammalian species. *Scand J Immunol* 1993;**37**:399–405.
23. Nilson B, Lögdeberg L, Kastern W, Björck L, Åkerström B. Purification of antibodies using protein L-binding framework structures in the light chain variable domain. *J Immunol Meth* 1993;**164**(1):33–40.
24. Kihlberg BM, Sjöbring U, Kastern W, Björck L. Protein LG: a hybrid molecule with unique immunoglobulin binding properties. *J Biol Chem* 1992;**267**:25583–8.
25. Svensson HG, Hoogenboom HR, Sjöbring U. Protein LA, a novel hybrid protein with unique single-chain Fv antibody- and Fab-binding properties. *Eur J Biochem* 1998;**258**:890–6.
26. Forsgren A, Grubb AO. Many bacterial species bind human IgD. *J Immunol* 1979;**122**:1468–72.
27. Akkoyunlu M, Ruan M, Forsgren A. Distribution of protein D, an immunoglobulin D-binding protein, in *Haemophilus* strains. *Infect Immun* 1991;**59**:1231–8.
28. Forsgren A, Brant M, Möllenkvist A, Muyombwe A, Janson H, Woin N, et al. Isolation and characterization of a novel IgD-binding protein from *Moraxella catarrhalis*. *J Immunol* 2001;**167**:2112–20.
29. Samuelsson M, Forsgren A, Riesbeck K. Purification of IgD from human serum—a novel application of recombinant *M. catarrhalis* IgD-binding protein (MID). *J Immunol Meth* 2006;**317**:31–7.
30. Zhang L, Jacobsson K, Vasi J, Lindberg M, Frykberg L. A second IgG-binding protein in *Staphylococcus aureus*. *Microbiology* 1998;**144**(Pt. 4):985–91.
31. Smith EJ, Visai L, Kerrigan SW, Speziale P, Foster TJ. The Sbi protein is a multifunctional immune evasion factor of *Staphylococcus aureus*. *Infect Immun* 2011;**79**:3801–9.
32. Haupt K, Reuter M, van den Elsen J, Burman J, Hälbich S, Richter J, et al. The *Staphylococcus aureus* protein Sbi acts as a complement inhibitor and forms a tripartite complex with host complement Factor H and C3b. *PLoS Pathog* 2008;**4**:e1000250.
33. Fagan PK, Reinscheid D, Gottschalk B, Chhatwal GS. Identification and characterization of a novel secreted immunoglobulin binding protein from group A streptococcus. *Infect Immun* 2001;**69**:4851–7.
34. Okamoto S, Terao Y, Hasuike K, Hamada S, Kawabata S. A novel streptococcal leucine zipper protein (Lzp) binds to human immunoglobulins. *Biochem Biophys Res Commun* 2008;**377**:1128–34.
35. Berge A, Björck L. Streptococcal cysteine proteinase releases biologically active fragments of streptococcal surface proteins. *J Biol Chem* 1995;**270**:9862–7.
36. Raeder R, Woischnik M, Podbielski A, Boyle MD. A secreted streptococcal cysteine protease can cleave a surface-expressed M1 protein and alter the immunoglobulin binding properties. *Res Microbiol* 1998;**149**:539–48.
37. Kilian M, Reinholdt J, Lomholt H, Poulsen K, Frandsen EV. Biological significance of IgA1 proteases in bacterial colonization and pathogenesis: critical evaluation of experimental evidence. *APMIS* 1996;**104**:321–38.
38. Takenouchi-Ohkubo N, Mortensen LM, Drasbek KR, Kilian M, Poulsen K. Horizontal transfer of the immunoglobulin A1 protease gene (IgA) from *Streptococcus* to *Gemella haemolysans*. *Microbiology* 2006;**152**:2171–80.
39. Bek-Thomsen M, Poulsen K, Kilian M. Occurrence and evolution of the paralogous zinc metalloproteases IgA1 protease, ZmpB, ZmpC, and ZmpD in *Streptococcus pneumoniae* and related commensal species. *MBio* 2012;**3**(5):e00303–12.
40. Fujiyama Y, Iwaki M, Hodohara K, Hosoda S, Kobayashi K. The site of cleavage in human alpha chains of IgA1 and IgA2:A2m(1) allotype paraproteins by the clostridial IGA protease. *Mol Immunol* 1986;**23**:147–50.
41. Kosowska K, Reinholdt J, Rasmussen LK, et al. The *Clostridium ramosum* IgA proteinase represents a novel type of metalloendopeptidase. *J Biol Chem* 2002;**277**:11987–94.
42. Pohlner J, Halter R, Beyreuther K, Meyer TF. Gene structure and extracellular secretion of *Neisseria gonorrhoeae* IgA protease. *Nature* 1987;**325**:458–62.
43. Poulsen K, Brandt J, Hjorth JP, Thøgersen HC, Kilian M. Cloning and sequencing of the immunoglobulin A1 protease gene (IgA) of *Haemophilus influenzae* serotype b. *Infect Immun* 1989;**57**:3097–105.
44. Poulsen K, Reinholdt J, Kilian M. Characterization of the *Streptococcus pneumoniae* immunoglobulin A1 protease gene (iga) and its translation product. *Infect Immun* 1996;**64**:3957–66.
45. Bender MH, Weiser JN. The atypical amino-terminal LPNTG-containing domain of the pneumococcal human IgA1-specific protease is required for proper enzyme localization and function. *Mol Microbiol* 2006;**61**:526–43.
46. Polissi A, Pontiggia A, Feger G, et al. Large-scale identification of virulence genes from *Streptococcus pneumoniae*. *Infect Immun* 1998;**66**:5620–9.
47. Hava DL, Camilli A. Large-scale identification of serotype 4 *Streptococcus pneumoniae* virulence factors. *Mol Microbiol* 2002;**45**:1389–406.

48. Kilian M, Poulsen K, Blomqvist T, Håvarstein LS, Bek-Thomsen M, Tettelin H, et al. Evolution of *Streptococcus pneumoniae* and its close commensal relatives. *PLoS ONE* 2008;**3**:e2683.
49. Chiavolini D, Memmi G, Maggi T, Iannelli F, Pozzi G, Oggioni MR. The three extra-cellular zinc metalloproteinases of *Streptococcus pneumoniae* have a different impact on virulence in mice. *BMC Microbiol* 2003;**3**:14.
50. Reinholdt J, Kilian M. Comparative analysis of immunoglobulin A1 protease activity among bacteria representing different genera, species, and strains. *Infect Immun* 1997;**65**:4452–9.
51. Vitovski S, Read RC, Sayers JR. Invasive isolates of *Neisseria meningitidis* possess enhanced immunoglobulin A1 protease activity compared to colonizing strains. *FASEB J* 1999;**13**:331–7.
52. Vitovski S, Dunkin KT, Howard AJ, Sayers JR. Nontypeable *Haemophilus influenzae* in carriage and disease: a difference in IgA1 protease activity levels. *JAMA* 2002;**287**:1699–705.
53. Plaut AG. The IgA1 proteases of pathogenic bacteria. *Annu Rev Microbiol* 1983;**37**:603–22.
54. Plaut AG, Qiu J, Grundy F, Wright A. Growth of *Haemophilus influenzae* in human milk: synthesis, distribution, and activity of IgA protease as determined by study of IgA^+ and mutant IgA^- cells. *J Infect Dis* 1992;**166**:43–52.
55. Sørensen CH, Kilian M. Bacterium-induced cleavage of IgA in nasopharyngeal secretions from atopic children. *Acta Pathol Microbiol Immunol Scand C* 1984;**92**:85–7.
56. Ahl T, Reinholdt J. Detection of immunoglobulin A1 protease-induced Fab alpha fragments on dental plaque bacteria. *Infect Immun* 1991;**59**:563–9.
57. Hedges SR, Mayo MS, Kallman L, Mestecky J, Hook EW, Russell MW. Evaluation of immunoglobulin A1 (IgA1) protease and IgA1 protease-inhibitory activity in human female genital infection with *Neisseria gonorrhoeae*. *Infect Immun* 1998;**66**:5826–32.
58. Kirkeby L, Rasmussen TT, Reinholdt J, Kilian M. Immunoglobulins in nasal secretions of healthy humans: structural integrity of secretory immunoglobulin A1 (IgA1) and occurrence of neutralizing antibodies to IgA1 proteases of nasal bacteria. *Clin Diagn Lab Immunol* 2000;**7**:31–9.
59. Cooper MD, McGee ZA, Mulks MH, Koomey JM, Hindman TL. Attachment to and invasion of human fallopian tube mucosa by an IgA1 protease-deficient mutant of *Neisseria gonorrhoeae* and its wild-type parent. *J Infect Dis* 1984;**150**:737–44.
60. Farley MM, Stephens DS, Mulks MH, Cooper MD, Bricker JV, Mirra SS, et al. Pathogenesis of IgA1 protease-producing and -nonproducing *Haemophilus influenzae* in human nasopharyngeal organ cultures. *J Infect Dis* 1986;**154**:752–9.
61. Johannsen DB, Johnston DM, Koymen HO, Cohen MS, Cannon JGA. *Neisseria gonorrhoeae* immunoglobulin A1 protease mutant is infectious in the human challenge model of urethral infection. *Infect Immun* 1999;**67**:3009–13.
62. Kilian M, Russell MW. Microbial evasion of IgA functions. In: Mestecky JF, Lamm EM, Strober W, Bienenstock J, McGhee RJ, editors. *Handbook of mucosal immunology*. San Diego, CA: Academic Press; 1999. p. 241–51.
63. Mansa B, Kilian M. Retained antigen-binding activity of Fab alpha fragments of human monoclonal immunoglobulin A1 (IgA1) cleaved by IgA1 protease. *Infect Immun* 1986;**52**:171–4.
64. Jarvis GA, Griffiss JM. Human IgA1 blockade of IgG-initiated lysis of *Neisseria meningitidis* is a function of antigen-binding fragment binding to the polysaccharide capsule. *J Immunol* 1991;**147**:1962–7.
65. Weiser JN, Bae D, Fasching C, Scamurra RW, Ratner AJ, Janoff EN. Antibody-enhanced pneumococcal adherence requires IgA1 protease. *Proc Natl Acad Sci USA* 2003;**100**:4215–20.
66. Kilian M, Reinholdt J. A hypothetical model for the development of invasive infection due to IgA1 protease-producing bacteria. *Adv Exp Med Biol* 1987;**216B**:1261–9.
67. Nizet V. Understanding how leading bacterial pathogens subvert innate immunity to reveal novel therapeutic targets. *J Allergy Clin Immunol* 2007;**120**:13–22.
68. Pawel-Rammingen von U, Johansson BP, Björck L. IdeS, a novel streptococcal cysteine proteinase with unique specificity for immunoglobulin G. *EMBO J* 2002;**21**:1607–15.
69. Pawel-Rammingen von U, Johansson B, Tapper H, Björck L. *Streptococcus pyogenes* and phagocytic killing. *Nat Med* 2002;**8**:1044–5.
70. Söderberg JJ, Pawel-Rammingen von U. The streptococcal protease IdeS modulates bacterial IgGFc binding and generates 1/2Fc fragments with the ability to prime polymorphonuclear leucocytes. *Mol Immunol* 2008;**45**:3347–53.
71. Pawel-Rammingen von U. Streptococcal IdeS and its impact on immune response and inflammation. *J Innate Immun* 2012;**4**:132–40.
72. Pawel-Rammingen von U, Björck L. IdeS and SpeB: immunoglobulin-degrading cysteine proteinases of *Streptococcus pyogenes*. *Curr Opin Microbiol* 2003;**6**:50–5.
73. Johansson BP, Shannon O, Björck L. IdeS: a bacterial proteolytic enzyme with therapeutic potential. *PLoS ONE* 2008;**3**:e1692.
74. Nandakumar KS, Johansson BP, Björck L, Holmdahl R. Blocking of experimental arthritis by cleavage of IgG antibodies *in vivo*. *Arthritis Rheum* 2007;**56**:3253–60.

75. Nandakumar K, Holmdahl R. Therapeutic cleavage of IgG: new avenues for treating inflammation. *Trends Immunol* 2008;**29**:173–8.
76. Kilian M. Degradation of immunoglobulins A2, A2, and G by suspected principal periodontal pathogens. *Infect Immun* 1981;**34**:757–65.
77. Döring G, Obernesser HJ, Botzenhart K. Extracellular toxins of *Pseudomonas aeruginosa*. II. Effect of two proteases on human immunoglobulins IgG, IgA and secretory IgA [author's transl.]. *Zentralbl Bakteriol A* 1981;**249**:89–98.
78. Heck LW, Alarcon PG, Kulhavy RM, Morihara K, Russell MW, Mestecky JF. Degradation of IgA proteins by *Pseudomonas aeruginosa* elastase. *J Immunol* 1990;**144**:2253–7.
79. Loomes LM, Senior BW, Kerr MA. A proteolytic enzyme secreted by *Proteus mirabilis* degrades immunoglobulins of the immunoglobulin A1 (IgA1), IgA2, and IgG isotypes. *Infect Immun* 1990;**58**:1979–85.
80. Loomes L, Kerr M, Senior B. The cleavage of immunoglobulin G *in vitro* and *in vivo* by a proteinase secreted by the urinary tract pathogen *Proteus mirabilis*. *J Med Microbiol* 1993;**39**:225–32.
81. Carroll RK, Musser JM. From transcription to activation: how group A streptococcus, the flesh-eating pathogen, regulates SpeB cysteine protease production. *Mol Microbiol* 2011;**81**:588–601.
82. Nelson DC, Garbe J, Collin M. Cysteine proteinase SpeB from *Streptococcus pyogenes*—a potent modifier of immunologically important host and bacterial proteins. *Biol Chem* 2011;**392**:1077–88.
83. Collin M, Olsén A. Effect of SpeB and EndoS from *Streptococcus pyogenes* on human immunoglobulins. *Infect Immun* 2001;**69**:7187–9.
84. Collin M, Svensson MD, Sjöholm AG, Jensenius JC, Sjöbring U, Olsén A. EndoS and SpeB from *Streptococcus pyogenes* inhibit immunoglobulin-mediated opsonophagocytosis. *Infect Immun* 2002;**70**:6646–51.
85. Rudd P, Elliott T, Cresswell P, Wilson I, Dwek R. Glycosylation and the immune system. *Science* 2001;**291**:2370–6.
86. Scanlan CN, Burton DR, Dwek RA. Making autoantibodies safe. *Proc Natl Acad Sci USA* 2008;**105**:4081–2.
87. Baenziger J, Kornfeld S. Structure of the carbohydrate units of IgA1 immunoglobulin. I. Composition, glycopeptide isolation, and structure of the asparagine-linked oligosaccharide units. *J Biol Chem* 1974;**249**:7260–9.
88. Mattu TS, Pleass RJ, Willis AC, Kilian M, Wormald MR, Lellouch AC, et al. The glycosylation and structure of human serum IgA1, Fab, and Fc regions and the role of N-glycosylation on Fc alpha receptor interactions. *J Biol Chem* 1998;**273**:2260–72.
89. Reinholdt J, Tomana M, Mortensen SB, Kilian M. Molecular aspects of immunoglobulin A1 degradation by oral streptococci. *Infect Immun* 1990;**58**:1186–94.
90. Collin M, Olsén A. EndoS, a novel secreted protein from *Streptococcus pyogenes* with endoglycosidase activity on human IgG. *EMBO J* 2001;**20**:3046–55.
91. Sjögren J, Okumura CYM, Collin M, Nizet V, Hollands A. Study of the IgG endoglycosidase EndoS in group A streptococcal phagocyte resistance and virulence. *BMC Microbiol* 2011;**11**:120.
92. Burton D, Dwek R. Immunology. Sugar determines antibody activity. *Science* 2006;**313**:627–8.
93. Lim P, Zouali M. Pathogenic autoantibodies: emerging insights into tissue injury. *Immunol Lett* 2006;**103**:17–26.
94. Colvin R, Smith R. Antibody-mediated organ-allograft rejection. *Nat Rev Immunol* 2005;**5**:807–17.
95. Lood C, Allhorn M, Lood R, Gullstrand B, Olin AI, Rönnblom L, et al. IgG glycan hydrolysis by endoglycosidase S diminishes the proinflammatory properties of immune complexes from patients with systemic lupus erythematosus: a possible new treatment?. *Arthritis Rheum* 2012;**64**:2698–706.
96. Benkhoucha M, Molnarfi N, Santiago-Raber M-L, Weber MS, Merkler D, Collin M, et al. IgG glycan hydrolysis by EndoS inhibits experimental autoimmune encephalomyelitis. *J Neuroinflammation* 2012;**9**:209.
97. Yang R, Otten MA, Hellmark T, Collin M, Björck L, Zhao M-H, et al. Successful treatment of experimental glomerulonephritis with IdeS and EndoS, IgG-degrading streptococcal enzymes. *Nephrol Dial Transplant* 2010;**25**:2479–86.
98. van Timmeren MM, van der Veen BS, Stegeman CA, Petersen AH, Hellmark T, Collin M, et al. IgG glycan hydrolysis attenuates ANCA-mediated glomerulonephritis. *J Am Soc Nephrol* 2010;**21**:1103–14.
99. Allhorn M, Briceño JG, Baudino L, Lood C, Olsson ML, Izui S, et al. The IgG-specific endoglycosidase EndoS inhibits both cellular and complement-mediated autoimmune hemolysis. *Blood* 2010;**115**:5080–8.
100. Allhorn M, Collin M. Sugar-free antibodies—the bacterial solution to autoimmunity? *Ann N Y Acad Sci* 2009;**1173**:664–9.
101. Albert H, Collin M, Dudziak D, Ravetch JV, Nimmerjahn F. *In vivo* enzymatic modulation of IgG glycosylation inhibits autoimmune disease in an IgG subclass-dependent manner. *Proc Natl Acad Sci USA* 2008;**105**:15005–9.
102. Collin M, Shannon O, Björck L. IgG glycan hydrolysis by a bacterial enzyme as a therapy against autoimmune conditions. *Proc Natl Acad Sci USA* 2008;**105**:4265–70.
103. Tradtrantip L, Ratelade J, Zhang H, Verkman AS. Enzymatic deglycosylation converts pathogenic neuromyelitis optica anti-aquaporin-4 IgG into therapeutic antibody. *Ann Neurol* 2012 [Epub ahead of print].

104. Collin M, Fischetti VA. A novel secreted endoglycosidase from *Enterococcus faecalis* with activity on human immunoglobulin G and ribonuclease B. *J Biol Chem* 2004;**279**:22558–70.
105. Garbe J, Sjögren J, Cosgrave E, Struwe WB, Bober M, Olin AI, et al. EndoE from *Enterococcus faecalis* cleaves the glycans of the biofilm inhibiting protein lactoferrin and is regulated via carbon catabolite repression. *PLoS ONE* [Under revision].
106. Collin M, Olsén A. Extracellular enzymes with immunomodulating activities: variations on a theme in *Streptococcus pyogenes*. *Infect Immun* 2003;**71**:2983–92.
107. Flock M, Frykberg L, Sköld M, Guss B, Flock J-I. Antiphagocytic function of an IgG glycosyl hydrolase from *Streptococcus equi* subsp. *equi* and its use as a vaccine component. *Infect Immun* 2012;**80**:2914–9.
108. Kilian M, Mestecky J, Kulhavy R, Tomana M, Butler WT. IgA1 proteases from *Haemophilus influenzae*, *Streptococcus pneumoniae*, *Neisseria meningitidis*, and *Streptococcus sanguis*: comparative immunochemical studies. *J Immunol* 1980;**124**:2596–600.
109. Frandsen EV. Carbohydrate depletion of immunoglobulin A1 by oral species of gram-positive rods. *Oral Microbiol Immunol* 1994;**9**:352–8.
110. Garbe J, Collin M. Bacterial hydrolysis of host glycoproteins—powerful protein modification and efficient nutrient acquisition. *J Innate Immun* 2012;**4**:121–31.
111. Genovese A, Borgia G, Björck L, Petraroli A, de Paulis A, Piazza M, et al. Immunoglobulin superantigen protein L induces IL-4 and IL-13 secretion from human FcγRI+ cells through interaction with the κ light chains of IgE. *J Immunol* 2003;**170**:1854–61.
112. Berge A, Kihlberg B-M, Sjöholm A, Björck L. Streptococcal protein H forms soluble complement-activating complexes with IgG, but inhibits complement activation by IgG-coated targets. *J Biol Chem* 1997;**272**:20774–81.
113. Fischetti VA. Streptococcal M protein: molecular design and biological behavior. *Clin Microbiol Rev* 1989;**2**:285–314.
114. Thern A, Stenberg L, Dahlbäck B, Lindahl G. Ig-binding surface proteins of *Streptococcus pyogenes* also bind human C4b-binding protein (C4BP), a regulatory component of the complement system. *J Immunol* 1995;**154**:375–86.
115. Russell-Jones GJ, Gotschlich EC, Blake MS. A surface receptor specific for human IgA on group B streptococci possessing the Ibc protein antigen. *J Exp Med* 1984;**160**:1467–75.
116. Gjörloff Wingren A, Hadzic R, Forsgren A, Riesbeck K. The novel IgD binding protein from *Moraxella catarrhalis* induces human B lymphocyte activation and Ig secretion in the presence of Th2 cytokines. *J Immunol* 2002;**168**:5582–8.
117. Ruan MR, Akkoyunlu M, Grubb A, Forsgren A. Protein D of *Haemophilus influenzae*. A novel bacterial surface protein with affinity for human IgD. *J Immunol* 1990;**145**:3379–84.
118. Plaut AG, Gilbert JV, Artenstein MS, Capra JD. *Neisseria gonorrhoeae* and *Neisseria meningitidis*: extracellular enzyme cleaves human immunoglobulin A. *Science* 1975;**190**:1103–5.
119. Mulks MH, Plaut AG. IgA protease production as a characteristic distinguishing pathogenic from harmless neisseriaceae. *N Engl J Med* 1978;**299**:973–6.
120. Kilian M, Mestecky J, Schrohenloher RE. Pathogenic species of the genus *Haemophilus* and *Streptococcus pneumoniae* produce immunoglobulin A1 protease. *Infect Immun* 1979;**26**:143–9.
121. Muramatsu H, Tachikui H, Ushida H, Song X-J, Qiu Y, Yamamoto S, et al. Molecular cloning and expression of endo-β-*N*-acetylglucosaminidase D, which acts on the core structure of complex type asparagine-linked oligosaccharides. *J Biochem* 2001;**129**:923–8.
122. Muramatsu T, Koide N, Maeyama K. Further studies on endo-β-*N*-acetylglucosaminidase D1. *J Biochem* 1978;**83**:363–70.
123. King SJ, Hippe KR, Weiser JN. Deglycosylation of human glycoconjugates by the sequential activities of exoglycosidases expressed by *Streptococcus pneumoniae*. *Mol Microbiol* 2006;**59**:961–74.
124. Burnaugh AM, Frantz LJ, King SJ. Growth of *Streptococcus pneumoniae* on human glycoconjugates is dependent upon the sequential activity of bacterial exoglycosidases. *J Bacteriol* 2008;**190**:221–30.
125. Renzi F, Manfredi P, Mally M, Moes S, Jenö P, Cornelis GR. The N-glycan glycoprotein deglycosylation complex (Gpd) from *Capnocytophaga canimorsus* deglycosylates human IgG. *PLoS Pathog* 2011;**7**:e1002118.

CHAPTER

19

Pathogenic Exploitation of Fc Activity

Scott B. Halstead

Dengue Vaccine Initiative, International Vaccine Institute, Seoul, Korea

INTRODUCTION

The phenomenon of antibody-dependent enhancement (ADE) underlies severe diseases across the entire spectrum of both microbes and vertebrates. Indeed, ADE could be classified as a fifth type of immunopathology (Table 19.1): Type I, IgE-mediated immediate hypersensitivity; Type II, IgG-mediated acute immune complex disease; Type III, IgG-mediated foreign antigen-complement-dependent immune complex disease; Type IV, cell-mediated immune and autoimmune diseases; and Type V, infectious immune complex enhancement of microbial infection in FcR-bearing cells.

Over the past four decades, different lines of scientific inquiry have coalesced to sharpen our understanding of antibody-mediated mechanisms that govern the severity of infections by a wide spectrum of microorganisms. Independent studies of host responses to acute and chronic human and animal infectious diseases have generated evidence that cross-linking of immune complexes with Fcγ receptors can increase intracellular infection and contribute to disease severity.[1,2] One of the earliest descriptions of this activity came from neutralization studies of Murray Valley encephalitis virus (MVEV), in which exposure to virus in the presence of dilute avian antibodies resulted in greater clearance of chick embryo fibroblast monolayers than virus-only controls.[3,4] While follow-up research in the 1960s suggested that this phenomenon resulted from the stabilization of MVEV by antibodies,[5] a different explanation emerged when sequential infections in humans with dengue viruses (DENVs) were shown to produce severe disease (dengue hemorrhagic fever, DHF).[6,7–10]

During initial studies on ADE it had been assumed that increased virus output, which in some cases approached 100- to 1000-fold, resulted from extrinsic phenomena, such as the avid attachment to monocytes and macrophage and increased internalization of infectious immune complexes via interactions with FcγI and FcγIIa receptors as compared to virus alone, which was observed in numerous systems.[9–15] However, this effect of IgG opsonization can be complemented by a complex phenomenon involving suppression of innate cellular immunity. Unexpectedly, the incubation of Ross River virus (RRV) with diluted RRV antiserum resulted in enhanced infection in mouse macrophage cell lines and in primary human monocytes/macrophages via innate

TABLE 19.1 The Five Types of Human Immunopathology

Type	Mechanism	Target
I	IgE antibodies	Antigens/mast cells
II	IgG antibodies	Autoantigens/tissue cells
III	IgG antibodies	Foreign antigens/PMNs
IV	Cell-mediated immunity	Tissue cells
"V"	IgG antibodies	Microbe/FcR-bearing cells

immune suppression involving reduced production of reactive nitrogen radicals via NOS2 and a downregulation of TNF-α and IFN-β production through abolished interferon regulatory factor 1 (IRF-1) and nuclear factor-κB gene expression. Remarkably, a marked increase in IL-10 gene transcription and protein production was observed.[16,17] Surprisingly, ligation of FcγR by zymosan–antibody complexes in the presence of RRV did not exhibit the same transcription patterns, indicating that features of the opsonized pathogen were involved in driving immune suppression.[17]

Similarly, many investigators showed that IgG bound to the surface of *Leishmania* amastigotes (the intracellular mammalian host-dwelling parasite stage) can induce the cytokine IL-10, which, in turn, can suppress the protective immune response to the parasite by downregulating inducible NO synthase (iNOS) and by inhibiting Th1 cell development and IFN-γ production.[18,19] Hence, the IgG response, which is usually protective, is usurped by the parasite for its survival. When T-cell immunity fails, in the presence of abundant IgG anti-amastigote antibodies, infection starts on a lethal course. Thus, ADE is a complex phenomenon in which antibody-mediated interactions with Fc receptors may be involved not only in altering pathogen uptake into macrophage or monocytes but also in the cellular response to internalized pathogen.

ADE IN VIRUSES

Antibody-enhanced viral infections require an initial adaptive immunological event, termed *sensitization*, which occurs in three settings: (1) Primary infections with naturally occurring heterotypic viruses of the same genera; (2) infection by viruses that create antigenic diversity by the rapid evolution of biologic or antigenic variants during the course of a chronic infection; and (3) immunizations that result in incomplete protective immunity (Table 19.2) (reviewed in Halstead[11,20,22] and Tirado and Yoon[21]). The ADE phenomenon has attracted wide interest in virology because many viruses replicate in macrophages *in vivo* and manifest antibody-enhanced infections/disease.[21,23,24]

Group 1: Dengue

The dengue viruses (DENVs) are a group of four closely related members of the *Flavivirus* genus. DENVs 1 through 4 share 60 to 70% genetic homology and are inoculated by the bite of an infected *Aedes aegypti* mosquito. Initial infections with any of the four DENVs raise protective but type-specific antibodies in addition to cross-reactive but non-neutralizing antibodies that may enhance infection by a different DENV type.[8,25–29] Indeed, infection-enhancing antibodies are a risk factor for enhanced dengue disease.[30] That infants regularly acquire severe dengue disease during their first dengue infection when maternal polyclonal dengue antibodies circulate below protective levels is a unique illustration of the ADE phenomenon in human medicine.[31–37] In humans, secondary dengue infections follow a stereotypical course with severe outcomes, including shock or gastrointestinal hemorrhage, accompanying vascular collapse that results from capillary permeability occurring around the time of defervescence.[38] High levels of viremia early in disease and high levels of

TABLE 19.2 Viruses Expressing ADE *In Vitro* or Producing Enhanced Disease

	Viruses	*In vitro* ADE	*In vivo* Enhanced Disease	Refs.
RNA Virus Group				
Picornaviridae	Coxsackie B	+	Animal model	Sauter and Hober[121]
Flaviviridae	Dengue	+	+	Halstead et al.,[7] Stueckemann et al.[122]
	LDH	+	–	
Coronaviridae	Feline infectious peritonitis	+	+	Weiss and Scott,[81] Olsen,[123] Yoon et al.[124]
	PRRSV	+	+	
	Simian HF	+	+	
Retroviridae	HIV	+	?	Burke,[125] Mdurvwa et al.,[126] Mealey et al.[127]
	Equine infectious anemia	+	+	
	Caprine arthritis	+	+	
DNA Virus Group				
Parvoviridae	Aleutian disease of mink	+	+	Porter et al.,[128] Kanno et al.,[129] Best and Bloom[130]
Asfarviridae	African swine fever			

Note: Sensitization results are from sequential or chronic infection with multiple naturally occurring antigenic types.

proinflammatory and immunomodulatory cytokines including IL-10 late in disease are associated with severe outcome.[39–41]

In vitro studies indicate that the major requirement for ADE activity is a sub-neutralizing antibody concentration.[22,42] In practice, antibodies directed at surface epitopes not involved in virus entry efficiently produce ADE.[43] In studies of ADE in the THP-1 cell model (human monocytic Fcγ receptor-bearing continuous cell line) intracellular DENV production was increased as a result of idiosyncratic Fcγ receptor signaling.[44] When immune complexes ligate FcγRI and FcγRIIA, at least two types of suppression pathways are expressed (Figure 19.1). Collectively, these pathways downregulate antiviral responses in ADE-infected target cells. As a result, ADE-infected THP-1 cells secreted reduced levels of type-I IFN and at the same time suppressed the transcription and translation of IL-12, IFN-γ and TNF-α, facilitating expression and synthesis of the antiinflammatory cytokines. ADE infection also suppressed the innate anti-DENV mediator, nitric oxide radicals, by disrupting the transcription of the iNOS gene transcription factor, IRF-1,[44] believed to be mediated by IL-10.[45] It can be concluded that *in vitro* ADE infection not only facilitates viral entry but also modifies innate and adaptive intracellular antiviral mechanisms resulting in enhanced DENV replication.

Critically, the same responses are observed *in vivo*. Genome-wide transcriptomes from peripheral blood mononuclear cells (PBMCs) collected during the acute phase from children with dengue fever (DF) or dengue hemorrhagic fever (DHF) indicated that patients with DHF had decreased levels of NO, reduced IFN transcript, and increased IL-10 blood levels compared to patients with milder illness.[46] In other

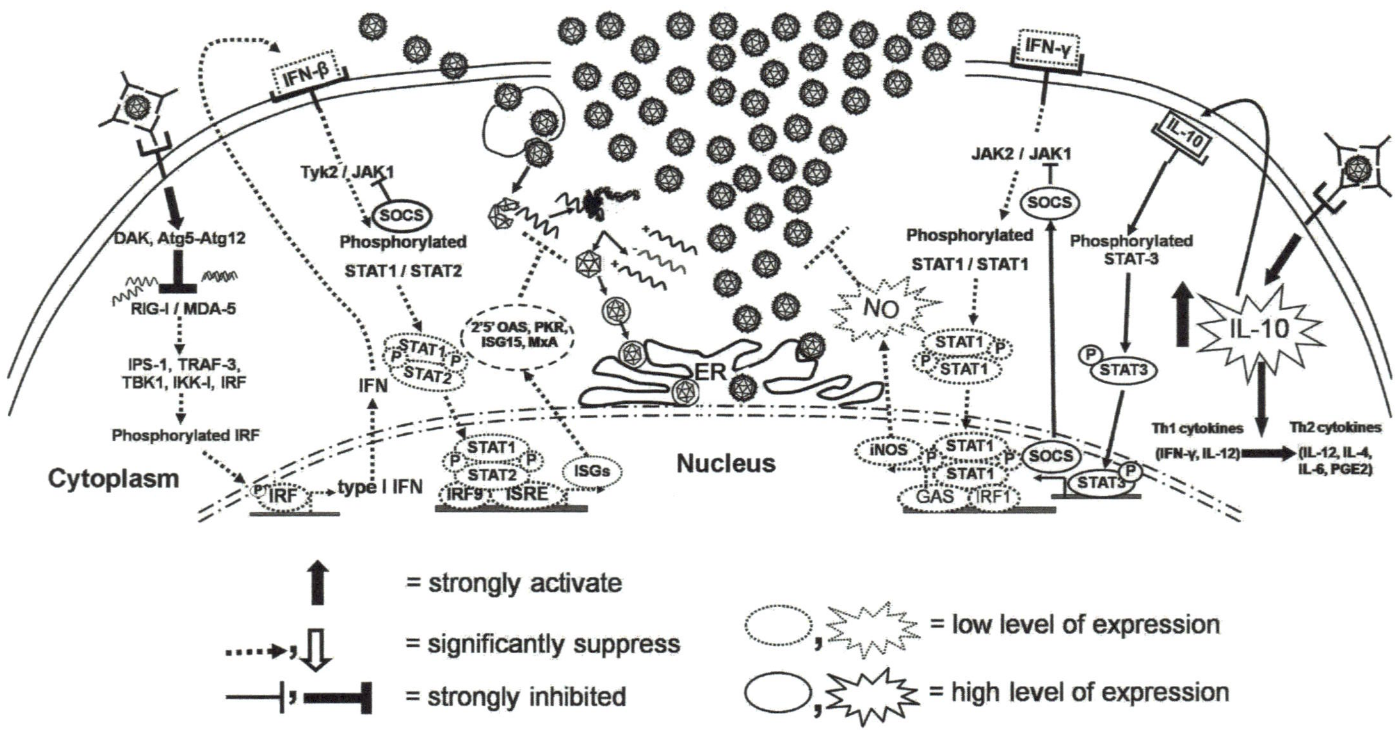

FIGURE 19.1 **The two-loop model of ADE.** Ligation of FcγR by infectious DENV-subneutralizing antibody complex induces suppression of innate immune responses: (1) By upregulation of negative regulators of pathogen pattern recognition, DAK, Atg5-Atg12, SARM, and TANK, that subsequently abolish expression of RLR and TLRs and its signaling pathway, resulting in decreased type-1 interferon and proinflammatory cytokines production. These serve to suppress interferon-mediated antiviral responses. (2) By early activation of IL-10, which potently activates the SOCS system suppressing the JAK/STAT signaling pathway and, in turn, the interferon-signaling pathway. IL-10 is known to promote type Th2 cytokines response, resulting in Th2-type cytokine biasing. These two loops of suppression switch off intracellular antiviral responses in DENV-ADE-infected cells, resulting in the production of high numbers of infectious virions. *(From Ubol, S. and Halstead, S.B.,* Clin. Vaccine Immunol., **17***(12), 1829–1835, 2010. With permission.)*

studies, during the acute stage of severe disease increased production of IL-10 and downregulation of multiple IFN regulatory genes were noted.[47–49] The protective role of IFN in moderating dengue infection has been demonstrated in a mouse model and suggested for humans with DF.[50–52] The precise role of immune complex-elicited IL-10 production on the clinical evolution of severe dengue infections is not well understood but may be responsible for the observed Th1 to Th2 shift observed in DHF.[53]

Results obtained by studying ADE in continuous human FcR-bearing cells are subject to a critical caveat: Are responses observed faithful to those occurring *in vivo*? When dengue ADE was studied in four different primary human myeloid cells derived from the same peripheral blood leukocyte (PBL) donors, viral infection and cytokine responses differed significantly.[54] Human monocytes, activated macrophages, and mature dendritic cells (DCs) support ADE, while immature DCs did not. Infection of macrophages by DENV 2 alone or as fully neutralized immune complexes stimulated high levels of α and β IFN, and these were downmodulated under ADE conditions and replaced by secretion of IL-6 and TNF-α. Type I IFNs were neither produced nor suppressed by ADE infection of monocytes with DENV 2.[54,55] However, during ADE infection of primary monocytes, IL-10 synthesis peaked at the same serum dilution that produced peak virus yield.[54] The precise mechanisms fueling enhanced production of dengue virus in monocytes and macrophages require further study, as neither the production of IL-10 nor suppression of type I interferon is critical to the ADE phenomenon. There is some evidence that the degree of antibody opsonization may impact FcγR interactions, resulting in differential processing of surface-bound virus. In particular, in the THP-1 model, large immune complexes have been found to stimulate FcγIIB, resulting in inhibition of cellular uptake.[56]

In considering the contribution of FcR-mediated phenomena during the course of acute infectious diseases it is important to note the differing kinetics of microbial invasion and response to infection. Infections in vertebrates can be divided into *afferent* and *efferent* events. *Afferent* events are those that relate to the invasion, propagation, and survival of infecting organisms. *Efferent* events are those contributing to reduce, retard, and eliminate infecting organisms. For those infections that produce disease, afferent events successfully predominate during the early stages, while efferent events may culminate in elimination of invading organism and cure. In the ADE phenomenon, IgG antibodies residual from a previous dengue infection, whether actively produced or passively acquired, act as powerful afferent events. IgM and, in the case of secondary dengue infections, IgG dengue antibodies play important roles in the efferent events of dengue infections, some of which include clearing extracellular virus, activating complement, and mediating ADCC.

In dengue-endemic countries, second heterotypic dengue infections are responsible for up to 95% of DHF, while primary dengue infections in infants account for the remainder.[57,58] The *in vitro* ADE literature makes it clear that antibodies to virtually any flavivirus can enhance dengue virus infection in FcR-bearing cells.[59] In Southeast Asia, the dengue viruses co-circulate with Japanese encephalitis (JE); in India, with JE and West Nile; in Pakistan, with West Nile; in Australia, with the Kunjin strain of West Nile; and, in most of the American region, yellow fever or use of yellow fever 17D vaccine. A direct examination of enhancement of DENV 2 infections in a human monocytic cell line by antibodies raised in humans who had experienced apparent wild-type JE infections was negative.[60] However, this study screened for ADE at just a single high dilution of serum. There have been no reports of enhancement of dengue infections by prior West Nile or yellow fever infections (or vaccination); however, recently it was observed that children in Thailand who had either had wild-type JE infections or were immunized with killed JE vaccine experienced a mild overt dengue disease at a higher frequency than when the same dengue virus infected susceptible individuals.[61] Not only did dengue infections in JE-immunes increase the frequency of mild overt dengue disease, but the ensuing illness lasted two times longer than dengue illnesses in susceptibles. Prior to this observation it was thought that JE vaccination actually reduced the severity of DHF accompanying a second dengue infection.[62]

Second DENV infections can occur in 12 combinations, at least 10 of which have been documented to result in hospitalized disease.[58] Human experimentation has established that there is a DENV infection refractory period of three months following an initial DENV infection. As presented briefly above, shortly after a primary DENV infection abundant heterotypic antibodies may form large immune aggregates that are neutralized in solution but not eliminated by standard phagocytic clearance by macrophages.[56] After the refractory period, second dengue infections occur and some are expressed as clinical illness. Varying amounts of heterotypic neutralizing antibodies are raised following a primary dengue infection. The natural histories of antibody responses following infection by DENVs 1, 2, 3, or 4 including heterotypic antibodies are essentially unknown. Heterotypic antibodies are critically important in modulation of a second DENV infection.[30] Low dilutions of preinfection sera from children who had unapparent secondary DENV 2 infections almost invariably reduced or neutralized DENV 2 in primary human monocytes, while preinfection sera from children who developed an illness requiring hospitalization had few or no detectable heterotypic neutralizing antibodies.[30] This observation suggests that low levels of heterotypic neutralizing antibodies (most were anti-DENV 1) did not prevent but downregulated DENV 2 clinical responses. Around one-fifth of monotypically dengue-immune schoolchildren lacked heterotypic DENV 2 antibodies and developed DHF when infected by DENV 2. This is virtually the same ratio for the occurrence of dengue shock syndrome (DSS) during sequential DENV 1 then DENV 2 in Rayong, Thailand.[63]

The sequence of infection may be highly determinative of disease severity. Only secondary DENV 2 infections were pathogenic in the 1980 cohort study at Rayong, Thailand.[63] The specific infection sequences associated with DSS cases were known from virus isolations in acute-phase sera and antibodies in pre-illness sera or by applying the original antigenic sin phenomenon to paired sera.[64] Although secondary DENV 1 infections were most common that year, DSS occurred only during secondary DENV 2 infections. Burmese workers came to a similar conclusion in their 1984 to 1988 longitudinal seroepidemiological study in Yangon, Myanmar.[65] By contrast, in an Indonesian study, DSS was associated with sequences ending in DENV 1, 3, and 4, but not DENV 2, even though secondary DENV 2 infections were common.[66] DENV 3 was associated with an outbreak of DHF/DSS on Tahiti in a population that had prior infection experience with DENV 1 and DENV 2.[67] Also on Tahiti in 2001, DENV 1 infections resulted in DHF/DSS in 4–11 year-old children who were immune to DENV 2.[68] Over time the pathogenicity of established DENV infection sequences may change. Notably, there was a rapid increase in pathogenic expression of secondary DENV 2 infections (in DENV 1-immunes) month to month in Cuba.[69] Complete and partial sequencing of DENV 2 viruses isolated from the beginning to the end of this outbreak identified no structural genetic mutations but consistent amino acid changes at position 69 in the NS1 protein.[70,71] A more complex study in Managua, Nicaragua, attributed year-to-year increases in disease pathogenic expression to a combination of genetic changes in DENV 2 and a waning DENV 1 immunity in the affected children.[72] Essentially none of these field observations has been subjected to study using cultures of primary human myeloid cells.

From the work cited above it must be concluded that ADE studies should not be performed on continuous human myeloid cells but instead on characterized primary human myeloid cells. To date, all research has been carried out using DENV 2. Studies of ADE should be extended as quickly as possible to the complete range of dengue viruses using type-specific polyclonal human antibodies rather than mouse or even human monoclonal antibodies. More observations on human dengue illnesses are needed to better understand the ADE phenomenon. In this context, understanding DHF in infants that accompanies primary DENV infections acquired during the latter half of the first year of life is important and has attracted recent research interest.[33,34] This unique clinical phenomenon illustrates not only the role played by dengue antibodies in modulating disease expression but also their bifurcated role—protection for several months after birth at high concentrations and enhancing infections some months later at sub-neutralizing concentrations. The contribution of immature DENV particles to ADE is of interest. Immature DEN virions are not infectious for human myeloid cells, but in the presence of enhancing dengue antibodies ADE infection occurs readily.[43,73] It has been surmised that immature DENV are released into circulation during human infections as antibodies to prM (immature DENV antigen) and are frequently observed.[43]

Note has been made above of the possible role of different Fcγ receptors in mediating ADE in macrophages in leishmania mouse models and the interesting observation suggesting that ligation of FcγRIIB may affect the fate of large immune complexes during the immune clearance phase of dengue infections. The real research challenge is to document the critical Fcγ receptors that are operative during human or veterinary clinical microbial disease enhancement episodes. But, more important will be to study the specific outcome of ADE infection by different wild-type dengue viruses—antibody combinations including appropriate genotype variants. The possibility that differing combinations of DENV and dengue antibodies (or, for that matter, antibodies to other flaviviruses) have uniquely different effects on monocyte/macrophage innate immunity requires careful study.

It is widely held that the process of eliminating dengue virus-infected cells generates a cascade of chemokines and cytokines that contribute to the pathophysiology of dengue disease syndromes. This has been termed "a perfect cytokine storm."[74] Given the evidence of increased infected cell mass in severe dengue infections, the cytokines generated by virus infection and by interactions between virus-infected cells and the host immune response would appear to be quantitatively proportional to viral load and not exaggerated or "abnormal." Because dengue is not a cytophilic virus, cellular infection proceeds until the infected cell is eliminated. A wide misconception is that peak viremia, which occurs early in infection, represents peak "viral load." In fact, the quantity of virus in blood during the course of infection only describes the kinetics of extracellular virus clearance. Using the sensitive technique of intrathoracic inoculation of *Toxorrhynchites splendens* mosquitoes,[40,75] it was observed that dengue virus could be detected in nearly all plasma samples collected within 72 hours of the onset of fever. The frequency of virus isolation declined rapidly and virus was usually not present at defervescence.[76] Viremia was of longer duration in individuals experiencing primary dengue virus infections than in those experiencing secondary dengue virus infections, and the slope of the decline in virus titer was greater in individuals with DHF than in those with DF.[40] The most important mechanism of extracellular virus clearance is thought to be IgM and IgG dengue antibodies, although T lymphocytes and antibody-dependent cell killing may contribute by attacking and destroying virus-infected cells. As discussed above, it is likely that elimination of dengue virus-infected cells continues well after onset of antibody production resulting in peak cellular infection (viral load) at around the time of defervescence and cellular infection is not eliminated until well after end of viremia. Of interest, a major effort failed to detect circulating CD8+ T cells during the late acute-illness phase of DHF patients.[77] This suggested to the authors that CD8+ T cells might be located only in the tissues where dengue virus replication had occurred. Alternatively, as in a Japanese encephalitis model, the antibody component of the adaptive immune response may play a much more important role in terminating dengue infections than heretofore thought.[78]

Groups 2 and 3

Feline infectious peritonitis virus (FIPV) is an example of Group 2/3 virus immunopathology involving ADE (Table 19.2). Feline coronaviruses circulate as two forms: Feline enteric coronavirus (FECV) is a pathogen of minor significance; however, a spontaneous mutation of this virus yields FIPV, which is capable of replicating in peritoneal macrophages and producing peritonitis and occasionally FIP, a fatal Arthus-like pyogranulomatous disease in kittens and cats. ADE has been incriminated as a disease-enhancing factor.[79–81] That antibodies are pathogenic is evidenced by observations that kittens who have acquired passive maternal FIPV antibodies develop a more rapid and fulminant disease following challenge with FIPV than do seronegatives.[81] Disease enhancement has been demonstrated in cats that were infected in the presence of vaccine-derived humoral immunity directed against the spike protein of FIPV (Table 19.3).[82] Similarly, cats immunized with a recombinant vaccinia virus

TABLE 19.3 Enhanced Viral Diseases Resulting from Sensitization by Administration of Vaccines

	Viruses	*In vitro* ADE	*In vivo* Enhanced Disease	Refs.
RNA Virus Group				
Orthomyxoviridae	Influenza A	+	+ (mouse model)	Webster and Askonas[131]
Paramyxoviridae	RSV	+	+	Chanock and Parrott,[132] Fulginiti et al.[133]
	Measles	+	+	
Rhabdoviridae	Rabies	+	+ (accelerated disease onset)	King et al.,[134] Prabhakar and Nathanson[135]
Coronaviridae	Feline infectious peritonitis	+	+	Tirado and Yoon,[21] Weiss and Scott,[81]
	PRRSV	+	+	Yoon et al.[124]
	Simian HF	+	+	
Retroviridae	HIV	+	?	Mdurvwa et al.,[126] Mealey et al.,[127] Burke[125]
	Equine infectious anemia	+	+	
	Caprine arthritis	+	+	
DNA Virus Group				
Parvoviridae	Aleutian disease of mink	+	+	Porter et al.[128]

expressing the spike protein of FIPV died earlier than control animals.[82] In adult cats, FIPV develops during chronic infections with feline coronaviruses after FECV mutates to FIPV, gaining macrophage tropism.[83] As antibody responses are mounted to FIPV, infection and disease severity are enhanced.[79] In summary, antibody responses to FIPV occurring during the course of infection, passive transfer of antibodies from natural infections, and immunization with killed or recombinant vaccines all have led to enhanced FIPV disease. Enhanced disease severity has been attributed largely to the presence of non-neutralizing antibodies.

ADE IN PROTOZOAN PARASITES OF MACROPHAGES: *LEISHMANIA*

Leishmaniasis is caused by protozoan parasites of the genus *Leishmania* which are transmitted by the bite of certain species of sandfly. Human infection is caused by about 21 of 30 *Leishmania* species that infect mammals. The disease exists in two major forms, cutaneous and visceral leishmaniasis. Visceral leishmaniasis (VL) is the most severe form of leishmaniasis and the second largest parasitic killer in the world after malaria, responsible for an estimated 500,000 cases each year worldwide. Leishmania are transmitted by sandflies as promastigotes, motile forms that parasitize macrophages and spread within hosts as amastigotes, which are obligate parasites of macrophages. In human hosts the responses to infection by *Leishmania* vary with species and the patient's immune reaction. Patients whose lymphocytes produce amounts of IFN-γ from Th1-type T cells often recover from cutaneous infection on their own and after recovery are immune to reinfection. Patients infected with visceral forms of the parasite make high levels of anti-parasite antibody that does not contribute to host defense. Without treatment, these patients are likely to succumb to VL. Mouse models exist for the study of cutaneous and VL. For example, normal BALB/c mice are susceptible to this disease and develop progressive non-healing lesions with numerous intracellular parasites within macrophages. Despite the presence of high levels of anti-parasite antibody, mimicking human VL, these parasites often disseminate to the liver, spleen, and bone marrow. *In vitro* models are also available—promastigote or amastigote infections in cultures of bone marrow or peritoneal macrophages from mice or in differentiated peripheral blood human monocytes.

During the 1980s and 1990s a number of mammalian cytokines were discovered; among them was mouse cytokine synthesis inhibitory factor produced by Th2 cells, later renamed IL-10.[84,85] IL-10 is a type II cytokine and the "founding" member of a family of cytokines that includes IL-19, IL-20, IL-22, IL-24, IL-26, IL-28, and IL-29.[86] All of these cytokines have similar intron–exon genomic organization, bind to receptors with similar structures and in some cases shared components, and all activate Janus kinase (JAK)/signal transducer and activator of transcription (STAT) signaling pathways. IL-10 is capable of inhibiting synthesis of pro-inflammatory cytokines such as IFN-γ, IL-2, IL-3, IL-12, TNF-α, and GM-CSF. IL-10 also displays a potent ability to suppress the antigen presentation capacity of antigen-presenting cells. There are, however, some settings in which IL-10 is not immunosuppressive. IL-10 can enhance NK and B-cell survival and B-cell antibody production.[87] IL-10 is made by macrophages, and a variety of T cells, including T reg, Th1, Th2, and Th17.[88]

IL-10 plays important roles in regulating immune responses and it can also increase host susceptibility to intracellular infections. In the mouse model of cutaneous leishmaniasis susceptibility of *Leishmania major* is associated with Th2 responses. $CD4^+$ T cells from susceptible BALB/c mice produced IL-4 and IL-10 when infected with *L. major*, while $CD4^+$ T cells from resistant C57BL/6 mice expressed IFN-γ and

IL-2.[89] The transient depletion of $CD4^+$ cells or the *in vivo* neutralization of IL-4 in BALB/c mice promoted the killing of intracellular parasites and healing of leishmanial lesions. IL-4 was not the only determinant of susceptibility, however, because susceptible BALB/c mice lacking IL-10 were fully resistant to infection.[18] Furthermore, in humans where the Th1/Th2 dichotomy is not as pronounced, IL-10 appears to be a major inducer of susceptibility. In humans with visceral leishmaniasis (VL), IL-10 levels in plasma directly correlate with disease severity.[90] IL-10 was identified in lymph nodes taken from patients with VL.[91] PBMCs from acute visceral leishmaniasis responded to stimulation with leishmania lysate by producing IL-10 mRNA. IL-10, when added to PBMCs, suppressed production of IFN-γ and IL-2 but after treatment with anti-IL-10 PBMCs from patients with acute VL demonstrated a marked increase in proliferative response to leishmania lysate. In *vitro* studies of *Leishmania*-infected peritoneal and bone marrow macrophages demonstrated that the intracellular killing of this organism by classically activated macrophages could be inhibited by the administration of exogenous IL-10[92,93] or by endogenous macrophage production of IL-10.[92]

Greater clarity was achieved when the reciprocal actions of IL-12 and IL-10 were recognized. The complementary cytokine IL-12 acts directly on $CD4^+$ T cells to enhance priming for IFN-γ production and reverse IL-4 priming.[94] The most potent cytokine for the induction of leishmanicidal activity in macrophages is IFN-γ.[95] The sustained production of IFN-γ in response to infection is commonly associated with the development of specific Th1 T-cell responses. Administration of IL-12 increased IFN-γ production and reduced the severity of *Leishmania major* infections in mice and potentiated vaccine-derived immunity and depressed IL-10 production.[96] However, exposure of macrophages from susceptible mice to opsonized *Leishmania* promastigotes suppressed the expression of IL-12.[97]

The importance of macrophage receptors in the generation of cytokines in *Leishmania*-infected macrophages was recognized when IL-12 production in BALB/c mouse bone marrow macrophages in response to LPS was suppressed after ligation of FcR, complement or scavenger receptors.[98] Both mRNA synthesis and protein secretion were diminished to near-undetectable levels following receptor ligation. Suppression was specific to IL-12 since TNF-α production was not inhibited. Also, the ligation of mouse FcγR with immune complexes was shown to enhance the production of IL-10.[99] Stimulation of mouse bone marrow macrophages by LPS resulted in some IL-10 production, but the addition of RBC opsonized with IgG antibodies dramatically enhanced IL-10 production. Immune complexes not only induce activated macrophages to produce IL-10 but also induce both macrophages and dendritic cells to switch off their production of IL-12.[98,100]

The modulation of IL-10 and IL-12 in macrophages results from different mechanisms.[101] Whereas the abrogation of IL-12 biosynthesis was a property shared by ligation of several macrophage receptors, the induction of IL-10 was specific to FcγRs. Additional evidence for the role of IL-10 in supporting chronicity of infection was obtained when normal BALB/c mice developed progressive non-healing lesions with numerous *Leishmania major* parasites while $IL-10^{-/-}$ BALB/c mice controlled disease progression and had relatively small lesions with 1000-fold fewer parasites at the fifth week of infection.[18] Furthermore, in established *L. donovani* visceral infection in normal mice, anti-IL-10 or anti-IL-10 receptor monoclonal antibody (mAb) treatment successfully induced intracellular parasite killing within liver macrophages.[102] These and other studies showed that amastigotes of *Leishmania* exploit an unusual and unexpected virulence factor, host IgG. When the surface of *Leishmania* amastigotes is coated with IgG, the resultant immune complexes allow them to ligate

Fcγ receptors on inflammatory macrophages, preferentially inducing the production of high amounts of IL-10. The IL-10 induction by IgG–amastigotes did not occur in macrophages from mice lacking the common gamma chain that signals through FcγRs 1, 3, and 4, indicating that one or all three of these receptors were involved. Subsequent studies using defined immune complexes demonstrated that all three of the FcγRs that signal through gamma were capable of signaling for IL-10 production in macrophages.[103] The implication from these studies is that in some settings IgG itself biases the immune response toward a Th2-type response. Indeed, for some species of *Leishmania*, chronicity of infection requires that amastigotes be coated with IgG.[104] This phenomenon is now very well established.[93,105,106]

That IL-10 induction by ligation of FcγR was a generic process was demonstrated with a non-microbial antigen.[107] Lipopolysaccharide-treated BALB/c mouse macrophages when exposed to ovalbumin (OVA) alone developed T-cell responses driven to Th-1 and characterized by the production of IFN-γ. When the same antigen was complexed with IgG anti-OVA, T-cell responses were driven to Th2 and produced IL-4. This Th2-like phenotype was stable and was retained when the T cells were subsequently restimulated under non-biasing conditions. Mice vaccinated with IgG-opsonized OVA made high levels of IgG Abs of the IgG_1 isotype. The T-cell biasing and its reversal via FcγR ligation was also observed *in vivo*. Using macrophages from gene knockout mice, the production of IFN-γ and IL-4 by T cells was shown to be controlled by the macrophage cytokines, IL-12 and IL-10, respectively. These and other studies demonstrate that the ligation of FcγR on activated macrophages reverses Th1 biasing that accompanies innate immune responses to microbial products.

Importantly, in patients with VL, high levels of anti-leishmanial antibodies correlate with peak parasitemia and with negative DTH responses.[93] Successful treatment of leishmaniasis with amphotericin resulted in decreased antibody titers and a restoration of DTH responses. Earlier observations identified polyclonal B-cell activation and high levels of immune complexes as well as rheumatoid factor in patients with VL.[108] Humans infected with *Leishmania donovani* had higher frequencies of rheumatoid arthritis.[109] In experimental models of VL, infected hamsters develop immune complex glomerulonephritis. These observations have been widely confirmed in mouse models. In addition to *Leishmania donovoni* and *L. major*, humoral immune responses against *L. mexicana* were not effective at killing organisms hiding in parasitophorous vacuoles because host IgG-coated amastigotes generated immunosuppressive IL-10 responses by infected macrophages.[19,110] A similar observation, although perhaps occurring by a different mechanism, may be involved in *L. amazonensis*-infected JhD mice in which infections were minimized in the absence of B cells or antibodies. When these immune elements were restored leishmania lesions progressed by a process thought to involve $CD4^+$ T cells.[111]

How do antibody-coated amastigotes result in the production of IL-10 by macrophages? Ligation of macrophage FcγR produces a rapid and enhanced activation of two MAPKs, ERK and p38.[112] The activation of ERK leads to the phosphorylation of serine 10 on histone H3 at the *IL-10* gene, making the promoter more accessible to transcription factors generated in response to p38 activation.[95] Activation of both MAPKs was required for IL-10 synthesis. In addition to ERK activation, an inflammatory stimulus, such as low-molecular-weight hyaluronic acid from the extracellular matrix, must also be present. The combination of these two signals resulted in the superinduction of IL-10.[113] Macrophages lacking FcγR, or macrophages treated with an inhibitor of spleen tyrosine kinase that is activated following FcγR ligation, failed to activate ERK and consequently failed to produce IL-10 following infection with *Leishmania* amastigotes.

Recently, however, it has been observed that IgG_1 and $IgG_{2a/c}$ induce IL-10 from mouse macrophages *in vitro* equally well but through different FcγR subtypes: IgG_1 through FcγRIII, and $IgG_{2a/c}$ through FcγRI primarily but also through FcγRIII. In sharp contrast, mice lacking IgG_1 develop earlier and stronger $IgG_{2a/c}$, IgG_3, and IgM responses to *Leishmania mexicana* infection and yet are more resistant to the infection.[114] Thus, IgG_1, but not $IgG_{2a/c}$ or IgG_3, is pathogenic *in vivo*, in agreement with prior studies indicating that FcγRIII is required for chronic disease. This calls into question the assumption that mouse macrophages, which should secrete IL-10 in response to both IgG_1 and $IgG_{2a/c}$ immune complexes, are the most important source of IL-10 generated by IgG–FcγR engagement in *L. mexicana* infection.

ADE IN OTHER INTRACELLULAR PARASITES AND BACTERIA

The possibility that FcR-mediated enhancement of disease occurs across a broad range of microorganisms has received little attention by research communities. The possibility that ADE contributes to severity or chronicity of disease exists because a large number of bacteria replicate partially or solely in human macrophages. Larger microorganisms that infect macrophages, "professional intracellular pathogens," often produce chronic infections. Indeed, one of the criteria of successful parasitism by microorganisms that produce systemic infections may be the ability to evade macrophage microbicidal mechanisms. These defensive mechanisms have been subject to intensive scrutiny.[115] Both chronic infections and an antigenic relatedness between microorganisms may contribute to the formation of pathogenic IgG immune complexes controlling microbial survival. Infections that may be analogous to the *Leishmania* model include *Mycobacterium tuberculosis* (Mtb), *Mycobacterium leprae*, *Legionella pneumophila*, *Listeria monocytogenes*, *Brucella* spp., *Salmonella* spp., *Shigella* spp., *Coxiella burnetii*, *Anaplasma phagocytophilum*, and *Ehrlichia chaffeensis*, as well as another protozoan, *Toxoplasma gondii*, and fungi (e.g., *Histoplasma capsulatum*).

The role of Fc receptors or immune complexes in mediating immunopathology has not been studied exhaustively for most of the organisms on the above list; however, interesting findings have been made in tuberculosis. Although studies on resistance to tuberculosis have centered on T-cell immunity, in a recent experiment C57BL/6 mice deficient in inhibitory FcγRIIB showed improved bacterial control and diminished pathology at 30 but not 20 days following aerosol challenge with *Mycobacterium tuberculosis*.[116] Enhanced production of IL-12p40 was observed in $Fc\gamma RIIB^{-/-}$ mice. IL-12 and IL-23 share the common subunit IL-12p40 and both promote the polarization of naive $CD4^+$ T cells into Th1 effectors.[117] Treatment of human macrophages with exogenous IL-12 combined with blockade of IL-27 reduced the burden of mycobacterial infection.[118] These infections were characterized by enhanced protective IFN-γ responses that coincided with heightened activation of macrophages. In humans, elevated levels of IL-10 correlate with the suppression of host defenses and exacerbation of infection.[119] In a model of reactivation tuberculosis the presence of macrophage-derived IL-10 in the lungs of infected transgenic mice permitted Th1 cells to efficiently express effector functions and secrete sufficient IFN-γ to induce classical macrophage activation characterized by expression of NOS2 and LRG-47.[120] However, mycobacteria survived and successfully proliferated within mouse macrophages with IL-10 production under control of a human CD68 promoter. Macrophage-derived IL-10 appears to override IFN-γ-dependent classical macrophage activation and other effector mechanisms against Mtb by inducing an alternatively activated phenotype. To date, an explicit contribution of Mtb–IgG antibody complexes toward modulation of infections in model systems has not been reported.

CONCLUDING THOUGHTS

Successful pathogens are armed with an array of weapons, including penetration and cell attachment factors and a galaxy of defenses against innate immune responses. Much is known and there is still much to learn about the offensive attributes of microbial pathogens. However, because of the ADE phenomena, antibodies very likely complement and contribute a generic and thus far poorly explored afferent disease mechanism for many infectious diseases in addition to the examples cited here. Cognizance of the need to balance protective and potentially harmful antibody activities remains an important concern in vaccine development.

References

1. Halstead SB, Mahalingam S, Marovich MA, Ubol S, Mosser DM. Intrinsic antibody-dependent enhancement of microbial infection in macrophages: disease regulation by immune complexes. *Lancet Infect Dis* 2010;**10**(10):712–22.
2. Ubol S, Halstead SB. How innate immune mechanisms contribute to antibody-enhanced viral infections. *Clin Vaccine Immunol* 2010;**17**(12):1829–35.
3. Hawkes RA. Enhancement of the infectivity of arboviruses by specific antisera produced in domestic fowls. *Aust J Exp Biol Med Sci* 1964;**42**:465–82.
4. Kliks S, Halstead SB. An explanation for enhanced virus plaque formation in chick embryo cells. *Nature* 1980;**285**:504–5.
5. Hawkes RA, Lafferty KJ. The enhancement of virus infectivity by antibody. *Virology* 1967;**33**:250–61.
6. Halstead SB, Nimmannitya S, Yamarat C, Russell PK. Hemorrhagic fever in Thailand; recent knowledge regarding etiology. *Jpn J Med Sci Biol* 1967;**20**(Suppl):96–103.
7. Halstead SB, Chow J, Marchette NJ. Immunologic enhancement of dengue virus replication. *Nat New Biol* 1973;**243**(122):24–6.
8. Halstead SB, O'Rourke EJ. Antibody-enhanced dengue virus infection in primate leukocytes. *Nature* 1977;**265**(5596):739–41.
9. Halstead SB, O'Rourke EJ. Dengue viruses and mononuclear phagocytes. I. Infection enhancement by non-neutralizing antibody. *J Exp Med* 1977;**146**:201–17.
10. Halstead SB, O'Rourke EJ, Allison AC. Dengue viruses and mononuclear phagocytes. II. Identity of blood and tissue leukocytes supporting *in vitro* infection. *J Exp Med* 1977;**146**:218–28.
11. Halstead SB. Immune enhancement of viral infection. *Prog Allergy* 1982;**31**:301–64.
12. Gollins SW, Porterfield JS. Flavivirus infection enhancement in macrophages: radioactive and biological studies on the effect of antibody on virus fate. *J Gen Virol* 1984;**65**:1261–72.
13. Gollins SW, Porterfield JS. Flavivirus infection enhancement in macrophages: an electron microscopic study of viral cellular entry. *J Gen Virol* 1985;**66**:1969–82.
14. Olsen C, Scott F. Evaluation of antibody-dependent enhancement of feline infectious peritonitis virus infectivity using *in situ* hybridization. *Microb Pathog* 1993;**14**(4):275–85.
15. Robinson Jr WE, Montefiori DC, Gillespie DH, Mitchell WM. Complement-mediated, antibody-dependent enhancement of HIV-1 infection *in vitro* is characterized by increased protein and RNA syntheses and infectious virus release. *JAIDS* 1989;**2**(1):33–42.
16. Lidbury BA, Mahalingam S. Specific ablation of antiviral gene expression in macrophages by antibody-dependent enhancement of ross river virus infection. *J Virol* 2000;**74**(18):8376–81.
17. Suhrbier A, La Linn M. Suppression of antiviral responses by antibody-dependent enhancement of macrophage infection. *Trends Immunol* 2003;**24**(4):165–8.
18. Kane MM, Mosser DM. The role of IL-10 in promoting disease progression in leishmaniasis. *J Immunol* 2001;**166**:1141–7.
19. Buxbaum LU, Scott P. Interleukin 10- and Fcgamma receptor-deficient mice resolve *Leishmania mexicana* lesions. *Infect Immun* 2005;**73**(4):2101–8.
20. Halstead SB. Antibody-dependent enhancement of infection: a mechanism for indirect virus entry into cells. In: Wimmer E, editor. *Cellular Receptors for Animal Viruses*. Cold Spring Harbor, NY: Cold Spring Harbor Laboratory Press; 1994. p. 493–515.
21. Tirado SM, Yoon KJ. Antibody-dependent enhancement of virus infection and disease. *Viral Immunol* 2003;**16**(1):69–86.
22. Halstead SB. Neutralization and antibody dependent enhancement of dengue viruses. *Adv Virus Res* 2003;**60**:421–67.
23. Sullivan NJ. Antibody-mediated enhancement of viral disease. *Curr Top Microbiol Immunol* 2001;**260**:145–69.

24. Huisman W, Martina BE, Rimmelzwaan GF, Gruters RA, Osterhaus AD. Vaccine-induced enhancement of viral infections. *Vaccine* 2009;**27**(4):505–12.
25. Halstead SB. Antibodies determine virulence in dengue. *Ann N Y Acad Sci* 2009;**1171**(Suppl. 1):E48–56.
26. Smith SA, Zhou Y, Olivarez NP, Broadwater AH, de Silva AM, Crowe Jr JE. Persistence of circulating B memory cell clones with potential for dengue virus disease enhancement for decades following infection. *J Virol* 2012;**86**(5):2665–75.
27. de Alwis R, Beltramello M, Messer WB, Sukupolvi-Petty S, Wahala WM, Kraus A, et al. In-depth analysis of the antibody response of individuals exposed to primary dengue virus infection. *PLoS Negl Trop Dis* 2011;**5**(6):e1188.
28. Beltramello M, Williams KL, Simmons CP, Macagno A, Simonelli L, Quyen NT, et al. The human immune response to dengue virus is dominated by highly cross-reactive antibodies endowed with neutralizing and enhancing activity. *Cell Host Microbe* 2010;**8**(3):271–83.
29. Wahala WM, Kraus AA, Haymore LB, Accavitti-Loper MA, de Silva AM. Dengue virus neutralization by human immune sera: role of envelope protein domain III-reactive antibody. *Virology* 2009;**392**(1):103–13.
30. Kliks SC, Nisalak A, Brandt WE, Wahl L, Burke DS. Antibody-dependent enhancement of dengue virus growth in human monocytes as a risk factor for dengue hemorrhagic fever. *Am J Trop Med Hyg* 1989;**40**(4):444–51.
31. Halstead SB, Nimmannitya S, Cohen SN. Observations related to pathogenesis of dengue hemorrhagic fever. IV. Relation of disease severity to antibody response and virus recovered. *Yale J Biol Med* 1970;**42**:311–28.
32. Kliks SC, Nimmannitya S, Nisalak A, Burke DS. Evidence that maternal dengue antibodies are important in the development of dengue hemorrhagic fever in infants. *Am J Trop Med Hyg* 1988;**38**(2):411–9.
33. Libraty DH, Acosta LP, Tallo V, Segubre-Mercado E, Bautista A, Potts JA, et al. A prospective nested case-control study of dengue in infants: rethinking and refining the antibody-dependent enhancement dengue hemorrhagic fever model. *PLoS Med* 2009;**6**(10):e1000171.
34. Simmons CP, Chau TN, Thuy TT, Tuan NM, Hoang DM, Thien NT, et al. Maternal antibody and viral factors in the pathogenesis of dengue virus in infants. *J Infect Dis* 2007;**196**(3):416–24.
35. Chau TN, Anders KL, Lien le B, Hung NT, Hieu LT, Tuan NM, et al. Clinical and virological features of dengue in Vietnamese infants. *PLoS Negl Trop Dis* 2010;**4**(4):e657.
36. Chau TN, Hieu NT, Anders KL, Wolbers M, Lien le B, Hieu LT, et al. Dengue virus infections and maternal antibody decay in a prospective birth cohort study of Vietnamese infants. *J Infect Dis* 2009;**200**(12):1893–900.
37. Chau TN, Quyen NT, Thuy TT, Tuan NM, Hoang DM, Dung NT, et al. Dengue in Vietnamese infants—results of infection-enhancement assays correlate with age-related disease epidemiology, and cellular immune responses correlate with disease severity. *J Infect Dis* 2008;**198**(4):516–24.
38. Cohen SN, Halstead SB. Shock associated with dengue infection. I. Clinical and physiologic manifestations of dengue hemorrhagic fever in Thailand, 1964. *J Pediatr* 1966;**68**:448–56.
39. Green S, Vaughn DW, Kalayanarooj S, Suntayakorn S, Nisalak A, Nimmannitya S, et al. Elevated plasma interleukin-10 levels in children with acute dengue 46th Meeting of the American Society of Tropical Medicine and Hygiene, Lake Buena Vista, FL, 7–11 December 1997. *Am J Trop Med Hyg* 1997;**57**(3, Suppl.):113.
40. Vaughn DW, Green S, Kalayanarooj S, Innis BL, Nimmannitya S, Suntayakorn S, et al. Dengue viremia titer, antibody response pattern, and virus serotype correlate with disease severity. *J Infect Dis* 2000;**181**(1):2–9.
41. Libraty DH, Endy TP, Houng HS, Green S, Kalayanarooj S, Suntayakorn S, et al. Differing influences of virus burden and immune activation on disease severity in secondary dengue-3 virus infections. *J Infect Dis* 2002;**185**(9):1213–21.
42. Halstead SB, Venkateshan CN, Gentry MK, Larsen LK. Heterogeneity of infection enhancement of dengue 2 strains by monoclonal antibodies. *J Immunol* 1984;**132**(3):1529–32.
43. Dejnirattisai W, Jumnainsong A, Onsirisakul N, Fitton P, Vasanawathana S, Limpitikul W, et al. Cross-reacting antibodies enhance dengue virus infection in humans. *Science* 2010;**328**(5979):745–8.
44. Chareonsirisuthigul T, Kalayanarooj S, Ubol S. Dengue virus (DENV) antibody-dependent enhancement of infection upregulates the production of anti-inflammatory cytokines, but suppresses anti-DENV free radical and pro-inflammatory cytokine production, in THP-1 cells. *J Gen Virol* 2007;**88**(Pt. 2):365–75.
45. Ubol S, Phuklia W, Kalayanarooj S, Modhiran N. Mechanisms of immune evasion induced by a complex of dengue virus and preexisting enhancing antibodies. *J Infect Dis* 2010;**201**(6):923–35.
46. Ubol S, Masrinoul P, Chaijaruwanich J, Kalayanarooj S, Charoensirisuthikul T, Kasisith J. Differences in global gene expression in peripheral blood mononuclear cells indicate a significant role of the innate responses in progression of dengue fever but not dengue hemorrhagic fever. *J Infect Dis* 2008;**197**(10):1459–67.

47. Chen LC, Lei HY, Liu CC, Shiesh SC, Chen SH, Liu HS, et al. Correlation of serum levels of macrophage migration inhibitory factor with disease severity and clinical outcome in dengue patients. *Am J Trop Med Hyg* 2006;**74**(1):142–7.
48. Simmons CP, Popper S, Dolocek C, Chau TN, Griffiths M, Dung NT, et al. Patterns of host genome-wide gene transcript abundance in the peripheral blood of patients with acute dengue hemorrhagic fever. *J Infect Dis* 2007;**195**(8):1097–107.
49. Nguyen TH, Lei HY, Nguyen TL, Lin YS, Huang KJ, Le BL, et al. Dengue hemorrhagic fever in infants: a study of clinical and cytokine profiles. *J Infect Dis* 2004;**189**(2):221–32.
50. Shresta S, Kyle JL, Snider HM, Basavapatna M, Beatty PR, Harris E. Interferon-dependent immunity is essential for resistance to primary dengue virus infection in mice, whereas T- and B-cell-dependent immunity are less critical. *J Virol* 2004;**78**(6):2701–10.
51. Shresta S, Sharar KL, Prigozhin DM, Snider HM, Beatty PR, Harris E. Critical roles for both STAT1-dependent and STAT1-independent pathways in the control of primary dengue virus infection in mice. *J Immunol* 2005;**175**(6):3946–54.
52. Navarro-Sanchez E, Despres P, Cedillo-Barron L. Innate immune responses to dengue virus. *Arch Med Res* 2005;**36**(5):425–35.
53. Chaturvedi UC, Raghupathy R, Pasca AS, Elbishbishi EA, Agarwal R, Nagar R, et al. Shift from a Th1-type response to Th1-type in dengue haemorrhagic fever. *Curr Sci* 1999;**76**:63–9.
54. Boonnak K, Dambach KM, Donofrio GC, Marovich MA. Cell type specificity and host genetic polymorphisms influence antibody dependent enhancement of dengue virus infection. *J Virol* 2011;**85**(4):1671–83.
55. Kou Z, Lim JY, Beltramello M, Quinn M, Chen H, Liu SN, et al. Human antibodies against dengue enhance dengue viral infectivity without suppressing type I interferon secretion in primary human monocytes. *Virology* 2011;**410**(1):240–7.
56. Chan KR, Zhang SL, Tan HC, Chan YK, Chow A, Lim AP, et al. Ligation of Fc gamma receptor IIB inhibits antibody-dependent enhancement of dengue virus infection. *Proc Natl Acad Sci USA* 2011;**108**(30):12479–84.
57. Halstead SB, Lan NT, Myint TT, Shwe TN, Nisalak A, Soegijanto S, et al. Infant dengue hemorrhagic fever: research opportunities ignored. *Emerg Infect Dis.* 2002;**12**:1474–9.
58. Gibbons RV, Kalanarooj S, Jarman RG, Nisalak A, Vaughn DW, Endy TP, et al. Analysis of repeat hospital admissions for dengue to estimate the frequency of third or fourth dengue infections resulting in admissions and dengue hemorrhagic fever, and serotype sequences. *Am J Trop Med Hyg* 2007;**77**(5):910–3.
59. Halstead SB, Porterfield JS, O'Rourke EJ. Enhancement of dengue virus infection in monocytes by flavivirus antisera. *Am J Trop Med Hyg* 1980;**29**(4):638–42.
60. Putvatana R, Yoksan S, Chayayodhin T, Bhamarapravati N, Halstead SB. Absence of dengue 2 infection enhancement in human sera containing Japanese encephalitis antibodies. *Am J Trop Med Hyg* 1984;**33**:288–94.
61. Anderson KB, Gibbons RV, Thomas SJ, Rothman AL, Nisalak A, Berkelman RL, et al. Preexisting Japanese encephalitis virus neutralizing antibodies and increased symptomatic dengue illness in a school-based cohort in Thailand. *PLoS Negl Trop Dis* 2011;**5**(10):e1311.
62. Hoke Jr CH, Nisalak A, Sangawhipa N, Jatanasen S, Laorakpongse T, Innis BL, et al. Protection against Japanese encephalitis by inactivated vaccines. *N Engl J Med* 1988;**319**:608–14.
63. Sangkawibha N, Rojanasuphot S, Ahandrik S, Viriyapongse S, Jatanasen S, Salitul V, et al. Risk factors in dengue shock syndrome: a prospective epidemiologic study in Rayong, Thailand. I. The 1980 outbreak. *Am J Epidemiol* 1984;**120**:653–69.
64. Halstead SB, Rojanasuphot S, Sangkawibha N. Original antigenic sin in dengue. *Am J Trop Med Hyg* 1983;**32**(1):154–6.
65. Thein S, Aung MM, Shwe TN, Aye M, Zaw A, Aye K, et al. Risk factors in dengue shock syndrome. *Am J Trop Med Hyg* 1997;**56**(5):566–72.
66. Graham RR, Juffrie M, Tan R, Hayes CG, Laksono I, Ma'roef C, et al. A prospective seroepidemiologic study on dengue in children four to nine years of age in Yogyakarta, Indonesia. I. Studies in 1995–1996. *Am J Trop Med Hyg* 1999;**61**(3):412–9.
67. Chungue E, Spiegel A, Roux J, Laudon F, Cardines R. Dengue-3 in French Polynesia: preliminary data. *Med J Aust* 1990;**152**:557–8.
68. Hubert B, Halstead SB. Dengue 1 virus and dengue hemorrhagic fever, French Polynesia, 2001. *Emerg Infect Dis* 2009;**15**(8):1265–70.
69. Guzman MG, Kouri G, Halstead SB. Do escape mutants explain rapid increases in dengue case-fatality rates within epidemics?. *Lancet* 2000;**355**(9218):1902–3.
70. Rodriguez-Roche R., Alvarez M., Gritsun T., Halstead S.B., Kouri G., Gould E.A., et al. Virus evolution during a severe dengue epidemic in Cuba, 1997. Virology. 2005; **334**: 154–159.
71. Rodriguez-Roche R, Sanchez L, Burgher Y, Rosario D, Alvarez M, Kouri G, et al. Virus role during intraepidemic increase in dengue disease severity. *Vector Borne Zoonotic Dis* 2011;**11**(6):675–81.
72. Ohainle M, Balmaseda A, Macalalad AR, Tellez Y, Zody MC, Saborio S, et al. Dynamics of dengue disease severity determined by the interplay between viral

genetics and serotype-specific immunity. *Sci Transl Med* 2011;**3**(114):114ra28.

73. Rodenhuis-Zybert IA, van der Schaar HM, Voorham JMD, van der Ende-Metselaar H, Lei HY, Wilschut J, et al. Immature dengue virus: a veiled pathogen? *PLoS Pathog* 2010;**6**(1):e1000718.
74. Pang T, Cardosa MJ, Guzman MG. Of cascades and perfect storms: the immunopathogenesis of dengue haemorrhagic fever-dengue shock syndrome (DHF/DSS). *Immunol Cell Biol* 2007;**85**(1):43–5.
75. Rosen L. The use of toxorhynchites mosquitoes to detect and propagate dengue and other arboviruses. *Am J Trop Med Hyg* 1981;**30**(10):177–83.
76. Vaughn DW, Green S, Kalayanarooj S, Innis BL, Nimmannitya S, Suntayakorn S, et al. Dengue in the early febrile phase: viremia and antibody responses. *J Infect Dis* 1997;**176**:322–30.
77. Dung NT, Duyen HT, Thuy NT, Ngoc TV, Chau NV, Hien TT, et al. Timing of CD8+ T cell responses in relation to commencement of capillary leakage in children with dengue. *J Immunol* 2010;**184**(12):7281–7.
78. Larena M, Regner M, Lee E, Lobigs M. Pivotal role of antibody and subsidiary contribution of CD8+ T cells to recovery from infection in a murine model of Japanese encephalitis. *J Virol* 2011;**85**(11):5446–55.
79. Pedersen NC. A review of feline infectious peritonitis virus infection: 1963–2008. *J Feline Med Surg* 2009;**11**(4):225–58.
80. Pedersen NC, Boyle JF. Immunologic phenomena in the effusive form of feline infectious peritonitis. *Am J Vet Res* 1980;**41**:868–76.
81. Weiss RC, Scott FW. Antibody-mediated enhancement of disease in feline infectious peritonitis: comparisons with dengue hemorrhagic fever. *Comp Immune Microbiol Infect Dis* 1981;**4**:175–88.
82. Vennema H, DeGroot RJ, Harbour DA, Dalderup M, Gruffydd-Jones T, Horzinek MC, Spaan WJM. Early death after feline infectious peritonitis challenge due to recombinant vaccinia virus immunization. *J Virol* 1990;**64**:1407–9.
83. Vennema H, Poland A, Foley J, Pedersen NC. Feline infectious peritonitis viruses arise by mutation from endemic feline enteric coronaviruses. *Virology* 1998;**243**(1):150–7.
84. Fiorentino DF, Bond MW, Mosmann TR. Two types of mouse T helper cell. IV. Th2 clones secrete a factor that inhibits cytokine production by Th1 clones. *J Exp Med* 1989;**170**(6):2081–95.
85. Moore KW, Vieira P, Fiorentino DF, Trounstine ML, Khan TA, Mosmann TR. Homology of cytokine synthesis inhibitory factor (IL-10) to the Epstein–Barr virus gene BCRFI. *Science* 1990;**248**(4960):1230–4.
86. Mosser DM, Zhang X. Interleukin-10: new perspectives on an old cytokine. *Immunol Rev* 2008;**226**:205–18.
87. Rousset F, Garcia E, Defrance T, Peronne C, Vezzio N, Hsu DH, et al. Interleukin 10 is a potent growth and differentiation factor for activated human B lymphocytes. *Proc Natl Acad Sci USA* 1992;**89**(5):1890–3.
88. O'Garra A, Vieira P. T(H)1 cells control themselves by producing interleukin-10. *Nat Rev Immunol* 2007;**7**(6):425–8.
89. Heinzel FP, Sadick MD, Mutha SS, Locksley RM. Production of interferon gamma, interleukin 2, interleukin 4, and interleukin 10 by CD4+ lymphocytes *in vivo* during healing and progressive murine leishmaniasis. *Proc Natl Acad Sci USA* 1991;**88**(16):7011–5.
90. Karp CL, el-Safi SH, Wynn TA, Satti MM, Kordofani AM, Hashim FA, et al. *In vivo* cytokine profiles in patients with kala-azar. Marked elevation of both interleukin-10 and interferon-gamma. *J Clin Invest* 1993;**91**(4):1644–8.
91. Ghalib HW, Piuvezam MR, Skeiky YA, Siddig M, Hashim FA, el-Hassan AM, et al. Interleukin 10 production correlates with pathology in human *Leishmania donovani* infections. *J Clin Invest* 1993;**92**(1):324–9.
92. Vieth M, Will A, Schroppel K, Rollinghoff M, Gessner A. Interleukin-10 inhibits antimicrobial activity against *Leishmania major* in murine macrophages. *Scand J Immunol* 1994;**40**(4):403–9.
93. Miles SA, Conrad SM, Alves RG, Jeronimo SM, Mosser DM. A role for IgG immune complexes during infection with the intracellular pathogen Leishmania. *J Exp Med* 2005;**201**(5):747–54.
94. Seder RA, Gazzinelli R, Sher A, Paul WE. Interleukin 12 acts directly on CD4+ T cells to enhance priming for interferon gamma production and diminishes interleukin 4 inhibition of such priming. *Proc Natl Acad Sci USA* 1993;**90**(21):10188–92.
95. Murray HW, Masur H, Keithly JS. Cell-mediated immune response in experimental visceral leishmaniasis. I. Correlation between resistance to *Leishmania donovani* and lymphokine-generating capacity. *J Immunol* 1982;**129**(1):344–50.
96. Heinzel FP, Schoenhaut DS, Rerko RM, Rosser LE, Gately MK. Recombinant interleukin 12 cures mice infected with *Leishmania major*. *J Exp Med* 1993;**177**(5):1505–9.
97. Carrera L, Gazzinelli RT, Badolato R, Hieny S, Muller W, Kuhn R, et al. Leishmania promastigotes selectively inhibit interleukin 12 induction in bone marrow-derived macrophages from susceptible and resistant mice. *J Exp Med* 1996;**183**(2):515–26.
98. Sutterwala FS, Noel GJ, Clynes R, Mosser DM. Selective suppression of interleukin-12 induction after macrophage receptor ligation. *J Exp Med* 1997;**185**(11):1977–85.
99. Sutterwala FS, Noel GJ, Salgame P, Mosser DM. Reversal of proinflammatory responses by ligating the macrophage Fcγreceptor type I. *J Exp Med* 1998;**188**(1):217–22.

100. Anderson CF, Lucas M, Gutierrez-Kobeh L, Field AE, Mosser DM. T cell biasing by activated dendritic cells. *J Immunol* 2004;**173**(2):955–61.
101. Gerber JS, Mosser DM. Stimulatory and inhibitory signals originating from the macrophage Fcgamma receptors. *Microbes Infect* 2001;**3**(2):131–9.
102. Murray HW, Moreira AL, Lu CM, DeVecchio JL, Matsuhashi M, Ma X, et al. Determinants of response to interleukin-10 receptor blockade immunotherapy in experimental visceral leishmaniasis. *J Infect Dis* 2003;**188**(3):458–64.
103. Ioan-Facsinay A, de Kimpe SJ, Hellwig SM, van Lent PL, Hofhuis FM, van Ojik HH, et al. FcγRI (CD64) contributes substantially to severity of arthritis, hypersensitivity responses, and protection from bacterial infection. *Immunity* 2002;**16**(3):391–402.
104. Kima PE, Constant SL, Hannum L, Colmenares M, Lee KS, Haberman AM, et al. Internalization of *Leishmania mexicana* complex amastigotes via the Fc receptor is required to sustain infection in murine cutaneous leishmaniasis. *J Exp Med* 2000;**191**(6):1063–8.
105. Padigel UM, Farrell JP. Control of infection with *Leishmania major* in susceptible BALB/c mice lacking the common γ-chain for FcR is associated with reduced production of IL-10 and TGF-β by parasitized cells. *J Immunol* 2005;**174**(10):6340–5.
106. Mosser DM. The many faces of macrophage activation. *J Leukoc Biol* 2003;**73**(2):209–12.
107. Anderson CF, Gerber JS, Mosser DM. Modulating macrophage function with IgG immune complexes. *J Endotoxin Res* 2002;**8**(6):477–81.
108. Pearson RD, Naidu TG, Young AC, de Alencar JE, Romito R, Davis JS. Circulating immune complexes and rheumatoid factors in visceral leishmaniasis. *J Infect Dis* 1983;**147**:1102.
109. Salama MM. Rheumatoid factor among several cases of visceral leishmaniasis. *J Egypt Soc Parasitol* 1990;**20**(2):837–9.
110. Buxbaum LU. A detrimental role for IgG and FcgammaR in *Leishmania mexicana* infection. *Immunol Res* 2008;**42**(1–3):197–209.
111. Wanasen N, Xin L, Soong L. Pathogenic role of B cells and antibodies in murine *Leishmania amazonensis* infection. *Int J Parasitol* 2008;**38**(3–4):417–29.
112. Lucas M, Zhang X, Prasanna V, Mosser DM. ERK activation following macrophage FcγR ligation leads to chromatin modifications at the IL-10 locus. *J Immunol* 2005;**175**(1):469–77.
113. Yang Z, Mosser DM, Zhang X. Activation of the MAPK, ERK, following *Leishmania amazonensis* infection of macrophages. *J Immunol* 2007;**178**(2):1077–85.
114. Buxbaum LU, Type I. IFNs promote the early IFN-gamma response and the IL-10 response in *Leishmania mexicana* infection. *Parasite Immunol* 2011;**32**(2):153–60.
115. Flannagan RS, Cosio G, Grinstein S. Antimicrobial mechanisms of phagocytes and bacterial evasion strategies. *Nat Rev Microbiol* 2009;**7**(5):355–66.
116. Maglione PJ, Xu J, Casadevall A, Chan J. Fc gamma receptors regulate immune activation and susceptibility during *Mycobacterium tuberculosis* infection. *J Immunol* 2008;**180**(5):3329–38.
117. Watford WT, Moriguchi M, Morinobu A, O'Shea JJ. The biology of IL-12: coordinating innate and adaptive immune responses. *Cytokine Growth Factor Rev* 2003;**14**(5):361–8.
118. Robinson CM, Nau GJ. Interleukin-12 and interleukin-27 regulate macrophage control of *Mycobacterium tuberculosis*. *J Infect Dis* 2008;**198**(3):359–66.
119. Almeida AS, Lago PM, Boechat N, Huard RC, Lazzarini LC, Santos AR, et al. Tuberculosis is associated with a down-modulatory lung immune response that impairs Th1-type immunity. *J Immunol* 2009;**183**(1):718–31.
120. Schreiber T, Ehlers S, Heitmann L, Rausch A, Mages J, Murray PJ, et al. Autocrine IL-10 induces hallmarks of alternative activation in macrophages and suppresses antituberculosis effector mechanisms without compromising T cell immunity. *J Immunol* 2009;**183**(2):1301–12.
121. Sauter P, Hober D. Mechanisms and results of the antibody dependent enhancement of viral infections and the role in the pathogenesis of coxsackievirus Binduced diseases. *Microbes Infect* 2009;**11**:443–51.
122. Stueckemann JA, Holth M, Swart WJ, Kowalchyk K, Smith MS, Wolstenholme AJ, et al. Replication of lactate dehydrogenase-elevating virus in macrophages. 2. Mechanism of persistent infection in mice and cell culture. *J Gen Virol* 1982;**59**(Pt. 2):263–72.
123. Olsen CW. A review of feline infectious peritonitis virus: molecular biology, immunopathogenesis, clinical aspects, and vaccination. *Vet Microbiol* 1993;**36**(1–2):1–37.
124. Yoon KJ, Wu LL, Zimmerman JJ, Hill HT, Platt KB. Antibody-dependent enhancement (ADE) of porcine reproductive and respiratory syndrome virus (PRRSV) infection in pigs. *Viral Immunol* 1996;**9**(1):51–63.
125. Burke DS. Human HIV vaccine trials: does antibody-dependent enhancement pose a genuine risk?. *Perspect Biol Med* 1992;**35**:511–30.
126. Mdurvwa EG, Ogunbiyi PO, Gakou HS, Reddy PG. Pathogenic mechanisms of caprine arthritis-encephalitis virus. *Vet Res Commun* 1994;**18**(6):483–90.
127. Mealey RH, Leib SR, Littke MH, Wagner B, Horohov DW, McGuire TC. Viral load and clinical disease enhancement associated with a lentivirus

cytotoxic T lymphocyte vaccine regimen. *Vaccine* 2009;**27**(18):2453–68.

128. Porter AD, Larsen AE, Porter HG. The pathogenesis of Aleutian disease of mink. II. Enhancement of tissue lesions following the administration of a killed virus vaccine or passive antibody. *J Immunol* 1972;**109**:1–7.
129. Kanno H, Wohlinbarger JB, Bloom ME. Aleutian mink disease parvovirus infection of mink macrophages and human macrophage cell line *937: demonstration of antibody-dependent enhancement of infection. *J Virol* 1993;**67**:7017–24.
130. Best SM, Bloom ME. Aleutian mink disease parvovirus. In: Kerr JR, Cotmore SF, Bloom ME, Linden RM, Parrish CR, editors. *The Parvoviruses*. London: Hodder Arnold; 2006. p. 457–71.
131. Webster RG, Askonas BA. Cross-protection and cross reactive cytotoxic T cells induced by influenza virus vaccines in mice. *Eur J Immunol* 1980;**10**:396–401.
132. Chanock RM, Parrott RH, Kapakian AZ. Possible role of immunological factors in pathogenesis of RS virus in lower respiratory tract disease. *Perspec Virol* 1968;**6**:125–35.
133. Fulginiti FA, Eller JJ, Downie AW, Kempe CH. Altered reactivity to measles virus. Atypical measles in children previously immunized with inactivated measles virus vaccines. *JAMA* 1967;**202**:1075–80.
134. King AA, Sands JJ, Porterfield JS. Antibody-mediated enhancement of rabies virus infection in a mouse macrophage cell line (P388D1). *J Gen Virol* 1984;**65**:1091–3.
135. Prabhakar BS, Nathanson N. Acute rabies deaths mediated by antibody. *Nature* 1981;**290**:590–1.

CHAPTER

20

Mechanisms of Immunoglobulin-Mediated Mucus Entrapment of Pathogens at Various Mucosal Surfaces

Shannon A. Allen[a] *and Thomas J. Hope*[b,*]

[a]Integrated Graduate Program, Department of Cell and Molecular Biology, Northwestern University Feinberg School of Medicine, Chicago, Illinois, [b]Department of Cell and Molecular Biology, Northwestern University Feinberg School of Medicine, Chicago, Illinois

INTRODUCTION

The mucosal epithelia and the mucus layer that cover it are responsible for protecting a highly organized internal environment from a chaotic and continually changing external environment. Many microorganisms that successfully invade the body enter through mucosal surfaces, including those that line gastrointestinal, respiratory, urinary, and reproductive tissues. Mucus-secreting epithelial surfaces are constantly exposed to potentially pathogenic and non-pathogenic microorganisms and must be continuously surveyed and protected. Pathogenic organisms include those that cause gastrointestinal, respiratory, urinary, and genital tract infections. Non-pathogenic microorganisms are harmless and can often be helpful to their host. Healthy human colonic mucosal tissues are exposed to thousands of species of commensal bacteria at any given time. Some of these bacteria aid in the further processing of indigestible food such as cellulose. In addition, these microflora can be beneficial by producing hydrogen peroxide in their micro-environment, a property that is unfavorable to many harmful pathogens.[1]

In normal cases, commensal bacteria do not elicit strong immune responses, as it would be counterproductive to generate aggressive immune responses to all microorganisms at mucosal surfaces. This process of selectively responding to some pathogens and not others is known as *immune tolerance*. However, in abnormal cases, such as with the inflammatory bowel disorder called Crohn's disease, there is a strong response to intestinal commensal bacteria with an inability to clear them from the mucus layer. Nevertheless, immune components at mucosal surfaces must differentiate

* Corresponding Author

between potentially dangerous agents and harmless or possibly helpful microorganisms.

STRUCTURE OF MUCUS

Specific specialized cells within mucosal epithelia secrete a viscous, gel-like fluid called *mucus*, which forms a protective mechanical barrier by physically impeding and trapping pathogens, preventing them from contacting mucosal epithelial cells. Mucus is primarily composed of water (about 95%) and mucins but also contains many defensive proteins, including immunoglobulins (Igs), defensins, and lysozymes, among others,[2] which constitute the barrier function of the mucus layer. The main protein components of mucus are large, complex, and highly glycosylated molecules called *mucins*. Thus far, a number of human mucins have been identified that can be divided into three separate categories: gel-forming mucins (MUC2, MUC5AC, MUC5AB, and MUC6), cell-surface mucins (MUC1, MUC3A/B, MUC4, MUC12, MUC13, MUC15, MUC16, MUC17, and MUC20), and secreted but non-gel forming mucins (MUC7). This chapter will focus on gel-forming mucins.

Gel-forming mucins consist mostly of domains of tandemly repeating amino acids with an abundance of proline, threonine, and serine (PTS) domains, which make up the core of the mucin monomer. The hydroxyl side-chains of the threonine and serine residues are bound to highly conjugated *O*-linked oligosaccharides and give the monomer a "bottle brush" appearance.[3] In addition, the N-terminal and C-terminal ends of mucin monomers (as well as other portions) contain regions that are similar to the structure of globular proteins with almost no *O*-linked oligosaccharides, minimal *N*-linked oligosaccharides, and cysteine-rich regions.[4] These cysteine-rich domains possess similarities to the cysteine-rich regions present in the von Willebrand factor (vWF) along with cysteine knots (CKs) at the carboxy-terminal end[5] and are involved in the formation of higher order mucin structures through disulfide bonds.[6] Interestingly, MUC2, the main gel-forming mucin in the intestine,[7] is autocatalytically cleaved at the C-terminus at low pH, generating a new C-terminal end that may covalently bind other proteins and glycans,[8] potentially anchoring these proteins to the mucus. For example, immunoglobulin G Fc gamma binding protein (FcγBP), present in intestinal mucus, was recently shown to be covalently linked to MUC2 in mice and humans.[8] Also, the secretory component bound to IgAs, the major protective Ig subtype in mucosal secretions, was shown to bind to mucus through its glycosylated domains in respiratory mucus.[7]

MECHANISMS OF IMMUNITY AT MUCOSAL SURFACES

Mammals are constantly under immune pressure from bacteria, viruses, and parasites, and the host immune system has to be able to regulate these pathogens. Antigens (bacterial, viral, or food) are for the most part sequestered on the lumenal side of mucosal epithelia. In order to generate an immune response, these antigens must cross the epithelia where they can be further processed and presented to immunocytes. Transport of antigens across the intestinal epithelia is mediated by microfold cells (M-cells). These specialized cells are located in the epithelia directly above organized mucosa-associated lymphoid tissues (O-MALTs) and release intact antigens into the subepithelial space where antigen-presenting cells (APCs) and lymphocytes reside.[9] Here, antigens are then processed by APCs and presented to T lymphocytes, which can become activated.[10] Activated APCs and T lymphocytes, through the secretion of specific cytokines, stimulate B cells to eventually become terminally differentiated into Ig-producing plasma cells.[11,12]

Located below the secretory epithelial layers are terminally differentiated B cells or plasma cells. These cells are devoted to producing secretory immunoglobulins (sIgs), including secretory IgM (sIgM) and IgA (sIgA), with sIgA being the most abundant sIg in mucosal secretions. SIgs are remarkably viable within the harsh mucosal environment and are typically more resistant to pathogen enzymatic degradation due to the Ig-associated proteins, secretory component (SC) and J-chain.[13] It has been shown that some sIgs of the same isotype are more resistant to proteolytic cleavage than others. For example, *Haemophilus influenzae*[14] and *Neisseria gonorrhoeae*,[15] two distinct but common mucosal pathogens, secrete enzymes that can cleave secretory IgA_1 but IgA_2 is resistant to proteolysis by the same enzymes. IgA_2 has a 13-amino-acid deletion that renders this Ig less prone to degradation.[16]

Local Production of Igs

The major class of Ig produced at mucosal surfaces is IgA. In the local immune system, IgA is produced by terminally differentiated plasma B-cells which typically produce dimeric IgA (dIgA) and pentameric IgM (pIgM). They also synthesize J-chain,[17] a 15-kDa protein that aids in the oligimerization of polymeric immunoglobulins (pIgs)[18] and is bound to an 18-amino-acid sequence in IgA and IgM. Although J-chain is not essential for polymerization of immunoglobulins,[19,20] it aids in proper pIg structure and translocation from the basal epithelia to the lumen and provides increased stability. An example of the importance of J-chain was demonstrated when J-chain-deficient mice were orally immunized with cholera toxin. Cholera toxin causes severe disease within the gut, and oral immunization can offer protection by inducing toxin-specific immunity.[21] Although serum toxin-specific IgAs were produced in J-chain-deficient mice, IgAs were not efficiently transported across the epithelia into mucosal secretions, causing susceptibility to disease. After gut cholera toxin challenge, toxin-specific secreted Igs were more protective than toxin-specific serum Igs. In this case, secreted Igs may have prevented attachment of the toxin to the epithelia.[22,23]

J-chain-containing pIgs, dIgA, and pIgM exit plasma B cells and must be transported across the secretory epithelia and into the mucosal secretions in order to interact with its antigen. For this to happen, J-chain of pIgs must first non-covalently interact with the polymeric immunoglobulin receptor (pIgR),[19] a 100-kDa five-domain transmembrane glycoprotein constitutively expressed on the basolateral side of the secretory epithelia. The resulting pIg/IgR complex is then endocytosed and transported through the secretory epithelial cells to the apical side. Once at the apical surface, partial cleavage of pIgR occurs and a portion (~80 kDa) of the pIgR, known as SC, becomes covalently bound to pIgs.[19] The complex is then released into the luminal secretions as sIgA or sIgM. The remaining cell-associated pIgR cleavage product at the apical surface is then targeted for degradation within the secretory epithelia.[24] The new secondary covalent linkage of SC and pIg, through J-chain, provides stability against proteolytic enzymes.[25] There is also evidence that Ig-free SC, or free SC, can be transported through the epithelia and released into mucosal secretions and may contribute to SC-mediated protection from invading pathogens.[26,27]

The presence of IgG has been extensively demonstrated in respiratory,[28] gut,[29] and genital[30] mucosal secretions; however, local production or systemic derivation responsible for its occurrence in mucosal secretions remains unclear. It has been shown that IgG levels are altered during the menstrual cycle[31] and during infections of the genital tract,[30] suggesting the possibility of an active transport of IgG. Receptor-mediated transport of the IgG across mucosal epithelial cells, specifically in the gut and genital tract, has been implicated.[32,33]

For example, in the gut of suckling rats, mucosal epithelia express a neonatal Fc-receptor (FcRn) on the apical side that can bind IgG ingested from IgG-rich breast milk. IgG is then transported to the basolateral side and released into the sub-epithelial space.[33,34] This process of ingesting Ig-rich milk is important in establishing the immune system for neonates. In murine genital tract studies, intravaginal delivery of biotin-labeled IgG resulted in the accumulation of labeled IgG in the serum of normal mice but not in that of FcRn knock-out mice.[33]

Experimental Analyses of Ig Protection at Mucosal Secretions

Mucosal immunoglobulins typically exert their protective properties through hindrance and entrapment within the mucus secretions that line various mucosal epithelia.[25] Mucus entrapment is defined as physically strengthening the association of pathogens to the luminal mucus. In short, mucus entrapment occurs by preventing the attachment, penetration, and colonization of potentially harmful or commensal microorganisms.[25,35–37] For example, two mucus layers have been identified in the intestine: A dense, tightly packed MUC2 network that makes up the inner mucus layer and a loose outer layer.[7,38] Commensal bacteria only reside in the outer layer via binding interactions, presumably with Igs, and cannot penetrate the dense inner layer, thereby protecting mucosal epithelia from bacterial ingress.[7,38,39]

Evidence of the ability of sIgA to prevent pathogenic colonization of mucosal epithelia has been extensively demonstrated.[35,40,41] A number of studies that investigated the ability of sIgA to prevent pathogen adherence have made use of murine dorsal "backpack" tumors. These are subcutaneous masses that continuously secrete pathogen-specific monoclonal IgAs into blood circulation, which subsequently enter mucosal secretions through transepithelial transport.[42] One such study used murine backpack tumors that secreted IgAs against an exposed carbohydrate, Sal4, on the surface of *Salmonella typhimurium*, a fatal disease-causing bacterium that infects the mouse liver and spleen.[40] Here, the sIgA against this epitope was protective in intestinal mucus secretions after oral challenge; however, when this epitope was mutated, the initially protective sIgA was no longer effective. A similar study used the backpack tumor system in which monoclonal IgAs were secreted against lipopolysaccharide surface proteins of *Vibrio cholerae*,[41] an enteric bacterium that causes severe diarrhea. The sIgA produced against this epitope was sufficient to protect neonatal mice from disease after multiple lethal dose oral challenges.

In addition to bacteria, penetration of mucosal epithelium by some viruses may be attenuated by sIgA.[42–44] For example, in a murine backpack tumor system, monoclonal IgAs directed against capsid protein, μ1c, of reovirus induced production of sIgA that was protective against oral challenge.[42] In another study, mice intraperitoneally injected with dIgA directed against the hemagglutinin H1 protein of respiratory disease-causing influenza virus resulted in transport of IgA into nasal secretions and protection from infection after intranasal challenge.[43] In addition, neonatal mice suckling from dams immunized with primate enteric rotavirus protein, SA-11, were protected against virus-induced diarrhea after oral inoculation,[44] presumably by the presence of sIgA.

As mentioned above, sIgA can prevent commensal and potentially harmful microorganisms from penetrating various epithelial surfaces within the body. This is thought to occur through the ability of sIgA to anchor the microorganisms to the mucus layer, which is likely mediated through binding of the carbohydrate residues of SC.[35] Evidence to support this claim was observed when deglycosylated SC of sIgA failed to protect against invasion of the respiratory bacterium *Shigella flexneri* in mice,[35] while normal SC elicited protection against colonization. In addition, free SC (SC that is not bound to Igs) within secretions may confer protection through these mechanisms. For example, free SC can bind to both enteric bacterium *Escherichia coli*[45] and *Clostridium difficile*[27] to reduce invasion in an Ig-independent manner.

Although there are clear results that IgA can interact with mucins through interactions mediated by SC, the situation is much less clear for IgG. Photobleaching-based mobility studies suggest that IgGs do not interact with mucins;[46] however, a potential role for IgG-mediated mucus entrapment and subsequent exclusion of pathogens from mucosal epithelia has been demonstrated in a variety of experiments.[47–50] For example, in rabbits immunized against human albumin and devoid of a secretory immune system, IgG antibodies were effective in excluding albumin from penetrating oral mucosal epithelia after the apical epithelia was exposed to albumin.[51]

Early evidence of pathogenic Ig-mediated mucus entrapment was demonstrated when *Nippostrongylus brasiliensis*, a type of intestinal parasitic nematode, was sequestered in the outer intestinal mucus layer of primed rats, preventing colonization of the intestinal epithelia.[48] This suggests the possibility of immune factors such as Igs in excluding parasites from establishing infection. In addition, intestinal mucus entrapment of parasitic *Trichinella spiralis* was established after immunization of parasite-specific IgGs in rats when compared to non-immunized rats. In the same study, productive intestinal epithelial infection was also reduced when parasites were precoated in specific IgG and fed to rats,[49] suggesting that IgG was responsible for entrapment of parasites. However, not all parasite-specific IgGs were effective at mucus entrapment as demonstrated when a panel of specific IgGs with varying epitopes were injected into rat suckling dams and only a few were protective,[50] suggesting that entrapment may be dependent upon Ig epitope specificity.

It is possible that the route of immunization plays a role in the efficiency of entrapment, as some intact IgGs promoted greater entrapment when administered orally; however, the same initially protective IgGs were ineffective when added directly to intestinal mucus.[50] Moreover, parasite trapping was observed even when only the variable region, the Fab, of parasite-specific protective IgGs was directly administered to mucus.[50]

The mechanism of IgG-mediated entrapment, within the intestinal mucus, has been investigated and described. As previously mentioned, healthy intestinal mucosal epithelia are blanketed by two layers of protective mucus: An outer loose layer where intestinal microorganisms reside and an inner firmly attached layer devoid of microorganisms.[7,38] The main gel-forming mucin expressed in intestinal mucus is MUC2, which has been shown to covalently bind to FcγBP,[8] a protein that binds the Fc region of IgG but not IgA, sIgA, or IgM.[52] Although the functional significance of the association of FcγBP with MUC2 has not yet been delineated, it is feasible that IgG-mediated mucus entrapment may occur through this mechanism. Here, FcγBP may stabilize IgG, and any IgG-bound pathogens would then become stationary within the intestinal mucus layer.

SUMMARY

It is becoming clear that the mucus layer covering mucosal surfaces has multiple mechanisms that provide barrier functions. It appears that adaptive immunity mediated by antibodies can further act to impede or entrap pathogens. Immunoglobulins may contribute to the mucus barrier function by binding to and impeding the transport of potentially harmful pathogenic microorganisms across the mucosal epithelia, as evidenced by the studies described above. IgA is known to interact with mucins through the secretory component. IgG has also been shown to influence pathogens at mucosal surfaces. Notably, most of these studies were published decades ago, and the potential role of IgG interactions with mucus has been explored sparsely since then. Given the prevalence of newer and emerging pathogens such as HIV, it is obvious that more investigation is needed because effective vaccines that block the acquisition of such pathogens have yet to be developed. Targeting vaccine-induced antibody responses to work in coordination with the mucus barrier may prove to be a critical component in the development of an effective vaccine.

Acknowledgments

We would like to acknowledge the NIH grants to SAA (T32AI060523) and TJH (R21AI094584, PO1AI082971), the Bill and Melinda Gates Foundation (OPP1031734, 38643), and the Rush Program Project Grant. We would also like to acknowledge Rosemary Clark, Shetha Shukair and Dan Stieh for their critical review of this text.

References

1. Eschenbach DA, Davick PR, Williams BL, Klebanoff SJ, Young-Smith K, Critchlow CM, et al. Prevalence of hydrogen peroxide-producing *Lactobacillus* species in normal women and women with bacterial vaginosis. *J Clin Microbiol* 1989;**27**(2):251–6.
2. Raj PA, Dentino AR. Current status of defensins and their role in innate and adaptive immunity. *FEMS Microbiol Lett* 2002;**206**(1):9–18.
3. Bansil R, Turner BS. Mucin structure, aggregation, physiological functions and biomedical applications. *Curr Opin Colloid Interface Sci* 2006;**11**:164–70.
4. Perez-Vilar J, Hill RL. The structure and assembly of secreted mucins. *J Biol Chem* 1999;**274**(45):31751–4.
5. Turner BS, Bhaskar KR, Hadzopoulou-Cladaras M, LaMont JT. Cysteine-rich regions of pig gastric mucin contain von Willebrand factor and cystine knot domains at the carboxyl terminal(1). *Biochim Biophys Acta* 1999;**1447**(1):77–92.
6. Bell SL, Xu G, Forstner JF. Role of the cystine-knot motif at the C-terminus of rat mucin protein Muc2 in dimer formation and secretion. *Biochem J* 2001;**357**(Pt. 1):203–9.
7. Johansson ME, Ambort D, Pelaseyed T, Schutte A, Gustafsson JK, Ermund A, et al. Composition and functional role of the mucus layers in the intestine. *Cell Mol Life Sci* 2011;**68**(22):3635–41.
8. Johansson ME, Thomsson KA, Hansson GC. Proteomic analyses of the two mucus layers of the colon barrier reveal that their main component, the Muc2 mucin, is strongly bound to the Fcgbp protein. *J Proteome Res* 2009;**8**(7):3549–57.
9. Neutra MR, Phillips TL, Mayer EL, Fishkind DJ. Transport of membrane-bound macromolecules by M cells in follicle-associated epithelium of rabbit Peyer's patch. *Cell Tissue Res* 1987;**247**(3):537–46.
10. Ermak TH, Owen RL. Differential distribution of lymphocytes and accessory cells in mouse Peyer's patches. *Anat Rec* 1986;**215**(2):144–52.
11. Brandtzaeg P, Johansen FE. Mucosal B cells: phenotypic characteristics, transcriptional regulation, and homing properties. *Immunol Rev* 2005;**206**:32–63.
12. Fagarasan S, Honjo T. Intestinal IgA synthesis: regulation of front-line body defences. *Nat Rev Immunol* 2003;**3**(1):63–72.
13. Kilian M, Mestecky J, Russell MW. Defense mechanisms involving Fc-dependent functions of immunoglobulin A and their subversion by bacterial immunoglobulin A proteases. *Microbiol Rev* 1988;**52**(2):296–303.
14. Mistry DV, Stockley RA. The cleavage specificity of an IgA1 protease from *Haemophilus influenzae*. *Virulence* 2011;**2**(2):103–10.
15. Plaut AG, Gilbert JV, Wistar Jr R. Loss of antibody activity in human immunoglobulin A exposed extracellular immunoglobulin A proteases of *Neisseria gonorrhoeae* and *Streptococcus sanguis*. *Infect Immun* 1977;**17**(1):130–5.
16. Frangione B, Wolfenstein-Todel C. Partial duplication in the "hinge" region of IgA1 myeloma proteins. *Proc Natl Acad Sci USA* 1972;**69**(12):3673–6.
17. Brandtzaeg P. Role of secretory antibodies in the defence against infections. *Int J Med Microbiol* 2003;**293**(1):3–15.
18. Johansen FE, Braathen R, Brandtzaeg P. The J chain is essential for polymeric Ig receptor-mediated epithelial transport of IgA. *J Immunol* 2001;**167**(9):5185–92.
19. Johansen FE, Braathen R, Brandtzaeg P. Role of J chain in secretory immunoglobulin formation. *Scand J Immunol* 2000;**52**(3):240–8.
20. Vaerman JP, Langendries A, Giffroy D, Brandtzaeg P, Kobayashi K. Lack of SC/pIgR-mediated epithelial transport of a human polymeric IgA devoid of J chain: *in vitro* and *in vivo* studies. *Immunology* 1998;**95**(1):90–6.
21. Svennerholm AM, Jertborn M, Gothefors L, Karim AM, Sack DA, Holmgren J. Mucosal antitoxic and antibacterial immunity after cholera disease and after immunization with a combined B subunit-whole cell vaccine. *J Infect Dis* 1984;**149**(6):884–93.
22. Lycke N, Erlandsson L, Ekman L, Schon K, Leanderson T. Lack of J chain inhibits the transport of gut IgA and abrogates the development of intestinal antitoxic protection. *J Immunol* 1999;**163**(2):913–9.
23. Uren TK, Wijburg OL, Simmons C, Johansen FE, Brandtzaeg P, Strugnell RA. Vaccine-induced protection against gastrointestinal bacterial infections in the absence of secretory antibodies. *Eur J Immunol* 2005;**35**(1):180–8.

24. Norderhaug IN, Johansen FE, Schjerven H, Brandtzaeg P. Regulation of the formation and external transport of secretory immunoglobulins. *Crit Rev Immunol* 1999;**19**(5–6):481–508.
25. Brandtzaeg P. Mucosal immunity in the female genital tract. *J Reprod Immunol* 1997;**36**(1–2):23–50.
26. Wold AE, Mestecky J, Tomana M, Kobata A, Ohbayashi H, Endo T, et al. Secretory immunoglobulin A carries oligosaccharide receptors for *Escherichia coli* type 1 fimbrial lectin. *Infect Immun* 1990;**58**(9):3073–7.
27. Dallas SD, Rolfe RD. Binding of *Clostridium difficile* toxin A to human milk secretory component. *J Med Microbiol* 1998;**47**(10):879–88.
28. Reynolds HY. Identification and role of immunoglobulins in respiratory secretions. *Eur J Respir Dis Suppl* 1987;**153**:103–16.
29. Samson RR, McClelland DB, Shearman DJ. Studies on the quantitation of immunoglobulin in human intestinal secretions. *Gut* 1973;**14**(8):616–26.
30. Haimovici F, Mayer KH, Anderson DJ. Quantitation of HIV-1-specific IgG, IgA, and IgM antibodies in human genital tract secretions. *J Acquir Immune Defic Syndr Hum Retrovirol* 1997;**15**(3):185–91.
31. Lu FX, Ma Z, Rourke T, Srinivasan S, McChesney M, Miller CJ. Immunoglobulin concentrations and antigen-specific antibody levels in cervicovaginal lavages of rhesus macaques are influenced by the stage of the menstrual cycle. *Infect Immun* 1999;**67**(12):6321–8.
32. Rodewald R, Kraehenbuhl JP. Receptor-mediated transport of IgG. *J Cell Biol* 1984;**99**(1, Pt. 2):159s–64s.
33. Li Z, Palaniyandi S, Zeng R, Tuo W, Roopenian DC, Zhu X. Transfer of IgG in the female genital tract by MHC class I-related neonatal Fc receptor (FcRn) confers protective immunity to vaginal infection. *Proc Natl Acad Sci USA* 2011;**108**(11):4388–93.
34. Ward ES, Ober RJ. Chapter 4: Multitasking by exploitation of intracellular transport functions the many faces of FcRn. *Adv Immunol* 2009;**103**:77–115.
35. Phalipon A, Cardona A, Kraehenbuhl JP, Edelman L, Sansonetti PJ, Corthesy B. Secretory component: a new role in secretory IgA-mediated immune exclusion *in vivo*. *Immunity* 2002;**17**(1):107–15.
36. Macpherson AJ, Slack E. The functional interactions of commensal bacteria with intestinal secretory IgA. *Curr Opin Gastroenterol* 2007;**23**(6):673–8.
37. Williams RC, Gibbons RJ. Inhibition of bacterial adherence by secretory immunoglobulin A: a mechanism of antigen disposal. *Science* 1972;**177**(4050):697–9.
38. Hansson GC, Johansson ME. The inner of the two Muc2 mucin-dependent mucus layers in colon is devoid of bacteria. *Gut Microbes* 2010;**1**(1):51–4.
39. Subramani DB, Johansson ME, Dahlen G, Hansson GC. *Lactobacillus* and *Bifidobacterium* species do not secrete protease that cleaves the MUC2 mucin which organises the colon mucus. *Benef Microbes* 2010;**1**(4):343–50.
40. Michetti P, Mahan MJ, Slauch JM, Mekalanos JJ, Neutra MR. Monoclonal secretory immunoglobulin A protects mice against oral challenge with the invasive pathogen *Salmonella typhimurium*. *Infect Immun* 1992;**60**(5):1786–92.
41. Winner III L, Mack J, Weltzin R, Mekalanos JJ, Kraehenbuhl JP, Neutra MR. New model for analysis of mucosal immunity: intestinal secretion of specific monoclonal immunoglobulin A from hybridoma tumors protects against *Vibrio cholerae* infection. *Infect Immun* 1991;**59**(3):977–82.
42. Kraehenbuhl JP, Neutra MR. Molecular and cellular basis of immune protection of mucosal surfaces. *Physiol Rev* 1992;**72**(4):853–79.
43. Hutchings AB, Helander A, Silvey KJ, Chandran K, Lucas WT, Nibert ML, et al. Secretory immunoglobulin A antibodies against the sigma1 outer capsid protein of reovirus type 1 Lang prevent infection of mouse Peyer's patches. *J Virol* 2004;**78**(2):947–57.
44. Renegar KB, Small Jr PA. Passive transfer of local immunity to influenza virus infection by IgA antibody. *J Immunol* 1991;**146**(6):1972–8.
45. Offit PA, Clark HF. Protection against rotavirus-induced gastroenteritis in a murine model by passively acquired gastrointestinal but not circulating antibodies. *J Virol* 1985;**54**(1):58–64.
46. de Oliveira IR, de Araujo AN, Bao SN, Giugliano LG. Binding of lactoferrin and free secretory component to enterotoxigenic *Escherichia coli*. *FEMS Microbiol Lett* 2001;**203**(1):29–33.
47. Saltzman WM, Radomsky ML, Whaley KJ, Cone RA. Antibody diffusion in human cervical mucus. *Biophys J* 1994;**66**(2, Pt. 1):508–15.
48. Miller HR, Huntley JF, Wallace GR. Immune exclusion and mucus trapping during the rapid expulsion of *Nippostrongylus brasiliensis* from primed rats. *Immunology* 1981;**44**(2):419–29.
49. Carlisle MS, McGregor DD, Appleton JA. The role of mucus in antibody-mediated rapid expulsion of *Trichinella spiralis* in suckling rats. *Immunology* 1990;**70**(1):126–32.
50. Carlisle MS, McGregor DD, Appleton JA. Intestinal mucus entrapment of *Trichinella spiralis* larvae induced by specific antibodies. *Immunology* 1991;**74**(3):546–51.
51. Brandtzaeg P, Tolo K. Mucosal penetrability enhanced by serum-derived antibodies. *Nature* 1977;**266**(5599):262–3.
52. Harada N, Iijima S, Kobayashi K, Yoshida T, Brown WR, Hibi T, et al. Human IgGFc binding protein (FcgammaBP) in colonic epithelial cells exhibits mucin-like structure. *J Biol Chem* 1997;**272**(24):15232–41.

Index

G

H

FSC
www.fsc.org
MIX
Papier | Fördert gute Waldnutzung
FSC® C083411

Kolibri 360 GmbH
Ferdinand-Jühlke-Straße 7
99095 Erfurt, Deutschland
produktsicherheit@kolibri360.de